PRINCIPLES OF MEDICAL TOXICOLOGY

Dr. Amit Kumar
Mrs. Shaik Aleesha
Dr. Narasimha Naik R
Dr. Ramesh Kumar Gupta
Mr. Sumit Kumar Gupta

ISBN: 9788198765796

Scan to view online

Editors

Dr. Amit Kumar

Mrs. Shaik Aleesha

Dr. Narasimha Naik R

Dr. Ramesh Kumar Gupta

Mr. Sumit Kumar Gupta

First Edition: 2025
ISBN: 9788198765796

Maximum Retail Price: Rs. 1000/- (Inclusive of all taxes)

Published by ThinkPlus Pharma Publications,
9-15/1, Indrapalem, Kakinada, AP-533006, India.
Website: www.books.jopir.in

Cover Page Illustration: Kiran Priyam Kumar Sarella

Printed at Tarangini Printing Works, Subhadra Arcade, Bhanugudi, Kakinada, AP-533003, India.

DEDICATION

This textbook represents not just a compilation of knowledge, but a bridge between theoretical understanding and practical application in saving lives. We dedicate this work to the healthcare professionals who face life-threatening emergencies daily, making split-second decisions that often mean the difference between life and death.

We offer this book as a guide in their journey through the complexities of medical toxicology to the students - past, present, and future - who approach this challenging field with enthusiasm and dedication. Their questions, curiosity, and desire to learn have been a constant source of inspiration in crafting this detailed yet accessible text. We hope this work serves as a reliable companion in their professional development and clinical practice.

Special dedication goes to the tireless workers in poison control centers worldwide, who provide crucial guidance and support around the clock. Their commitment to public health and safety, often working behind the scenes, forms the backbone of toxicology emergency response systems.

Finally, we dedicate this work to our families, whose unwavering support and understanding have made this endeavor possible. Through their sacrifices and encouragement, we found the strength to persevere in creating a resource that we hope will contribute meaningfully to the field of medical toxicology and, ultimately, to patient care.

CONTENTS

ACKNOWLEDGMENTS

The creation of this textbook has been a collaborative journey that would not have been possible without the support and contributions of numerous individuals and organizations. We extend our heartfelt gratitude to all those who have played a role in bringing this project to fruition.

We are deeply indebted to our academic mentors whose guidance and wisdom have shaped our understanding of toxicology and pharmaceutical sciences. Their expertise and knowledge have been invaluable in ensuring the accuracy and relevance of the content presented in this book.

Our sincere appreciation goes to the review team comprising experienced clinicians, toxicologists, and academicians who provided constructive feedback and suggestions that significantly enhanced the quality of this work.

We are grateful to our colleagues and the various professional associations that have provided platforms for discussion and exchange of ideas. Their support in validating concepts and sharing experiences has enriched the content of this book.

Our appreciation extends to the editorial team for their meticulous attention to detail and commitment to maintaining high standards of quality throughout the development of this book.

Finally, we express our deepest gratitude to our families for their patience, understanding, and unwavering support throughout this challenging but rewarding journey.

CHAPTER 1

INTRODUCTION TO MEDICAL TOXICOLOGY

Author

Mrs. Bhagyamma Tholla, Assistant Professor, Department of Pharmacology, Sultan-ul-Uloom College of Pharmacy, Banjara Hills, Hyderabad, Telangana, India

Abstract

Medical toxicology has evolved from ancient observations of poisonous substances to a sophisticated medical specialty addressing diverse toxic exposures. Its origins trace back to Egyptian, Greek, and Roman civilizations, with significant advancements marked by Paracelsus's principle that "the dose makes the poison." The discipline encompasses the study, diagnosis, management, and prevention of adverse effects from medications, occupational chemicals, environmental toxins, and biological agents. Core principles include dose-response relationships, routes of exposure, mechanisms of action, and systematic approaches to risk assessment. Medical toxicologists serve crucial roles across healthcare settings—managing poisonings in emergency departments, providing consultation for complex cases, conducting surveillance of emerging threats, advising on pharmaceutical safety, and contributing to environmental and occupational health policies. The field continues to adapt to contemporary challenges including novel pharmaceuticals, designer drugs, environmental pollutants, and chemical threats. This multidisciplinary specialty bridges clinical medicine, pharmacology, biochemistry, and public health to address the increasing complexity of toxic exposures in modern society.

Keywords: *Medical Toxicology, Poisoning, Toxic Exposure, Paracelsus, Risk Assessment*

Learning Objectives

After completion of the chapter, the learners should be able to:

- Describe the historical evolution of toxicology from ancient civilizations to modern medical practice.
- Define the scope of medical toxicology and differentiate it from related medical specialties.
- Explain the fundamental principle of dose-response relationships and its importance in toxicological assessment.
- Identify the key principles of toxicokinetics and toxicodynamics in the context of poisoning.
- Analyze the multidisciplinary role of medical toxicology across various healthcare settings including emergency medicine, occupational health, and public health.
- Evaluate current challenges and future directions in medical toxicology related to emerging toxins and changing exposure patterns

HISTORICAL PERSPECTIVE

Medical toxicology has evolved over centuries, from empirical observations of poisonings to a sophisticated clinical discipline. The earliest recorded toxicological knowledge appears in ancient Egyptian papyri dated circa 1500 BCE, including descriptions of various poisons and their effects. In classical antiquity, notable figures like Hippocrates documented clinical manifestations of toxic exposures, while Dioscorides compiled the first systematic treatise on poisons in his work "De Materia Medica" in the first century CE.

Remember

Medical toxicology evolved from ancient observations to a modern medical specialty, with Paracelsus's principle that "the dose makes the poison" serving as a foundational concept

The Middle Ages witnessed both regression and advancement in toxicological understanding. Poisoning became a political tool, exemplified by the notorious Borgia family, while Persian physician Avicenna contributed significantly through his "Canon of Medicine," which included detailed accounts of various toxins and their treatments. The Renaissance period brought more systematic approaches to toxicology, with Paracelsus (1493-1541) establishing the fundamental principle that "the dose makes the poison"—recognizing that substances harmful at high doses might be benign or even beneficial at lower concentrations.

The foundations of modern toxicology emerged in the 19th century through the work of Mathieu Orfila, often considered the father of modern toxicology. His treatise "Traité des Poisons" (1814) established toxicology as a distinct scientific discipline, introducing systematic methods for detecting poisons in biological specimens. The Industrial Revolution generated new challenges as exposure to industrial chemicals created novel toxicological concerns, prompting the development of occupational toxicology.

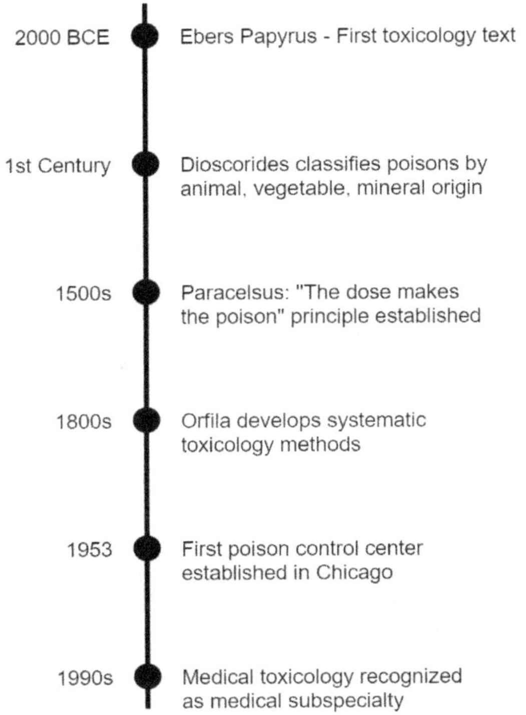

Figure 1.1: Historical Developments in Medical Toxicology

The 20th century witnessed exponential growth in toxicological knowledge and its clinical applications. Following World War II, a surge in pharmaceutical development necessitated more sophisticated safety testing. The thalidomide tragedy of the late 1950s, resulting in thousands of birth defects, highlighted the critical importance of toxicological evaluation and led to strengthened regulatory frameworks worldwide. The establishment of poison control centers beginning in the 1950s marked a pivotal advancement in clinical toxicology, providing specialized consultation services and surveillance capabilities.

The latter half of the 20th century saw the emergence of medical toxicology as a recognized medical subspecialty, with formal certification programs established in many countries. Today's medical toxicology integrates biochemical, pharmacological, and clinical principles to address an ever-expanding range of toxic exposures in both clinical and public health contexts.

SCOPE AND DEFINITION

Medical toxicology encompasses the study, diagnosis, management, and prevention of adverse effects from exposure to drugs, chemicals, biological agents, and environmental toxicants. Unlike traditional toxicology, which broadly addresses harmful effects of chemicals on all organisms, medical toxicology specifically focuses on human health implications. This specialized discipline operates at the intersection of clinical medicine, pharmacology, biochemistry, and environmental science.

Table 1.1: Core Domains of Medical Toxicology Practice

Domain	Primary Activities	Settings
Clinical Care	Direct patient management for poisonings and overdoses	Emergency departments, ICUs, inpatient toxicology services
Consultation	Remote expertise for complex cases	Poison centers, telemedicine, hospital consultation services
Prevention	Education, policy development, surveillance	Public health agencies, healthcare systems, schools
Research	Mechanisms of toxicity, antidote development, epidemiology	Academic centers, government agencies, industry
Education	Training healthcare providers, public education	Medical schools, residency programs, community outreach
Regulatory	Risk assessment, exposure standards, regulations	Government agencies, industry compliance

The scope of medical toxicology extends across several domains. Clinically, it addresses acute poisonings, chronic toxic exposures, addiction medicine, and adverse drug reactions. From a public health perspective, medical toxicology includes surveillance, disaster preparedness, risk assessment, and preventive strategies for population-level exposures. In the research domain, medical toxicologists investigate toxic mechanisms, develop novel detection methods, devise innovative treatment approaches, and contribute to toxicovigilance systems.

Medical toxicology's reach extends to legal guidelines through forensic toxicology, providing expertise in medicolegal investigations involving toxic substances.

> Remember
>
> **The scope includes diagnosis, management, and prevention of adverse effects from medications, chemicals, occupational exposures, environmental toxins, and biological agents**

Additionally, the regulatory aspects of the field contribute to pharmaceutical safety assessment, chemical regulation, and occupational exposure standards. The educational dimension encompasses professional training, public awareness campaigns, and risk communication strategies.

As a medical subspecialty, medical toxicology requires practitioners to possess comprehensive knowledge of pharmacokinetics, pathophysiology, critical care medicine, and analytical techniques. Medical toxicologists must remain current with an ever-expanding array of potential toxicants, including pharmaceutical agents, illicit substances, industrial chemicals, environmental pollutants, natural toxins, and emerging threats such as novel psychoactive substances and nanomaterials

BASIC PRINCIPLES

Several fundamental principles underpin the practice of medical toxicology. The toxicokinetic principle emphasizes understanding how toxicants enter, distribute within, metabolize, and exit the body—processes that determine the intensity and duration of toxic effects. The toxicodynamic principle focuses on how toxicants interact with biological systems at molecular, cellular, and organ levels to produce adverse effects, accounting for mechanisms ranging from receptor interactions to enzyme inhibition.

The dose-response relationship constitutes another core principle, recognizing that the severity of toxic effects typically correlates with exposure concentration, though this relationship may follow various patterns including linear, threshold, hormetic, or idiosyncratic responses. Time-course considerations acknowledge that toxic manifestations evolve over time, with initial presentations potentially differing substantially from delayed effects.

Risk assessment frameworks provide structured approaches to evaluating potential hazards, incorporating hazard identification, dose-response assessment, exposure assessment, and risk characterization.

> **Remember**
>
> **Core principles include dose-response relationships, toxicokinetics/toxicodynamics, and systematic approaches to risk assessment**

These assessments inform both individual patient management and broader public health interventions. The individual variation principle recognizes that genetic factors, age, pre-existing conditions, and concurrent exposures substantially modify susceptibility to toxicants.

Table 1.2: Fundamental Principles of Medical Toxicology

Principle	Description	Clinical Application
Dose-response relationship	Effects vary with exposure quantity	Guides risk assessment and treatment decisions
Toxicokinetics	How the body processes toxins	Determines treatment timing and duration
Toxicodynamics	How toxins affect body systems	Explains clinical manifestations and complications
Risk-benefit assessment	Weighing treatment risks vs. toxicity	Guides antidote use and intervention timing
Supportive care primacy	Basic physiological support as foundation	Applies across all toxicological emergencies
Multi-organ system approach	Toxins often affect multiple systems	Requires comprehensive assessment beyond presenting symptoms
Time-course consideration	Toxicity evolves over predictable patterns	Anticipatory management prevents complications

The diagnostic approach in medical toxicology relies on recognition of toxidromes—characteristic clusters of signs and symptoms associated with specific classes of toxicants. This pattern recognition, combined with exposure history and targeted laboratory testing, guides clinical decision-making. Treatment strategies follow the principle of therapeutic hierarchy, prioritizing life-sustaining measures, followed by toxicant elimination, antidote administration when available, and supportive care.

Prevention principles emphasize primary prevention (avoiding exposure), secondary prevention (early detection and intervention), and tertiary prevention (minimizing complications after exposure). The environmental principle recognizes that toxic exposures occur within ecological contexts, necessitating consideration of environmental persistence, bioaccumulation potential, and ecosystem effects

ROLE IN HEALTHCARE

Medical toxicology serves diverse and essential functions within healthcare systems. In emergency departments and intensive care units, medical toxicologists provide crucial expertise in managing acute poisonings and overdoses, developing protocols, guiding decontamination procedures, recommending antidotes, and supporting critical care management. Through poison control centers, toxicologists offer 24-hour consultation services, coordinate care for poisoned patients, maintain surveillance systems for toxic exposures, and collect valuable epidemiological data.

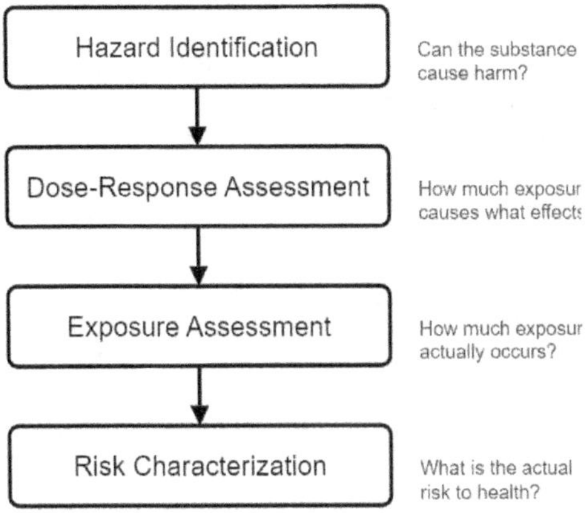

Figure 1.2: Toxicological Risk Assessment

In outpatient settings, medical toxicologists evaluate and manage patients with chronic toxic exposures, occupational illnesses, and adverse drug reactions, often serving as consultants for complex diagnostic challenges. Their expertise extends to public health agencies, where they contribute to outbreak investigations, environmental health assessments, disaster response planning, and policy development regarding chemical threats.

> **Remember**
>
> **Medical toxicologists serve in multiple healthcare settings including emergency departments, poison centers, occupational health, public health agencies, pharmaceutical industry, and forensic investigations**

Medical toxicologists play vital roles in medication safety programs within healthcare institutions, participating in adverse drug event monitoring, developing prevention strategies, and creating institutional guidelines for high-risk medications. They provide essential education to healthcare professionals, patients, and the public about toxic hazards, prevention strategies, and appropriate response to exposures.

The research contributions of medical toxicologists advance clinical practice through investigating toxic mechanisms, developing novel treatment approaches, evaluating antidote efficacy, and refining diagnostic methods. In legal contexts, they serve as expert witnesses in cases involving poisonings, substance abuse, environmental exposures, and product liability.

Medical toxicologists often collaborate with regulatory agencies to evaluate pharmaceutical safety, establish workplace exposure limits, assess environmental contaminants, and develop warning systems for emerging toxicological threats. Their role in addiction medicine has grown increasingly important, contributing expertise to substance use disorder treatment programs, medication-assisted treatment initiatives, and harm reduction strategies.

As healthcare systems continue to evolve, medical toxicologists increasingly participate in interprofessional teams addressing complex health challenges, including environmental justice issues, climate change impacts, emerging pharmaceutical technologies, and global chemical safety. Through this multifaceted involvement across healthcare domains, medical toxicology serves as a critical discipline for addressing the diverse toxic challenges facing contemporary society

Summary

Medical toxicology examines the adverse effects of chemicals, pharmaceuticals, and biological substances on human health. Its origins trace from ancient poison recognition through medieval applications to modern scientific approaches established in the 20th century. The discipline encompasses acute poisonings, chronic exposures, environmental toxins, occupational hazards, pharmaceutical adverse effects, and substance abuse. Core principles include dose-response relationships demonstrating how effects vary with exposure levels, toxicokinetics describing how substances move through the body, and toxicodynamics explaining mechanisms of toxicity at molecular and cellular levels. Medical toxicologists function across diverse settings—treating poisoned patients in emergency departments, providing consultation through poison centers, conducting surveillance for emerging threats, establishing workplace safety standards, evaluating pharmaceutical safety, and supporting legal proceedings. The field continues to evolve with new challenges from novel drugs, environmental pollutants, and changing exposure patterns, requiring ongoing adaptation of assessment tools, treatment protocols, and preventive strategies. This integrative discipline combines principles from pharmacology, biochemistry, emergency medicine, and public health to address the complex interplay between chemical exposures and human health.

Self-Assessment Questions

1. Discuss the historical evolution of toxicology as a medical discipline, highlighting key contributors and milestone events that shaped the field.
2. Explain how Paracelsus's principle that "the dose makes the poison" relates to modern concepts of therapeutic windows and safety margins in pharmaceutical use.
3. Compare and contrast the roles of medical toxicologists in emergency department settings versus occupational health environments.
4. Describe how toxidromes aid in the recognition and management of poisoned patients when the specific agent is unknown.
5. Analyze the multidisciplinary nature of medical toxicology and how it intersects with other medical specialties including emergency medicine, occupational medicine, and preventive medicine.
6. Evaluate the importance of poison control centers in modern healthcare systems and their contributions to both clinical care and public health surveillance.
7. Explain how risk assessment principles in toxicology inform regulatory decisions about environmental chemicals, occupational exposures, and pharmaceutical safety.
8. Describe the challenges in diagnosing and managing toxicity from emerging substances such as novel psychoactive substances or new pharmaceutical agents.
9. Discuss how medical toxicology principles apply to mass casualty scenarios involving chemical exposures or bioterrorism events.
10. Analyze current trends in poisoning epidemiology and how these patterns influence both clinical practice and preventive strategies in medical toxicology.

Bibliography

1. Hoffman RS, Howland MA, Lewin NA, Nelson LS, Goldfrank LR. Goldfrank's toxicologic emergencies. 11th ed. New York: McGraw-Hill Education; 2019.
2. Barceloux DG. Medical toxicology: diagnosis and treatment of human poisoning. New York: Elsevier; 2012.
3. Brent J, Burkhart K, Dargan P, Hatten B, Megarbane B, Palmer R, White J, editors. Critical care toxicology: diagnosis and management of the critically poisoned patient. 2nd ed. Cham: Springer International Publishing; 2017.
4. Dart RC, editor. Medical toxicology. 3rd ed. Philadelphia: Lippincott Williams & Wilkins; 2004.
5. Wax PM, Stolbach A. The changing roles of medical toxicologists: response to the opioid epidemic. J Med Toxicol. 2021;17(2):125-131.
6. Nelson LS, Perrone J, DeRoos F, Stork C, Hoffman RS. Poison control centers and emergency departments: partners in toxicosurveillance and public health. J Med Toxicol. 2019;15(2):126-130.
7. Gummin DD, Mowry JB, Beuhler MC, Spyker DA, Bronstein AC, Rivers LJ, et al. 2020 Annual Report of the American Association of Poison Control Centers' National Poison Data System (NPDS): 38th Annual Report. Clin Toxicol (Phila). 2021;59(12):1282-1501.
8. Curry SC, Beuhler MC, Finnell JT, Rice PJ, Donovan JW, Kunisaki TA, et al. Update on the core content of medical toxicology. J Med Toxicol. 2019;15(4):238-247.
9. Brent J. Critical care toxicology. Crit Care Clin. 2005;21(4):1-7.
10. Wax PM, Donovan JW. Fellowship training in medical toxicology: characteristics, employment patterns, and career satisfaction of fellows. Clin Toxicol (Phila). 2006;44(1):25-28

CHAPTER 2

TOXICOKINETICS AND TOXICODYNAMICS

Author

Mr. Mushraff Ali Khan M, Associate Professor, Department of Pharmaceutics, Sultan-ul-Uloom College of Pharmacy, Banjara Hills, Hyderabad, Telangana, India

Abstract

The knowledge about how the toxic substances enter, distribute through, transform within, and exit the body is fundamental to predicting, preventing, and treating poisonings. Toxicokinetics is the study about absorption of xenobiotics through gastrointestinal, dermal, pulmonary, and parenteral routes, each with distinct characteristics affecting the rate and extent of entry into circulation. Once absorbed, distribution is influenced by factors including protein binding, lipid solubility, and specialized barriers such as the blood-brain and placental interfaces. Metabolism, primarily occurring in the liver, encompasses Phase I (functionalization) and Phase II (conjugation) reactions that can either detoxify harmful substances or bioactivate relatively innocuous compounds into toxic metabolites. Excretion pathways—renal, biliary, pulmonary, and others—complete the ADME process, with parameters like half-life and clearance rate determining how long toxins persist. Toxicodynamics addresses mechanisms by which substances produce adverse effects, including receptor interactions, enzyme inhibition, protein and DNA adduct formation, oxidative stress, and disruption of cellular homeostasis. These principles provide the mechanistic foundation for clinical toxicology, explaining why certain exposures produce specific symptoms and guiding the development of targeted therapeutic interventions.

Keywords: *Toxicokinetics, Toxicodynamics, Biotransformation, Bioactivation, Xenobiotic Metabolism, Cellular Toxicity*

Learning Objectives

After completion of the chapter, the learners should be able to:

- Differentiate between toxicokinetic and toxicodynamic processes and explain their interrelationship in determining toxic responses.
- Compare the absorption characteristics of toxic substances across different routes of exposure and identify factors that enhance or inhibit absorption.
- Analyze how distribution factors including protein binding, tissue affinity, and specialized barriers affect the toxicity of substances.
- Explain the role of Phase I and Phase II metabolic pathways in both detoxification and bioactivation of xenobiotics.
- Evaluate the primary excretion mechanisms for toxic substances and calculate parameters such as half-life and clearance rates.
- Identify the major cellular and molecular mechanisms of toxicity and relate them to specific clinical manifestations of poisoning

ABSORPTION

The entry of toxicants into the body initiates the toxicokinetic process, with absorption dynamics significantly influencing the ultimate toxic impact. Various routes of exposure present distinct absorption profiles that determine the bioavailability of toxicants and their subsequent systemic effects.

Gastrointestinal Absorption

Gastrointestinal absorption represents the most common route for toxicant entry, whether through intentional ingestion, accidental exposure, or contaminated food and water. The complex physiology of the gastrointestinal tract creates variable absorption environments throughout its length. Gastric absorption occurs primarily with weak acids that remain predominantly in their non-ionized form in the acidic environment of the stomach (pH 1-3), allowing passive diffusion across the gastric mucosa. The small intestine, with its extensive surface area enhanced by villi and microvilli, serves as the principal site of absorption for most toxicants. Its relatively alkaline environment (pH 5-7) favors absorption of weakly basic compounds that become non-ionized in this milieu. The specialized enterocytes lining the intestinal wall employ multiple transport mechanisms, including passive diffusion, facilitated diffusion, active transport, and pinocytosis, depending on the physicochemical properties of the toxicant.

Several factors modulate gastrointestinal absorption. Food presence generally delays gastric emptying, potentially reducing absorption rates of concurrent toxicants, though high-fat meals may enhance absorption of lipophilic compounds.

> **Remember**
>
> **Absorption varies significantly by route of exposure, with inhalation typically providing the most rapid systemic exposure, followed by intravenous, intramuscular, subcutaneous, oral, and dermal routes.**

Gastrointestinal motility alterations, whether accelerated or decreased, significantly impact toxicant transit time and absorption opportunity. Pathological conditions affecting mucosal integrity, such as inflammatory bowel disease or celiac disease, may enhance absorption of compounds normally restricted by intact epithelial barriers. First-pass metabolism, particularly in the liver, can substantially reduce bioavailability of orally ingested toxicants through biotransformation before they reach systemic circulation.

Table 2.1: Factors Affecting Toxicant Absorption

Route	Major Factors	Examples of Modifying Factors
Oral	Gastric pH, food presence, formulation	Antacids increase lead absorption
	First-pass metabolism, gastric emptying	Alcohol accelerates chloral hydrate absorption
Dermal	Molecular weight, lipid solubility	Solvents enhance pesticide absorption
	Skin integrity, anatomical location	Damaged skin increases all absorption
Inhalation	Particle size, solubility	Exercise increases respiratory absorption
	Respiratory rate, airway pathology	Asthma enhances inhaled toxin absorption
Parenteral	Tissue vascularity, injection site	IV administration bypasses absorption barriers
	Formulation (solution vs. suspension)	IM depot formulations delay absorption

Pulmonary Absorption

The respiratory system provides an extensive absorption surface with immediate access to the bloodstream, bypassing hepatic first-pass metabolism. Gases, vapors, and fine particulates can reach the alveolar surfaces, where the extremely thin alveolar-capillary membrane (0.2-0.5 μm) facilitates rapid exchange. Gaseous toxicants dissolve in the alveolar lining fluid before diffusing into pulmonary circulation, with more soluble compounds generally achieving higher blood concentrations. Particle size fundamentally determines the deposition site within the respiratory tract: large particles (>10 μm) typically deposit in the upper airways, medium particles (2.5-10 μm) reach the tracheobronchial region, while fine (<2.5 μm) and ultrafine (<0.1 μm) particles can penetrate to alveolar spaces.

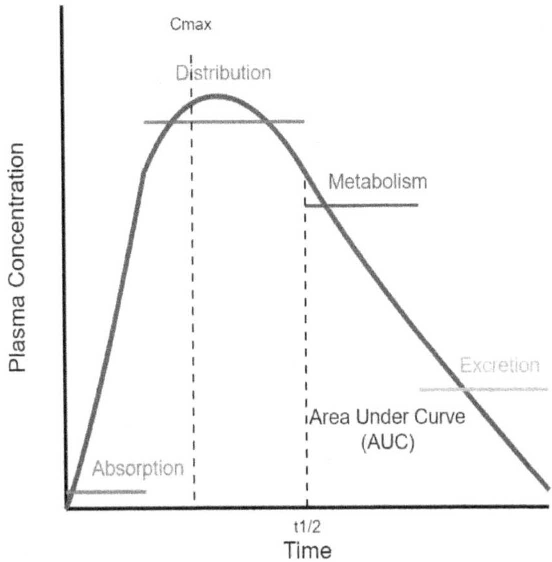

Figure 2.1 Various Phases in Toxicokinetics

Ventilation rate significantly influences absorption kinetics, with increased respiratory rate and depth during physical exertion enhancing toxic exposure. Pre-existing pulmonary conditions, such as chronic obstructive pulmonary disease or asthma, may alter airflow patterns and deposition of inhaled toxicants. The pulmonary epithelium contains specialized defense mechanisms, including ciliated cells and mucus secretion, which can trap and eliminate particles through mucociliary clearance, though these defenses may become overwhelmed with high-concentration exposures or compromised by concurrent respiratory conditions.

Dermal Absorption

The skin, while serving as a protective barrier, permits absorption of certain toxicants, particularly lipophilic compounds. The stratum corneum, composed of dead keratinocytes embedded in a lipid matrix, represents the rate-limiting barrier to percutaneous absorption. Toxicants must traverse this hydrophobic layer before reaching viable epidermis and ultimately dermal blood vessels. The physicochemical properties of compounds significantly determine their skin penetration potential, with molecular weight under 500 Da, moderate lipophilicity (log P between 1-3), and adequate water solubility favoring absorption.

Regional variations in skin thickness and composition create different absorption potentials across the body. Thin-skinned areas with rich vascularization, such as the face, scrotum, and forehead, demonstrate enhanced absorption compared to thicker regions like the palms and soles. Skin condition dramatically affects barrier function, with abrasions, lacerations, inflammation, or diseases like psoriasis or eczema potentially increasing absorption rates by orders of magnitude. Environmental conditions, particularly increased temperature and humidity, enhance percutaneous absorption by increasing blood flow, hydrating the stratum corneum, and potentially expanding intercellular channels. Occlusion, whether from clothing, gloves, or specialized transdermal delivery systems, creates a microenvironment of increased hydration and temperature that can significantly enhance absorption.

Other Absorption Routes

Several specialized absorption routes present unique toxicological considerations. Parenteral administration bypasses absorption barriers, with intravenous injection delivering toxicants directly to systemic circulation, while intramuscular and subcutaneous routes provide slower absorption through tissue diffusion before reaching bloodstream. Ocular exposure permits absorption through the cornea and conjunctiva, with lipophilic substances penetrating the corneal epithelium and hydrophilic compounds traversing conjunctival blood vessels. The blood-brain barrier generally restricts direct central nervous system absorption, though lipophilic toxicants and compounds utilizing specific transporters can cross this specialized interface. Transplacental transfer occurs primarily via passive diffusion, active transport, or facilitated diffusion, with lipophilic, low-molecular-weight, un-ionized compounds most readily crossing the placental barrier and potentially affecting fetal development.

DISTRIBUTION

Following absorption, toxicants undergo distribution throughout the body, a process governed by physiological and physicochemical factors that determine tissue concentrations and potential sites of toxic action.

Physiological Determinants of Distribution

Blood flow fundamentally influences toxicant distribution, with highly perfused organs like the brain, liver, and kidneys receiving disproportionately large fractions of cardiac output and consequently experiencing initial high toxicant concentrations.

> Remember
>
> **Distribution of toxins depends on factors including protein binding, lipid solubility, volume of distribution, and specialized barriers such as the blood-brain and placental barriers.**

Plasma protein binding significantly affects distribution patterns, as only unbound (free) fractions of toxicants can traverse capillary membranes and interact with target tissues. Albumin primarily binds acidic compounds, while α1-acid glycoprotein preferentially binds basic substances. Binding affinity varies substantially between compounds, from negligible to exceeding 99% of circulating toxicant. Competition for binding sites can occur when multiple toxicants or medications simultaneously occupy circulation, potentially increasing free concentrations of displaced substances.

Tissue permeability barriers selectively restrict toxicant distribution to protected compartments. The blood-brain barrier, formed by tight junctions between cerebrovascular endothelial cells and astrocyte foot processes, limits penetration to lipophilic compounds, small uncharged molecules, and substances utilizing specific transporters. Similarly, the blood-testis barrier protects germinal epithelium, while the placental barrier offers partial protection to developing fetuses, though many toxicants can traverse these specialized interfaces to varying degrees. Body fluid compartments influence distribution patterns, with water-soluble toxicants primarily distributing within extracellular fluids, while lipophilic compounds may extensively penetrate cell membranes and distribute throughout total body water.

Table 2.2: Toxicant Distribution Determinants and Clinical Implications

Factor	Description	Clinical Example
Protein binding	Binding to albumin and other proteins reduces active toxin	Highly protein-bound drugs (warfarin) displaced by competitors
Volume of distribution	Apparent space in which toxin distributes	Lipophilic substances (TCAs) with large Vd resist removal
Blood flow	Rate of delivery to tissues	Shock reduces peripheral tissue distribution
Lipid solubility	Ability to cross membranes and enter tissues	Lipophilic toxins (organophosphates) penetrate CNS rapidly
pKa and pH	Ionization affects membrane crossing	Alkalization "traps" salicylates in blood, enhancing elimination
Tissue affinity	Selective concentration in specific organs	Lead stored in bone creates ongoing exposure source
Barriers	Blood-brain, placental, other selective barriers	Lipophilic substances cross BBB, causing neurotoxicity

Physicochemical Aspects of Distribution

Lipophilicity represents a critical determinant of distribution patterns. Highly lipophilic toxicants readily cross cell membranes and tend to accumulate in adipose tissue, creating potential reservoirs for prolonged release and extended toxic effects. Ionization state significantly affects distribution, as ionized molecules generally demonstrate reduced membrane permeability compared to their un-ionized counterparts. The pH partition theory explains how weakly acidic toxicants accumulate in relatively alkaline compartments, while weakly basic compounds concentrate in more acidic environments, creating potential ion trapping in specific tissues. Molecular size influences distribution capabilities, with smaller molecules (<500 Da) generally exhibiting broader distribution compared to larger compounds that may face restricted passage across certain biological membranes.

Volume of Distribution

The volume of distribution (Vd) represents a fundamental pharmacokinetic parameter reflecting the theoretical volume required to contain the total amount of a toxicant at the same concentration measured in blood plasma. This parameter does not represent an actual physiological space but rather describes the apparent space into which a toxicant distributes. Toxicants primarily confined to the vascular compartment, such as highly protein-bound compounds or large molecules, typically exhibit low Vd values approximating blood volume (0.07-0.08 L/kg). Substances distributing throughout total body water demonstrate moderate Vd values around 0.6 L/kg, while extensively tissue-bound toxicants may present very high Vd values (>10 L/kg), indicating significant sequestration in tissues compared to plasma. Volume of distribution calculations inform estimates of total body burden, guide dosing of antidotes or chelating agents, and help predict the potential effectiveness of elimination techniques such as hemodialysis.

Redistribution Phenomena

Dynamic changes in distribution patterns occur throughout the toxicokinetic process. Initial distribution often follows blood flow patterns, with highly perfused organs receiving disproportionate toxicant concentrations. Subsequent redistribution may occur as tissue binding sites become saturated or as toxicants move from central circulation to peripheral compartments. This redistribution explains the biphasic clinical course observed with some toxicants, particularly lipophilic central nervous system depressants, where initial improvement followed by secondary deterioration reflects redistribution from brain tissue back to circulation upon decreased blood concentrations. Postmortem redistribution presents particular challenges for forensic toxicology, as concentrations measured after death may not accurately reflect antemortem levels due to passive diffusion from highly concentrated tissues into surrounding blood vessels, particularly with lipophilic basic drugs

METABOLISM

Biotransformation of toxicants, primarily occurring in the liver but also in other tissues, represents a critical determinant of toxicity duration, intensity, and character. These metabolic processes typically render lipophilic compounds more hydrophilic, facilitating their eventual elimination.

Phase I Reactions

Phase I metabolic reactions introduce or expose functional groups on toxicant molecules, generally increasing their polarity and reactivity. Cytochrome P450 (CYP) enzymes, a superfamily of heme-containing monooxygenases embedded in the endoplasmic reticulum, catalyze the majority of oxidative biotransformations. These microsomal enzymes incorporate one oxygen atom from molecular oxygen into the substrate while reducing the other oxygen atom to water. The human genome encodes approximately 57 CYP enzymes, with CYP1A2, CYP2C9, CYP2C19, CYP2D6, CYP2E1, and CYP3A4 accounting for the metabolism of most xenobiotics. Each isoenzyme demonstrates distinct substrate specificity, though considerable overlap exists between some forms.

> **Remember**
>
> **Metabolism can either detoxify harmful substances (most Phase II reactions) or bioactivate relatively innocuous compounds into toxic metabolites (certain Phase I reactions), with the liver serving as the primary site.**

Oxidation reactions catalyzed by CYP enzymes include aromatic and aliphatic hydroxylation, N-dealkylation, O-dealkylation, S-oxidation, and deamination. These reactions generally increase hydrophilicity by introducing hydroxyl groups or exposing polar functional groups previously masked by alkyl substituents. Non-CYP oxidative enzymes also contribute to toxicant metabolism, including flavin-containing monooxygenases (FMOs), which primarily oxidize nucleophilic nitrogen, sulfur, and phosphorus heteroatoms, alcohol dehydrogenase, which catalyzes the oxidation of alcohols to aldehydes, and aldehyde dehydrogenase, which further oxidizes aldehydes to carboxylic acids.

Reduction reactions, though less common than oxidations, play important roles in metabolizing certain toxicants, particularly those containing carbonyl, azo, nitro, and sulfoxide groups. These reactions often occur in low-oxygen environments through the action of reductases including NADPH-cytochrome P450 reductase and NADPH:quinone oxidoreductase. Hydrolytic reactions, catalyzed by esterases, amidases, and epoxide hydrolases, cleave esters, amides, and epoxides respectively through the addition of water across susceptible bonds.

Phase II Reactions

Phase II conjugation reactions involve the attachment of endogenous hydrophilic moieties to toxicants or their phase I metabolites, substantially increasing molecular weight and water solubility while typically reducing biological activity.

Table 2.3: Major Metabolic Pathways in Toxicology

Pathway	Process	Examples	Clinical Significance
Phase I: Oxidation	Addition of oxygen or removal of hydrogen	Cytochrome P450 metabolism of alcohols	Can produce toxic metabolites (acetaminophe n → NAPQI)
Phase I: Reduction	Addition of hydrogen or removal of oxygen	Reduction of nitro compounds	Can activate certain prodrugs
Phase I: Hydrolysis	Cleavage by addition of water	Esterase hydrolysis of organophosphat es	Can detoxify or activate compounds
Phase II: Glucuronidatio n	Conjugatio n with glucuronic acid	Morphine, acetaminophen, TCA metabolism	Enhances water solubility for excretion
Phase II: Sulfation	Addition of sulfate group	Acetaminophen, steroid hormones	Alternate pathway when primary routes saturated
Phase II: Glutathione conjugation	Binding to glutathione	Detoxifies reactive intermediates	Depletion can lead to increased toxicity
Phase II: Acetylation	Addition of acetyl group	Isoniazid, sulfonamides	Genetic polymorphism s affect toxicity risk

These synthetic reactions require specific transferase enzymes and high-energy cofactors. Glucuronidation, mediated by UDP-glucuronosyltransferases (UGTs), represents the most common conjugation pathway, attaching glucuronic acid to substrates containing hydroxyl, carboxyl, amino, or sulfhydryl groups. The resulting glucuronides exhibit enhanced water solubility and are predominantly excreted in bile or urine.

Sulfation, catalyzed by sulfotransferase enzymes, transfers a sulfonyl group from 3'-phosphoadenosine-5'-phosphosulfate (PAPS) to hydroxyl or amino groups, creating highly polar sulfate conjugates efficiently eliminated in urine. Glutathione conjugation, performed by glutathione S-transferases (GSTs), facilitates nucleophilic attack by reduced glutathione on electrophilic carbon, nitrogen, or sulfur atoms in toxicants, forming thioether bonds. This mechanism provides critical protection against reactive electrophilic compounds that might otherwise form covalent adducts with cellular macromolecules.

Additional phase II pathways include amino acid conjugation, primarily glycine and glutamine, with carboxylic acid groups, acetylation of aromatic amines and hydrazines through N-acetyltransferases, and methylation reactions catalyzed by methyltransferases, which transfer methyl groups to oxygen, nitrogen, or sulfur atoms in substrate molecules. Unlike most conjugation reactions, methylation typically decreases hydrophilicity but may facilitate subsequent conjugation steps.

Factors Affecting Metabolism

Genetic polymorphisms in metabolizing enzymes create substantial interindividual variation in biotransformation capacity, ranging from minimal to extremely rapid metabolism of specific substrates. Clinically significant polymorphisms affect numerous enzymes including CYP2D6, CYP2C9, CYP2C19, UGT1A1, and N-acetyltransferase 2, creating important population differences in toxicant susceptibility. Age profoundly influences metabolic capacity, with neonates exhibiting reduced activity of many enzymes that gradually increases during development, while elderly individuals often demonstrate decreased hepatic metabolism due to reduced liver mass and blood flow rather than specific enzyme deficiencies.

Sex differences in metabolism arise from hormonal influences on enzyme expression, with females generally showing higher CYP3A4 activity and males exhibiting greater CYP1A2 function. Nutritional status affects biotransformation through multiple mechanisms: protein malnutrition can reduce synthesis of metabolizing enzymes, certain dietary components like cruciferous vegetables can induce specific CYP isoforms, and vitamin cofactors are required for optimal enzyme function. Pre-existing disease states, particularly hepatic disorders like cirrhosis or hepatitis, can significantly impair metabolic capacity by reducing functional hepatocyte mass, altering blood flow patterns, or disrupting enzyme synthesis.

Enzyme induction and inhibition represent critical mechanisms of toxicokinetic interactions. Induction involves increased enzyme synthesis through receptor-mediated gene transcription, typically requiring days to reach maximal effect and potentially persisting for similar periods after inducer removal. Common inducers include rifampin (CYP3A4, CYP2C9), phenobarbital (multiple CYPs), cigarette smoke (CYP1A2), and ethanol (CYP2E1). Conversely, enzyme inhibition occurs more rapidly through competitive binding to active sites, structural inactivation, or reduced enzyme synthesis. Notable inhibitors include cimetidine (multiple CYPs), ciprofloxacin (CYP1A2), fluconazole (CYP2C9), and grapefruit juice compounds (CYP3A4).

Metabolic Activation

While metabolism often decreases toxicity through detoxification, certain compounds undergo bioactivation, where metabolic processes generate intermediates with greater toxicity than the parent compound. These reactive metabolites may include electrophiles, free radicals, or compounds with enhanced receptor affinity. Classical examples include acetaminophen, whose CYP-mediated oxidation produces the reactive metabolite N-acetyl-p-benzoquinone imine (NAPQI) that depletes glutathione and forms protein adducts leading to hepatocellular necrosis; carbon tetrachloride, which undergoes reductive metabolism to generate trichloromethyl free radicals causing lipid peroxidation; and certain pyrrolizidine alkaloids, activated to pyrrolic derivatives that alkylate cellular macromolecules.

The balance between activating and detoxifying pathways critically determines toxic outcomes. Competitive metabolism pathways may lead different proportions of a toxicant through activation versus detoxification routes. Saturation kinetics can shift metabolism from high-affinity detoxification pathways to alternative routes generating reactive intermediates at higher doses. Depletion of conjugating agents, particularly glutathione, may allow accumulation of reactive metabolites normally neutralized through conjugation. Understanding these complex metabolic interactions provides the foundation for rational antidote development, such as N-acetylcysteine for acetaminophen poisoning, which replenishes glutathione stores and provides alternative conjugation capacity

EXCRETION

The elimination of toxicants and their metabolites represents the final phase of toxicokinetics, with multiple organ systems contributing to their removal from the body.

Renal Excretion

The kidneys serve as the primary excretory organs for most water-soluble toxicants and metabolites. Renal elimination encompasses three fundamental processes: glomerular filtration, tubular secretion, and tubular reabsorption. Glomerular filtration allows passage of unbound toxicants with molecular weights below approximately 60,000 Da through the glomerular filtration barrier into the tubular lumen. The filtration rate, normally about 120 mL/min in adults, can be significantly altered by changes in renal blood flow, as occurs in shock, heart failure, or with vasoconstrictive agents.

Tubular secretion involves active transport of toxicants from peritubular capillaries into tubular fluid, primarily occurring in the proximal tubule. Two major transport systems facilitate this process: the organic anion transporters (OATs), which secrete acidic compounds and their conjugates, and the organic cation transporters (OCTs), which handle basic substances. These carrier-mediated systems demonstrate saturable kinetics and competitive inhibition between substrates, creating potential toxicokinetic interactions. Probenecid, for instance, competitively inhibits organic anion secretion, potentially prolonging the half-life of compounds utilizing this pathway.

Tubular reabsorption occurs primarily through passive diffusion across tubular epithelium, with lipophilic, un-ionized compounds most readily reabsorbed into circulation. This process follows principles of pH partition theory, where urinary pH significantly influences reabsorption of weakly acidic or basic compounds. Alkalinization of urine increases ionization of weak acids, reducing their reabsorption and enhancing elimination (ion trapping) – a principle exploited in treating salicylate poisoning through sodium bicarbonate administration. Conversely, acidification of urine enhances elimination of weak bases like amphetamines and phencyclidine.

Several factors modulate renal excretion efficiency. Renal blood flow, representing approximately 25% of cardiac output, determines delivery of toxicants to kidney tissues, with reduced flow in shock states compromising elimination. Glomerular filtration rate directly affects filtration-dependent elimination, with age-related declines or pathological reductions in kidney disease substantially prolonging toxicant half-lives. Competitive transport interactions at secretory sites can reduce elimination rates of affected compounds, as observed with probenecid-penicillin or cimetidine-procainamide interactions.

Hepatobiliary Excretion

The liver excretes numerous compounds into bile, particularly larger molecular weight (>300 Da) substances, including glucuronide and glutathione conjugates. This process involves active transport across the canalicular membrane of hepatocytes into bile canaliculi through specialized transport proteins including P-glycoprotein, multidrug resistance-associated proteins (MRPs), and organic anion-transporting polypeptides (OATPs). Biliary excretion demonstrates saturable kinetics and competitive interactions between substrates sharing transport systems.

Enterohepatic circulation significantly influences the toxicokinetics of many compounds excreted in bile. This process occurs when biliary metabolites reach the intestinal lumen and undergo deconjugation by bacterial enzymes, regenerating more lipophilic compounds that can be reabsorbed and returned to the liver via portal circulation. This recycling can substantially prolong toxicant presence in the body, creating sustained exposure and delayed elimination curves. Interrupting enterohepatic circulation through administration of binding resins like cholestyramine can enhance elimination of compounds undergoing this recycling, as demonstrated in the treatment of T4 thyroid hormone overdose.

Hepatobiliary excretion efficiency depends on several factors. Hepatic blood flow, representing approximately 25% of cardiac output, determines delivery of toxicants to hepatocytes for potential biliary excretion. Transport protein expression and function significantly influence biliary secretion capacity, with certain genetic polymorphisms or drug interactions potentially altering this process. Bile flow rates affect the volume available for toxicant dilution, with cholestasis potentially reducing elimination of biliary-excreted compounds. Intestinal transit time influences reabsorption probability during enterohepatic circulation, with diarrhea potentially reducing recycling and enhancing elimination.

Pulmonary Excretion

The lungs primarily eliminate volatile substances and gases, with the large surface area of alveolar-capillary interface facilitating rapid exchange. Pulmonary elimination efficiency correlates with several physicochemical properties: volatility (vapor pressure) determines tendency to transition from liquid to gas phase; blood:gas partition coefficient reflects the relative solubility in these phases, with lower values favoring more rapid pulmonary elimination; and molecular size influences diffusion rates across alveolar membranes.

Volatile anesthetics exemplify compounds primarily eliminated through pulmonary excretion, with their elimination rates largely determined by their blood:gas partition coefficients. Similarly, carbon monoxide, hydrogen cyanide, and ethanol partially undergo pulmonary elimination. Alveolar ventilation rate directly influences elimination efficiency, with hyperventilation enhancing removal of volatile compounds—a principle employed in treating carbon monoxide poisoning through high-flow oxygen administration, which both displaces carbon monoxide from hemoglobin and increases its pulmonary elimination.

Other Routes of Excretion

Several additional pathways contribute to toxicant elimination. Salivary excretion occurs through passive diffusion of lipophilic compounds and active transport of certain substances into saliva, though most swallowed toxicants undergo intestinal reabsorption rather than true elimination through this route. Sweat contains various toxicants reaching skin glands through passive diffusion, particularly lipophilic compounds, though the quantitative contribution to total elimination remains relatively minor for most substances.

Breast milk represents an important excretion pathway for lipophilic compounds, creating potential exposure concerns for nursing infants. The mammary epithelium allows passage of un-ionized, lipophilic substances, with the relatively high fat content of milk creating a favorable partition coefficient for such compounds. Toxicants documented in breast milk include persistent organic pollutants like polychlorinated biphenyls, numerous pharmaceuticals, and drugs of abuse including cocaine and cannabis metabolites.

Hair incorporates various toxicants during its formation, creating a historical record of exposure that forms the basis for retrospective toxicological analyses. Incorporation occurs primarily at the hair follicle level during formation, with melanin binding particularly relevant for basic compounds. The hair matrix preserves toxicants for extended periods, allowing detection months or even years after exposure, though external contamination and variability in incorporation rates complicate interpretation

MECHANISMS OF TOXICITY

Toxicants produce adverse effects through diverse mechanisms that disrupt normal physiological functions at molecular, cellular, and organ system levels.

Receptor-Mediated Toxicity

Many toxicants exert their effects through interactions with specific cellular receptors, either mimicking endogenous ligands (agonists) or preventing normal receptor activation (antagonists). Neurotransmitter receptors represent common toxicological targets. Organophosphate and carbamate insecticides inhibit acetylcholinesterase, preventing acetylcholine breakdown and causing cholinergic overstimulation. Opioids bind μ-opioid receptors, producing respiratory depression and analgesia. Antipsychotic drugs antagonize dopamine D2 receptors, potentially causing extrapyramidal symptoms through disrupted basal ganglia function.

Hormone receptors provide another important target class. Endocrine disrupting chemicals like bisphenol A interact with estrogen receptors, potentially altering reproductive development and function. Dioxins activate the aryl hydrocarbon receptor, inducing expression of cytochrome P450 enzymes and producing wasting syndrome, immunotoxicity, and developmental abnormalities. Peroxisome proliferator-activated receptor gamma (PPARγ) agonists like thiazolidinediones affect glucose metabolism and adipogenesis, while potentially causing fluid retention and cardiac complications.

Ion channels, which regulate electrochemical gradients across cell membranes, represent critical toxicological targets. Tetrodotoxin and saxitoxin block voltage-gated sodium channels, preventing action potential generation and causing paralysis. Batrachotoxin and pyrethroids keep sodium channels in open conformation, causing persistent depolarization. Calcium channel blockers like verapamil inhibit voltage-dependent calcium channels, reducing cardiac contractility and peripheral vascular resistance.

Receptor-mediated toxicity exhibits several characteristic features. Specificity typically manifests as effects corresponding to the receptor's normal physiological role. Stereoselectivity often appears, with different stereoisomers demonstrating variable receptor affinities. Competitive interactions between toxicants targeting the same receptor may produce antagonistic effects. Tolerance and adaptation frequently develop through receptor downregulation, desensitization, or compensatory mechanisms with prolonged exposure.

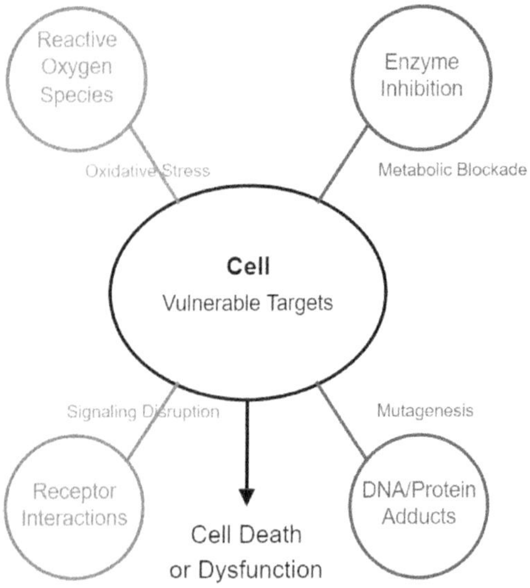

Figure 2.2 Mechanisms of Toxicity

Enzyme Inhibition and Induction

Numerous toxicants disrupt enzymatic processes through various mechanisms. Competitive inhibition occurs when toxicants structurally resemble normal substrates and occupy enzyme active sites without undergoing transformation, as exemplified by methotrexate's inhibition of dihydrofolate reductase. Noncompetitive inhibition involves toxicant binding at allosteric sites, altering enzyme conformation and reducing catalytic efficiency without directly competing with substrates, as seen with lead inhibition of delta-aminolevulinic acid dehydratase in heme synthesis.

Irreversible inhibition results from covalent modification of essential enzyme components, permanently inactivating them until new protein synthesis occurs. Organophosphate insecticides exemplify this mechanism through phosphorylation of acetylcholinesterase's active site serine residue. Mercury compounds irreversibly inhibit numerous enzymes by binding to sulfhydryl groups in active sites. Carbon monoxide produces irreversible inhibition of cytochrome oxidase through binding to heme iron, disrupting mitochondrial electron transport.

Enzyme induction represents another significant toxicological mechanism, typically occurring through increased gene transcription and protein synthesis. Phenobarbital induces multiple cytochrome P450 enzymes through constitutive androstane receptor (CAR) activation. Polycyclic aromatic hydrocarbons induce CYP1A1/1A2 via aryl hydrocarbon receptor binding. Ethanol induces CYP2E1 through protein stabilization and increased synthesis. Such induction can accelerate metabolism of co-administered substances, potentially reducing therapeutic efficacy or increasing formation of toxic metabolites.

Oxidative Stress

Oxidative stress represents a fundamental mechanism underlying numerous toxic effects, occurring when reactive oxygen species (ROS) production exceeds cellular antioxidant defenses. Primary ROS include superoxide anion ($O_2\bullet-$), hydrogen peroxide (H_2O_2), hydroxyl radical ($OH\bullet$), and singlet oxygen ($1O_2$). These highly reactive species damage cellular components through lipid peroxidation, protein oxidation, and DNA modification.

Several mechanisms generate oxidative stress in toxicological contexts. Redox cycling compounds like paraquat and doxorubicin undergo repetitive reduction and re-oxidation, continuously generating superoxide during this process. Mitochondrial electron transport chain disruption by toxicants like rotenone and cyanide increases electron leakage and superoxide formation. Metal-catalyzed oxidation by redox-active metals such as iron and copper promotes hydroxyl radical generation through Fenton chemistry. Depletion of antioxidant defenses, including reduced glutathione, vitamin E, and catalase, sensitizes cells to oxidative damage.

Lipid peroxidation represents a principal consequence of oxidative stress, particularly affecting polyunsaturated fatty acids in cell membranes. This self-propagating chain reaction produces lipid hydroperoxides and reactive aldehydes like malondialdehyde and 4-hydroxynonenal that damage membrane integrity and form protein adducts. Protein oxidation includes carbonylation, thiol oxidation, and tyrosine nitration, potentially altering enzymatic function, signal transduction, and structural integrity. DNA oxidation produces base modifications, strand breaks, and cross-links that may lead to mutations, genomic instability, or cell death if inadequately repaired.

Cellular antioxidant defenses include enzymatic systems such as superoxide dismutase, catalase, and glutathione peroxidase, as well as non-enzymatic molecules including glutathione, vitamin C, vitamin E, and ubiquinol. These defenses operate as coordinated networks that become overwhelmed during severe oxidative stress. Oxidative stress contributes to the toxicity of numerous agents including heavy metals, pesticides, air pollutants, and pharmaceutical agents, and plays roles in carcinogenesis, neurodegenerative disorders, and cardiovascular disease.

Covalent Binding and Adduct Formation

Many toxicants or their reactive metabolites form covalent bonds with cellular macromolecules, creating adducts that can disrupt structural and functional integrity. Electrophilic compounds or metabolites react with nucleophilic centers in proteins and nucleic acids, including sulfhydryl, amino, hydroxyl, and phosphate groups. Such adducts may alter enzyme function, disrupt signal transduction, form neoantigens triggering autoimmune responses, or damage DNA potentially initiating carcinogenesis.

Protein adduction illustrates the diversity of toxicological consequences. Acetaminophen's reactive metabolite NAPQI forms protein adducts in hepatocytes after glutathione depletion, contributing to cellular dysfunction and hepatotoxicity. Isocyanates in diisocyanates and methyl isocyanate (Bhopal disaster) form adducts with proteins, creating hapten-carrier complexes that elicit hypersensitivity reactions. Heavy metals including mercury, lead, and arsenic bind to protein sulfhydryl groups, potentially disrupting enzymatic function and cellular structure.

DNA adduction represents a particularly significant mechanism in chemical carcinogenesis. Polycyclic aromatic hydrocarbons form DNA adducts after metabolic activation to diol epoxides, potentially causing mutations if unrepaired. Aflatoxin B1's epoxide metabolite creates guanine adducts associated with hepatocellular carcinoma development. Alkylating agents like nitrogen mustards form crosslinks between DNA strands, disrupting replication and transcription. Such DNA damage activates repair mechanisms, with unrepaired or misrepaired lesions potentially leading to mutations, chromosomal aberrations, or cell death.

Mitochondrial Toxicity

Mitochondrial dysfunction represents a critical mechanism in various toxicological scenarios, given these organelles' central role in energy production, calcium homeostasis, and apoptosis regulation. Several mechanisms contribute to mitochondrial toxicity. Electron transport chain inhibition occurs with numerous toxicants targeting specific complexes: rotenone and MPP+ (complex I), antimycin A (complex III), cyanide and carbon monoxide (complex IV). Such inhibition reduces ATP production while potentially increasing reactive oxygen species generation.

Uncoupling of oxidative phosphorylation dissociates electron transport from ATP synthesis by increasing inner membrane permeability to protons, as observed with compounds like 2,4-dinitrophenol, pentachlorophenol, and carbonyl cyanide mchlorophenylhydrazone (CCCP). Such uncoupling causes energy dissipation as heat rather than ATP production. Inhibition of fatty acid β-oxidation, demonstrated by valproic acid, aspirin, and certain antiretroviral drugs, prevents utilization of fatty acids for energy production, potentially causing microvesicular steatosis and hypoglycemia.

Mitochondrial DNA (mtDNA) damage particularly affects mitochondrial function due to limited repair mechanisms and absence of protective histones. Nucleoside reverse transcriptase inhibitors inhibit mitochondrial DNA polymerase γ, reducing mtDNA replication and potentially causing depletion syndromes. Mitochondrial permeability transition involves opening of a non-specific pore in the inner mitochondrial membrane, dissipating membrane potential and releasing pro-apoptotic factors. This mechanism contributes to acetaminophen, carbon tetrachloride, and ischemia-reperfusion toxicity.

Consequences of mitochondrial dysfunction include ATP depletion leading to energy failure, calcium dysregulation causing activation of degradative enzymes, excessive reactive oxygen species production damaging cellular components, and initiation of apoptotic or necrotic cell death depending on the severity of dysfunction and ATP availability.

Cell Death Pathways

Toxicants can trigger various forms of cell death, with the specific pathway influenced by the nature of the toxicant, cellular energy status, and intensity of damage. Apoptosis represents a programmed, energy-dependent process characterized by cell shrinkage, chromatin condensation, membrane blebbing, and formation of apoptotic bodies subsequently phagocytosed without inflammatory response. Intrinsic apoptotic pathways initiate at the mitochondria, where various stressors cause release of cytochrome c, which forms the apoptosome complex and activates caspase cascades. Extrinsic pathways begin with activation of death receptors like Fas and tumor necrosis factor receptor by their respective ligands, triggering caspase-8 activation.

Necrosis typically occurs under severe toxic insult or energy depletion, characterized by cellular swelling, plasma membrane rupture, organelle degradation, and cellular content release triggering inflammation. While historically considered unregulated, evidence indicates that certain forms of necrosis follow regulated pathways, including necroptosis involving receptor-interacting protein kinases. Autophagy, primarily a cytoprotective process involving degradation and recycling of cellular components, can contribute to cell death under certain circumstances, particularly when extensive or dysregulated.

Various toxicants preferentially induce specific death pathways.

Dioxins trigger apoptosis through aryl hydrocarbon receptor-mediated gene expression. Heavy metals like cadmium and mercury can cause apoptosis at lower concentrations but necrosis at higher doses. Carbon tetrachloride typically induces necrosis through massive lipid peroxidation and membrane damage.

Genotoxicity and Carcinogenesis

Chemical carcinogenesis typically progresses through multiple stages, with various toxicants potentially acting as initiators, promoters, or progressors in this process. Genotoxic carcinogens directly damage DNA through mechanisms including formation of DNA adducts, oxidative damage, or strand breaks. These genetic alterations, if incompletely or incorrectly repaired, may produce mutations in critical genes regulating cell growth, differentiation, or genomic stability. Alkylating agents like ethylene oxide form DNA adducts at nucleophilic sites. Aromatic amines undergo metabolic activation to form DNA-reactive nitrenium ions. Aflatoxins create guanine adducts after epoxidation, potentially causing characteristic G→T transversions in the p53 tumor suppressor gene.

Non-genotoxic carcinogens operate through mechanisms that do not directly involve DNA damage. These include receptor-mediated effects, such as dioxin activation of the aryl hydrocarbon receptor; epigenetic alterations modifying gene expression without sequence changes; endocrine disruption affecting hormone-dependent tissues; immunosuppression reducing surveillance against transformed cells; inflammatory responses creating reactive oxygen and nitrogen species; and cytotoxicity with regenerative hyperplasia increasing mutation opportunities during enhanced DNA replication.

Several testing strategies assess carcinogenic potential. Bacterial mutagenicity assays, particularly the Ames test using Salmonella typhimurium strains, detect mutations caused by test compounds. Mammalian cell assays evaluate chromosomal aberrations, micronuclei formation, or specific locus mutations. *In vivo* genotoxicity assays examine DNA damage in exposed animal tissues. Chronic bioassays, typically two-year rodent studies, remain the gold standard for carcinogenicity assessment despite limitations including high cost, lengthy duration, and species extrapolation challenges. evidence of carcinogenicity derives from epidemiological studies, with occupational cohorts often providing the strongest evidence linking specific chemical exposures to cancer outcomes. Established human carcinogens include benzene (leukemia), vinyl chloride (angiosarcoma), asbestos (mesothelioma and lung cancer), and arsenic (skin and lung cancer), among others identified through epidemiological investigation and supported by mechanistic understanding.

Summary

Toxicokinetics and toxicodynamics form the mechanistic foundation for understanding how toxic substances interact with the body. Toxicokinetics describes the absorption, distribution, metabolism, and excretion (ADME) processes determining a toxin's fate. Absorption varies significantly by exposure route, with inhalation providing rapid uptake through the extensive alveolar surface area, while gastrointestinal absorption depends on factors including pH, motility, and chemical properties. Dermal absorption occurs primarily with lipophilic compounds. Once absorbed, distribution is influenced by blood flow, protein binding, lipid solubility, and anatomical barriers including the blood-brain and placental interfaces. Metabolism, predominantly occurring in the liver, involves Phase I (functionalization) and Phase II (conjugation) reactions that can either detoxify harmful substances or activate relatively harmless compounds into toxic metabolites. Excretion primarily occurs through renal filtration, with additional pathways including biliary excretion, pulmonary exhalation, and minor routes such as sweat and breast milk. Toxicodynamics examines the biochemical and molecular mechanisms by which toxins produce adverse effects, including receptor interactions (agonism, antagonism, allosteric modulation), enzyme inhibition or induction, disruption of ion channels and membrane function, protein and DNA adduct formation, oxidative stress generation, and disturbance of cellular homeostasis. Understanding these processes allows prediction of toxic effects, development of targeted treatments, and establishment of biomarkers for exposure and effect.

Self-Assessment Questions

1. Describe how gastric pH, food presence, and gastrointestinal motility affect the absorption of toxins following oral ingestion.
2. Explain the concept of volume of distribution and how it influences the effectiveness of various elimination techniques for different toxins.
3. Compare and contrast Phase I and Phase II metabolic reactions, providing examples of toxins that undergo each type of transformation.
4. Analyze how protein binding affects the toxicity, distribution, and elimination of xenobiotics, with examples of highly protein-bound toxins.
5. Describe the first-pass effect and its significance in determining the bioavailability and toxicity of orally ingested substances.
6. Discuss how age-related changes in absorption, distribution, metabolism, and excretion modify toxin responses in pediatric and geriatric populations.
7. Explain the process of enterohepatic recirculation and how it can prolong the effects of certain toxins in the body.
8. Analyze the mechanisms and clinical significance of receptor antagonism as both a toxic mechanism and therapeutic strategy in poisoning cases.
9. Describe how oxidative stress serves as a common pathway for cellular damage across different classes of toxins.
10. Evaluate the pharmacokinetic principles that determine whether a toxin is likely to be effectively removed by hemodialysis

Bibliography

1. Roberts DM, Buckley NA. Pharmacokinetic considerations in clinical toxicology: clinical applications. Clin Pharmacokinet. 2007;46(11):897-939.
2. Rowland M, Tozer TN. Clinical pharmacokinetics and pharmacodynamics: concepts and applications. 4th ed. Philadelphia: Lippincott Williams & Wilkins; 2010.
3. Linder MW, Prough RA, Valdes R. Pharmacogenetics: a laboratory tool for optimizing therapeutic efficiency. Clin Chem. 1997;43(2):254-266.
4. Curry SC, Watts DJ, Katz KD, Bikin D, Bukhari AF. The effect of single-dose activated charcoal on the apparent half-life of intravenous phenobarbital. J Med Toxicol. 2019;15(1):1-7.
5. Leung N, Wexler D, Yaksh TL, Hanson LR, Satyanarayana P, Bao H, et al. Prediction of systemic toxicity and pulmonary toxicity in chemical exposures: extrapolation beyond species and route of exposure. Toxicol Sci. 2019;172(2):237-245.
6. Liu X, Guo Z, Sun H, Chen Y, Chen X. Comprehensive insights into metabolism and metabolic regulation of drug-drug interactions: application of physiologically based pharmacokinetic modeling. Drug Metab Rev. 2022;54(1):51-76.
7. Dinis-Oliveira RJ. Metabolic profiles of propofol and fospropofol: clinical and forensic interpretative aspects. Biomed Res Int. 2018;2018:6852857.
8. Zanger UM, Schwab M. Cytochrome P450 enzymes in drug metabolism: regulation of gene expression, enzyme activities, and impact of genetic variation. Pharmacol Ther. 2013;138(1):103-141.
9. Mégarbane B, Deye N, Baud F. Folinic acid administration for methotrexate poisoning: a critical reappraisal. Basic Clin Pharmacol Toxicol. 2020;127(2):113-114.
10. Gosselin S, Hoegberg LC, Hoffman RS, Graudins A, Stork CM, Thomas SH, et al. Evidence-based recommendations on the use of intravenous lipid emulsion therapy in poisoning. Clin Toxicol (Phila). 2016;54(10):899-923.

CHAPTER 3

DOSE-RESPONSE RELATIONSHIPS

Author

Miss Reethu Metilda Manukonda, PG Scholar,
Department of Pharmacology, Sri Vasavi Institute of Pharmaceutical Sciences, Tadepalligudem, Andhra Pradesh, India

Abstract

Dose-response relationships represent the cornerstone of toxicological assessment, quantifying how biological systems react to varying exposure levels of toxic substances. These relationships help determine whether effects follow threshold or non-threshold models, with threshold responses occurring only above specific dose levels while non-threshold effects theoretically possible at any exposure. The concept of hormesis—where low doses produce opposite effects from high doses—further complicates these patterns. Toxicologists establish critical reference points including NOAEL (No-Observed-Adverse-Effect Level), LOAEL (Lowest-Observed-Adverse-Effect Level), TD50 (Toxic Dose affecting 50% of population), and LD50 (Lethal Dose for 50%). Safety margins derive from these values through application of uncertainty factors accounting for interspecies differences, human variability, data limitations, and exposure duration. The resulting reference doses and acceptable daily intakes guide regulatory standards and clinical decision-making. Risk assessment integrates these principles through a structured four-stage process: hazard identification, dose-response assessment, exposure assessment, and risk characterization. Individual variations due to genetics, age, health status, and other factors create significant response differences, necessitating population-protective approaches when establishing safety standards for environmental toxins, pharmaceuticals, and occupational exposures.

Keywords: *Dose-response, Threshold, Risk Assessment, Uncertainty Factors, NOAEL, Reference Dose*

Learning Objectives

After completion of the chapter, the learners should be able to:

- Differentiate between threshold and non-threshold dose-response relationships and explain the concept of hormesis.
- Calculate and interpret key toxic dose parameters including NOAEL, LOAEL, TD50, and LD50.
- Apply uncertainty factors appropriately to establish safety margins and reference doses for various exposure scenarios.
- Construct and analyze dose-response curves to predict toxicological outcomes at different exposure levels.
- Perform a structured risk assessment following the four-stage process of hazard identification, dose-response assessment, exposure assessment, and risk characterization.
- Evaluate how individual variations including genetic polymorphisms, age, and health status modify dose-response relationships and influence risk assessment.

THRESHOLD CONCEPTS

The relationship between exposure dose and resulting biological effect forms the cornerstone of toxicological science, with threshold concepts providing essential frameworks for understanding when toxic responses emerge.

Fundamental Principles

The threshold concept represents a foundational principle in toxicology, proposing that for many toxic effects, a critical dose exists below which no adverse response occurs. This concept derives from the biological reality that organisms possess compensatory mechanisms capable of managing limited toxic insults without manifesting detectable dysfunction. These adaptive capacities include detoxification enzymes, antioxidant systems, DNA repair mechanisms, and cellular regenerative capabilities that collectively establish a buffer zone between exposure and observable harm. The threshold dose, therefore, represents the point at which these defensive and adaptive systems become overwhelmed, allowing the toxic effect to manifest.

Thresholds operate at multiple biological levels. At the molecular level, covalent binding of reactive metabolites to cellular macromolecules may remain inconsequential until a critical number of adducts forms. At the cellular level, oxidative stress may be effectively neutralized by glutathione and antioxidant enzymes until these defenses become saturated. At the tissue level, cellular death may be compensated by regeneration until the rate of cell loss exceeds replacement capacity. At the organismal level, physiological compensatory mechanisms may maintain function despite underlying damage until a critical mass of dysfunction accumulates.

> Remember
>
> **Threshold models propose that adverse effects occur only above specific exposure levels, while non-threshold models suggest some risk exists at any dose, with concepts like hormesis describing beneficial effects at low doses of otherwise toxic substances.**

The manifestation of thresholds in dose-response relationships typically produces sigmoidal curves when response magnitude is plotted against logarithmic dose. These curves display a no-effect region at low doses, a transition zone where response begins and increases rapidly with small dose increments, and a plateau region at high doses where maximum response is approached. This pattern reflects the biological reality that most toxicological processes involve multiple steps with saturable components, creating non-linear relationships between exposure and effect.

Threshold Types

Different conceptual threshold models apply to various toxicological contexts. The true threshold model proposes an absolute dose below which no adverse effect occurs in any individual within a population. This model typically applies to non-genotoxic effects where clear mechanistic grounds exist for expecting a threshold, such as irritation requiring a minimum concentration to overcome epithelial barriers or enzyme inhibition requiring a minimum percentage of inhibition before functional consequences emerge.

The practical threshold model acknowledges that while theoretical responses might occur at very low doses, they remain undetectable using available methods or become indistinguishable from background variation. This concept proves particularly relevant for endpoints with high spontaneous incidence rates or substantial intra-individual variability, where subtle toxicant-induced changes may be masked by normal biological fluctuations.

The population threshold model addresses inter-individual variability, recognizing that while thresholds exist for individuals, they vary across populations due to genetic polymorphisms, pre-existing conditions, age-related differences, and other susceptibility factors. This distribution of individual thresholds means that as dose increases, an increasing proportion of the population manifests effects, creating an apparent dose-response relationship even when each individual possesses a discrete threshold.

The hormetic threshold model describes biphasic responses where low doses produce effects opposite to those seen at higher doses, often reflecting adaptive responses beneficial to the organism. Examples include radiation hormesis, where low doses may stimulate DNA repair mechanisms, and chemical hormesis, where mild oxidative stress might upregulate protective antioxidant pathways. This model challenges linear extrapolations and suggests that biological responses to toxicants may be fundamentally non-monotonic.

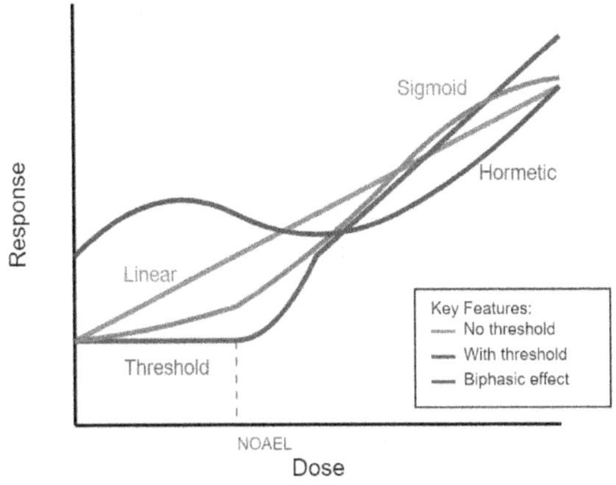

Figure 3.1 Types of Dose-Response Curves

Non-Threshold Models

Certain toxicological effects, particularly carcinogenesis initiated by genotoxic agents, are traditionally considered non-threshold phenomena. This perspective derives from the theoretical premise that a single DNA mutation in a critical gene could potentially initiate the carcinogenic process, and that even a single molecule of a DNA-reactive compound could cause such a mutation. This one-hit model suggests that no absolutely safe dose exists for genotoxic carcinogens, with risk decreasing but never reaching zero as dose approaches zero.

The linear no-threshold (LNT) model represents the practical application of non-threshold concepts in regulatory toxicology, assuming proportionality between dose and response down to the lowest doses. While this model provides a conservative approach to risk management, it remains controversial due to limited empirical evidence at extremely low doses and emerging understanding of adaptive responses, DNA repair efficiency, and the multi-stage nature of carcinogenesis that may introduce practical thresholds even for genotoxic agents.

Several factors complicate the no-threshold paradigm for carcinogenesis. Background DNA damage from endogenous processes, including oxidative metabolism and spontaneous hydrolysis, continuously produces levels of DNA lesions far exceeding those from typical environmental exposures to genotoxic chemicals. Efficient DNA repair systems preferentially address certain lesions, potentially creating practical thresholds below which damage is effectively repaired. Immune surveillance mechanisms recognize and eliminate transformed cells, providing another defense layer that may introduce threshold-like effects in the carcinogenic process.

Recent advances in molecular toxicology suggest alternatives to the strict non-threshold model even for genotoxic carcinogens. The margin of exposure approach acknowledges potential practical thresholds while maintaining conservative assessments. The key events dose-response framework evaluates thresholds at each stage of a toxicological process, recognizing that even for carcinogenesis, rate-limiting steps with threshold characteristics may exist within the overall process.

Threshold Determination Methods

Establishing threshold values involves multiple experimental approaches and statistical methods. The No Observed Adverse Effect Level (NOAEL) represents the highest experimental dose producing no statistically significant increase in frequency or severity of adverse effects compared to controls. This empirical approach relies on the experimental dose spacing, sample size, and statistical power of the study design, potentially overestimating the true threshold if the study lacks sensitivity or appropriate dose selection.

The Lowest Observed Adverse Effect Level (LOAEL) identifies the lowest experimental dose producing statistically significant adverse effects, providing an upper bound for the threshold when a clear NOAEL cannot be established. The Benchmark Dose (BMD) methodology addresses limitations of the NOAEL/LOAEL approach by modeling the entire dose-response curve to estimate the dose associated with a predefined level of response (typically 5% or 10% above background). This approach maximizes use of all experimental data, quantifies uncertainty, and reduces dependency on experimental dose selection.

For non-threshold effects, mathematical models facilitate low-dose extrapolation from observable effect ranges to environmentally relevant exposures. Linear models assume proportionality between dose and response throughout the extrapolation range. Multi-stage models incorporate biological concepts of carcinogenesis requiring multiple sequential events. Physiologically based toxicokinetic (PBTK) models integrate absorption, distribution, metabolism, and excretion data to estimate internal doses at target tissues, potentially revealing nonlinear relationships between external exposure and internal effective dose.

The threshold of toxicological concern (TTC) provides a generic threshold approach when chemical-specific data are limited, establishing exposure thresholds below which risk remains negligible based on structural categories and existing toxicological databases. This pragmatic approach enables preliminary risk assessment for substances lacking complete toxicological profiles, though it requires careful consideration of applicability domains and exclusion of highly potent substance classes.

TOXIC DOSES

Quantitative expression of toxicant potency through defined dose metrics enables systematic comparison between compounds and informs risk management decisions across regulatory frameworks.

Dose Metrics and Definitions

The quantification of toxic potency requires precise dose metrics adapted to various exposure scenarios and toxicological endpoints. Administered dose represents the amount of toxicant provided to an organism, typically expressed as mg/kg body weight for acute exposures or mg/kg/day for repeated exposures. This most basic metric provides a standardized comparison across different body sizes but does not account for toxicokinetic differences between species or compounds. For airborne toxicants, concentration-time products (Ct) express the relationship between exposure concentration and duration, recognizing that these factors often demonstrate reciprocity in determining toxic outcomes.

Absorbed dose refines this concept by quantifying the fraction of administered dose actually entering systemic circulation, accounting for incomplete absorption across exposure barriers. For oral exposures, first-pass hepatic metabolism may substantially reduce bioavailability compared to other routes. Internal dose further specifies the amount reaching a specific organ, tissue, or cellular target, incorporating distribution factors. Biologically effective dose represents the most precise metric, measuring the amount actually interacting with critical molecular targets to initiate toxic responses, such as DNA adduct formation or enzyme inhibition.

Table 3.1: Types of Dose-Response Relationships

Type	Characteristics	Examples	Implications
Linear	Direct proportionality between dose and effect	Many carcinogens, radiation effects	No safe threshold assumed
Threshold	No effects below specific dose level	Most non-cancer endpoints	NOAEL/LOAEL can be established
Hormetic	Beneficial effects at low doses, harmful at high doses	Some essential elements, radiation	Complicates risk assessment
Sigmoid	S-shaped curve with plateau at high doses	Many pharmacological effects	Defines ED50, LD50 parameters
Bell-shaped	Increasing then decreasing effect with dose	Some immunological, endocrine effects	Maximum effect at intermediate doses
U-shaped	Adverse effects at both low and high doses	Some vitamins and minerals	Optimal range between extremes

Remember

Critical dose parameters include NOAEL (No-Observed-Adverse-Effect Level), LOAEL (Lowest-Observed-Adverse-Effect Level), TD50 (Toxic Dose affecting 50%), and LD50 (Lethal Dose affecting 50%).

Several specialized dose concepts address specific toxicological contexts. The minimum lethal dose (MLD) identifies the lowest dose causing death in a test species. The absolutely lethal dose (ALD) represents the dose causing death in all exposed individuals. Maximum tolerated dose (MTD) defines the highest dose producing toxicity without significantly affecting survival, often used as the high dose in carcinogenicity bioassays. Human equivalent dose (HED) translates animal dosing to predicted human exposures, incorporating allometric scaling or physiologically based models to account for interspecies differences in toxicokinetics and toxicodynamics.

Lethal Dose Determinations

Median lethal dose (LD50) historically provided the standard acute toxicity metric, representing the statistically derived dose estimated to cause death in 50% of a test population under specified conditions. While ethically controversial and now largely replaced by alternative approaches, LD50 determinations historically involved administering graded doses to animal groups, recording mortality over a defined observation period (typically 14 days), and calculating the median lethal point through probit analysis, moving average, or other statistical methods.

Table 3.2: Critical Dose Concepts in Toxicology

Term	Definition	Application	Limitations
LD50	Dose lethal to 50% of test population	Comparing relative acute toxicity	Limited human relevance
ED50	Dose producing effect in 50% of population	Determining effective dose range	Varies by endpoint measured
TD50	Dose producing toxic effect in 50%	Establishing toxic dose range	Depends on toxicity definition
NOAEL	No Observed Adverse Effect Level	Regulatory safety assessment	Depends on study design sensitivity
LOAEL	Lowest Observed Adverse Effect Level	Used when NOAEL unavailable	Contains some adverse effects
BMD	Benchmark Dose producing defined response	Statistical approach to dose-response	Requires quality dose-response data
MOS	Margin of Safety between exposure and toxic dose	Risk characterization	Judgment required for "adequate" margin

Route of administration significantly affects LD50 values, with intravenous administration typically yielding lower values than oral routes due to bypassing absorption barriers and first-pass metabolism.

Vehicle selection influences absorption characteristics, potentially altering apparent toxicity. Observation period duration affects outcomes, particularly with delayed-action toxicants. Animal strain differences, nutritional status, age, sex, and environmental conditions all contribute to variability in LD50 determinations, necessitating standardized protocols for meaningful comparisons.

Contemporary approaches emphasize alternative methods minimizing animal use and suffering while maintaining scientific value. The fixed dose procedure uses predefined dose levels and fewer animals, focusing on signs of toxicity rather than death as endpoints. The acute toxic class method categorizes toxicity by determining whether mortality exceeds defined thresholds at specific doses. The up-and-down procedure sequentially tests individual animals, with each dose selection informed by the previous animal's outcome, substantially reducing animal numbers while providing comparable precision for LD50 estimation.

Regulatory classification schemes translate lethal dose determinations into hazard categories guiding handling, transportation, and labeling requirements. The Globally Harmonized System of Classification and Labelling of Chemicals (GHS) defines acute toxicity categories based on LD50 ranges, with Category 1 representing the most toxic compounds (LD50 $\leq$ 5 mg/kg oral) and Category 5 the least toxic (LD50 > 2000 mg/kg oral). These standardized categories facilitate international consistency in hazard communication.

Nonlethal Toxic Doses

Various dose metrics characterize nonlethal toxicity, addressing the reality that many significant toxic effects occur at doses well below those causing mortality. The effective dose (ED50) represents the dose producing a defined effect in 50% of the test population, providing a standardized potency metric for specific nonlethal endpoints such as enzyme inhibition, behavioral changes, or physiological alterations. Toxic dose (TD50) specifically refers to doses producing adverse effects, distinguished from doses causing pharmacological effects that might be beneficial in therapeutic contexts.

Specialized nonlethal metrics address specific contexts. The teratogenic dose (TeD50) measures induction of birth defects, while the tumorigenic dose (TD50) in carcinogenicity studies represents the dose inducing tumors in 50% of test animals over their lifetime. The immunotoxic dose (ID50) quantifies immune system suppression or inappropriate activation. These specialized metrics enable focused evaluation of particular concern areas independent of general toxicity or lethality.

For repeated exposure scenarios, distinct metrics apply. The lowest observed adverse effect level (LOAEL) identifies the lowest tested dose producing statistically or biologically significant increases in frequency or severity of adverse effects. The no observed adverse effect level (NOAEL) represents the highest tested dose producing no significant adverse effects compared to controls. The benchmark dose (BMD) and its lower confidence limit (BMDL) derive from mathematical modeling of the dose-response relationship, identifying doses corresponding to predefined response levels (typically 5% or 10% change from background).

Collective metrics comparing beneficial and harmful dose ranges provide important perspectives for therapeutic compounds or essential nutrients. The therapeutic index (TI) or margin of safety represents the ratio between median lethal dose and median effective dose (LD50/ED50), quantifying the separation between therapeutic and toxic ranges. Compounds with low therapeutic indices require careful dosing and monitoring to prevent toxicity. The certain safety factor extends this concept by comparing the highest dose causing no deaths with the lowest dose reliably producing the desired effect (LD0/ED100), providing a more conservative safety estimate.

Comparative Toxicity

Systematic comparison of toxic potencies between compounds facilitates prioritization of regulatory attention and development of structure-activity relationships. The conventional toxicity classification system ranks compounds from "practically non-toxic" (LD50 > 15 g/kg) to "supertoxic" (LD50 < 5 mg/kg), creating a framework for relative hazard assessment. However, this classification applies primarily to acute lethality and may not reflect chronic toxicity potential, carcinogenicity, or other specialized concerns.

Comparative potency metrics enable direct quantitative comparison between compounds. Toxic potency value (TPV) expresses potency as the reciprocal of the ED50, with higher values indicating greater potency. Toxic equivalency factors (TEFs) relate the potency of similar compounds within a chemical class to a reference compound, as used for dioxins and dioxin-like compounds relative to 2,3,7,8-tetrachlorodibenzo-p-dioxin (TCDD). These approaches facilitate cumulative risk assessment for mixtures containing multiple compounds with similar mechanisms.

Structure-activity relationships link molecular features to toxic potency, enabling prediction of toxicity for untested compounds and guiding rational design of safer alternatives. Quantitative structure-activity relationships (QSARs) develop mathematical correlations between molecular descriptors (physicochemical properties, structural features, or calculated parameters) and toxicity metrics. These models identify toxicophores (structural features conferring toxicity) and predict relative potencies based on molecular modifications. Successful QSAR applications include prediction of acute aquatic toxicity based on octanol-water partition coefficients, respiratory sensitization potential from protein reactivity parameters, and skin irritation from membrane disruption properties.

Read-across approaches leverage toxicity data from structurally similar compounds to estimate properties of data-poor substances, implementing a chemical category approach that maximizes existing knowledge while minimizing additional testing requirements. This methodology forms a cornerstone of modern regulatory toxicology, addressing the practical impossibility of comprehensive testing for all industrial and environmental chemicals while maintaining protection against significant hazards

SAFETY MARGINS

The inherent uncertainty in extrapolating from experimental models to human populations necessitates safety margins that provide buffers between demonstrated effect levels and permissible human exposures.

Safety and Uncertainty Factors

Safety factors, also termed uncertainty factors, address specific knowledge gaps in the risk assessment process.

> **Remember**
>
> **Safety margins are established by applying uncertainty factors to account for interspecies differences, human variability, data limitations, and exposure duration when extrapolating from experimental data to human risk assessment.**

Interspecies extrapolation factors, typically 10-fold, account for potential differences in susceptibility between test animals and humans arising from variations in toxicokinetics (absorption, distribution, metabolism, excretion) and toxicodynamics (tissue responsiveness). This factor acknowledges that humans may prove more sensitive than test species due to differences in detoxification capacity, receptor binding affinities, or compensatory mechanisms.

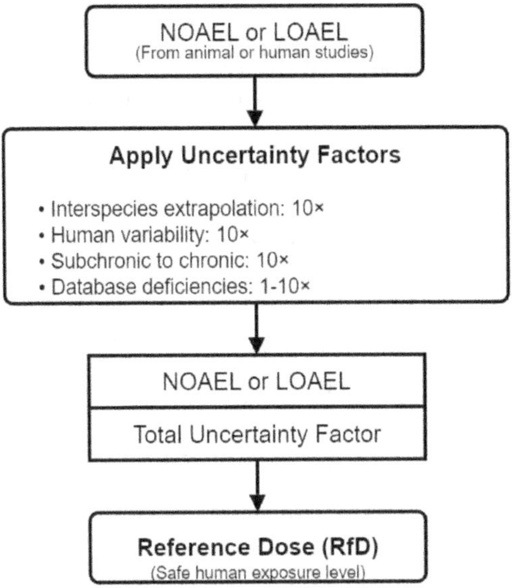

Figure 3.2: Safety Factor Derivation in Risk Assessment

Intraspecies variability factors, conventionally 10-fold, address heterogeneity within human populations, including genetic polymorphisms affecting metabolizing enzymes, age-related differences in physiological functions, pre-existing health conditions, and lifestyle factors influencing susceptibility. This factor specifically aims to protect sensitive subpopulations who may respond more severely than the typical individual. When combined, these two traditional factors create a 100-fold safety margin commonly applied in regulatory assessments.

Additional factors address specific data limitations. The subchronic-to-chronic extrapolation factor (typically 3-10 fold) applies when deriving chronic exposure limits from shorter-term studies, acknowledging that longer exposures may reveal effects not apparent in abbreviated testing. The LOAEL-to-NOAEL conversion factor (typically 3-10 fold) provides a margin when a clear no-effect level was not established in available studies. Database deficiency factors (typically 3-10 fold) compensate for missing studies addressing particular endpoints or life stages, explicitly acknowledging knowledge gaps requiring conservative assessment.

The application of these factors follows either a default approach using standard values or a chemical-specific approach incorporating data-derived adjustment factors when sufficient information exists regarding particular uncertainty components. The composite application of multiple factors reflects the multiplicative nature of various uncertainty sources, potentially creating very large margins between experimental effect levels and acceptable human exposures, particularly for data-poor substances.

Table 3.3: Safety and Uncertainty Factors in Risk Assessment

Factor	Typical Value	Application	Rationale
Interspecies	10×	Animal to human extrapolation	Physiological differences between species
Intraspecies	10×	Human variability	Genetic, age, health status differences
Subchronic to chronic	10×	Study duration inadequacy	Accounting for effects requiring longer exposure
LOAEL to NOAEL	10×	When NOAEL unavailable	Extrapolating to no-effect level
Database deficiency	1-10×	Incomplete toxicity data	Addressing potential unknown effects
Children's safety	10×	Special vulnerability	FQPA requirement for certain pesticides
Chemical-specific	Variable	Based on mechanistic data	Replaces default factors when data available
Composite UF	10-3000×	Combined factors (product)	Typically capped at 3000× to avoid overconservatism

Acceptable Daily Intakes

The acceptable daily intake (ADI) represents a toxicologically derived estimate of the amount of a substance that can be ingested daily over a lifetime without appreciable health risk. This concept, initially developed for food additives and pesticide residues, derives from applying appropriate safety factors to the most sensitive relevant NOAEL or BMDL from animal studies or, when available, human epidemiological data. The ADI incorporates the assumption of threshold effects and addresses chronic, lifetime exposure scenarios.

Several analogous concepts serve specific regulatory contexts while maintaining similar methodological approaches. The reference dose

(RfD) used by the U.S. Environmental Protection Agency applies principally to non-carcinogenic effects of environmental contaminants. The tolerable daily intake (TDI) typically addresses unavoidable contaminants rather than intentionally added substances. The provisional tolerable weekly intake (PTWI) applies to contaminants with bioaccumulative properties where weekly averaging provides more appropriate risk characterization than daily limits. Each approach divides a point of departure (typically a NOAEL or BMDL) by appropriate uncertainty factors to derive an exposure limit with reasonable assurance of safety.

These health-based guidance values serve multiple functions in risk management. They provide scientific foundations for establishing regulatory standards for environmental media, food, and consumer products. They enable risk characterization for actual exposure scenarios by comparing estimated intakes to these toxicologically derived benchmarks. They guide prioritization of risk management interventions when exposures approach or exceed these values. They inform design of biomonitoring programs focused on substances with exposures potentially approaching critical levels.

For non-threshold effects, particularly genotoxic carcinogenesis, alternative approaches typically apply. The margin of exposure (MOE) approach compares the point of departure from animal studies (typically a benchmark dose) with estimated human exposure levels, with larger margins indicating lower concern levels. The negligible risk approach defines acceptably low lifetime cancer risk levels, typically between 10^-4 and 10^-6, and derives corresponding exposure limits through mathematical modeling. These approaches acknowledge the theoretical absence of absolutely safe exposure levels while providing practical frameworks for risk management decisions.

Exposure Limits in Occupational Settings

Occupational exposure limits apply specific safety margin concepts to workplace environments, where higher exposures may be permitted compared to general population scenarios due to the adult, generally healthy worker population, limited exposure duration (working lifetime rather than entire lifetime), and implementation of monitoring programs and medical surveillance. These limits typically derive from applying smaller uncertainty factors (often 10-fold total) to toxicological points of departure, reflecting the more controlled exposure circumstances and more homogeneous exposed population.

Various jurisdictions establish different types of occupational limits. The threshold limit value-time weighted average (TLV-TWA) represents the time-weighted average concentration for a conventional 8-hour workday and 40-hour workweek to which nearly all workers may be repeatedly exposed without adverse effects. The permissible exposure limit (PEL) serves as the legally enforceable standard in U.S. workplaces. The recommended exposure limit (REL) provides guidance from research organizations like the National Institute for Occupational Safety and Health. These values apply primarily to airborne exposures and typically address local effects on the respiratory system as well as systemic effects following inhalation.

Supplementary limit types address specific exposure scenarios. Short-term exposure limits (STELs) specify maximum allowable average concentrations during 15-minute periods, addressing acute effects not controlled by time-weighted averages. Ceiling limits (C) identify concentrations that should never be exceeded, even momentarily, typically applied to rapidly acting or highly dangerous substances. Biological exposure indices (BEIs) specify acceptable levels of chemicals or their metabolites in biological samples from workers, reflecting the integrated exposure across all routes and accounting for individual differences in absorption and metabolism.

Several factors influence the implementation and interpretation of occupational exposure limits. Mixtures of workplace chemicals may produce additive, synergistic, or antagonistic effects not predicted by individual substance limits. Extended work shifts beyond conventional 8-hour schedules require adjustment of time-weighted limits to maintain equivalent protection. Physical factors including temperature, humidity, and workload can significantly affect breathing rates and thus inhaled doses. Individual susceptibility factors like genetic polymorphisms in metabolizing enzymes may create subpopulations with greater vulnerability to certain exposures despite remaining within established limits.

Special Populations

Conventional safety margins may prove insufficient for populations with enhanced susceptibility or exposure patterns not addressed in standard scenarios. Children represent a particularly vulnerable subpopulation due to developmental processes susceptible to disruption, higher exposure rates relative to body weight, immature metabolic detoxification systems, distinctive exposure pathways (e.g., hand-to-mouth behavior), and longer remaining lifetime for chronic disease development. These concerns have led to the application of additional child-specific safety factors in certain regulatory frameworks and development of specialized risk assessment approaches for developmental exposures.

Pregnant women require special consideration due to potential impacts on the developing fetus, which may be more sensitive than the maternal system to certain toxicants. The placenta, while providing some protective function, remains permeable to many environmental chemicals, particularly lipophilic compounds. Physiological changes during pregnancy, including increased respiratory rate, cardiac output, and glomerular filtration, can alter toxicokinetics and potentially increase susceptibility to certain exposures. Specific developmental windows display heightened vulnerability to particular toxicants, potentially resulting in permanent structural or functional alterations even at exposure levels below maternal toxicity thresholds.

Elderly populations present distinctive risk factors including reduced physiological reserve capacity, altered toxicokinetics due to reduced renal and hepatic function, increased prevalence of pre-existing health conditions, potential medication interactions, and accumulated body burden of persistent compounds. These factors may necessitate additional safety considerations beyond standard uncertainty factors, particularly for exposures predominantly affecting the elderly population or compounds with excretion pathways highly dependent on renal clearance.

Genetic polymorphisms in metabolism and transport proteins create subpopulations with dramatically different susceptibilities to specific toxicants. The classic example involves variable expression of cytochrome P450 2D6, creating populations of poor, intermediate, extensive, and ultrarapid metabolizers with substantially different responses to affected drugs and environmental chemicals. Similarly, variations in paraoxonase activity create differential susceptibility to organophosphate pesticides. As toxicogenomic knowledge advances, increasing recognition of genetic susceptibility factors will likely drive more individualized approaches to safety margin application, potentially moving from population-based to genotype-specific risk assessments for certain exposures.

RISK ASSESSMENT

Risk assessment integrates hazard identification, dose-response assessment, exposure assessment, and risk characterization to provide structured evaluation of potential health threats from toxicant exposures.

Hazard Identification

Hazard identification determines a substance's inherent capacity to cause harm, drawing evidence from multiple sources to characterize the spectrum of potential adverse effects. Epidemiological studies provide direct evidence of human health effects associated with specific exposures, offering particular value for hazard identification despite limitations including confounding factors, exposure misclassification, and limited statistical power for detecting rare outcomes. Strong epidemiological evidence typically derives from cohort studies tracking exposed populations over time, case-control studies comparing exposure histories between affected and unaffected individuals, and cross-sectional studies examining current exposure and health status relationships.

Animal bioassays offer controlled experimental assessment of toxicological endpoints across exposure ranges exceeding typical human exposures. These studies systematically evaluate endpoints including acute toxicity, repeated-dose toxicity, developmental and reproductive effects, genotoxicity, immunotoxicity, neurotoxicity, and carcinogenicity. While providing the backbone of toxicological hazard identification, animal studies require careful extrapolation to human contexts, considering interspecies differences in physiology, metabolism, and susceptibility.

In vitro and alternative testing methods increasingly contribute to hazard identification. Cell culture systems provide insights into cytotoxicity mechanisms, receptor interactions, and cellular pathway perturbations. High-throughput screening approaches test thousands of compounds across multiple assay systems, identifying potential hazards for further investigation. Computational toxicology employs structure-activity relationships, molecular modeling, and pathway analysis to predict toxicological properties based on chemical structure and physicochemical characteristics. These alternative approaches offer advantages in efficiency, cost, and reduced animal use, though correlation with *in vivo* outcomes requires ongoing validation.

The weight of evidence approach integrates diverse information sources, considering factors including consistency across studies, biological plausibility, dose-response relationships, temporal associations, and coherence with existing knowledge. This approach acknowledges that no single study or data type provides definitive hazard characterization, particularly for complex endpoints like carcinogenicity or developmental toxicity. Structured frameworks like the Bradford Hill criteria guide causal inference from observational data, while systematic review methodologies provide transparent evaluation of evidence quality and consistency across available studies.

Dose-Response Assessment

Dose-response assessment quantifies the relationship between exposure level and effect probability or severity, establishing the foundation for subsequent risk characterization. For threshold effects, this assessment typically identifies point-of-departure (POD) values, including the NOAEL, LOAEL, or benchmark dose (BMD), which serve as reference points for calculating acceptable exposure levels. Selection between these approaches depends on data quality, study design, and regulatory context, with the BMD approach increasingly preferred for its statistical rigor and maximal use of dose-response information.

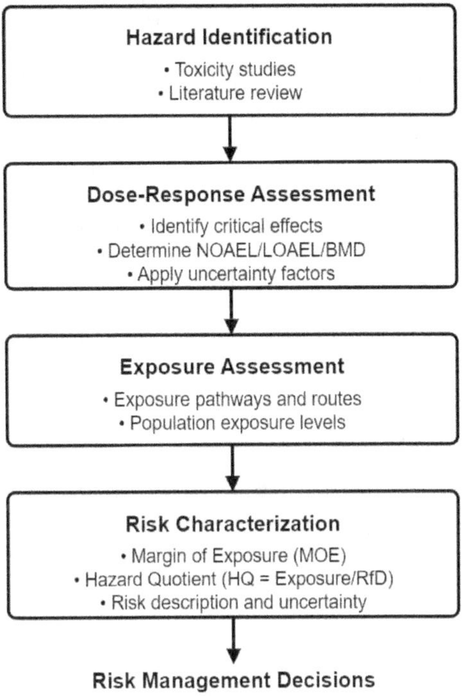

Figure 3.3: Risk Assessment Process

Special consideration applies to dose-response assessment for carcinogens. For genotoxic carcinogens operating through DNA-reactive mechanisms, linear non-threshold models traditionally apply, assuming proportionality between dose and cancer risk down to the lowest doses. The multistage model, reflecting the biological reality of carcinogenesis requiring multiple sequential steps, frequently provides the mathematical framework for this extrapolation. For non-genotoxic carcinogens operating through mechanisms like receptor activation, enzyme induction, or cytotoxicity with regenerative hyperplasia, threshold approaches may be scientifically justified based on understanding of the specific mode of action.

Mathematical modeling plays an essential role in dose-response assessment, particularly for extrapolation beyond the observable data range. Model selection significantly influences outcome, with options including linear, quadratic, logistic, probit, Weibull, and specialized models for particular endpoints. Contemporary approaches emphasize model averaging techniques that incorporate predictions from multiple models weighted by goodness-of-fit criteria, reducing dependency on single model selection. Physiologically based toxicokinetic (PBTK) modeling enhances dose-response assessment by translating external exposures to internal doses at target tissues, potentially revealing nonlinear relationships masked in analyses based solely on administered doses. variability in dose-response relationships arises from multiple sources, including genetic polymorphisms affecting metabolizing enzymes and receptors, age-related differences in physiological functions, sex-based variations in toxicokinetics and target tissue susceptibility, pre-existing health conditions altering baseline function of affected systems, and nutritional status affecting protective mechanisms. Population-based dose-response assessments must account for this variability, either through explicit modeling of different susceptibility groups or application of uncertainty factors providing margins of safety for sensitive subpopulations.

Assessment of Exposure

Exposure assessment characterizes the magnitude, frequency, duration, and routes of human contact with toxicants, employing various methodologies to estimate actual or potential exposure levels. Environmental monitoring directly measures toxicant concentrations in relevant media including air, water, soil, food, and consumer products. These measurements, combined with contact rates and absorption factors, enable calculation of potential intake doses. Stationary monitors provide continuous data at fixed locations, while personal monitors worn by individuals capture actual exposure concentrations in their breathing zones or immediate environments.

Biomonitoring directly measures toxicants or their metabolites in biological specimens including blood, urine, hair, nails, breast milk, or adipose tissue. These measurements integrate exposure across all routes, account for individual absorption and metabolism differences, and reflect the biologically relevant internal dose. Interpretation requires understanding of toxicokinetics, including half-lives and clearance rates, to relate measured levels to exposure timing and intensity. Reference ranges from population studies provide context for individual measurements, while biomonitoring equivalents relate biomarker levels to existing health-based guidance values.

Exposure modeling estimates doses through mathematical representations of environmental fate, transport, and human interaction with contaminated media. These models incorporate emission sources, environmental persistence, movement between media compartments, degradation processes, and human activity patterns to predict exposure levels across populations or geographic regions. Model complexity ranges from simple deterministic calculations to sophisticated probabilistic approaches incorporating parameter distributions rather than single values. Validation against measured data remains essential for establishing model reliability and defining appropriate application domains.

Exposure scenarios characterize distinctive patterns among different population segments. Occupational scenarios typically involve higher concentrations but adult populations and limited durations. Residential scenarios feature lower concentrations but extended durations and diverse population demographics including sensitive subgroups. Consumer product exposure occurs intermittently through direct contact with manufactured items. Dietary exposure follows consumption patterns varying by cultural, regional, and individual preferences. Accurate exposure assessment requires scenario-specific consideration of relevant pathways, activities, and populations to avoid systematic underestimation or overestimation of actual contact with toxicants.

Risk Characterization

Risk characterization integrates findings from hazard identification, dose-response assessment, and exposure assessment to express the nature and magnitude of risk to individuals or populations. For threshold effects, risk characterization typically compares estimated exposure levels with health-based guidance values like reference doses or acceptable daily intakes. The resulting hazard quotient (exposure divided by reference value) indicates potential concern when exceeding unity. For multiple substances affecting similar endpoints, hazard index approaches sum the individual quotients to address cumulative effects from mixture exposures.

For non-threshold effects, particularly carcinogenesis, risk characterization typically expresses probability of adverse outcome, often as excess lifetime cancer risk. This quantitative representation reflects the likelihood of developing cancer beyond background rates due to specific exposure, typically expressed in scientific notation (e.g., 10^-6 representing one additional case per million exposed individuals). Regulatory frameworks establish acceptable or negligible risk levels, generally between 10^-4 and 10^-6 lifetime excess cancer risk, though specific contexts may employ different criteria depending on exposure voluntariness, affected population characteristics, and uncertainty levels.

Uncertainty and variability analysis forms an essential component of comprehensive risk characterization. Uncertainty reflects incomplete knowledge about parameters, models, or assumptions, potentially addressable through additional research. Variability represents inherent heterogeneity in populations or environments that cannot be reduced through additional study. Deterministic approaches address these factors through explicit uncertainty factors applying numerical safety margins to central estimates. Probabilistic approaches employ techniques like Monte Carlo simulation, incorporating parameter distributions rather than point estimates to generate risk distributions rather than single values, providing more nuanced understanding of both central tendency and high-end risks across populations.

Effective risk characterization communicates findings to diverse stakeholders including regulators, industry, and the public. This communication must balance technical accuracy with accessibility, presenting complex probabilistic concepts in comprehensible terms while maintaining scientific integrity. Transparent presentation of assumptions, uncertainties, and limitations provides essential context for interpreting risk estimates and making informed decisions. Comparative risk perspectives, relating assessed risks to familiar contexts or alternative scenarios, help stakeholders integrate technical risk information with broader value considerations necessary for balanced risk management decisions

Summary

Dose-response relationships provide the quantitative foundation for toxicological assessment by describing how biological effects change with varying exposure levels. This relationship typically follows predictable patterns, from no observable effect at low doses through increasing response severity as doses rise. Threshold concepts distinguish between threshold effects, which occur only after exposure exceeds a specific level, and non-threshold effects (particularly carcinogenesis), where theoretical risk exists at any dose. The hormesis phenomenon further complicates this model by demonstrating beneficial effects at low doses of otherwise toxic substances. Establishing toxic dose parameters involves determining the NOAEL (No-Observed-Adverse-Effect Level), LOAEL (Lowest-Observed-Adverse-Effect Level), TD50 (Toxic Dose affecting 50% of subjects), and LD50 (Lethal Dose affecting 50%). These values, traditionally derived from animal studies, require careful extrapolation to human risk assessment. Safety margins incorporate uncertainty factors to account for interspecies differences (typically 10x), human variability (10x), data limitations, and exposure duration differences. These factors combine to establish reference doses and acceptable daily intakes for chronic exposures. Risk assessment integrates dose-response data with exposure information through a four-stage process: hazard identification determining a substance's potential to cause harm, dose-response assessment quantifying the relationship between dose and effect, exposure assessment determining population contact levels, and risk characterization synthesizing this information to guide regulatory and clinical decisions. Individual variations in susceptibility create significant response differences based on genetics, age, health status, and environmental factors.

Self-Assessment Questions

1. Describe the concept of hormesis and discuss examples where low doses of toxic substances may produce beneficial or adaptive responses.
2. Explain how NOAEL and LOAEL values are determined in toxicological studies and their limitations in risk assessment.
3. Analyze how uncertainty factors are applied in developing reference doses from animal toxicity data, providing rationale for each factor commonly used.
4. Compare and contrast threshold versus non-threshold dose-response models, discussing which toxicological endpoints are commonly associated with each.
5. Describe how individual variations in metabolism, excretion, and target organ sensitivity influence population dose-response relationships.
6. Evaluate the advantages and limitations of using LD50 as a measure of acute toxicity compared to other toxicity endpoints.
7. Discuss how dose-response assessments for developmental toxicants differ from those for adult toxicity, considering critical windows of exposure.
8. Explain the concept of the therapeutic index and how it relates to safety considerations in pharmaceutical development and clinical practice.
9. Analyze how exposure assessment methodologies integrate with dose-response data to characterize risk in different population groups.
10. Describe how dose-response principles inform both acute poisoning management decisions and long-term regulatory standards for environmental and occupational exposures.

Bibliography

1. Calabrese EJ, Baldwin LA. Hormesis: the dose-response revolution. Annu Rev Pharmacol Toxicol. 2003;43:175-197.
2. Eaton DL, Gilbert SG. Principles of toxicology. In: Klaassen CD, editor. Casarett and Doull's toxicology: the basic science of poisons. 8th ed. New York: McGraw-Hill Education; 2013. p. 13-48.
3. Clewell HJ, Gearhart JM, Gentry PR, Covington TR, VanLandingham CB, Crump KS, et al. Evaluation of the uncertainty in an oral reference dose for methylmercury due to interindividual variability in pharmacokinetics. Risk Anal. 1999;19(4):547-558.
4. Rhomberg LR, Goodman JE, Haber LT, Dourson M, Andersen ME, Klaunig JE, et al. Linear low-dose extrapolation for noncancer health effects is the exception, not the rule. Crit Rev Toxicol. 2011;41(1):1-19.
5. Crump KS, Hoel DG, Langley CH, Peto R. Fundamental carcinogenic processes and their implications for low dose risk assessment. Cancer Res. 1976;36(9 pt.1):2973-2979.
6. Wignall JA, Shapiro AJ, Wright FA, Woodruff TJ, Chiu WA, Guyton KZ, et al. Standardizing benchmark dose calculations to improve science-based decisions in human health assessments. Environ Health Perspect. 2014;122(5):499-505.
7. Rietjens IMCM, Alink GM. Future of toxicology—low-dose toxicology and risk-benefit analysis. Chem Res Toxicol. 2006;19(8):977-981.
8. Allen BC, Kavlock RJ, Kimmel CA, Faustman EM. Dose-response assessment for developmental toxicity: II. Comparison of generic benchmark dose estimates with no observed adverse effect levels. Fundam Appl Toxicol. 1994;23(4):487-495.
9. Slikker W Jr, Andersen ME, Bogdanffy MS, Bus JS, Cohen SD, Conolly RB, et al. Dose-dependent transitions in mechanisms of toxicity: case studies. Toxicol Appl Pharmacol. 2004;201(3):226-294.
10. Rodricks JV, Levy JI. Science and decisions: advancing toxicology to improve risk assessment. Toxicol Sci. 2013;131(1):1-8.

CHAPTER 4

DIAGNOSTIC METHODS

Author

Mr. Gourab Saha, Associate Professor,
Department of Pharmaceutics, College of Pharmaceutical Sciences, Berhampur, Mohada, Odisha, India

Abstract

Accurate diagnosis of toxic exposures requires a systematic approach combining thorough clinical assessment with appropriate laboratory investigations. The diagnostic process begins with a detailed history addressing the substance involved, time of exposure, quantity, route, and intent, while recognizing challenges like altered mental status or intentional deception. Physical examination focuses on vital signs, pupil size, mucous membrane appearance, skin findings, and neurological status, with special attention to characteristic toxidromes that suggest specific poisonings. Laboratory testing includes both routine tests (electrolytes, glucose, renal and liver function, arterial blood gases) and toxin-specific assays. Toxicological screening employs immunoassays for rapid detection of common substances, though these have important limitations including cross-reactivity and false results. Definitive testing uses sophisticated analytical methods including gas and liquid chromatography, mass spectrometry, and specialized techniques for metals and other toxins. Interpretation requires understanding detection windows, metabolites, specimen selection, and confirmation thresholds. Integration of clinical findings with appropriate laboratory investigations remains essential, as testing must be guided by the clinical presentation rather than performed indiscriminately, with recognition that absence of a substance on screening does not exclude significant toxicity from agents not included in standard panels.

Keywords: *Toxicology Screening, Toxidromes, Analytical Methods, Chromatography, Mass Spectrometry, Clinical Assessment*

Learning Objectives

After completion of the chapter, the learners should be able to:

- Conduct a comprehensive toxicological history and physical examination to identify potential toxic exposures and guide diagnostic testing.
- Recognize and differentiate major toxidromes based on clinical presentation and vital sign patterns.
- Select appropriate laboratory tests based on suspected toxic exposures and interpret results within clinical context.
- Explain the principles, applications, and limitations of immunoassay-based toxicology screening methods.
- Compare analytical techniques including gas chromatography, liquid chromatography, and mass spectrometry for toxicological analysis, identifying appropriate applications for each.
- Evaluate specimen selection considerations for toxicological testing including detection windows, chain of custody requirements, and potential sources of false results

CLINICAL ASSESSMENT

The systematic evaluation of potentially poisoned patients begins with comprehensive clinical assessment, combining focused history-taking, physical examination, and recognition of toxidrome patterns to guide subsequent management decisions.

History Taking

History acquisition in toxicological cases presents unique challenges due to altered mental status, intentional deception, uncertainty regarding exposure, or multiple concurrent toxicants.

> Remember
>
> **Clinical assessment remains the cornerstone of toxicological diagnosis, with toxidromes (characteristic constellations of signs and symptoms) often providing critical clues to specific poisonings even before laboratory confirmation.**

The toxicological history extends beyond standard medical interviewing to incorporate specific elements crucial for exposure characterization. Exposure circumstances require detailed documentation, including timing (onset, duration, and progression), route of exposure (ingestion, inhalation, dermal, ocular, parenteral), estimated quantity, formulation (liquid, solid, extended-release), and concurrent substances. For intentional exposures, psychiatric history, previous suicide attempts, and precipitating factors provide essential context, while unintentional exposures necessitate environmental assessment of the exposure setting.

Table 4.1: Core Components of Toxicological Clinical Assessment

Assessment Component	Elements	Clinical Significance
History	Substance identity, amount, time, intent	Directs diagnostic testing and treatment
Exposure circumstances	Route, co-ingestants, sequential timing	Determines absorption and intervention priorities
Symptom timeline	Onset, progression, fluctuation	Helps identify toxin and predict clinical course
Physical examination	Vital signs, mental status, pupillary response	Identifies toxidromes and severity indicators
Toxidrome recognition	Constellation of signs and symptoms	Narrows differential even without exposure history
Focused organ system assessment	Targeted exam based on suspected toxin	Identifies complications requiring intervention
Response to therapy	Effect of diagnostic interventions (e.g., naloxone)	Can confirm suspected toxin

Multiple collateral information sources supplement patient reports. Family members or witnesses often provide crucial details regarding pre-hospital symptoms, exposure timing, and observed substances. First responder observations, including environmental conditions, container information, household chemicals, and medication inventories prove invaluable for exposure identification. Pre-hospital treatment documentation helps distinguish iatrogenic effects from the primary toxidrome. Prescription databases may reveal undisclosed medications, patterns of misuse, or multiple provider prescribing. Poison control center consultation facilitates rapid access to toxicant-specific information and management guidance, particularly for unusual or complex exposures.

Past medical history takes on particular significance in toxicological assessment. Pre-existing conditions may predispose to toxic effects (e.g., renal insufficiency reducing elimination), mimic toxic syndromes (e.g., diabetic ketoacidosis resembling toxic alcohol poisoning), or complicate management (e.g., cardiac conduction abnormalities exacerbated by cardiotoxic agents). Medication history must include prescription medications, over-the-counter products, supplements, herbal preparations, and recreational substances, with particular attention to agents affecting cardiac conduction, seizure threshold, thermoregulation, and metabolic pathways relevant to the suspected exposure.

Occupational and environmental histories provide crucial context for certain exposures. Occupational assessment includes industry type, specific job duties, chemical exposures, protective equipment usage, coworker symptoms, and temporal relationship between work and symptom onset. Environmental evaluation covers home conditions, nearby industrial facilities, water source, recent renovations, heating systems, vector control measures, and potential hobbies involving toxicant exposure. Travel history may suggest exotic toxin exposures including unfamiliar plants, marine organisms, or endemic venomous species in recently visited regions.

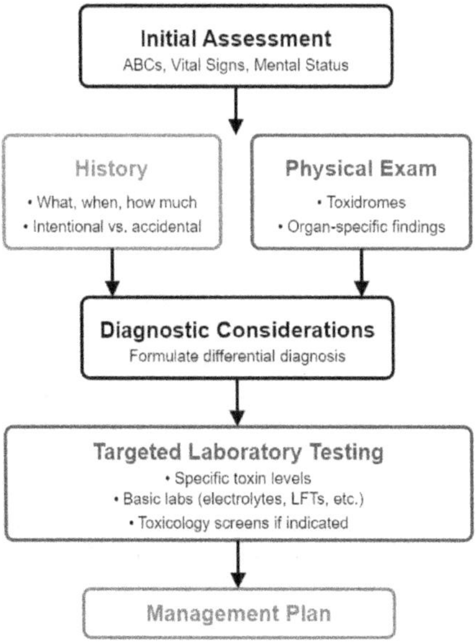

Figure 4.1: Clinical Assessment Algorithm

Physical Examination

Physical examination in toxicological cases emphasizes vital sign abnormalities and systematic evaluation for toxidrome features. Vital signs often provide the earliest indicators of significant toxicity, with characteristic patterns suggesting specific exposures. Hyperthermia accompanies sympathomimetic, anticholinergic, serotonergic, and malignant hyperthermia-inducing agents. Hypothermia suggests sedative-hypnotics, alcohols, opioids, or hypoglycemic agents. Tachycardia characterizes sympathomimetics, anticholinergics, and withdrawal states, while bradycardia suggests cholinergics, cardiac glycosides, calcium channel blockers, beta-blockers, and certain antiarrhythmics. Hypertension occurs with sympathomimetics, anticholinergics, and serotonergic agents, while hypotension suggests antihypertensives, tricyclic antidepressants, sedative-hypnotics, and opioids. Tachypnea compensates for metabolic acidosis or responds to salicylate stimulation of the respiratory center, while bradypnea typically indicates opioid, sedative-hypnotic, or intracranial pressure effects.

Neurological examination provides particularly valuable toxicological insights. Pupillary assessment distinguishes between miosis (opioids, cholinergics, sympatholytics) and mydriasis (sympathomimetics, anticholinergics, serotonergic agents). Mental status evaluation reveals characteristic patterns: agitation and hypervigilance with sympathomimetics, anticholinergics, and hallucinogens; sedation and confusion with opioids, sedative-hypnotics, and anticonvulsants. Neuromuscular findings include hyperreflexia and clonus in serotonergic toxicity, fasciculations with cholinergics, rigidity with neuroleptic malignant syndrome, and distinctive movement disorders with specific toxicants. Cerebellar function assessment may reveal signs of alcohol, anticonvulsant, or heavy metal intoxication.

Dermatological manifestations provide visible evidence of certain exposures. Cyanosis suggests methemoglobinemia or hydrogen sulfide poisoning. Flushing occurs with niacin, calcium channel blockers, vancomycin, carcinoid syndrome, and scombroid poisoning. Bullae formation accompanies barbiturate or carbon monoxide-induced pressure necrosis. Alopecia develops following thallium or radiation exposure. Characteristic odors emanating from the patient often suggest specific toxicants: garlic (organophosphates, arsenic), bitter almonds (cyanide), acetone (isopropanol, diabetic ketoacidosis), fruity (ethanol, isopropanol), wintergreen (methyl salicylate), and rotten eggs (hydrogen sulfide).

Comprehensive systems review extends beyond these characteristic findings. Cardiac examination may reveal dysrhythmias, conduction abnormalities, or hemodynamic compromise. Respiratory assessment distinguishes upper airway obstruction from parenchymal or neuromuscular pathology. Abdominal examination evaluates for hepatotoxicity, gastroenteritis, or ileus. Careful documentation of response to initial interventions, particularly naloxone, thiamine, glucose, and oxygen, provides both diagnostic and therapeutic information while establishing baseline for monitoring clinical progression.

Toxidrome Recognition

Toxidromes represent characteristic constellations of signs and symptoms that suggest specific toxicant classes, providing crucial diagnostic frameworks when specific agent identification remains uncertain. The anticholinergic toxidrome presents with hyperthermia, tachycardia, mydriasis, flushed dry skin, urinary retention, decreased bowel sounds, and altered mental status ranging from agitation to delirium. This constellation results from antagonism of muscarinic acetylcholine receptors by agents including antihistamines, antipsychotics, tricyclic antidepressants, and plants containing belladonna alkaloids. The classic descriptive mnemonic "hot as a hare, blind as a bat, dry as a bone, red as a beet, mad as a hatter" captures key features, while hyperthermia often represents the most immediately life-threatening component requiring aggressive intervention.

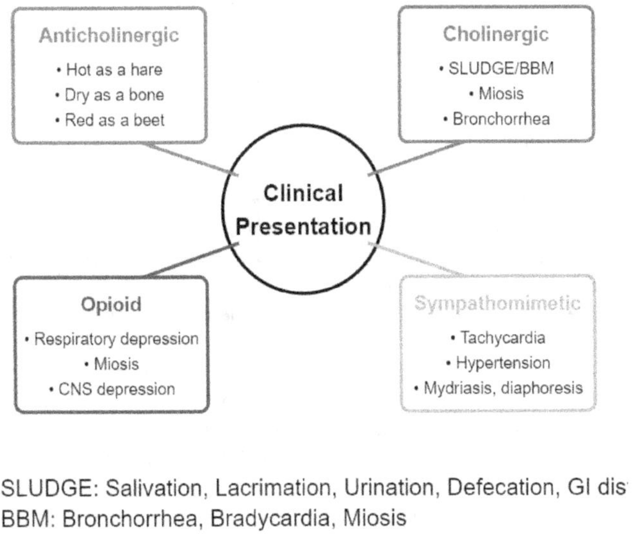

Figure 4.2. Recognition of Toxidromes

The cholinergic toxidrome manifests with bronchorrhea, bronchospasm, bradycardia, miosis, lacrimation, salivation, diaphoresis, urination, and gastrointestinal hyperactivity. This presentation reflects excessive cholinergic stimulation from organophosphate and carbamate insecticides, nerve agents, or certain mushrooms containing muscarine. Nicotinic effects, including fasciculations, weakness, and paradoxical tachycardia, may accompany muscarinic manifestations particularly with organophosphate poisoning. The SLUDGE mnemonic (Salivation, Lacrimation, Urination, Defecation, Gastrointestinal distress, Emesis) captures major features, while respiratory secretions often present the most immediate threat through airway compromise.

The sympathomimetic toxidrome features hyperthermia, tachycardia, hypertension, mydriasis, diaphoresis, and agitation. This presentation results from excessive adrenergic stimulation through direct receptor activation, increased neurotransmitter release, or reuptake inhibition. Common causative agents include cocaine, amphetamines, synthetic cathinones ("bath salts"), and pseudoephedrine. Complications include hyperthermia-induced rhabdomyolysis, seizures, dysrhythmias, and intracerebral hemorrhage. Distinguishing features from the similar anticholinergic toxidrome include the presence of diaphoresis and hyperactive bowel sounds in sympathomimetic toxicity.

The opioid toxidrome classically presents with the triad of respiratory depression, central nervous system depression, and miosis, though pupillary response may be inconsistent with certain synthetic opioids or in the setting of severe hypoxia. Additional features include hypotension, bradycardia, hypothermia, and decreased bowel sounds. This constellation results from mu-opioid receptor agonism by natural, semisynthetic, or synthetic opioids including heroin, oxycodone, fentanyl, and methadone. Naloxone responsiveness provides both diagnostic confirmation and therapeutic intervention, though increasingly potent synthetic opioids may require multiple or higher doses than historically needed.

The sedative-hypnotic toxidrome manifests with central nervous system depression, respiratory depression, hypotension, hypothermia, and ataxia. This presentation results from gamma-aminobutyric acid (GABA) potentiation by benzodiazepines, barbiturates, nonbenzodiazepine hypnotics, and ethanol. Distinguishing features from opioid toxicity include normal or slightly dilated pupils and lack of naloxone response. Flumazenil can reverse benzodiazepine effects but carries seizure risk particularly in patients with benzodiazepine dependence or mixed ingestions including proconvulsant agents.

Several additional toxidromes require recognition. The serotonin syndrome presents with autonomic instability, neuromuscular abnormalities (hyperreflexia, clonus, rigidity), and altered mental status, resulting from excessive serotonergic activity typically following therapeutic combinations or overdoses of serotonergic medications. The hallucinogenic toxidrome features perceptual distortions, synesthesia, mydriasis, and sympathetic activation without severe hyperthermia, caused by agents including LSD, psilocybin, and mescaline. Withdrawal syndromes, particularly from ethanol, benzodiazepines, and opioids, present distinct constellations requiring specific recognition and management approaches.

Table 4.2: Common Toxidromes and Their Clinical Features

Toxidrome	Vital Signs	Mental Status	Pupils	Examples
Anticholinergic	↑HR, ↑BP, ↑Temp	Agitation, delirium	Mydriasis	Antihistamines, atropine
Cholinergic	↓HR, variable BP	Confusion, seizures	Miosis	Organophosphates, carbamates
Opioid	↓HR, ↓BP, ↓RR	Sedation, coma	Miosis	Heroin, fentanyl, oxycodone
Sympathomimetic	↑HR, ↑BP, ↑Temp	Agitation, psychosis	Mydriasis	Cocaine, amphetamines
Sedative-hypnotic	↓HR, ↓BP, ↓RR	Sedation, coma	Normal	Benzodiazepines, barbiturates
Serotonergic	↑HR, ↑BP, ↑Temp	Agitation, confusion	Variable	SSRIs, MAOIs, MDMA
Hallucinogenic	↑HR, ↑BP	Hallucinations	Mydriasis	LSD, psilocybin

Diagnostic Challenges

Several factors complicate toxicological diagnosis despite systematic clinical assessment. Polypharmacy exposures create mixed presentations that obscure classic toxidrome recognition. For instance, combined opioid-stimulant ("speedball") ingestion may produce counteracting pupillary effects, while anticholinergic-cholinergic combinations can generate unpredictable clinical pictures. Time-released formulations create delayed onset toxicity that may manifest after initial assessment appears reassuring, particularly problematic with modified-release calcium channel blockers, beta-blockers, and certain antipsychotics. Unknown substances, particularly novel psychoactive substances and designer drugs, often produce effects incompletely characterized in medical literature, requiring syndrome-based rather than agent-specific management.

Comorbid conditions frequently confound toxicological assessment. Pre-existing neurological conditions, including dementia, psychiatric illness, intellectual disability, or previous stroke, complicate mental status evaluation. Baseline autonomic dysfunction from diabetic neuropathy or congenital disorders affects vital sign interpretation. Underlying hepatic or renal impairment alters toxicant metabolism and elimination, potentially exacerbating and prolonging effects. Distinguishing acute toxicant effects from decompensated chronic disease often requires careful integration of history, physical findings, and targeted testing.

Specific populations present unique diagnostic challenges. Pediatric patients manifest toxicant effects differently, with more rapid deterioration due to limited physiological reserve, altered body composition affecting distribution, developmental differences in biotransformation capacity, and distinctive exposure patterns often involving household products or medications with appealing characteristics. Geriatric patients demonstrate increased susceptibility due to reduced metabolic capacity, polypharmacy creating complex interactions, altered body composition, and decreased homeostatic reserve. Pregnancy alters toxicokinetics through increased plasma volume, enhanced renal clearance, and delayed gastric emptying, while raising concerns about fetal effects that influence management decisions.

Dynamic clinical evolution characterizes many poisonings, requiring serial reassessment rather than single evaluation. Initial sympathetic activation from certain toxicants may progress to delayed cardiovascular collapse. Hepatotoxic agents like acetaminophen typically produce minimal initial symptoms despite impending severe toxicity. Carbon monoxide victims may appear recovered after oxygen therapy yet develop delayed neuropsychiatric sequelae days or weeks later. These temporal patterns emphasize the importance of observation periods, scheduled reassessments, and anticipatory management based on known toxicant kinetics rather than solely responding to current clinical status.

LABORATORY TESTING

Laboratory investigations complement clinical assessment in poisoned patients, aiding diagnosis, guiding management, and assessing complications through both routine and specialized testing methods.

General Laboratory Evaluation

Basic laboratory studies provide essential information in toxicological cases, often revealing diagnostic patterns and identifying complications before specific toxicant confirmation. Electrolyte assessment identifies characteristic disturbances associated with specific toxicants: hypokalemia with beta-adrenergic agonists, theophylline, and barium; hyperkalemia with digoxin, potassium supplements, and succinylcholine; hyponatremia with ecstasy (MDMA), carbamazepine, and water intoxication; hypernatremia with salt poisoning or excessive sodium bicarbonate administration. The anion gap calculation (Na^+ - [Cl^- + HCO_3^-]) helps identify presence of unmeasured anions, with elevation suggesting toxic alcohols, salicylates, metformin, or certain anticonvulsants. The osmolal gap, representing the difference between measured serum osmolality and calculated osmolality (2[Na^+] + glucose/18 + BUN/2.8), increases with alcohols (ethanol, methanol, isopropanol, ethylene glycol), acetone, and mannitol.

Renal function tests assess both injury from nephrotoxic substances and elimination capacity for renally cleared toxicants. Blood urea nitrogen and creatinine elevations may reflect pre-renal causes from volume depletion, intrinsic renal toxicity from agents like NSAIDs or aminoglycosides, or post-renal obstruction from crystal formation with certain medications. Urinalysis provides valuable toxicological information, revealing myoglobinuria in rhabdomyolysis (dark urine positive for blood without erythrocytes), crystal formation with ethylene glycol (calcium oxalate) or acyclovir (needle-shaped crystals), or direct tissue toxicity manifesting as sterile pyuria.

Hepatic function tests identify hepatotoxicity and inform metabolic capacity assessment. Transaminase elevations suggest direct hepatocellular damage from acetaminophen, Amanita phalloides mushrooms, or volatile hydrocarbons. Bilirubin fractionation distinguishes predominantly direct (conjugated) hyperbilirubinemia in hepatocellular or cholangiocellular toxicity from indirect (unconjugated) elevation in hemolytic processes. Coagulation studies, particularly prothrombin time and international normalized ratio (INR), provide sensitive indicators of hepatic synthetic function, with early prolongation preceding other clinical manifestations of severe hepatotoxicity.

Hematological assessment reveals characteristic abnormalities including methemoglobinemia (decreased oxygen-carrying capacity from oxidized hemoglobin) from dapsone, local anesthetics, or nitrites; hemolysis from oxidant stressors including naphthalene or copper; and bone marrow suppression from chemotherapeutics, anticonvulsants, or colchicine. Complete blood count with differential provides baseline assessment for monitoring progression and evaluating complications like infection secondary to toxicant-induced immunosuppression.

Table 4.3: Toxicological Laboratory Testing Approaches

Test Type	Applications	Limitations
Qualitative screens	Drug of abuse detection, unknown exposure	Limited substance panel, false positives/negatives
Quantitative levels	Specific toxin measurement, therapy guidance	Availability, turnaround time
Therapeutic drug monitoring	Medication overdose assessment	Limited to selected pharmaceuticals
Metabolic panels	Detect secondary effects of toxins	Nonspecific, often late changes
Anion/osmol gaps	Identify presence of unmeasured substances	Low sensitivity, multiple causes
Arterial blood gases	Assess acid-base status, oxygenation	Requires arterial puncture
Imaging studies	Detect pill concretions, complications	Limited direct toxin detection
Electrocardiography	Cardiotoxicity assessment	Many toxins affect the ECG similarly

Arterial blood gases provide crucial information about acid-base status and respiratory function. Metabolic acidosis characterizes numerous toxicants, with increased anion gap acidosis suggesting toxic alcohols, salicylates, or metformin; normal anion gap acidosis occurring with toluene exposure or diarrheal fluid losses; and mixed acid-base disturbances frequently accompanying complex poisonings. The calculated alveolar-arterial oxygen gradient assesses pulmonary oxygen transfer efficiency, helping distinguish respiratory failure etiologies in toxicant exposure.

Specific Toxicant Assays

Therapeutic drug monitoring techniques have been adapted for toxicological applications, providing quantitative assessment of drug concentrations in biological matrices. These assays typically employ immunoassay or chromatographic techniques targeted at specific agents where concentration data guides management decisions. Acetaminophen levels correlate with hepatotoxicity risk when plotted on the Rumack-Matthew nomogram, requiring measurement at least 4 hours post-ingestion for accurate risk stratification. Salicylate concentrations help determine treatment intensity, with levels above 100 mg/dL in acute overdose typically indicating need for hemodialysis. Lithium levels guide management decisions, with concentrations above 4 mEq/L generally warranting hemodialysis consideration even in asymptomatic patients due to potential for delayed toxicity.

Several additional agents warrant specific quantitative analysis. Carbamazepine toxicity assessment benefits from direct measurement due to nonlinear kinetics at higher concentrations. Valproic acid levels correlate with neurological depression, hyperammonemia, and metabolic abnormalities. Digoxin concentrations help distinguish toxicity from therapeutic effect and guide digoxin-specific antibody fragment dosing. Iron level determination helps assess poisoning severity, with concentrations above 500 μg/dL suggesting significant toxicity requiring chelation. These quantitative assays require careful interpretation considering timing relative to ingestion, distribution phases, protein binding variations, active metabolites, and laboratory methodological limitations.

Toxic alcohol assays provide crucial management guidance for methanol and ethylene glycol poisonings, where early intervention prevents metabolic conversion to toxic metabolites. Gas chromatography represents the gold standard methodology for these measurements, though limited availability in many facilities creates problematic delays. Surrogate markers including osmolal gap, anion gap metabolic acidosis, and characteristic crystal formation (calcium oxalate in ethylene glycol poisoning) often guide initial management pending definitive testing. Serial ethanol measurements assess both toxic effects and therapeutic administration when ethanol serves as competitive substrate inhibitor in toxic alcohol poisonings.

Carbon monoxide poisoning assessment requires specialized carboxyhemoglobin measurement, typically through co-oximetry rather than standard pulse oximetry which cannot distinguish oxyhemoglobin from carboxyhemoglobin. Levels correlate imperfectly with symptoms due to individual susceptibility factors, though measurements above 25% generally indicate significant toxicity. Heavy metal testing provides essential diagnostic information for exposures including lead, arsenic, and mercury, typically employing atomic absorption spectroscopy or inductively coupled plasma mass spectrometry to achieve necessary sensitivity and specificity for these determinations.

Diagnostic Imaging

Radiographic studies provide valuable toxicological information in selected scenarios. Plain radiography identifies radio-opaque substances including heavy metals (lead, iron, bismuth), certain medications (chloral hydrate, enteric-coated aspirin), and foreign bodies. The pneumonic "CHIPES" captures major radio-opaque categories: Chloral hydrate, Heavy metals, Iron, Phenothiazines, Enteric-coated tablets, and Sustained-release preparations. Abdominal radiographs may reveal tablet contours, concretions, or characteristic patterns like the "string of pearls" appearance in iron overdose. Chest radiography assesses pulmonary complications including non-cardiogenic pulmonary edema from salicylates or opioids, aspiration pneumonitis, or hydrocarbon pneumonitis.

Computed tomography (CT) provides enhanced resolution for specific toxicological applications. CT abdomen may identify radio-dense tablets not visible on plain films, detect early signs of hepatic injury, or evaluate suspected body packing in drug traffickers who have ingested drug-filled packets. CT brain without contrast remains the preferred neuroimaging modality for altered mental status evaluation, identifying cerebral edema from toxic exposures, excluding structural lesions mimicking toxidromes, or detecting ischemic changes from carbon monoxide or cyanide exposures. CT angiography helps assess potential vascular complications from vasoactive substances including cocaine and sympathomimetics.

Magnetic resonance imaging offers superiority for specific toxicant-related pathologies. MRI brain demonstrates characteristic findings in certain poisonings, including bilateral basal ganglia hyperintensities in carbon monoxide exposure, restricted diffusion in hypoxic injury from respiratory depressants, or white matter changes in solvent abuse. MR spectroscopy can identify metabolite abnormalities in certain toxicant exposures, including lactate elevation in mitochondrial toxins and myoinositol changes in hepatic encephalopathy secondary to hepatotoxins.

Several specialized imaging techniques offer diagnostic advantages in specific contexts. Doppler ultrasound helps assess vascular complications including thromboembolic events from cocaine or ergot derivatives. Echocardiography evaluates cardiac function in cardiotoxic exposures including calcium channel blockers and beta-blockers. Nuclear medicine studies, particularly technetium-99m lung scans, can identify inhalation injuries from caustic gases or smoke exposure. Dual-energy CT improves detection of low atomic number materials that may be indistinguishable from soft tissue on conventional CT, enhancing identification of certain drug concretions.

Electrocardiography and Other Functional Studies

Electrocardiography provides critical information regarding cardiovascular effects of numerous toxicants. QRS prolongation (>100 ms) suggests sodium channel blockade from tricyclic antidepressants, antiarrhythmics, or cocaine, correlating with seizure and ventricular dysrhythmia risk. QT interval prolongation (QTc >470 ms in males, >480 ms in females) indicates potassium channel blockade from numerous agents including antipsychotics, methadone, and antiarrhythmics, predisposing to torsades de pointes. The terminally peaked T wave morphology of hyperkalemia appears in digitalis glycoside toxicity and potassium supplement overdose. U waves emerge with hypokalemia from diuretics or beta-agonists. Specific dysrhythmias provide diagnostic clues, including bidirectional ventricular tachycardia suggesting digitalis toxicity and polymorphic ventricular tachycardia indicating QT-prolonging agents.

Several ECG patterns suggest specific toxicants. The Brugada pattern (right bundle branch block with ST elevation in right precordial leads) appears with sodium channel blockers, particularly at higher concentrations. The "terminal 40ms right axis deviation" or rightward shift of the terminal QRS complex in aVR suggests cyclic antidepressant toxicity. Osborn waves (J-point elevation) appear in hypothermia from ethanol, sedatives, or environmental exposure. First-degree AV block progressing to higher-grade blocks suggests nodal blocking agents including calcium channel blockers, beta-blockers, and digitalis glycosides.

Additional functional studies provide valuable assessment in selected poisonings. Pulmonary function testing quantifies bronchospasm in cholinergic or irritant gas exposures and identifies restrictive patterns in parenchymal toxicity from agents like paraquat. Spirometry trends monitor progression and treatment response in these exposures. Carbon monoxide diffusion capacity testing helps assess persistent impairment following significant inhalational exposures. Nerve conduction studies identify delayed neuropathies from organophosphates, heavy metals, and industrial solvents, though changes typically emerge days to weeks after acute exposure, limiting utility in initial assessment.

Electroencephalography assists evaluation of altered mental status, seizures, or encephalopathy from toxicant exposure. Characteristic patterns include diffuse slowing in metabolic encephalopathy from hepatotoxins, triphasic waves in hepatic or uremic encephalopathy, epileptiform discharges with proconvulsant toxicants like isoniazid or tricyclic antidepressants, and burst suppression in severe sedative-hypnotic exposure. Continuous EEG monitoring provides particular value in patients with persistent altered consciousness after seizure-inducing toxicant exposure, identifying subclinical seizure activity requiring treatment

TOXICOLOGICAL SCREENING

Systematic toxicological analysis enables detection of unknown substances in biological samples, providing crucial diagnostic information when history remains unclear or clinical presentation suggests unidentified exposures.

Immunoassay Techniques

Immunoassay screening provides rapid qualitative or semi-quantitative detection of substance classes based on antibody-antigen binding principles. These tests serve as frontline screening tools in emergency settings due to their speed, automation capability, and widespread availability, though they provide presumptive rather than definitive identification. Enzyme-linked immunosorbent assays (ELISA) employ enzyme-labeled antibodies or antigens that generate colorimetric changes when target substances are present. Fluorescence polarization immunoassay (FPIA) measures changes in polarized light rotation when fluorescent-labeled antigens bind to antibodies. Cloned enzyme donor immunoassay (CEDIA) utilizes genetically engineered enzyme fragments that regain activity when drug-antibody binding occurs.

> **Remember**
>
> **Immunoassay-based toxicology screens offer rapid results but have significant limitations including cross-reactivity, limited substance coverage, and inability to detect many clinically important toxins.**

Conventional immunoassay panels typically include several substance categories. Opioid screens primarily detect morphine and its natural derivatives, with variable sensitivity for semisynthetic and synthetic opioids, and frequent false negatives for fentanyl, buprenorphine, and oxycodone due to structural differences from morphine. Benzodiazepine assays detect most agents in this class but may miss clonazepam, lorazepam, or designer benzodiazepines depending on antibody specificity. Amphetamine screens detect amphetamine and methamphetamine but show inconsistent cross-reactivity with MDMA, pseudoephedrine, and synthetic cathinones. Cocaine assays detect benzoylecgonine (primary cocaine metabolite) rather than cocaine itself, offering longer detection windows but requiring metabolism for positive results.

Immunoassay limitations require careful interpretation. Cross-reactivity with structurally similar compounds causes false positives, exemplified by diphenhydramine or doxylamine triggering tricyclic antidepressant screens, or ranitidine producing false-positive amphetamine results. Detection thresholds typically exceed therapeutic concentrations, potentially missing clinically significant levels particularly with dilute samples. Limited substance coverage leaves numerous toxicologically significant substances undetected, including synthetic cannabinoids, novel psychoactive substances, and many prescription medications. These limitations necessitate understanding which substances can and cannot be reliably detected before using results to guide management decisions.

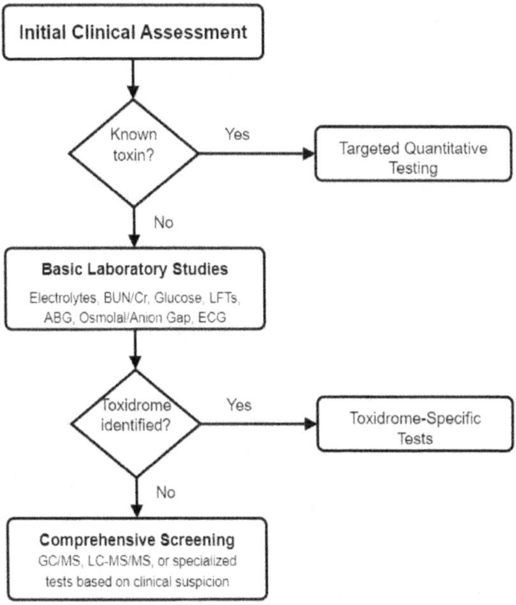

Figure 4.3: Laboratory Testing Decision Algorithm

Several methodological factors affect interpretation. Sample type influences detection windows, with urine offering longer detection periods (days) compared to serum (hours), though blood better reflects current intoxication status. Detection cutoffs, established to minimize false positives in workplace testing, may exceed clinically relevant concentrations in emergency settings. Semi-quantitative results provide approximate concentration ranges rather than precise values, requiring confirmation for accurate quantification. Point-of-care immunoassay devices offer convenience but typically demonstrate lower sensitivity and specificity compared to laboratory-based systems, creating particular challenges in interpretation at concentration ranges near cutoff thresholds.

Chromatographic Techniques

Chromatographic methods separate complex mixtures into individual components based on differential migration through a stationary phase under the influence of a mobile phase. These techniques provide significantly greater specificity than immunoassays, serving as confirmatory methods and enabling detection of substances not covered by conventional screening panels. Thin-layer chromatography, while largely replaced by instrumental methods in developed countries, continues to serve in resource-limited settings due to low cost and minimal equipment requirements. This technique separates compounds based on migration distance on adsorbent-coated plates, with identification based on retention factor values and visualization under specific light conditions or with chemical reagents.

Gas chromatography (GC) separates volatile and semi-volatile compounds vaporized in a heated injection port and carried through a capillary column by inert carrier gas. Separation occurs based on partitioning between gaseous mobile phase and liquid or solid stationary phase, with elution time (retention time) providing provisional identification. Detection systems include flame ionization detectors offering broad sensitivity to carbon-containing compounds, electron capture detectors with particular sensitivity for halogenated compounds, and nitrogen-phosphorus detectors selectively responding to nitrogen and phosphorus-containing substances. GC excels in analyzing volatile substances including alcohols, inhalants, and anesthetic gases, but requires derivatization for many non-volatile compounds.

High-performance liquid chromatography (HPLC) separates compounds based on interactions between liquid mobile phase, solid stationary phase, and sample components, accommodating thermally labile and non-volatile substances unsuitable for GC analysis. Various detector types include ultraviolet-visible spectrophotometers detecting compounds absorbing specific wavelengths, fluorescence detectors for naturally fluorescent substances or derivatized compounds, and electrochemical detectors for readily oxidized or reduced substances.

HPLC applications include analysis of non-volatile drugs, drug metabolites, and endogenous compounds affected by toxic exposures.

Hyphenated techniques combining chromatographic separation with spectroscopic identification provide definitive substance identification rather than presumptive results. Gas chromatography-mass spectrometry (GC-MS) couples the separation capabilities of GC with mass spectral identification, fragmenting compounds into characteristic charged particles that generate distinctive spectral patterns serving as molecular fingerprints. This technique represents the traditional gold standard for definitive toxicological confirmation. Liquid chromatography-tandem mass spectrometry (LC-MS/MS) offers similar capabilities for non-volatile compounds, with enhanced sensitivity permitting detection at sub-nanogram levels. These methods enable comprehensive unknown screening against reference libraries containing thousands of compounds, though remain limited by available reference spectra, particularly for novel substances.

Systematic Screening

Systematic toxicological analysis methods balance breadth of coverage against analytical complexity, resource requirements, and turnaround time. Tiered approaches typically begin with immunoassay screening for common substance classes, followed by confirmatory testing of positive results and expanded testing based on clinical suspicion when initial screens prove negative despite suggestive presentation. Targeted analysis directed by clinical findings provides efficiency by focusing on substances consistent with observed toxidrome features, though potentially missing unexpected or multiple toxicants. Broad spectrum screening employs chromatographic methods with mass spectral detection to identify substances across numerous classes without predetermined targets, providing maximal coverage but requiring greater technical resources and expertise.

Sample selection significantly influences detection capability and interpretation. Urine provides the preferred matrix for comprehensive screening due to concentrated metabolite presence, extended detection windows (typically days after exposure), and non-invasive collection. Blood or serum better reflects current intoxication status and permits estimation of toxicant burden, particularly valuable for substances with established toxic concentration thresholds. Gastric contents enable detection of substances not yet absorbed, potentially identifying exposures before systemic distribution occurs. Alternative matrices including hair (providing historical exposure information over months), oral fluid (reflecting recent exposure with collection advantages), and vitreous humor (resistant to postmortem changes) serve specialized contexts including forensic investigations and workplace monitoring.

Clinical and analytical factors guide selection of appropriate testing methods. Clinical urgency dictates acceptable turnaround times, with critically ill patients requiring rapid results to guide immediate interventions while stable patients permit more comprehensive analysis. Laboratory capabilities vary substantially between facilities, from limited point-of-care immunoassay panels to comprehensive reference laboratory capabilities including high-resolution mass spectrometry. Resource allocation considerations become particularly relevant in mass casualty scenarios, where focused testing for specific threats provides greater public health value than exhaustive analysis of individual cases. Retrospective analysis may supplement initial restricted testing when clinical course diverges from expectations based on preliminary results.

Interpretation of comprehensive screening results requires integration of analytical findings with clinical context. Identified substances must be evaluated for pharmacological plausibility in explaining observed symptoms, with consideration of confounding factors including post-collection stability, detection timing relative to exposure and symptom onset, and potential for undetected co-ingestants. Negative results never completely exclude exposure possibilities due to inherent methodological limitations, substances falling below detection thresholds, novel compounds absent from reference libraries, or testing performed outside substance detection windows. These interpretive limitations underscore the principle that toxicological testing serves to complement rather than replace thorough clinical assessment in poisoned patients.

Novel Substances and Analytical Challenges

The proliferation of novel psychoactive substances (NPS) presents significant analytical challenges for toxicological screening. These compounds, designed to mimic effects of controlled substances while circumventing legal restrictions, undergo continuous structural modification to evade regulation and detection. Synthetic cannabinoids acting on cannabis receptors with greater potency than THC include hundreds of structurally diverse compounds marketed as "Spice" or "K2." Synthetic cathinones stimulating monoamine release include derivatives like mephedrone, methylone, and alpha-PVP ("bath salts" or "flakka"). Novel opioids, particularly fentanyl analogs with extreme potency, contribute substantially to overdose mortality. Designer benzodiazepines, phenethylamines, and tryptamines further expand this continuously evolving landscape.

Conventional screening methods demonstrate significant limitations for novel substance detection. Immunoassays typically lack cross-reactivity with structurally modified analogs, creating false negative results despite significant toxicity. Even chromatographic methods with mass spectral detection face challenges when reference standards and spectral libraries lack entries for newly emerged compounds. The rapid proliferation of novel substances outpaces development of validated analytical methods, creating persistent detection gaps between substance emergence and analytical capability development.

Advanced analytical approaches address some of these challenges. High-resolution mass spectrometry enables molecular formula determination through accurate mass measurement, providing structural information even without reference standards. Fragmentation pattern analysis through tandem mass spectrometry generates structural information enabling classification of unknown compounds into pharmacological categories. Metabolite identification helps detect parent compounds already eliminated from circulation, particularly valuable when metabolism produces more persistent or more easily detected derivatives. Activity-based assays measuring biological effects rather than specific chemical structures can detect previously uncharacterized substances with particular receptor activities.

Coordinated response systems enhance detection capabilities for novel substances. Early warning networks connecting clinical toxicologists, analytical laboratories, law enforcement, and public health agencies facilitate rapid information sharing about emerging threats. Bio-analytical gathering projects collect and analyze samples from various sources including drug seizures, anonymous drug checking services, and clinical cases to identify novel substances entering circulation. International collaboration through organizations like the United Nations Office on Drugs and Crime enables global monitoring of substance trends and dissemination of analytical protocols. These systematic approaches, while not eliminating detection challenges, reduce delays between substance emergence and detection capability development

ANALYTICAL METHODS

Specialized analytical techniques provide definitive identification and quantification of toxicants, supporting clinical management, public health surveillance, and forensic investigations.

Sample Collection and Preparation

Proper specimen collection and handling critically influence analytical reliability in toxicological testing. Collection timing significantly affects interpretation, with blood samples reflecting current intoxication, urine demonstrating recent exposure (typically within days), and hair or nails providing historical information over weeks to months. Volume requirements vary by analytical method, from microliters for some immunoassays to several milliliters for comprehensive screening. Documentation must include patient identifiers, collection time, specimen type, preservatives added, chain of custody information when legally relevant, and clinical information guiding analysis selection.

> **Remember**
>
> **Definitive analytical methods including gas chromatography-mass spectrometry and liquid chromatography-mass spectrometry provide specific identification and quantification but are more resource-intensive and time-consuming.**

Specific collection considerations apply to different specimen types. Blood collection requires attention to site preparation, as alcohol-based antiseptics can contaminate samples for ethanol analysis, necessitating alternative disinfectants. Anticoagulant selection affects stability, with EDTA or oxalate-fluoride tubes preferred for most toxicological analyses, the latter providing metabolic inhibition particularly important for alcohol samples. Urine collection benefits from witnessed provision when adulteration concerns exist, with temperature verification providing immediate authenticity assessment. Post-collection processing includes centrifugation to separate serum or plasma from cellular components and refrigeration or freezing for specimens awaiting analysis beyond a few hours.

Sample preparation techniques extract and concentrate analytes while removing potentially interfering substances. Liquid-liquid extraction separates compounds based on differential solubility between immiscible phases, typically aqueous sample and organic solvent, with pH adjustment enhancing extraction efficiency for ionizable compounds. Solid-phase extraction employs sorbent materials selectively retaining analytes while allowing interferents to pass through, followed by elution with appropriate solvents. Precipitation methods, particularly protein precipitation in blood samples, remove macromolecules that might interfere with analysis through addition of organic solvents, acids, or metal salts causing protein denaturation.

Sample preparation for specific analytical techniques may require additional steps. Derivatization chemically modifies analytes to enhance volatility for gas chromatography, improve detector response, or add distinctive functional groups aiding identification. Hydrolysis procedures, either enzymatic or chemical, cleave conjugated metabolites back to parent compounds, potentially increasing detection sensitivity for substances extensively metabolized before excretion. Internal standard addition provides reference compounds enabling quantitative analysis through comparison of analyte-to-standard response ratios, ideally using isotopically labeled versions of target compounds that demonstrate identical extraction and detection characteristics while remaining chromatographically distinguishable.

Mass Spectrometry

Mass spectrometry provides the gold standard for toxicant identification through generation and analysis of charged particles (ions) created from sample components. This technique measures the mass-to-charge ratio (m/z) of ionized molecules and their fragmentation products, creating distinctive spectral patterns serving as molecular fingerprints for definitive identification. Various ionization methods accommodate different compound classes and analytical requirements. Electron ionization (EI) bombards vaporized samples with high-energy electrons, creating reproducible fragmentation patterns ideal for library matching. Electrospray ionization (ESI) nebulizes liquid samples in an electric field, producing multiply charged ions from larger molecules with minimal fragmentation. Atmospheric pressure chemical ionization (APCI) uses gas-phase chemical reactions to transfer charge to analyte molecules, accommodating less polar compounds than ESI.

Mass analyzers separate ions based on their mass-to-charge ratios through various physical principles. Quadrupole analyzers use oscillating electric fields between four parallel rods to selectively transmit ions of specific m/z values to the detector. Time-of-flight (TOF) analyzers measure the time required for accelerated ions to traverse a flight tube, with lighter ions reaching the detector before heavier ones. Ion trap analyzers capture ions within a three-dimensional electric field, selectively ejecting them based on m/z for detection. Orbitrap analyzers trap ions in orbital motion around a central electrode, with m/z values determined from oscillation frequencies. Each analyzer type offers different strengths regarding resolution, mass accuracy, scan speed, and dynamic range.

Tandem mass spectrometry (MS/MS) provides enhanced specificity through multiple stages of mass analysis. This approach typically selects specific ions from the first mass analyzer, subjects them to collision-induced dissociation with inert gas molecules, and analyzes resulting fragments in a second mass analyzer. The combination of precursor ion selection and fragment pattern analysis dramatically increases specificity compared to single-stage methods. Multiple reaction monitoring (MRM) focuses on specific precursor-fragment transitions characteristic of target compounds, enabling highly selective detection even in complex matrices. Data-dependent acquisition automatically triggers MS/MS analysis when target compounds are detected, while data-independent acquisition fragments all ions within specified mass ranges regardless of abundance.

High-resolution mass spectrometry distinguishes ions differing by very small mass differences, enabling determination of molecular formulas through exact mass measurement. This capability proves particularly valuable for identifying unknown compounds without reference standards, as molecular formula constraints dramatically narrow structural possibilities. Instruments achieving resolutions exceeding 50,000 (measured as m/z divided by peak width) can distinguish compounds with identical nominal masses but different elemental compositions. When combined with chromatographic retention time data, isotope pattern analysis, and fragmentation information, high-resolution mass spectrometry provides powerful tools for identifying novel or unexpected toxicants that would remain undetected or misidentified by conventional targeted approaches.

Spectroscopic Methods

Spectroscopic techniques analyze interactions between electromagnetic radiation and matter, providing structural information and quantitative measurement capabilities for toxicological analysis. Ultraviolet-visible spectrophotometry measures absorption of light in the ultraviolet (190-400 nm) and visible (400-800 nm) regions by compounds containing chromophores—functional groups with π electrons or non-bonding electrons that can undergo electronic transitions when absorbing specific wavelengths. Each compound demonstrates characteristic absorption spectra determined by its molecular structure, enabling both identification and quantification through Beer-Lambert law relationships between absorbance and concentration. This technique finds particular application in therapeutic drug monitoring, colorimetric screening tests, and detector systems for liquid chromatography.

Infrared spectroscopy examines absorption of infrared radiation (750 nm to 1 mm wavelength) causing molecular vibrations including stretching and bending of chemical bonds. The resulting spectrum provides a molecular fingerprint reflecting functional group composition and arrangement, enabling identification through comparison with reference spectra. Fourier transform infrared spectroscopy (FTIR) enhances sensitivity and resolution through simultaneous measurement of all wavelengths. This technique proves particularly valuable for identifying pharmaceuticals, illicit drugs, and unknown powders or tablets without requiring sample dissolution or extensive preparation, though matrix effects from biological specimens limit direct application to unaided clinical samples.

Nuclear magnetic resonance (NMR) spectroscopy analyzes the behavior of certain atomic nuclei in magnetic fields, providing detailed structural information unattainable through other methods. This technique observes energy absorption and release when nuclei transition between energy states in an applied magnetic field, with resulting spectral patterns reflecting the electronic environment surrounding each nucleus. Proton (^{1}H) NMR provides information about hydrogen atom distribution and connectivity, while carbon (^{13}C) NMR reveals carbon skeleton structure. Two-dimensional techniques establish correlations between different nuclei, enabling determination of complex molecular structures. While historically limited by sensitivity requirements, advanced techniques including cryoprobe technology and higher field strengths increasingly enable NMR application to toxicological samples at physiologically relevant concentrations.

Raman spectroscopy analyzes inelastic light scattering when monochromatic light interacts with molecules, causing energy transitions in molecular vibrations. The resulting spectrum reflects molecular structure similarly to infrared spectroscopy but through complementary selection rules, often providing information about symmetric vibrations poorly observed in infrared analysis. Surface-enhanced Raman spectroscopy (SERS) dramatically increases sensitivity through interaction with metallic nanostructures, enabling detection at significantly lower concentrations. Non-destructive analysis capability, minimal sample preparation requirements, and ability to analyze aqueous solutions make Raman spectroscopy particularly valuable for rapid identification of unknown substances, including through-container analysis without opening packaging—a significant advantage for suspicious materials.

Summary

Diagnostic approaches in toxicology require integration of clinical assessment with strategic laboratory investigations. The clinical assessment begins with a detailed history addressing substance identification, time of exposure, quantity, route, intent, and existing medical conditions, though this information may be limited by patient capacity or reliability. Physical examination focuses on vital signs, mental status, pupillary responses, skin findings, gastrointestinal activity, and neurological function, with special attention to toxidromes—characteristic constellations of signs and symptoms associated with specific toxin classes. Laboratory testing encompasses both general studies (complete blood count, electrolytes, renal and hepatic function tests, coagulation studies, arterial blood gases) and toxin-specific assays. Toxicological screening employs immunoassay-based methods for rapid detection of common substances, though these have significant limitations including cross-reactivity, limited substance coverage, and semi-quantitative results requiring confirmation. Definitive analytical methods include gas chromatography, liquid chromatography, and mass spectrometry, which provide both qualitative identification and quantitative measurement of specific substances. Additional specialized techniques address unique toxins like metals, gases, and biological agents. Interpretation requires understanding detection windows, metabolite patterns, specimen selection considerations, and confirmation thresholds. The optimal diagnostic approach considers the clinical context, resource availability, and time constraints, recognizing that management decisions often cannot await comprehensive toxicological analysis and must proceed based on clinical presentation and presumptive diagnosis.

Self-Assessment Questions

1. Describe the key components of a comprehensive toxicological history and explain how clinicians should approach situations where history is limited or unreliable.
2. Compare and contrast the major toxidromes (anticholinergic, cholinergic, sympathomimetic, opioid, and sedative-hypnotic), including their clinical features and characteristic substances.
3. Analyze the advantages and limitations of different biological specimens (blood, urine, saliva, hair) for toxicological testing, including detection windows and specific applications.
4. Explain the principle of immunoassay-based drug screening, discussing sources of false positive and false negative results with clinical examples.
5. Describe how gas chromatography-mass spectrometry works in toxicological analysis and its advantages over screening immunoassays.
6. Evaluate the clinical utility of specific quantitative assays (such as acetaminophen, salicylate, and digoxin levels) in guiding management decisions for potentially toxic exposures.
7. Discuss the challenges in detecting and quantifying novel psychoactive substances and designer drugs using conventional toxicology screening methods.
8. Analyze how anion gap, osmolal gap, and other laboratory findings can provide indirect evidence of specific toxic exposures when direct testing is unavailable.
9. Explain the concept of "chain of custody" in forensic toxicology testing and how it differs from clinical toxicology procedures.
10. Describe strategies for rational and cost-effective use of toxicological testing in emergency settings, balancing the need for diagnostic certainty against resource constraints.

Bibliography

1. Holstege CP, Borek HA. Toxidromes. Crit Care Clin. 2012;28(4):479-498.
2. Wu AHB, McKay C, Broussard LA, Hoffman RS, Kwong TC, Moyer TP, et al. National Academy of Clinical Biochemistry laboratory medicine practice guidelines: recommendations for the use of laboratory tests to support poisoned patients who present to the emergency department. Clin Chem. 2003;49(3):357-379.
3. Gummin DD, Mowry JB, Beuhler MC, Spyker DA, Bronstein AC, Rivers LJ, et al. 2020 Annual Report of the American Association of Poison Control Centers' National Poison Data System (NPDS): 38th Annual Report. Clin Toxicol (Phila). 2021;59(12):1282-1501.
4. Drummer OH. Postmortem toxicology of drugs of abuse. Forensic Sci Int. 2004;142(2-3):101-113.
5. Moeller KE, Kissack JC, Atayee RS, Lee KC. Clinical interpretation of urine drug tests: what clinicians need to know about urine drug screens. Mayo Clin Proc. 2017;92(5):774-796.
6. Lynch KL, Breaud AR, Vandenberghe H, Wu AHB, Clarke W. Performance evaluation of three liquid chromatography mass spectrometry methods for broad spectrum drug screening. Clin Chem. 2010;56(9):1436-1441.
7. Smith MP, Bluth MH. Forensic toxicology: an introduction. Clin Lab Med. 2016;36(4):753-759.
8. Schulz M, Iwersen-Bergmann S, Andresen H, Schmoldt A. Therapeutic and toxic blood concentrations of nearly 1,000 drugs and other xenobiotics. Crit Care. 2012;16(4):R136.
9. Brent J, Kulig K, Rumack BH, Dart RC. An analysis of the types of intravenous fluids administered in poisonings: an enhanced role for poison centers. Vet Hum Toxicol. 1990;32(2):110-112.
10. Mégarbane B, Oberlin M, Alvarez JC, Balen F, Beaune S, Bédry R, et al. Management of pharmaceutical and recreational drug poisoning. Ann Intensive Care. 2020;10(1):157.

CHAPTER 5

TREATMENT PRINCIPLES

Author

Prof. Dr. Suresh V Chennupati, Principal and Professor, Chennupati Indo-American School of Pharmacy, Andhra Pradesh India

Abstract

Management of toxic exposures follows systematic principles aimed at reducing further absorption, enhancing elimination, administering specific antidotes when available, and providing supportive care. Gastrointestinal decontamination methods include activated charcoal, which adsorbs many toxins but is contraindicated for caustic ingestions, hydrocarbons, and patients with unprotected airways. Once widely used, gastric lavage and induced emesis now have limited roles due to efficacy and safety concerns. Whole bowel irrigation may benefit in specific scenarios like sustained-release medication or body packer ingestions. Antidotal therapy directly counteracts toxic mechanisms through various actions including receptor antagonism, chelation, substrate competition, and metabolic interventions. Well-established antidotes include N-acetylcysteine for acetaminophen, naloxone for opioids, and various chelating agents for heavy metals, though many poisonings lack specific antidotes. Supportive care forms the cornerstone of management for most exposures, focusing on maintaining vital functions, treating symptoms, and preventing complications. Enhanced elimination techniques—including multiple-dose activated charcoal, urinary alkalinization, and extracorporeal methods like hemodialysis—can significantly reduce toxin burden for selected substances with appropriate pharmacokinetic properties. Treatment decisions must balance potential benefits against risks while considering individual patient factors including age, comorbidities, and exposure characteristics.

Keywords: *Decontamination, Antidotes, Activated Charcoal, Enhanced Elimination, Hemodialysis, Supportive Care*

Learning Objectives

After completion of the chapter, the learners should be able to:

- Evaluate the indications, contraindications, and efficacy of various gastrointestinal decontamination methods for different toxic exposures.
- Select appropriate antidotes for specific poisonings and explain their mechanisms of action, dosing, and administration routes.
- Implement comprehensive supportive care measures for toxic exposures lacking specific antidotes.
- Determine when enhanced elimination techniques are indicated based on toxin properties and patient factors.
- Compare the efficacy of different elimination methods including multiple-dose activated charcoal, urinary alkalinization, and extracorporeal techniques for specific toxins.
- Develop treatment plans that integrate decontamination, antidotal therapy, supportive care, and enhanced elimination based on specific poisoning scenarios and patient characteristics.

DECONTAMINATION METHODS

Decontamination procedures aim to reduce toxicant absorption and systemic burden through removal from exposure sites, with approach selection guided by route of exposure, toxicant properties, and time since exposure.

Gastrointestinal Decontamination

Gastric lavage, historically a mainstay of poisoning management, involves placement of a large-bore orogastric tube (36-40 French for adults) and sequential instillation and withdrawal of small aliquots (200-300 mL) of warm water or normal saline until returning fluid appears clear. This procedure demonstrates greatest efficacy when performed within one hour of ingestion, after which gastric emptying significantly reduces potential yield.

Modern practice has substantially restricted gastric lavage indications due to limited proven benefit and significant potential complications. Absolute contraindications include corrosive ingestion due to perforation risk, hydrocarbon ingestion due to aspiration concern, and unstable patient condition unless airway is secured. Potential complications include aspiration pneumonitis, hypoxemia, laryngospasm, esophageal perforation, and fluid/electrolyte imbalances, particularly with repeated lavage attempts. Current positioning restricts lavage consideration to life-threatening poisonings presenting within one hour where no safer alternatives exist, and only by properly trained personnel with capacity for airway management.

> **Remember**
>
> **Activated charcoal effectively adsorbs many toxins when administered within 1-2 hours of ingestion, but is contraindicated with caustic substances, hydrocarbons, and in patients with unprotected airways or gastrointestinal obstruction.**

Activated charcoal administration represents the most widely employed gastrointestinal decontamination strategy, acting through adsorption of toxicants to its extensive internal surface area (1000-2000 m^2/g), preventing their absorption into systemic circulation. Standard adult dosing provides 1 g/kg (typically 50-100 g), administered as an aqueous slurry, ideally within one hour of ingestion, though potentially beneficial up to 4 hours post-ingestion for certain sustained-release preparations or drugs undergoing enterohepatic circulation. Activated charcoal demonstrates greatest efficacy for compounds with high charcoal affinity, including many pharmaceuticals, plant toxins, and mycotoxins. Important exceptions include alcohols, hydrocarbons, metals, corrosives, and lithium, which bind poorly to charcoal. Contraindications include unprotected airway in obtunded patients, gastrointestinal perforation risk, and corrosive ingestions where endoscopic evaluation may be compromised by charcoal presence. Complications include aspiration with subsequent pneumonitis, constipation, bowel obstruction with multiple-dose regimens, and reduced absorption of concurrently administered therapeutic medications.

Whole bowel irrigation employs large volumes of polyethylene glycol electrolyte solution (typically 1-2 L/hour in adults) administered orally or via nasogastric tube until rectal effluent becomes clear. This procedure mechanically flushes intestinal contents through the gastrointestinal tract, reducing toxicant absorption without relying on adsorptive binding. Primary indications include ingestions poorly adsorbed by activated charcoal, particularly sustained-release preparations, toxic metals including iron and lithium, and illicit drug packets in body packers. The isotonic, non-absorbable solution minimizes fluid and electrolyte disturbances compared to older cathartic approaches. Contraindications include gastrointestinal perforation or obstruction, significantly compromised hemodynamics, and uncontrolled vomiting. Absolute completion of the procedure requires many hours, potentially delaying alternative interventions, though toxicant binding and movement through the gastrointestinal tract begins immediately upon solution administration.

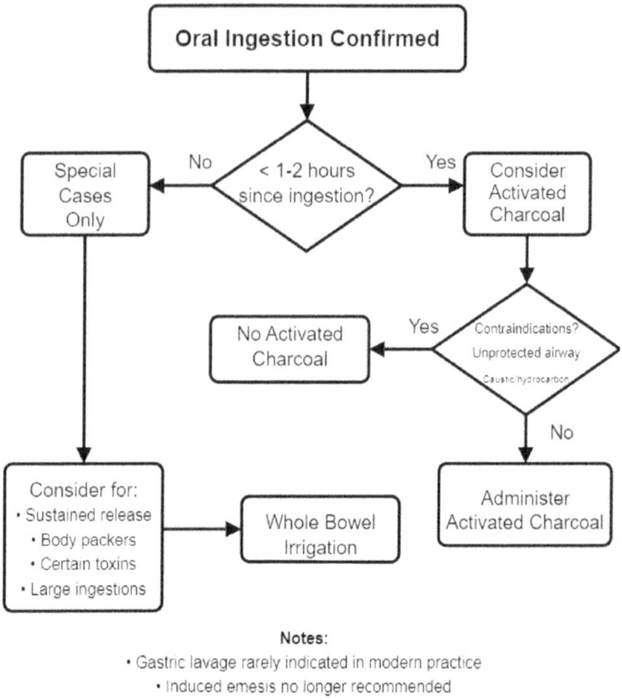

Figure 5.1: Gastrointestinal Decontamination Algorithm

Cathartics, including sorbitol, magnesium citrate, and magnesium sulfate, historically accompanied activated charcoal administration under the theoretical premise of accelerating gastrointestinal transit and reducing toxicant absorption time. Contemporary evidence indicates minimal benefit from this practice while introducing potential complications including fluid/electrolyte disturbances, excessive intestinal cramping, and hypotension from third-spacing of fluids. Current guidelines discourage routine cathartic use, particularly repeated doses or administration to pediatric or elderly patients. Syrup of ipecac, previously recommended for home use to induce emesis, has been abandoned in modern practice due to limited efficacy, potential for delayed administration of more effective interventions, aspiration risk, and persistent vomiting potentially interfering with oral antidote administration.

Table 5.1: Gastrointestinal Decontamination Methods

Method	Indications	Contraindications	Timing
Activated charcoal	Most oral poisonings	Caustics, hydrocarbons, altered mental status without airway protection	Most effective <1 hour, consider up to 4 hours for some toxins
Gastric lavage	Life-threatening ingestions when benefits outweigh risks	Caustics, hydrocarbons, absent gag reflex without intubation	<1 hour post-ingestion
Whole bowel irrigation	Sustained-release medications, body packers, heavy metals, iron	Bowel obstruction, perforation, ileus, hemodynamic instability	Effective for up to 12-24 hours for certain substances
Multiple-dose activated charcoal	Carbamazepine, phenobarbital, theophylline, salicylates	Same as single-dose charcoal	Can start later than single dose
Cathartics	No longer recommended as sole therapy	Bowel obstruction, diarrhea, electrolyte imbalances	N/A

Dermal Decontamination

Dermal decontamination procedures aim to remove toxicants from skin surfaces before significant absorption occurs, with effectiveness highly dependent on prompt initiation. Initial measures include removal of contaminated clothing, which may harbor substantial toxicant reservoirs, particularly with liquid exposures. Garments should be removed carefully to prevent secondary contamination of unaffected areas, with cutting rather than pulling over the head when feasible. Removed clothing requires proper containment and disposal according to hazardous materials protocols, particularly with pesticidal, chemical warfare, or radiological contamination.

Water lavage represents the principal dermal decontamination method, rapidly diluting and removing water-soluble toxicants while physically dislodging particulate matter. Irrigation should commence immediately and continue for 15-20 minutes with tepid, gentle-pressure water. Attention to irrigation runoff disposal prevents secondary contamination, particularly in mass casualty scenarios. High-pressure irrigation mechanisms may paradoxically enhance toxicant absorption by damaging skin barrier function or driving particulate matter deeper into tissues. Temperature extremes should be avoided, as hot water enhances percutaneous absorption through vasodilation and cold water may induce hypothermia with prolonged irrigation, particularly in pediatric patients.

Special considerations apply to specific toxicant classes. Oils, tars, and resins adherent to skin may require initial wiping with mineral oil or petroleum jelly before water irrigation, as these lipophilic substances resist water removal. Water-reactive compounds including elemental sodium, potassium, lithium, and certain metal hydrides necessitate initial dry brushing to remove visible material before cautious wet decontamination, as premature water application may generate exothermic reactions or caustic byproducts. Powdered caustic materials benefit from brushing before irrigation to prevent heat generation upon hydration. Hydrofluoric acid exposures require specialized decontamination with calcium gluconate gel (2.5-10%) to prevent fluoride ion penetration and subsequent tissue destruction through calcium sequestration.

Ocular decontamination follows similar principles but demands particular care given the eye's vulnerability to both toxicants and improper decontamination techniques. Initial irrigation should commence immediately using copious tepid water or saline, ideally through a Morgan lens or eyewash station allowing continuous flow while eyelids are manually held open. Irrigation should continue for at least 15-20 minutes, with pH testing of tears guiding prolonged irrigation needs after chemical exposures. Contact lenses must be removed early in decontamination to prevent trapping of toxicants against corneal surfaces. Particulate matter may require gentle saline lavage or careful removal with moistened cotton-tipped applicators. Petroleum-based products resistant to water irrigation may require special surfactant solutions. All significant ocular exposures warrant ophthalmological evaluation after initial decontamination to assess corneal damage and need for further intervention.

Inhalational Decontamination

Inhalational exposures require immediate removal from the contaminated environment to terminate ongoing toxicant absorption.

Rescuer safety remains paramount, with appropriate respiratory protection and hazardous materials protocols implemented before entry into contaminated areas, particularly with highly toxic gases including hydrogen sulfide, cyanide, or carbon monoxide. Patients capable of spontaneous respiration should be relocated to fresh air immediately, while those requiring rescue breathing or resuscitation should be removed from the contaminated area first to prevent rescuer exposure during airway management. Initial decontamination should occur outside healthcare facilities when feasible to prevent secondary contamination of hospital environments and staff.

Oxygen administration represents the primary intervention for most inhalational toxicants, addressing both hypoxemia from alveolar-capillary diffusion impairment and competitive displacement of toxicants from binding sites. High-flow oxygen (100% if available) should be administered immediately while avoiding positive pressure ventilation when possible with pulmonary irritants that may have caused alveolar damage. Carbon monoxide poisoning specifically requires high-flow oxygen to accelerate displacement from hemoglobin binding sites, with consideration of hyperbaric oxygen therapy for severe poisonings. Special oxygen delivery systems including Venturi masks and high-flow nasal cannulas provide precise oxygen titration capabilities for specific scenarios.

Removal of contaminated clothing and thorough skin decontamination remain essential complementary measures, as chemicals on clothing or skin surfaces may continue off-gassing, creating ongoing inhalational exposure. Particular attention to hair decontamination is warranted as the large surface area can trap significant toxicant quantities. Healthcare personnel should wear appropriate personal protective equipment during decontamination to prevent secondary contamination, with level of protection determined by toxicant properties and exposure risk.

Airway management considerations for inhalational exposures include recognition of potentially rapid progression of airway edema following irritant gas exposure. Early endotracheal intubation may be warranted with signs of impending airway compromise, including stridor, respiratory distress, or facial/oropharyngeal edema, particularly with exposures to highly water-soluble gases like ammonia or chlorine that create immediate upper airway injury. Bronchodilator therapy addresses bronchospasm common with irritant gas exposures, while corticosteroids may reduce inflammatory airway edema though evidence for their efficacy remains limited. Positive end-expiratory pressure may improve oxygenation in non-cardiogenic pulmonary edema resulting from less water-soluble irritants like phosgene or nitrogen dioxide that primarily affect distal airways and alveoli.

Special Decontamination Scenarios

Specific toxicant classes and exposure scenarios require specialized decontamination approaches extending beyond standard protocols. Chemical warfare agent exposures including nerve agents (sarin, VX), vesicants (sulfur mustard), and pulmonary agents (chlorine, phosgene) necessitate specialized decontamination procedures. Initial dry decontamination using absorbent materials removes gross contamination before wet decontamination to minimize spread of agent through runoff. Military decontamination kits containing specialized adsorbents and neutralizing solutions may provide superior efficacy compared to water alone. Rapid initiation is critical, particularly with nerve agents where minutes can significantly affect outcome. Mass casualty incidents require decontamination corridors with separate lanes for ambulatory and non-ambulatory patients to maximize throughput, with attention to wastewater containment and provider protection through appropriate personal protective equipment.

Radioactive contamination presents unique challenges requiring specialized approach. External contamination assessment utilizes radiation detectors (Geiger-Muller counters) to identify contaminated body regions requiring focused decontamination. Removal and contained disposal of clothing eliminates approximately 80-90% of external contamination in most scenarios. Gentle washing with tepid water and mild soap removes most remaining external contamination, with careful attention to skin folds, hair, and orifices where particulate matter may concentrate. Wound decontamination requires separate collection of irrigation fluid to prevent spread of contamination, with radiation monitoring between decontamination cycles. Internal contamination with radioisotopes may require specific decorporation agents including Prussian blue (cesium, thallium), calcium DTPA (plutonium, americium), or potassium iodide (radioactive iodine) to reduce systemic burden.

Body packing and body stuffing, involving ingestion of drug-filled packets for concealment or transportation, require specialized management. Body packers typically ingest professionally prepared, multiple-layer packages containing large quantities of illicit drugs intended for smuggling, while body stuffers hastily ingest poorly wrapped drugs to evade imminent law enforcement detection. Decontamination approaches vary based on package characteristics and clinical presentation. Asymptomatic body packers with professionally wrapped packages typically receive whole bowel irrigation without activated charcoal, which might obscure packet visualization. Surgical intervention becomes necessary with signs of packet rupture, bowel obstruction, or prolonged intestinal transit. Body stuffers with poorly wrapped packages face higher rupture risk, often warranting activated charcoal administration alongside whole bowel irrigation, with lower threshold for surgical intervention with symptom development.

Pediatric poisoning cases require decontamination modifications reflecting developmental and physiological differences. Children's proportionally larger body surface area relative to weight increases dermal absorption risk, necessitating particular attention to thorough skin decontamination. Gastric lavage rarely proves indicated due to small tube diameter requirements and poor risk-benefit ratio. Activated charcoal dosing follows weight-based guidelines (1 g/kg), with attention to palatability through flavoring agents or administration via nasogastric tube when necessary. Fluid-electrolyte balance requires careful monitoring during decontamination procedures due to children's reduced physiological reserve. Attention to maintaining normothermia during prolonged irrigation procedures remains essential given children's increased hypothermia risk from high surface area to mass ratio and underdeveloped thermoregulatory capacity.

ANTIDOTES

Specific pharmacological antagonists or binding agents targeting particular toxicants or toxicant classes can dramatically alter poisoning outcomes when appropriately selected and administered.

Receptor Antagonists

Receptor antagonists competitively or non-competitively block toxicant interactions with specific cellular receptors, preventing or reversing toxic effects. Naloxone, an opioid receptor antagonist, competitively displaces opioids from μ-receptors, rapidly reversing respiratory depression, miosis, and central nervous system depression. Initial adult dosing typically begins at 0.4 mg intravenously, with subsequent dose escalation up to 10 mg if needed for partial response, particularly with potent synthetic opioids like fentanyl analogs. The short half-life (30-90 minutes) relative to many opioids necessitates repeated dosing or continuous infusion (starting at two-thirds the effective bolus dose per hour) to maintain reversal. Potential complications include precipitation of withdrawal in opioid-dependent individuals, sympathetic surge with hypertension and dysrhythmias, and pulmonary edema, though the latter more likely represents underlying toxicity unmasked by reversal rather than direct antagonist effect.

Flumazenil antagonizes benzodiazepines at the GABA-A receptor complex, reversing sedation, respiratory depression, and amnesia through competitive binding at the benzodiazepine recognition site.

Initial dosing begins at 0.2 mg intravenously, with titration up to a cumulative dose of 3-5 mg. Despite demonstrated efficacy, flumazenil use remains controversial due to seizure risk, particularly in patients with benzodiazepine dependence, mixed overdoses involving proconvulsant agents (especially tricyclic antidepressants), or underlying seizure disorders. Additional concerns include the potentially short duration of action relative to the offending benzodiazepine and precipitation of benzodiazepine withdrawal, which may prove life-threatening. These risks confine appropriate use to iatrogenic oversedation scenarios and limited diagnostic applications rather than routine management of undifferentiated overdose.

Table 5.2: Major Antidotes and Their Applications

Antidote	Toxin(s)	Mechanism
N-acetylcysteine	Acetaminophen	Glutathione precursor, free radical scavenging
Naloxone	Opioids	Competitive opioid receptor antagonist
Flumazenil	Benzodiazepines	Competitive GABA receptor antagonist
Digoxin Fab	Digoxin, other cardiac glycosides	Binds free digoxin
Fomepizole	Methanol, ethylene glycol	Alcohol dehydrogenase inhibitor
Atropine	Organophosphates, carbamates	Competitive antagonist at muscarinic receptors
Pralidoxime	Organophosphates	Reactivates acetylcholinesterase
Hydroxocobalamin	Cyanide	Forms cyanocobalamin
Deferoxamine	Iron	Chelates iron
Physostigmine	Anticholinergic agents	Acetylcholinesterase inhibitor

Atropine antagonizes muscarinic acetylcholine receptors, counteracting excessive parasympathetic stimulation in cholinergic toxicity from organophosphates, carbamates, and muscarinic mushrooms. Unlike typical antidotes requiring weight-based dosing, atropine administration follows physiological endpoints, with initial doses of 1-2 mg in adults doubled every 3-5 minutes until resolution of bronchorrhea and bronchospasm.

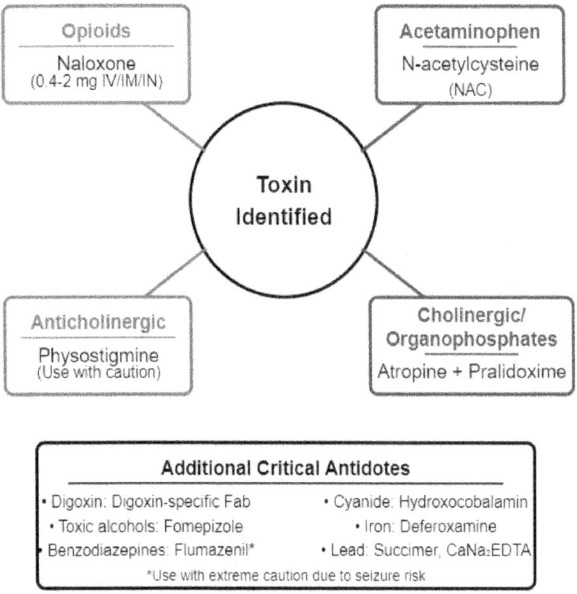

Figure 5.2: Antidote Selection

Severe organophosphate poisonings may require hundreds of milligrams over the treatment course. Treatment adequacy is assessed through pulmonary secretion control rather than pupillary response or heart rate. Atropine addresses only muscarinic manifestations of cholinergic excess without affecting nicotinic symptoms including muscle fasciculations and weakness, necessitating concurrent oxime therapy for organophosphate poisonings to reactivate inhibited acetylcholinesterase.

Several additional receptor antagonists serve specialized toxicological applications. Physostigmine, a reversible acetylcholinesterase inhibitor, treats antimuscarinic syndrome by increasing acetylcholine availability at receptor sites, addressing both peripheral and central anticholinergic manifestations. Its use remains reserved for severe cases with dangerous hyperthermia, agitation, or cardiac conduction abnormalities due to potential adverse effects including seizures and asystole. Cyproheptadine, a serotonin receptor antagonist with additional antihistamine and anticholinergic properties, treats serotonin syndrome, particularly addressing hyperthermia and neuromuscular hyperactivity. Pralidoxime reactivates phosphorylated acetylcholinesterase in organophosphate poisoning before aging occurs, particularly addressing nicotinic manifestations including muscle weakness and respiratory failure.

Metabolic Antagonists and Enzyme Inhibitors

Metabolic antagonists interfere with toxicant biotransformation pathways that generate harmful metabolites, preventing or reducing toxicity. N-acetylcysteine (NAC) serves as the definitive antidote for acetaminophen poisoning through multiple mechanisms. Primarily, it replenishes glutathione stores depleted by the reactive metabolite N-acetyl-p-benzoquinone imine (NAPQI), allowing continued detoxification and preventing covalent binding to hepatocellular proteins. Secondary mechanisms include direct NAPQI scavenging, enhanced sulfate conjugation, and antioxidant effects. Oral administration follows a 72-hour protocol beginning with a loading dose of 140 mg/kg followed by 70 mg/kg every 4 hours for 17 additional doses. Intravenous administration employs a 21-hour protocol with 150 mg/kg over 60 minutes, followed by 50 mg/kg over 4 hours, and 100 mg/kg over 16 hours. Treatment initiation timing significantly influences efficacy, with maximal benefit within 8-10 hours post-ingestion, though benefit persists even with delayed administration in patients with established hepatotoxicity.

Ethanol competitively inhibits alcohol dehydrogenase, the initial metabolic enzyme in both methanol and ethylene glycol biotransformation pathways, preventing formation of their toxic metabolites (formic acid and glycolic/oxalic acids, respectively). This competitive inhibition occurs because ethanol demonstrates approximately 10-fold higher affinity for the enzyme compared to methanol or ethylene glycol. Therapeutic regimens target blood ethanol concentrations of 100-150 mg/dL, requiring loading doses of 7-10 mL/kg of 10% ethanol solution intravenously or 1.8 mL/kg of 95% ethanol orally, followed by maintenance infusions adjusted based on serum level monitoring. Concurrent hemodialysis necessitates substantially increased maintenance rates due to ethanol's removal during the procedure. While largely replaced by fomepizole in developed countries, ethanol remains an important alternative where fomepizole is unavailable or unaffordable, though challenges include complex dosing requirements, need for intensive monitoring, hypoglycemia risk, and central nervous system depression.

> Remember
>
> **Specific antidotes exist for relatively few toxins, with key examples including N-acetylcysteine for acetaminophen, naloxone for opioids, digoxin-specific antibodies for digoxin, and various chelating agents for heavy metals.**

Fomepizole (4-methylpyrazole) provides more selective alcohol dehydrogenase inhibition without ethanol's sedative effects or complex pharmacokinetics. Indicated for both methanol and ethylene glycol poisoning, fomepizole follows a fixed dosing schedule beginning with 15 mg/kg loading dose, followed by 10 mg/kg every 12 hours for four doses, then 15 mg/kg every 12 hours until toxicant levels decrease below 20 mg/dL. Hemodialysis necessitates dose adjustment to every 4 hours due to fomepizole's dialyzability. Advantages over ethanol include predictable pharmacokinetics, minimal adverse effects, elimination of intensive monitoring requirements, and avoidance of central nervous system depression. The principal disadvantage remains high acquisition cost, though overall treatment costs may prove lower when accounting for reduced monitoring requirements and complications compared to ethanol therapy.

Sodium nitrite and sodium thiosulfate compose the traditional cyanide antidote kit, addressing different aspects of cyanide's toxicodynamics. Sodium nitrite oxidizes hemoglobin to methemoglobin, which binds cyanide with greater affinity than cytochrome oxidase, shifting cyanide away from its site of toxicity in the mitochondrial electron transport chain. Sodium thiosulfate provides substrate for the enzyme rhodanese, enhancing conversion of cyanide to the less toxic thiocyanate subsequently excreted in urine. Contemporary practice increasingly favors hydroxocobalamin (vitamin B12a), which directly binds cyanide forming cyanocobalamin (vitamin B12) without forming methemoglobin, providing particular advantage in smoke inhalation victims with concurrent carbon monoxide exposure and pre-existing methemoglobinemia.

Chelating Agents

Chelating agents form stable, water-soluble complexes with metal ions, reducing free metal concentration, enhancing urinary elimination, and preventing interaction with cellular targets. Deferoxamine specifically chelates ferric iron (Fe^{3+}), forming the water-soluble complex ferrioxamine subsequently excreted by kidneys. Indicated for significant iron poisoning, particularly with serum iron levels exceeding 500 μg/dL or signs of systemic toxicity, administration typically employs continuous intravenous infusion at 15 mg/kg/hour, not exceeding 24 hours when possible due to infectious complications with prolonged therapy. The characteristic vin rosé urine coloration indicates ferrioxamine excretion but not necessarily treatment adequacy. Potential adverse effects include hypotension with rapid infusion, histamine release, pulmonary toxicity with prolonged high-dose therapy, and enhanced growth of certain microorganisms including Yersinia enterocolitica due to the siderophore properties of ferrioxamine.

Heavy metal chelation employs several agents with different metal affinities and administration routes. Dimercaprol (British Anti-Lewisite, BAL) chelates arsenic, mercury, and lead, administered as deep intramuscular injection in a peanut oil vehicle, with significant adverse effects including hypertension, tachycardia, and painful injection sites. Succimer (2,3-dimercaptosuccinic acid, DMSA) provides oral chelation for lead, arsenic, and mercury, with superior safety profile compared to dimercaprol, particularly for outpatient lead chelation in pediatric patients with blood lead levels between 45-70 μg/dL. Calcium disodium EDTA chelates lead and other divalent and trivalent metals, administered intravenously or intramuscularly, with nephrotoxicity representing the primary adverse effect. Prussian blue (ferric hexacyanoferrate) serves as an oral chelator for thallium and cesium, acting within the gastrointestinal tract to trap these metals in an ion-exchange process, interrupting their enterohepatic circulation.

Chelation therapy requires careful consideration of indications, timing, and potential adverse effects. Treatment generally proves most effective when initiated early before significant cellular damage occurs, though remains indicated even in delayed presentations with ongoing systemic toxicity. Symptomatic patients with confirmed significant exposure or elevated biological measurements of metal burden typically warrant treatment, with specific thresholds varying by agent and clinical context. Empiric chelation in suspected but unconfirmed exposures generally requires risk-benefit analysis considering chelator toxicity versus potential benefit. Inappropriate chelation carries risks including essential metal depletion, redistribution of toxic metals to sensitive tissues including brain, and direct chelator toxicity to kidneys and other organs.

Each chelator demonstrates distinct pharmacological properties requiring individualized application. Metal specificity varies substantially, with some chelators demonstrating higher affinity for specific metals while others chelate multiple metals with different affinities. Distribution characteristics determine which body compartments the chelator can access, with lipophilic agents like dimercaprol penetrating cell membranes and blood-brain barrier more effectively than hydrophilic agents like EDTA. Elimination routes affect both efficacy and toxicity, with renally excreted chelators potentially concentrating in damaged kidneys and causing further injury. These pharmacological considerations guide selection, with combination therapy sometimes providing synergistic benefit by addressing different compartments or binding sites.

Antitoxins and Antibodies

Antitoxins and specific antibody preparations neutralize circulating toxins before they reach target tissues, providing particular benefit for toxins with delayed cellular effects. Digoxin-specific antibody fragments (Fab) bind circulating digoxin and digitoxin molecules, creating complexes subsequently eliminated through renal filtration. Derived from ovine immunoglobulin, these fragments demonstrate smaller size and reduced immunogenicity compared to intact antibodies. Indications include life-threatening dysrhythmias, progressive bradycardia unresponsive to atropine, serum potassium exceeding 5.5 mEq/L, and serum digoxin concentration above 10 ng/mL. Dosing employs either empiric administration based on clinical scenario (typically 5-10 vials in life-threatening cases) or calculated dosing based on ingested amount or serum concentration when available. Potential complications include allergic reactions (less common with fragments than whole antibodies), hypokalemia from rapid reversal, and returning digitalis toxicity as fragments are eliminated before the redistributed digoxin in severe poisonings.

Crotalidae polyvalent immune Fab (CroFab) and Crotalidae immune $F(ab')_2$ (Anavip) neutralize venom components from North American pit vipers including rattlesnakes, copperheads, and cottonmouths. These antivenom preparations contain antibody fragments that bind and neutralize various venom components including hemorrhagins, myotoxins, and neurotoxins. Indications include progressive local tissue injury, coagulopathy, systemic effects including hypotension or neurotoxicity, and elevated creatine kinase suggesting rhabdomyolysis. Initial dosing typically involves 4-6 vials with additional doses guided by clinical response. The two preparations differ in duration of effect, with $F(ab')_2$ fragments demonstrating longer half-life and reduced recurrence phenomena compared to Fab fragments. Potential adverse effects include acute hypersensitivity reactions and delayed serum sickness, though modern purified preparations show substantially reduced immunogenicity compared to older whole-immunoglobulin products.

Botulinum antitoxin neutralizes circulating botulinum toxin before internalization into nerve terminals, preventing progression of paralysis though unable to reverse existing deficits. Two preparations currently exist: Heptavalent botulinum antitoxin for adult cases, covering all seven botulinum toxin serotypes (A-G); and Human Botulism Immune

Globulin (BabyBIG) for infant botulism, derived from human donors with high botulinum antibody titers. Administration should occur as early as possible after clinical diagnosis without awaiting laboratory confirmation, as delay significantly reduces efficacy once toxin enters neurons. Potential adverse effects include hypersensitivity reactions, serum sickness, and theoretical infectious disease transmission risk with human-derived products, though modern purification techniques have minimized this concern.

Antivenoms for other venomous creatures follow similar principles with specific applications. Black widow spider antivenom (Latrodectus mactans antivenom) addresses severe systemic effects of envenomation including intractable pain, autonomic instability, and hypertension unresponsive to conventional therapy. Hypersensitivity risk has limited use to severe cases, with alternative treatments including benzodiazepines, calcium, and opioids appropriate for milder envenomations. Coral snake antivenom (Micrurus fulvius) neutralizes neurotoxic components that produce progressive paralysis, though limited availability has created therapeutic challenges. Investigation continues into potential cross-reactivity with similar elapid antivenoms when specific coral snake antivenom remains unavailable.

SUPPORTIVE CARE

Supportive management involves physiological derangements and maintains vital functions while specific antidotes act or natural elimination proceeds, often representing the principal therapeutic approach for toxicants lacking specific antidotes.

Airway and Breathing Management

Airway protection represents a primary concern in poisoned patients, particularly those with altered mental status, respiratory depression, or caustic exposures affecting upper airway structures. Coma without protective airway reflexes creates aspiration risk, necessitating careful monitoring of gag reflex, ability to handle secretions, and Glasgow Coma Scale trends. Endotracheal intubation provides definitive airway management when indicated, with rapid sequence induction typically employing etomidate or ketamine for hemodynamic stability in potentially unstable poisoned patients. Succinylcholine remains appropriate for most toxicological scenarios despite theoretical concerns regarding potassium elevation in specific poisonings (organophosphates, strychnine) where fasciculations might exacerbate existing hyperkalemia. Post-intubation sedation typically employs benzodiazepines with or without opioids, recognizing potential synergistic respiratory and central nervous system depression with certain toxicants.

Ventilation methods must address specific toxicant-induced pathophysiology. Opioid and sedative-hypnotic overdoses typically produce direct respiratory center depression requiring ventilatory support until clearance occurs or pharmacological reversal succeeds. Organophosphate poisoning creates complex respiratory compromise through bronchorrhea, bronchospasm, respiratory muscle weakness, and central respiratory depression, necessitating high positive end-expiratory pressure (PEEP) to maintain alveolar recruitment despite increased secretions. Salicylate toxicity induces respiratory center stimulation resulting in respiratory alkalosis, with mechanical ventilation potentially eliminating this compensatory mechanism and worsening acidosis unless hyperventilation is maintained. Toxic inhalations require careful consideration of optimal PEEP to balance recruitment of damaged alveoli against potential barotrauma to already compromised lung tissue.

Oxygenation support extends beyond standard approaches in specific toxicological scenarios. Carbon monoxide poisoning requires 100% oxygen administration to accelerate carboxyhemoglobin dissociation, with hyperbaric oxygen therapy considered for severe poisonings (carboxyhemoglobin levels >25%, neurological abnormalities, cardiac ischemia, pregnancy with fetal distress). Cyanide poisoning produces profound cellular hypoxia despite adequate blood oxygen content due to mitochondrial cytochrome oxidase inhibition, necessitating specific antidote therapy alongside maximized oxygen delivery. Methemoglobinemia reduces oxygen-carrying capacity through conversion of hemoglobin to its oxidized form, requiring methylene blue administration rather than simply increased inspired oxygen when levels exceed 20-30% or symptomatic presentation occurs.

Pulmonary complications requiring specific management include non-cardiogenic pulmonary edema from opioids, salicylates, and inhalational toxicants; aspiration pneumonitis from hydrocarbons and gastric contents during altered consciousness; and bronchospasm from irritant gas exposure or sympatholytic poisoning. Management follows general critical care principles with syndrome-specific modifications. Bronchodilator therapy employs β-agonists for bronchospasm, recognizing potentially limited response in β-blocker poisoning. Corticosteroids show limited evidence in most toxicant-induced lung injuries despite theoretical benefits, with clearer indications in caustic inhalations and chlorine gas exposure. Extracorporeal membrane oxygenation (ECMO) provides rescue therapy in severe respiratory failure unresponsive to conventional ventilation strategies, particularly valuable in poisonings with reversible toxicity but severe temporary pulmonary compromise.

Cardiovascular Support

Hemodynamic management in poisoned patients frequently addresses hypotension resulting from various pathophysiological mechanisms. Vasodilatory shock from calcium channel blockers, ACE inhibitors, or phenothiazines requires vasopressor support, typically beginning with norepinephrine targeting mean arterial pressure above 65 mmHg. Vasopressin provides particular advantage in severe vasodilatory states refractory to catecholamines. Cardiogenic shock from cardiotoxic agents including calcium channel blockers, beta-blockers, and tricyclic antidepressants may require inotropic support with agents like epinephrine, dobutamine, or milrinone alongside vasopressors. Hypovolemic shock from gastrointestinal fluid losses or third-spacing requires volume resuscitation with crystalloid solutions, typically beginning with 20 mL/kg boluses while monitoring response. Mixed shock pictures frequently occur in severe poisonings, necessitating combined approaches and careful hemodynamic monitoring to guide therapy.

Dysrhythmia management follows advanced cardiac life support principles with toxicant-specific modifications. Sodium channel blockade from tricyclic antidepressants or class 1 antiarrhythmics produces QRS prolongation and ventricular dysrhythmias responsive to sodium bicarbonate administration (1-2 mEq/kg IV bolus followed by infusion titrated to QRS normalization and serum pH 7.5-7.55). Torsades de pointes from QT-prolonging agents including antipsychotics, methadone, and class III antiarrhythmics responds to magnesium sulfate (2 g IV over 10 minutes) and correction of contributing factors including hypokalemia and hypomagnesemia. Digitalis-induced dysrhythmias including bidirectional ventricular tachycardia require digoxin-specific antibody fragments rather than standard antiarrhythmic approaches. Bradydysrhythmias from beta-blockers, calcium channel blockers, and cholinergic agents may require external pacing when pharmacological approaches prove insufficient.

Specific cardiovascular toxicities necessitate tailored interventional approaches. High-dose insulin euglycemia therapy (HIET) addresses calcium channel blocker and beta-blocker poisonings through positive inotropy, improved myocardial glucose utilization, and vasodilation of peripheral vascular beds. Protocol typically begins with 1 unit/kg regular insulin bolus followed by infusion starting at 0.5-1 unit/kg/hour, titrated up to 10 units/kg/hour in severe cases, with concurrent dextrose administration and frequent glucose monitoring. Calcium administration (calcium chloride 10-20 mg/kg or calcium gluconate 30-60 mg/kg) addresses hypocalcemia and provides inotropic support, particularly valuable in calcium channel blocker poisoning. Lipid emulsion therapy (1.5 mL/kg bolus followed by 0.25 mL/kg/minute infusion) stabilizes cardiovascular collapse from lipophilic drug toxicity through proposed mechanisms including lipid sink effect sequestering toxicants, enhanced myocardial energy supply, and direct inotropic effects.

Mechanical circulatory support provides rescue therapy for refractory cardiovascular collapse unresponsive to pharmacological interventions. Intra-aortic balloon pumps reduce afterload and augment coronary perfusion in cardiogenic shock from cardiotoxic agents. Venoarterial extracorporeal membrane oxygenation (VA-ECMO) provides complete cardiopulmonary support during profound cardiovascular collapse, particularly valuable in poisonings with reversible toxicity but temporary severe cardiac dysfunction, including tricyclic antidepressants, beta-blockers, calcium channel blockers, and cardiotoxic plants. Cardiopulmonary bypass similarly maintains circulation during severe intoxication, though with more limited duration capability compared to ECMO. These advanced modalities support patients through the period of greatest toxicity until clearance occurs or specific antidotes take effect, with high survival rates reported in toxicological applications despite severe initial presentations.

Neurological Management

Central nervous system effects in poisoned patients range from sedation and coma to agitation, seizures, and movement disorders, requiring targeted management approaches. Altered mental status assessment begins with glucose measurement and thiamine administration, addressing common underlying etiologies before attributing neurological depression exclusively to toxicant effect. Coma management includes regular neurological assessments, positioning to prevent aspiration, vigilance for sequelae including rhabdomyolysis from prolonged immobility, and recognition that conventional intracranial pressure concerns may not apply to metabolic coma from most toxicants. Neurological recovery often follows predictable time courses based on toxicant pharmacokinetics, though post-hypoxic injury may complicate the clinical picture in cases involving respiratory depression or cardiac arrest.

Seizure management in toxicological contexts addresses both clinical and subclinical seizure activity, with potential for status epilepticus carrying high morbidity and mortality. First-line therapy typically employs benzodiazepines at standard or increased doses, recognizing potential resistance in certain toxicant-induced seizures including theophylline, isoniazid, or tricyclic antidepressants. Second-line agents include phenobarbital or propofol, with phenytoin generally avoided due to limited efficacy in toxicant-induced seizures and potential exacerbation of cardiac toxicity with certain agents. Isoniazid-induced seizures specifically require pyridoxine (vitamin B6) in gram-for-gram equivalence to the ingested isoniazid dose, addressing the underlying GABA depletion mechanism. Refractory status epilepticus may necessitate general anesthesia with continuous EEG monitoring to confirm seizure suppression, particularly important in neurotoxic poisonings where motor manifestations may be masked by neuromuscular blockade.

Agitation management must balance behavioral control against risks of excessive sedation, particularly respiratory depression in patients with potential multi-substance ingestion. Initial approaches employ verbal de-escalation and environmental modification where feasible, recognizing that agitation often reflects sympathomimetic toxicity, anticholinergic delirium, withdrawal syndromes, or hypoxemia rather than purely psychiatric etiology. Pharmacological management typically begins with benzodiazepines, providing sedation, anxiolysis, and specific therapeutic benefit for stimulant toxicity, alcohol withdrawal, and serotonin syndrome. Butyrophenone antipsychotics including haloperidol provide alternative or adjunctive therapy, though potential QT prolongation warrants caution with certain coingestants. Physical restraints, when necessary, require continuous monitoring, regular repositioning, padding to prevent injury, and protocols for earliest possible discontinuation once chemical restraint achieves effect or agitation resolves.

Hyperthermia management proves particularly critical in several toxicological syndromes including sympathomimetic excess, serotonin syndrome, neuroleptic malignant syndrome, and anticholinergic toxicity. External cooling measures include ice packs applied to groin and axillae, mist and fan techniques utilizing evaporative cooling, and cooling blankets. Severe hyperthermia (>40-41°C) may require endovascular cooling devices or cold intravenous fluid administration. Pharmacological approaches target underlying mechanisms: benzodiazepines for sympathomimetic excess and serotonin syndrome; dantrolene for malignant hyperthermia; and cyproheptadine for serotonin syndrome. Antipyretics demonstrate minimal efficacy in these scenarios as temperature elevation reflects dysregulated heat production rather than hypothalamic setpoint adjustment. Neuromuscular blockade with mechanical ventilation may become necessary in refractory cases where muscular activity significantly contributes to heat generation, though this approach masks physical examination findings and necessitates continuous EEG monitoring to detect subclinical seizures.

Renal and Metabolic Support

Fluid and electrolyte management addresses common toxicant-induced disturbances while supporting renal function and enhancing toxicant elimination. Fluid resuscitation employs crystalloid solutions targeting euvolemia, with additional considerations in specific poisonings. Lithium toxicity management requires careful attention to sodium levels, as hyponatremia enhances lithium-induced neurotoxicity, while hypernatremia may exacerbate nephrogenic diabetes insipidus associated with chronic lithium therapy. Salicylate toxicity creates substantial insensible fluid losses through hyperpnea and hyperthermia, requiring aggressive replacement to prevent dehydration that would otherwise enhance salicylate entry into the central nervous system. Toxic alcohols (methanol, ethylene glycol) create profound metabolic acidosis necessitating substantial bicarbonate therapy, with attendant fluid volume expansion requiring monitoring for overload in patients with compromised cardiac or renal function.

Acid-base disturbances require both supportive correction and consideration of therapeutic manipulation. Metabolic acidosis treatment addresses underlying mechanisms through specific antidotes where available, while sodium bicarbonate provides symptomatic correction for severe acidemia (pH <7.2) compromising cardiac function or vasopressor responsiveness. Salicylate poisoning presents complex acid-base disturbances typically beginning with respiratory alkalosis and developing mixed respiratory alkalosis/metabolic acidosis as toxicity progresses. Management maintains respiratory alkalosis (through mechanical ventilation if necessary) while administering sodium bicarbonate to achieve serum pH 7.5-7.55, enhancing salicylate ionization that reduces central nervous system penetration. Metabolic alkalosis from diuretic overdose or massive antacid ingestion typically responds to volume repletion and potassium correction, with acidifying agents including ammonium chloride rarely required.

Electrolyte abnormalities in poisoned patients often reflect both direct toxicant effects and compensatory mechanisms. Hypokalemia from β-agonists, caffeine, or theophylline requires aggressive replacement, recognizing potential for rapid intracellular potassium shifts with treatment of the underlying toxicity. Hyperkalemia from digoxin, β-blockers, or angiotensin-converting enzyme inhibitors follows standard management protocols including calcium administration (contraindicated in digoxin toxicity due to "stone heart" phenomenon), insulin-glucose therapy, sodium bicarbonate, and potassium-binding resins, with hemodialysis reserved for life-threatening elevations unresponsive to conventional therapy. Sodium abnormalities from water intoxication, ecstasy (MDMA), or lithium require careful correction targeting no more than 8-10 mEq/L increase over 24 hours to prevent osmotic demyelination syndrome, particularly when hyponatremia has developed chronically.

Renal supportive care addresses both toxicant-induced renal injury and the kidney's role in toxicant elimination. Rhabdomyolysis from sympathomimetics, serotonergic agents, or prolonged immobility creates risk for acute kidney injury through multiple mechanisms including myoglobin nephrotoxicity, tubular obstruction, and renal vasoconstriction. Management includes aggressive fluid resuscitation targeting urine output >2 mL/kg/hour, with consideration of urinary alkalinization (target pH >6.5) to reduce myoglobin precipitation though evidence remains limited. Direct nephrotoxicity from aminoglycosides, NSAIDs, or contrast agents benefits from volume expansion and discontinuation of additional nephrotoxic agents. Renal replacement therapy provides both supportive care for renal failure and enhanced elimination for certain toxicants, with indications including refractory acidosis, electrolyte abnormalities, fluid overload unresponsive to diuretics, uremia, and removal of dialyzable toxicants including lithium, salicylates, metformin, and toxic alcohols

ENHANCED ELIMINATION

Interventions accelerating toxicant clearance beyond normal elimination rates provide valuable adjuncts when toxicity severity, prolonged duration, or limited natural clearance threaten significant morbidity or mortality.

Toxicokinetic Manipulation

Enhanced elimination techniques exploit toxicokinetic principles to accelerate removal beyond endogenous clearance mechanisms. Distribution volume fundamentally influences elimination enhancement potential, with small-volume distributions (<1 L/kg) typically permitting more effective intervention as larger proportions of the toxicant remain in the vascular compartment accessible to extracorporeal removal or enhanced excretion. Protein binding affects elimination techniques differently: highly protein-bound toxicants resist renal elimination enhancement through alkalinization or forced diuresis, while hemodialysis primarily removes unbound fractions, limiting efficacy for substances with binding exceeding 80-90%. Molecular weight constraints apply particularly to membrane-based techniques, with conventional hemodialysis efficiently removing substances below 500-1000 daltons while larger molecules require high-flux membranes or alternative approaches.

Determination of enhanced elimination benefit requires balanced assessment of potential advantages against associated risks and resource utilization. Toxicant characteristics supporting consideration include established serious toxicity, anticipated prolonged duration of effect, limited efficacy of supportive care and available antidotes, and established efficacy of enhanced elimination for the specific agent.

Table 5.3: Enhanced Elimination Techniques

Method	Mechanism	Applications	Contraindications
Urinary alkalinization	Traps ionized weak acids in urine	Salicylates, phenobarbital, chlorpropamide	Renal failure, cerebral edema, pulmonary edema
Hemodialysis	Direct removal across semipermeable membrane	Toxic alcohols, salicylates, lithium, valproic acid	Hemodynamic instability (relative)
Hemoperfusion	Direct adsorption to cartridge material	Theophylline, carbamazepine, barbiturates	Thrombocytopenia, bleeding disorders
Continuous renal replacement therapy	Prolonged but less efficient filtration	When conventional dialysis unavailable or poorly tolerated	Few absolute contraindications
Exchange transfusion	Removes toxin with blood replacement	Severe methemoglobinemia, hemolytic poisons	Limited availability, transfusion reactions
Plasmapheresis	Removes plasma containing toxin	Protein-bound toxins (amatoxins, immune complexes)	Hemodynamic instability, difficult vascular access
Lipid emulsion therapy	Sequesters lipophilic toxins	Local anesthetics, calcium channel blockers, other lipophilic drugs	Allergy to components

Patient factors influencing decisions include severity of presentation, comorbidities affecting natural clearance including renal or hepatic dysfunction, and contraindications to specific techniques. Practical implementations require consideration of clearance rate relative to toxicant burden, with techniques providing marginal enhancement over natural elimination offering limited benefit despite theoretical appeal. These determinations often employ the extracorporeal removal ratio, comparing elimination through the enhanced technique against simultaneous endogenous clearance to assess meaningful contribution.

Various mathematical parameters quantify enhanced elimination efficacy. Extraction ratio represents the fraction of toxicant removed during a single passage through the elimination device, calculated as the arterial-venous concentration difference divided by arterial concentration. Clearance quantifies the volume of blood completely cleared of toxicant per unit time, reflecting extraction ratio multiplied by blood flow rate through the elimination system. Toxicant half-life reduction provides the most clinically relevant assessment, comparing elimination rates with and without intervention. Significant half-life reduction typically requires clearance rates approaching or exceeding endogenous elimination, with greater impact for toxicants normally exhibiting prolonged half-lives due to limited natural clearance.

The timing of enhanced elimination initiation significantly influences efficacy, with earlier intervention typically providing greater benefit by addressing higher plasma concentrations before extensive tissue distribution occurs. However, redistribution phenomena must be considered, as rapid removal from plasma may establish concentration gradients driving toxicant movement from tissue reservoirs back into circulation. This redistribution effect creates rebound increases in plasma concentrations after discontinuation of elimination procedures, potentially necessitating repeated or prolonged interventions particularly for toxicants with large distribution volumes. For toxicants undergoing bioactivation to harmful metabolites, enhanced elimination of the parent compound before metabolism provides particular advantage, potentially preventing toxicity rather than simply addressing established effects.

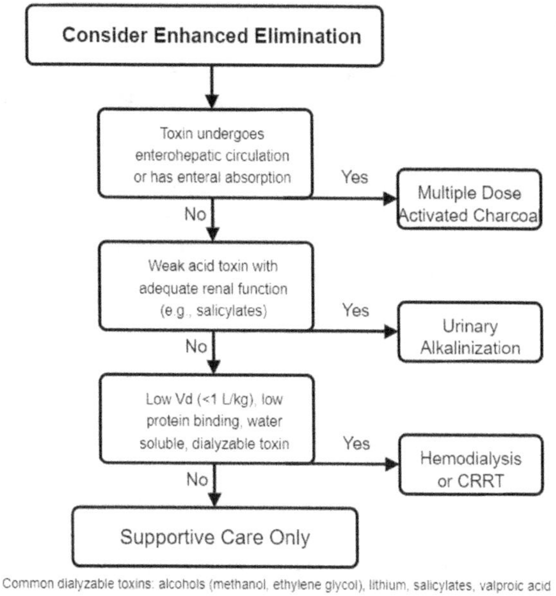

Figure 5.3: Enhanced Elimination Techniques Decision Tree

Urinary Manipulation

Urinary alkalinization enhances elimination of weak acids through ion trapping, increasing ionization of these compounds in alkaline urine and thereby preventing reabsorption across tubular epithelium. This technique involves intravenous sodium bicarbonate administration targeting urinary pH above 7.5-8.0, typically beginning with 1-2 mEq/kg bolus followed by continuous infusion titrated to urinary pH measurements. While conceptually applicable to numerous weak acids with pKa values between 3.0 and the physiological pH of 7.4, established clinical efficacy remains limited primarily to salicylates, with possible benefit for phenobarbital, chlorpropamide, fluoride, methotrexate, and chlorophenoxy herbicides. Contraindications include significant volume overload, heart failure, renal failure, cerebral edema, and hypocalcemia, with relative contraindication in mixed overdoses containing both acids and bases where alkalinization might enhance central nervous system penetration of basic compounds.

Urinary acidification, the theoretical counterpart enhancing elimination of weak bases through the same ion trapping mechanism, carries excessive risk-to-benefit ratio in most clinical scenarios. Acidifying agents including ammonium chloride or ascorbic acid theoretically enhance elimination of basic compounds including amphetamines, phencyclidine, and quinidine by increasing ionization and reducing reabsorption. However, practical limitations include difficulty achieving substantial pH reduction, risks of worsening acidosis in already acidemic patients, and enhanced renal toxicity risk for rhabdomyolysis-associated compounds through increased myoglobin precipitation at acidic pH. These considerations have essentially eliminated urinary acidification from contemporary clinical practice despite theoretical applications in certain poisonings.

Forced diuresis involves administration of intravenous fluids and sometimes diuretics to increase urine flow rate beyond normal values, theoretically enhancing elimination through reduced transit time in renal tubules and decreased concentration gradients for reabsorption. Historical practice employed high-volume fluid administration targeting urine output of 3-6 mL/kg/hour, sometimes with furosemide or mannitol to maintain diuresis. Contemporary evidence suggests limited efficacy for most toxicants, with risks including fluid overload, electrolyte abnormalities, and pulmonary edema outweighing modest elimination enhancement. Current practice generally restricts forced diuresis to scenarios where enhanced elimination provides established benefit but more advanced techniques remain unavailable, primarily for lithium and potentially for certain water-soluble medications with limited protein binding and significant renal elimination.

Multiple factors influence urinary manipulation efficacy beyond simple pH or flow rate considerations. Protein binding limits filtration at the glomerulus, with only free fractions available for enhanced elimination regardless of urinary conditions. Toxicant location within renal structures affects accessibility to manipulation, with substances undergoing substantial active tubular secretion or extensive reabsorption generally showing greater response to urinary manipulation than those with primarily glomerular filtration. Renal perfusion significantly affects all urinary elimination processes, with hypotension reducing efficacy of enhancement techniques and potentially exacerbating toxicity through prolonged exposure. Pre-existing kidney disease or toxicant-induced nephrotoxicity similarly limits potential benefit while increasing complication risks from fluid and electrolyte shifts associated with these techniques.

Extracorporeal Techniques

Hemodialysis represents the most widely employed extracorporeal elimination technique, using concentration gradients across semipermeable membranes to remove toxicants from bloodstream into dialysate solution. Diffusive clearance through conventional hemodialysis effectively removes small (<500 daltons), water-soluble compounds with limited protein binding and distribution volumes. High-efficiency and high-flux membranes expand capabilities to larger molecules and protein-bound compounds through increased surface area, enhanced permeability, and convective transport mechanisms. Vascular access typically employs large-bore temporary dialysis catheters in acute poisoning scenarios, with blood flow rates of 200-400 mL/minute maximizing clearance efficiency. Contemporary devices permit simultaneous correction of acid-base and electrolyte abnormalities alongside toxicant removal, providing both enhanced elimination and supportive care benefits in critically ill poisoned patients.

Toxicant characteristics predicting hemodialysis efficacy include molecular weight below 500-1000 daltons, water solubility, limited protein binding (<80%), small volume of distribution (<1 L/kg), and limited endogenous clearance. Specific toxicants with established hemodialysis benefit include lithium, salicylates, toxic alcohols (methanol, ethylene glycol), valproic acid, metformin, and certain barbiturates. Indications beyond simple concentration-based thresholds incorporate clinical severity assessment, recognizing that laboratory values alone inadequately predict individual patient outcomes. For instance, lithium dialysis indications include severe neurotoxicity regardless of level, renal failure limiting natural elimination, and levels exceeding 4 mEq/L even in asymptomatic patients due to delayed distribution kinetics. Potential complications include hypotension, hemorrhage from anticoagulation, electrolyte shifts, dialysis disequilibrium syndrome, and vascular access complications.

Hemoperfusion passes blood through cartridges containing adsorbent materials, typically activated charcoal or resins, that bind toxicants through various physicochemical interactions. This technique effectively removes larger molecular weight, hydrophobic, or highly protein-bound substances that dialysis membranes cannot efficiently extract. Historical applications included tricyclic antidepressants, barbiturates, carbamazepine, and certain pesticides. Contemporary practice has largely replaced hemoperfusion with high-efficiency hemodialysis or combination modalities due to several limitations: cartridge saturation requiring replacement during prolonged procedures, significant platelet consumption and hemorrhage risk, inability to simultaneously correct electrolyte and acid-base abnormalities, and reduced availability of cartridges and technical expertise in many centers. Selected applications remain primarily for specific toxicants with high charcoal affinity but poor dialyzability, including theophylline, carbamazepine, and certain mushroom toxins.

Continuous renal replacement therapies (CRRT) provide slower but sustained toxicant removal through extended treatment periods, typically 24-72 hours.

Remember

Enhanced elimination techniques (multiple-dose activated charcoal, urinary alkalinization, hemodialysis) are effective only for toxins with specific pharmacokinetic properties and should be considered based on severity, toxin characteristics, and patient condition.

Modalities include continuous venovenous hemofiltration (CVVH) employing convective clearance through pressure gradients, continuous venovenous hemodialysis (CVVHD) utilizing diffusive clearance across dialysis membranes, and combination approaches (CVVHDF) incorporating both mechanisms. The main advantages include hemodynamic stability due to slower fluid shifts, sustained elimination without rebound phenomena common after intermittent procedures, and simultaneous management of fluid overload and electrolyte abnormalities. Limitations include slower toxicant removal rates compared to conventional hemodialysis, technical complexity requiring specialized nursing expertise, and continuous anticoagulation requirements. CRRT proves particularly valuable for hemodynamically unstable patients requiring both enhanced elimination and critical care support, and for toxicants with large distribution volumes where sustained removal addresses tissue redistribution phenomena.

Several specialized extracorporeal techniques address specific toxicological scenarios. Therapeutic plasma exchange removes protein-bound toxicants by separating and replacing patient plasma, providing particular benefit for substances with binding exceeding 95% that resist conventional extracorporeal approaches. Applications include levothyroxine overdose and certain mushroom poisonings. Molecular adsorbent recirculating system (MARS) incorporates albumin dialysis to remove protein-bound toxicants, primarily used for hepatic failure but with potential application in poisonings involving highly protein-bound compounds. Exchange transfusion, though rarely employed in modern practice, remains a consideration in severe methemoglobinemia unresponsive to methylene blue and in certain pediatric poisonings where other techniques prove technically challenging. Each specialized approach requires individualized risk-benefit assessment considering institutional capabilities, alternative options, and specific toxicokinetic parameters of the involved toxicant.

Multiple-Dose Activated Charcoal

Multiple-dose activated charcoal (MDAC) enhances elimination of certain toxicants through repetitive binding in the gastrointestinal tract, interrupting enterohepatic circulation, and creating concentration gradients that promote diffusion from bloodstream back into intestinal lumen ("gut dialysis"). This approach typically involves activated charcoal administration every 2-6 hours for extended periods, with adult doses ranging from 25-50 g per administration after an initial larger loading dose. The technique proves most effective for toxicants with significant enterohepatic circulation, small volumes of distribution, prolonged absorption phases, or local intestinal secretion. Established efficacy exists for carbamazepine, dapsone, phenobarbital, quinine, and theophylline, with possible benefit for salicylates, digoxin, nadolol, phenylbutazone, and certain cardiac glycosides from plants.

Several mechanisms contribute to enhanced elimination beyond simple prevention of ongoing absorption. Binding of toxicants that undergo biliary excretion prevents reabsorption and interrupts enterohepatic circulation, promoting fecal elimination rather than recirculation. Enhanced elimination through intestinal secretion occurs when concentration gradients favor movement from bloodstream into intestinal lumen, where charcoal binding prevents reabsorption and maintains the gradient for continued clearance. This mechanism operates most effectively for toxicants with small volumes of distribution and good gastrointestinal diffusion characteristics. These combined effects may reduce toxicant half-lives by 50-80% for susceptible compounds, representing significant clinical benefit in serious poisonings.

Patient selection for MDAC requires careful consideration of potential benefits, contraindications, and practical implementation challenges. Contraindications include unprotected airway in obtunded patients, gastrointestinal obstruction or perforation risk, corrosive ingestions, and absence of bowel sounds suggesting ileus. Relative contraindications include concurrent need for oral antidotes or therapeutic medications that charcoal might adsorb, reducing their efficacy. Complications include aspiration pneumonitis, constipation, intestinal obstruction, and electrolyte abnormalities, with mortality reported in rare cases of charcoal aspiration or intestinal perforation. These risks necessitate thorough assessment of risk-benefit ratio, particularly in patients with altered mental status or compromised gastrointestinal function.

Practical implementation considerations affect both efficacy and safety. Palatability challenges often limit voluntary consumption of multiple doses, necessitating nasogastric administration in many cases.

Cathartics, historically administered with initial charcoal doses to accelerate intestinal transit, should generally be avoided with multiple-dose regimens due to potential fluid and electrolyte complications from repeated administration. Concurrent sorbitol with initial dose may be considered if not contraindicated. Monitoring during therapy should include regular abdominal examination for developing tenderness or distension suggesting ileus or obstruction, stool output assessment, and electrolyte measurements particularly with prolonged therapy. Concurrent antiemetics may improve tolerability when nausea limits administration. Treatment duration typically continues until clinical improvement occurs and toxicant levels (when measurable) demonstrate substantial reduction, generally 24-48 hours for most applications.

Evidence quality supporting MDAC varies substantially between toxicants, with volunteer studies demonstrating kinetic enhancement that may not directly translate to clinical outcome benefits in actual poisonings. The most robust evidence supports application for carbamazepine, dapsone, phenobarbital, quinine, and theophylline, where significant reductions in half-life and improved clinical outcomes have been demonstrated. For other toxicants including salicylates, phenytoin, and digoxin, conflicting evidence exists regarding meaningful clinical benefit despite theoretical applications. Contemporary practice increasingly restricts MDAC to scenarios with clear evidence of benefit, significant clinical toxicity, and absence of safer alternatives, representing substantial practice evolution from historical approaches that employed this technique more broadly across toxicological presentations.

Summary

Treatment of toxic exposures follows systematic principles designed to prevent further toxin absorption, administer specific antidotes when available, enhance elimination when indicated, and provide comprehensive supportive care. Gastrointestinal decontamination begins with activated charcoal, which effectively adsorbs many toxins when administered within 1-2 hours of ingestion, though it is contraindicated with caustic ingestions, hydrocarbons, and compromised airways. Gastric lavage and induced emesis now have limited roles due to efficacy and safety concerns. Whole bowel irrigation using polyethylene glycol solution can benefit patients with sustained-release medication or packet ingestions. Specific antidotes counteract toxins through various mechanisms: competitive receptor antagonism (naloxone for opioids), chelation of metals (deferoxamine for iron), metabolic protection (N-acetylcysteine for acetaminophen), physiologic counteraction (atropine for cholinergic toxicity), and enzyme reactivation (pralidoxime for organophosphates). However, many common poisonings lack specific antidotes, necessitating supportive care as the cornerstone of management. This includes airway protection, hemodynamic support, seizure control, temperature regulation, and management of specific organ dysfunctions. Enhanced elimination techniques accelerate toxin clearance when substances have specific pharmacokinetic properties. Multiple-dose activated charcoal interrupts enterohepatic circulation for certain substances, while urinary alkalinization enhances elimination of weak acids through ion trapping. Extracorporeal methods including hemodialysis and hemoperfusion can rapidly remove toxins with low volume of distribution, low protein binding, and water solubility. Treatment decisions must balance potential benefits against risks while considering the specific toxin, timing, patient factors, and available resources.

Self-Assessment Questions

1. Evaluate the current evidence regarding gastric lavage in toxicology, discussing specific scenarios where it might still be considered and contraindications to its use.
2. Explain the mechanism of action, indications, dosing considerations, and potential adverse effects of N-acetylcysteine in acetaminophen toxicity.
3. Compare and contrast the pharmacology, indications, and administration techniques for the opioid antagonists naloxone, naltrexone, and nalmefene.
4. Analyze the factors that determine whether a specific toxin is likely to be effectively removed by hemodialysis, providing examples of toxins that are good candidates for this intervention.
5. Describe the mechanism, indications, contraindications, and administration of multiple-dose activated charcoal, with examples of toxins for which this approach is particularly effective.
6. Discuss the principle of urinary alkalinization (ion trapping) and how it enhances elimination of weak acids, with specific examples of toxins amenable to this approach.
7. Explain the mechanisms of action, indications, and administration considerations for various chelating agents used in heavy metal poisoning.
8. Analyze the role of lipid emulsion therapy in toxicology, including proposed mechanisms, indications, administration techniques, and current evidence regarding efficacy.
9. Describe the supportive care approach to managing a patient with tricyclic antidepressant overdose, focusing on cardiovascular, neurological, and respiratory management.
10. Evaluate the evidence for and against various decontamination approaches for dermal exposures to different classes of toxins

Bibliography

1. Benson BE, Hoppu K, Troutman WG, Bedry R, Erdman A, Höjer J, et al. Position paper update: gastric lavage for gastrointestinal decontamination. Clin Toxicol (Phila). 2013;51(3):140-146.
2. Chyka PA, Seger D, Krenzelok EP, Vale JA; American Academy of Clinical Toxicology; European Association of Poisons Centres and Clinical Toxicologists. Position paper: single-dose activated charcoal. Clin Toxicol (Phila). 2005;43(2):61-87.
3. Heard K. Gastrointestinal decontamination. Med Clin North Am. 2005;89(6):1067-1078.
4. Mokhlesi B, Leikin JB, Murray P, Corbridge TC. Adult toxicology in critical care: part II: specific poisonings. Chest. 2003;123(3):897-922.
5. Bateman DN, Dear JW, Thanacoody HK, Thomas SH, Eddleston M, Sandilands EA, et al. Reduction of adverse effects from intravenous acetylcysteine treatment for paracetamol poisoning: a randomised controlled trial. Lancet. 2014;383(9918):697-704.
6. Ghannoum M, Hoffman RS, Gosselin S, Nolin TD, Lavergne V, Roberts DM. Use of extracorporeal treatments in the management of poisonings. Kidney Int. 2018;94(4):682-688.
7. Juurlink DN, Buckley NA, Stanbrook MB, Isbister GK, Bennett M, McGuigan MA. Hyperbaric oxygen for carbon monoxide poisoning. Cochrane Database Syst Rev. 2005;(1):CD002041.
8. Lavonas EJ, Buchanan J, Auerbach PS, Dart RC, Scaglione M, Lewis B, et al. Year 3 of bite treatment with a new F(ab')2 antivenom for North American pit viper envenomation: quicker initial therapeutic response and decreased hospitalization. Wilderness Environ Med. 2015;26(4):488-495.
9. Eddleston M, Juszczak E, Buckley NA, Senarathna L, Mohamed F, Dissanayake W, et al. Multiple-dose activated charcoal in acute self-poisoning: a randomised controlled trial. Lancet. 2008;371(9612):579-587.
10. Roberts DM, Yates C, Megarbane B, Winchester JF, Maclaren R, Gosselin S, et al. Recommendations for the role of extracorporeal treatments in the management of acute methanol poisoning: a systematic review and consensus statement. Crit Care Med. 2015;43(2):461-472.

CHAPTER 6

EMERGENCY TOXICOLOGY

Author

Dr. Shannumukha Sainath A, Assistant Professor,
Department of Pharmacy Practice, Nirmala College of Pharmacy,
Ukkayapalli, Kadapa, Andhra Pradesh, India

Abstract

Managing toxic emergencies requires a systematic approach beginning with rapid stabilization followed by specific interventions. Initial management follows the ABCDE (Airway, Breathing, Circulation, Disability, Exposure) framework, with particular attention to securing compromised airways, supporting ventilation, establishing vascular access, and addressing life-threatening dysrhythmias or hypotension. Simultaneously, attempts to identify the toxin involve examining vital sign patterns, recognizing toxidromes, and gathering exposure history from patients, bystanders, or prehospital personnel. Critical care management addresses organ system complications including hepatotoxicity, nephrotoxicity, cardiotoxicity, neurotoxicity, and metabolic disturbances. Targeted interventions for specific toxins are initiated while monitoring progresses from basic vital signs to advanced parameters including continuous ECG, capnography, invasive hemodynamic measurements, and serial laboratory studies tailored to the suspected agent. Particular toxins require specialized monitoring such as QRS duration in sodium channel blocker toxicity or anion gap in toxic alcohol ingestions. Comprehensive documentation encompasses initial presentation, interventions, response to treatment, consultation with poison centers or toxicologists, laboratory and diagnostic findings, and disposition decisions. This structured approach optimizes outcomes in poisoned patients while facilitating continuity of care, quality improvement, risk management, and potential medicolegal review.

Keywords: *Toxidromes, Critical Care, Antidotal Therapy, Toxicological Monitoring, Airway Management, Toxicology*

Learning Objectives

After completion of the chapter, the learners should be able to:

- Apply the ABCDE approach to initial stabilization of acutely poisoned patients with emphasis on toxin-specific airway and hemodynamic considerations.
- Recognize common toxidromes and vital sign patterns to guide early management decisions and toxin identification.
- Implement appropriate critical care interventions for organ-specific toxic effects including hepatotoxicity, nephrotoxicity, cardiotoxicity, and neurotoxicity.
- Select appropriate monitoring parameters for specific toxic exposures and interpret findings to guide ongoing management.
- Develop comprehensive documentation of toxic exposures that captures essential elements for clinical care, quality improvement, and potential legal proceedings.
- Formulate disposition plans for poisoned patients based on clinical stability, toxin characteristics, anticipated clinical course, and available monitoring capabilities.

INITIAL MANAGEMENT

The approach to acutely poisoned patients demands systematic assessment and intervention, addressing life-threatening complications while establishing foundations for definitive care.

Triage and Risk Assessment

Effective triage of potentially poisoned patients requires structured evaluation focusing on exposure characteristics, presenting symptoms, and risk factors for severe outcomes. Initial telephone triage, often conducted through poison control centers, evaluates exposure circumstances, substance identity and quantity, time elapsed since exposure, current symptoms, and pre-existing conditions affecting risk. This preliminary assessment determines whether home observation with monitoring suffices or healthcare facility evaluation becomes necessary. For patients presenting directly to healthcare facilities, rapid triage assessment focuses on vital sign abnormalities, level of consciousness, specific high-risk symptoms like seizures or dysrhythmias, and exposure to substances associated with delayed toxicity or rapid deterioration.

Risk stratification incorporates both toxicant-specific and patient-specific factors. High-risk substances include calcium channel blockers, beta-blockers, cyclic antidepressants, opioids, hypoglycemic agents, and toxins with delayed onset of life-threatening effects like acetaminophen, certain mushrooms, and paraquat. High-risk exposure characteristics include large estimated doses, sustained-release formulations, multiple substance exposure, and unusual routes like injection or inhalation that bypass normal protective barriers. Patient risk factors include extremes of age, pregnancy, significant comorbidities affecting metabolic or eliminative functions, and lack of reliable observation capability for home management plans. This multifactorial assessment guides both triage categorization and initial resource allocation, including immediate bedside evaluation, continuous monitoring requirements, and anticipatory preparation for potential deterioration.

Table 6.1: Initial Management in Toxicological Emergencies

Priority	**Actions**	**Potential Complications**
Airway	Assessment, positioning, intubation if needed	Aspiration, respiratory arrest
Breathing	Oxygen, ventilatory support	Hypoxemia, hypercarbia
Circulation	IV access, fluid resuscitation, vasopressors if needed	Hypotension, dysrhythmias
Decontamination	Appropriate method based on route and timing	Aspiration, further absorption
Enhanced elimination	Consider in severe cases of dialyzable toxins	Complications of procedure
Targeted antidotes	Administration when indicated	Adverse effects of antidotes
Diagnostic testing	Targeted based on clinical presentation	Delayed diagnosis, missed toxins

Triage systems for poisoned patients increasingly incorporate structured toxicological triage tools alongside general emergency severity indices. The Poisoning Severity Score categorizes cases from asymptomatic (grade 0) through mild (grade 1), moderate (grade 2), and severe (grade 3), based on standardized criteria across multiple organ systems. Additional standardized assessment tools evaluate specific toxidrome presentations, pediatric poisoning severity, and risk for delayed toxicity manifestation. These structured approaches enhance consistency in initial assessment and disposition decision-making across providers with varying toxicological experience levels.

Communication with regional poison centers provides critical triage support and management guidance, particularly valuable for uncommon exposures or complex scenarios. These centers maintain comprehensive toxicant databases, case registries documenting previous similar exposures, and specialists experienced in risk assessment for diverse poisonings. Early poison center consultation enables appropriate resource utilization through evidence-based recommendations regarding necessary observation periods, laboratory evaluations, and interventions based on specific toxicant characteristics and exposure circumstances. This collaboration enhances both individual patient care and public health surveillance for emerging toxicological threats or product hazards.

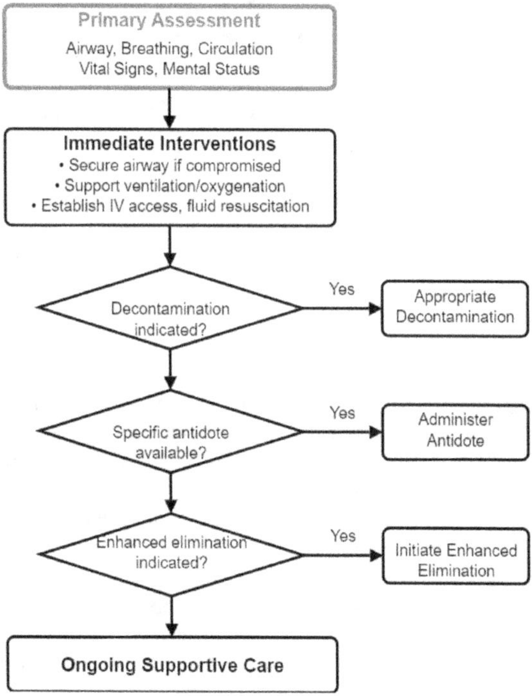

Figure 6.1: Initial Management Algorithm for Toxicological Emergencies

Resuscitation Priorities

Initial stabilization of poisoned patients follows modified advanced life support principles addressing toxicant-specific pathophysiology. Airway assessment carries particular importance given the frequency of mental status alteration and protective reflex impairment in toxicological emergencies. Indications for early intubation include Glasgow Coma Scale below 8, inability to maintain patent airway, progressive deterioration in respiratory status, severe agitation requiring sedation, and anticipation of complications requiring airway protection based on specific toxicant properties. Rapid sequence intubation protocols for poisoned patients typically employ etomidate or ketamine for induction, minimizing additional hemodynamic compromise in potentially unstable patients, with special consideration for potential drug interactions with specific toxicants.

> **Remember**
>
> **Initial management of poisoned patients follows the ABCDE approach (Airway, Breathing, Circulation, Disability, Exposure) with emphasis on early airway protection in patients with decreased consciousness or risk of aspiration**

Respiratory support addresses multiple pathophysiological processes including central respiratory depression from sedative-hypnotics or opioids, bronchospasm from cholinergic or irritant exposures, and non-cardiogenic pulmonary edema from various toxicants including salicylates and opioids. Oxygen administration targets saturation above 94% in most scenarios, with 100% oxygen indicated for carbon monoxide poisoning to accelerate carboxyhemoglobin dissociation. Ventilation strategies require toxicant-specific modifications, particularly in salicylate poisoning where hyperventilation provides compensatory alkalosis that should be maintained during mechanical ventilation to prevent paradoxical acidosis and increased central nervous system toxicity.

Circulatory support begins with establishing reliable vascular access, typically through two large-bore peripheral intravenous lines, with central venous access considered for patients requiring vasopressor support or specialized monitoring. Hypotension management follows a stepwise approach beginning with crystalloid fluid resuscitation (typically 20 mL/kg initially), followed by vasopressor support if inadequate response occurs. Vasopressor selection considers toxicant-specific mechanisms: norepinephrine for distributive shock from vasodilatory toxins, epinephrine for bradycardia-associated hypotension from beta-blockers or calcium channel blockers, and pure alpha-agonists like phenylephrine for toxicants causing both vasodilation and tachycardia. Specific antidotal therapy often proves more effective than conventional hemodynamic support alone, exemplified by calcium, glucagon, and high-dose insulin therapy for calcium channel blocker and beta-blocker toxicity.

Neurological emergencies in poisoned patients require aggressive management, with seizures representing a common complication of numerous toxicants. Initial treatment employs benzodiazepines at standard or increased doses, recognizing that toxicant-induced seizures often prove more resistant to standard anticonvulsant regimens. Second-line agents include phenobarbital or propofol rather than phenytoin, which shows limited efficacy against most toxicant-induced seizures. Specific antidotal therapy addresses underlying mechanisms in certain poisonings, exemplified by pyridoxine administration for isoniazid-induced seizures refractory to conventional anticonvulsants. Status epilepticus unresponsive to standard measures may require rapid progression to general anesthesia with continuous electroencephalogram monitoring, particularly when neuromuscular blockade masks motor manifestations of ongoing seizure activity.

Diagnosis

Initial diagnostic evaluation incorporates focused history-taking, physical examination targeting toxidrome recognition, and selected laboratory and imaging studies guided by clinical presentation. History acquisition, often challenging in poisoned patients due to altered mental status or intentional deception, emphasizes toxicant identification, quantity, timing, coingestants, and available medical history. Collateral information sources including family members, emergency medical services personnel, prescription databases, and scene observations often provide critical details unavailable from the patient. Physical examination focuses on vital sign patterns and characteristic toxidrome manifestations, with particular attention to pupillary response, mucous membrane moisture, bowel sounds, skin characteristics, and neuromuscular findings that may suggest specific toxicant classes.

Laboratory evaluation begins with essential studies indicated for most significant poisonings: comprehensive metabolic panel assessing electrolytes, renal and hepatic function; complete blood count; coagulation studies; arterial blood gas analysis; urinalysis; and pregnancy testing for women of childbearing potential. Toxicant-specific testing follows a targeted approach guided by clinical presentation and suspected exposures. Quantitative levels for specific toxicants like acetaminophen, salicylates, digoxin, lithium, iron, carbamazepine, and valproic acid provide critical management guidance when corresponding toxicity is suspected. Toxicology screening may include immunoassay-based urine drug screens for common substances of abuse, recognizing the significant limitations in sensitivity, specificity, and substance coverage of these tests. Expanded toxicological testing requires consultation with laboratory services and consideration of send-out testing to reference laboratories when results would meaningfully impact management.

Electrocardiography provides essential assessment in suspected poisonings, with specific attention to rate, rhythm, intervals, and morphological abnormalities suggesting particular toxicants. QRS prolongation (>100 ms) suggests sodium channel blockade from agents like tricyclic antidepressants or class Ia antiarrhythmics. QT prolongation indicates potassium channel effects from numerous medications including antipsychotics, methadone, and class III antiarrhythmics. Specific dysrhythmias may suggest particular toxicants: bidirectional ventricular tachycardia suggesting digitalis glycoside toxicity; torsades de pointes indicating QT-prolonging agents; and bradydysrhythmias suggesting beta-blockers, calcium channel blockers, or cholinergic excess. Serial electrocardiograms provide valuable trending information, particularly for cardiotoxic substances with delayed manifestations.

Imaging studies serve targeted purposes in selected poisoning scenarios. Abdominal radiographs may identify radio-opaque tablets, foreign body ingestions, or characteristic patterns like the "string of pearls" appearance in iron tablet ingestion. Chest radiography evaluates for aspiration pneumonitis, non-cardiogenic pulmonary edema, and pneumothorax from inhalational exposures. Computed tomography of the brain remains the preferred neuroimaging modality for altered mental status evaluation, excluding structural lesions mimicking toxicological presentations and identifying complications like cerebral edema in specific poisonings. Bedside ultrasonography increasingly provides valuable assessment of cardiac function in cardiotoxic exposures, volume status in conditions with significant fluid shifts, and presence of foreign bodies in selected ingestions.

Early Interventions

Time-sensitive interventions often prove critical in poisoned patients, with early administration of certain antidotes substantially improving outcomes. Naloxone administration for suspected opioid toxicity presenting with respiratory depression follows a titrated approach, beginning with 0.4 mg intravenously in adults with escalation as needed to restore adequate respiratory status without precipitating severe withdrawal in opioid-dependent individuals. Higher initial doses (2-4 mg) may be warranted with suspected potent synthetic opioid exposures like fentanyl analogs. Dextrose administration (25 g intravenously in adults) addresses hypoglycemia, a common contributor to altered mental status either independently or concurrent with toxicant exposure. Thiamine supplementation (100 mg intravenously) should precede dextrose administration in malnourished or alcoholic patients to prevent precipitation of Wernicke's encephalopathy.

Table 6.2: Critical Toxicological Syndromes Requiring Immediate Intervention

Syndrome	Priority Interventions	Monitoring Parameters
Severe sympathomimetic toxicity	Benzodiazepines, cooling, fluid resuscitation	Temperature, BP, HR, CK, renal function
Opioid overdose	Airway management, naloxone, ventilatory support	Respiratory rate, oxygen saturation, level of consciousness
Organophosphate poisoning	Atropine, pralidoxime, benzodiazepines	Secretions, respiratory status, cholinesterase levels
Calcium channel blocker toxicity	Calcium, high-dose insulin euglycemia therapy, vasopressors	BP, HR, glucose, calcium, cardiac output
Toxic alcohol poisoning	Fomepizole, bicarbonate, hemodialysis	Anion gap, osmolal gap, pH, methanol/ethylene glycol levels
Salicylate toxicity	Alkalinization, fluid resuscitation, hemodialysis in severe cases	Salicylate level, pH, mental status, temperature
Cyanide toxicity	Hydroxocobalamin or sodium thiosulfate	Lactate, vital signs, pH, cardiac function

Decontamination procedures, when indicated, require prompt implementation for maximal effectiveness. Activated charcoal administration (typically 1 g/kg orally or via nasogastric tube) provides greatest benefit when administered within 1-2 hours of ingestion for most toxicants, with possibly extended efficacy for sustained-release preparations or substances undergoing enterohepatic circulation.

Appropriate patient selection requires assessment of mental status, protective airway reflexes, absence of corrosive or hydrocarbon ingestion, and contraindications including intestinal obstruction or perforation risk. Enhanced elimination procedures like urinary alkalinization for salicylate poisoning demonstrate greater efficacy when initiated early, before extensive tissue distribution occurs. External decontamination for dermal or ocular exposures should commence immediately, recognizing that even brief delays may substantially reduce effectiveness for rapidly absorbed toxicants.

Toxicant-specific antidotes require early recognition and administration in appropriate scenarios. N-acetylcysteine for acetaminophen poisoning shows substantially greater hepatoprotective efficacy when administered within 8-10 hours of ingestion, though benefit persists even with delayed administration. Digoxin-specific antibody fragments rapidly reverse life-threatening digitalis toxicity manifestations, with dosing based on ingested amount, serum concentration, or empiric administration in unstable patients. Fomepizole or ethanol therapy for toxic alcohol ingestions prevents formation of toxic metabolites most effectively when administered before significant metabolism occurs. Cyanide antidotes including hydroxocobalamin demonstrate greatest efficacy when given before prolonged cellular hypoxia produces irreversible damage. These time-dependent interventions necessitate both rapid recognition of potential indications and systems ensuring prompt availability of necessary antidotes, particularly for less commonly used agents.

Critical care anticipation requires early recognition of poisonings likely to require intensive monitoring or intervention despite initially stable presentations. Calcium channel blocker and beta-blocker ingestions frequently demonstrate delayed deterioration, particularly with sustained-release formulations, warranting proactive intensive care unit admission and preparation of specific therapies including high-dose insulin, calcium, glucagon, and potentially extracorporeal support. Acetaminophen ingestions with concerning serum levels require N-acetylcysteine therapy and hepatic function monitoring in appropriate settings, recognizing that clinical manifestations of toxicity typically lag behind early laboratory changes. Cyclic antidepressant overdoses necessitate continuous cardiac monitoring and observation for at least 6-12 hours given the potential for delayed dysrhythmias or seizures. This anticipatory approach to potential deterioration enables appropriate resource allocation and preparation before decompensation occurs, potentially improving outcomes in high-risk poisonings.

CRITICAL CARE

Management of severely poisoned patients in intensive care settings addresses complex physiological derangements while providing extended monitoring and specialized interventions for toxicant-specific complications.

Advanced Airway and Ventilation

Airway management in critically ill poisoned patients extends beyond initial intubation to include ongoing optimization addressing toxicant-specific respiratory pathophysiology. Post-intubation care includes confirmation of endotracheal tube placement through multiple methods (capnography, chest radiography, and auscultation), recognition of potential tube displacement during seizures or agitated states, and prevention of ventilator-associated pneumonia through head elevation and oral care protocols. Sedation management requires careful consideration of potential interactions between sedative medications and the underlying toxicant, with preference for short-acting agents like propofol or dexmedetomidine that permit regular neurological reassessment in toxicants with fluctuating or improving effects over time.

Ventilation strategies must address specific toxicant-induced pathophysiology rather than applying standard approaches uniformly. Salicylate poisoning creates particular challenges, as the normal respiratory alkalosis these patients develop compensates for metabolic acidosis and reduces central nervous system salicylate penetration. Mechanical ventilation must maintain this compensatory hyperventilation through higher minute ventilation settings, as loss of respiratory alkalosis may precipitate rapid clinical deterioration through increased brain salicylate levels. Paraquat poisoning presents the opposite challenge, where supplemental oxygen may paradoxically worsen pulmonary injury through enhanced free radical generation, necessitating careful oxygen titration to maintain saturation between 85-90% rather than conventional targets. Inhalational toxicant exposures often create heterogeneous lung injury patterns requiring personalized ventilator settings with careful attention to preventing ventilator-induced lung injury through lung-protective strategies.

Specialized ventilation approaches address specific toxicological scenarios. Extracorporeal membrane oxygenation (ECMO) provides rescue therapy for profound respiratory failure unresponsive to conventional ventilation, particularly valuable in poisonings with reversible toxicity but severe temporary pulmonary compromise. High-frequency oscillatory ventilation may benefit patients with significant inhalational injuries causing severe hypoxemia despite conventional approaches. Inhaled pulmonary vasodilators including nitric oxide and prostacyclin analogues address ventilation-perfusion mismatching and pulmonary hypertension in selected toxicant-induced lung injuries. Airway pressure release ventilation provides alternative management for poisonings producing acute respiratory distress syndrome with refractory hypoxemia despite conventional protective ventilation strategies.

Weaning from mechanical ventilation requires systematic assessment of multiple factors including resolution of the underlying toxic effect, reversal of specific complications like pulmonary edema or pneumonitis, adequate neuromuscular function, and hemodynamic stability without significant vasopressor support. Spontaneous breathing trials assess readiness for extubation, with modified parameters sometimes necessary based on residual toxicant effects. Premature extubation carries particular risks in certain poisonings, including recurrent respiratory depression from redistribution of lipophilic substances like tricyclic antidepressants or prolonged-release opioid formulations. Conversely, unnecessarily prolonged intubation increases complications including ventilator-associated pneumonia, deconditioning, and sedation-related delirium. This balance requires regular reassessment guided by understanding of specific toxicant pharmacokinetics and anticipated recovery timelines.

Hemodynamic Support

Advanced hemodynamic management in toxicological critical care addresses diverse mechanisms of cardiovascular dysfunction through targeted interventions beyond conventional approaches. Distributive shock from vasodilatory toxicants (phenothiazines, calcium channel blockers, ACE inhibitors) typically requires vasopressor support, with norepinephrine generally preferred as first-line agent due to combined alpha and beta effects. Vasopressin (0.01-0.04 units/minute) provides particular advantage in refractory vasodilatory shock through a non-catecholamine mechanism less affected by acidosis. Pure alpha-agonists like phenylephrine may benefit patients with toxicant-induced tachycardia that worsens with mixed alpha/beta agents. Cardiogenic shock from cardiotoxic agents (beta-blockers, calcium channel blockers, antiarrhythmics) may require inotropic support with agents like dobutamine, milrinone, or epinephrine alongside vasopressors, with selection guided by specific hemodynamic parameters and toxicant properties.

Specific toxicant-directed therapies frequently prove more effective than conventional hemodynamic support alone. High-dose insulin euglycemia therapy (HIET) addresses cardiogenic shock from beta-blocker and calcium channel blocker poisoning through positive inotropy, improved myocardial glucose utilization, and vasodilation. Protocol typically begins with 1 unit/kg regular insulin bolus followed by infusion starting at 0.5-1 unit/kg/hour, titrated up to 10 units/kg/hour in severe cases, with concurrent dextrose administration to maintain euglycemia. Calcium administration (calcium chloride 10-20 mg/kg or calcium gluconate 30-60 mg/kg) addresses both hypocalcemia and calcium channel antagonism, particularly valuable in calcium channel blocker poisoning where repeated doses often prove necessary. Glucagon (5-10 mg bolus followed by 1-5 mg/hour infusion) provides positive chronotropic and inotropic effects through non-beta-receptor-mediated cAMP increases, particularly useful in beta-blocker toxicity though limited by frequent tachyphylaxis.

> **Remember**
>
> **Cardiac monitoring is essential for many toxins, with particular attention to QRS duration (sodium channel blockers), QT interval (multiple toxins), and conduction blocks (calcium channel blockers, beta-blockers).**

Mechanical circulatory support provides rescue therapy for refractory cardiovascular collapse unresponsive to pharmacological interventions. Intra-aortic balloon pumps reduce afterload and augment coronary perfusion in cardiogenic shock from cardiotoxic agents. Venoarterial extracorporeal membrane oxygenation (VA-ECMO) provides complete cardiopulmonary support during profound cardiovascular collapse, particularly valuable in poisonings with reversible toxicity but temporary severe cardiac dysfunction. Case series demonstrate survival rates exceeding 80% with VA-ECMO for severe calcium channel blocker and beta-blocker poisonings despite initial cardiovascular collapse refractory to conventional therapies. Timing of initiation remains critical, ideally before prolonged end-organ hypoperfusion causes irreversible damage, necessitating early consultation with ECMO specialists when managing potentially eligible poisonings. Specialized centers have developed protocols for rapid ECMO deployment in toxicological emergencies, recognizing the potentially favorable risk-benefit profile compared to standard indications due to the often-reversible nature of toxicant-induced cardiac dysfunction.

Advanced hemodynamic monitoring guides therapy selection and titration in complex poisonings. Central venous pressure measurements help assess volume status and right heart function, particularly valuable in toxicants causing venodilation or myocardial depression. Arterial line placement provides continuous blood pressure monitoring and facilitates repeated arterial blood gas sampling. Echocardiography offers direct assessment of ventricular function, valvular competence, and pericardial effusion, with point-of-care ultrasonography increasingly available for serial evaluations. Pulmonary artery catheters, while less commonly employed in contemporary critical care, may provide particular value in differentiating mechanisms of shock in complex poisonings with mixed cardiogenic and distributive components or in guiding therapy for toxicants with complex hemodynamic effects like tricyclic antidepressants. These advanced monitoring modalities enable precision in both diagnosis and therapeutic titration, potentially improving outcomes in hemodynamically unstable poisoned patients.

Advanced Toxin-Specific Interventions

Critical care management of severely poisoned patients frequently requires specialized interventions addressing specific toxicological mechanisms beyond standard supportive care. Lipid emulsion therapy addresses cardiovascular collapse from lipophilic drug toxicity through proposed mechanisms including lipid sink effect sequestering toxicants, enhanced myocardial energy supply, and direct inotropic effects. Administration typically involves 1.5 mL/kg bolus of 20% lipid emulsion followed by 0.25 mL/kg/minute infusion for 30-60 minutes, with potential repeated boluses for persistent cardiovascular instability. Indications include local anesthetic systemic toxicity, cardiovascular collapse from lipophilic medications including calcium channel blockers, beta-blockers, and tricyclic antidepressants refractory to conventional therapy. Potential complications include pancreatitis, hypersensitivity reactions, and interference with laboratory testing, though overall safety profile remains favorable in life-threatening scenarios.

Sodium bicarbonate therapy serves multiple purposes in toxicological critical care beyond simple acid-base correction. For sodium channel blocking agents including tricyclic antidepressants and certain antiarrhythmics, bicarbonate administration (1-2 mEq/kg bolus followed by infusion) increases serum pH to 7.5-7.55, reducing the fraction of drug bound to sodium channels through both increased protein binding of the toxicant and alteration of sodium channel conformation. This intervention decreases QRS prolongation and reduces risk of ventricular dysrhythmias and hypotension. For salicylate poisoning, bicarbonate therapy addresses metabolic acidosis while creating serum and urine alkalinization that reduces central nervous system penetration through ion trapping and enhances urinary elimination. In metformin-associated lactic acidosis, bicarbonate addresses severe acidemia that might otherwise compromise cardiac function and vasopressor responsiveness, though with careful attention to avoiding fluid overload in potentially volume-sensitive patients.

Enhanced elimination techniques implemented in critical care settings address toxicants with life-threatening effects and prolonged duration of action. Hemodialysis provides definitive management for lithium poisoning with severe neurotoxicity or levels exceeding 4 mEq/L, with extended or repeated sessions often necessary due to redistribution from tissue stores after initial treatment. Toxic alcohols (methanol, ethylene glycol) typically require both antidotal therapy with fomepizole or ethanol and hemodialysis for severe poisonings with significant metabolic acidosis, end-organ damage, or levels exceeding treatment thresholds (typically >50 mg/dL if asymptomatic). Continuous renal replacement therapies provide alternative enhanced elimination for hemodynamically unstable patients unable to tolerate conventional hemodialysis, offering slower but sustained toxicant removal with better cardiovascular tolerance. Implementation requires close collaboration between toxicology, nephrology, and critical care teams, with specialized prescription modifications often necessary to optimize elimination of specific toxicants.

Hyperbaric oxygen therapy addresses selected poisonings through mechanisms including enhanced oxygen delivery, competitive displacement of toxicants, and modulation of inflammatory pathways. Carbon monoxide poisoning represents the primary toxicological indication, with treatment typically considered for patients with loss of consciousness, neurological abnormalities, cardiac ischemia, pregnancy with elevated carboxyhemoglobin, or levels exceeding 25%, ideally within 6-12 hours of exposure. Treatment protocols typically involve 2.5-3.0 atmospheres absolute for 90-120 minutes, with potential repeated treatments for severe cases. Additional potential applications include cyanide poisoning (particularly with concurrent carbon monoxide exposure from smoke inhalation), hydrogen sulfide exposure, and severe methemoglobinemia unresponsive to methylene blue. Implementation challenges include limited availability in many regions, transportation risks for unstable patients, and difficulties managing critically ill patients in the confined chamber environment, necessitating careful risk-benefit assessment and early consultation with hyperbaric specialists when considering this intervention.

Management of Multisystem Complications

Toxicological critical care frequently addresses multiple organ system complications occurring simultaneously or sequentially as poisoning evolves. Renal failure may result directly from nephrotoxic agents (aminoglycosides, ethylene glycol metabolites, heavy metals) or secondarily from complications like rhabdomyolysis, hemodynamic instability, or contrast administration. Management includes meticulous fluid balance, electrolyte correction, avoidance of additional nephrotoxic insults, and renal replacement therapy when indicated by conventional criteria (refractory hyperkalemia, severe acidosis, uremic complications, or fluid overload unresponsive to diuretics). Timing of initiation follows critical care principles, with some evidence suggesting potential benefit from earlier intervention in selected toxicological scenarios with severe acid-base or electrolyte derangements.

Hepatotoxicity represents a common critical care challenge in various poisonings, most notably acetaminophen but also including Amanita phalloides mushrooms, carbon tetrachloride, and numerous pharmaceutical agents. Management begins with specific antidotes when available (N-acetylcysteine for acetaminophen, silibinin for Amanita) and continues with supportive care addressing complications of hepatic dysfunction. Coagulopathy management may require vitamin K, fresh frozen plasma, or prothrombin complex concentrates based on severity and bleeding manifestations. Encephalopathy necessitates ammonia-lowering strategies including lactulose, rifaximin, and protein restriction. Monitoring for infection proves essential given impaired immune function. Severe cases unresponsive to conventional management may require consideration of liver transplantation, with toxicant-specific modifications to standard listing criteria reflecting potentially favorable recovery trajectories for certain poisonings compared to other causes of acute liver failure.

Rhabdomyolysis frequently complicates poisonings involving prolonged immobility, muscle hyperactivity, or direct myotoxicity, with examples including sympathomimetics, serotonergic agents, neuroleptic malignant syndrome, and certain venoms or mushrooms. Critical care management includes aggressive fluid resuscitation targeting urine output above 2 mL/kg/hour, with consideration of urinary alkalinization (target pH >6.5) to reduce myoglobin precipitation though evidence remains limited. Electrolyte management requires particular attention to hyperkalemia, hyperphosphatemia, hypocalcemia, and hyperuricemia. Compartment syndrome monitoring and early surgical consultation for concerning extremity findings remain essential, as fasciotomy delays significantly increase morbidity. Continuous renal replacement therapy may offer advantages over intermittent hemodialysis for patients with rhabdomyolysis-associated renal failure and hemodynamic instability, providing more gradual correction of electrolyte abnormalities and better volume management flexibility.

Neurological complications requiring critical care management include status epilepticus, elevated intracranial pressure, and prolonged altered mental status. Refractory status epilepticus from toxicants like isoniazid, tricyclic antidepressants, or theophylline may require progression to general anesthesia with midazolam, propofol, or ketamine infusions titrated to seizure suppression on continuous electroencephalogram monitoring. Intracranial pressure management follows neurointensive care principles, though with recognition that many toxicant-induced cerebral edema patterns respond differently than traumatic or ischemic etiologies, potentially modifying indications for invasive monitoring or aggressive interventions. Prolonged altered mental status management includes prevention of complications through positioning, mobilization when feasible, aspiration precautions, and vigilance for development of withdrawal syndromes or unmasked traumatic injuries as toxicant effects resolve. Neurocognitive assessment during recovery aids both prognostication and identification of rehabilitation needs, particularly for toxicants associated with delayed or incomplete neurological recovery

MONITORING

Systematic observation of poisoned patients detects evolving toxicity, guides intervention timing, and assesses treatment efficacy through integrated physiological and laboratory surveillance.

Vital Sign Monitoring

Vital sign patterns in poisoned patients provide both diagnostic clues and critical indicators of clinical progression or improvement. Continuous cardiac monitoring detects both rate and rhythm disturbances, with specific attention to intervals and morphological changes suggesting particular toxicities. QRS prolongation beyond 100 ms indicates sodium channel blockade, warranting intervention with sodium bicarbonate when associated with hemodynamic instability or progression beyond 120 ms even in stable patients. QT prolongation (QTc >500 ms) identifies increased risk for torsades de pointes, requiring enhanced monitoring, electrolyte optimization, and consideration of magnesium prophylaxis. PR prolongation suggests calcium channel blockade, digitalis effect, or beta-blockade. ST segment and T wave abnormalities may indicate myocardial ischemia from coronary vasospasm in stimulant toxicity or direct myocardial injury in cardiotoxic exposures.

Blood pressure monitoring strategies vary based on poisoning severity and expected clinical course. Noninvasive measurements at 15-30 minute intervals suffice for stable patients with low-risk exposures, while continuous intraarterial monitoring provides beat-to-beat assessment in hemodynamically unstable poisonings or those receiving vasoactive infusions. Specific attention to pulse pressure may reveal additional information, with widening suggesting vasodilation or aortic insufficiency (as in severe theophylline toxicity) and narrowing indicating decreased stroke volume or increased peripheral resistance. Postural measurements detect occult volume depletion in appropriate patients, particularly valuable in poisonings with significant gastrointestinal fluid losses or vasodilation.

Table 6.3: Monitoring Parameters for Major Toxicological Emergencies

Parameter	Toxins Requiring Special Attention	Critical Values Requiring Intervention
Vital signs	Sympathomimetics, calcium channel blockers, beta-blockers, sedative-hypnotics	Systolic BP <90 mmHg, HR <50 or >150 bpm, RR <8 or >30, Temp >40°C
ECG	TCA, antipsychotics, sodium channel blockers, potassium channel blockers	QRS >120 ms, QTc >500 ms, significant dysrhythmias
Pulse oximetry	Carbon monoxide, methemoglobin producers, respiratory depressants	SpO_2 <90% (unreliable in CO or methemoglobinemia)
Blood glucose	Insulin, oral hypoglycemics, beta-blockers, salicylates, alcohols	<70 mg/dL or >250 mg/dL
Electrolytes	Diuretics, alcohols, salicylates, lithium	K^+ <3.0 or >6.0 mEq/L, Na^+ <125 or >150 mEq/L
Renal function	NSAIDs, lithium, ethylene glycol, rhabdomyolysis-causing agents	Cr increase >0.3 mg/dL in 48h, BUN:Cr ratio >20:1
Hepatic function	Acetaminophen, mushrooms, carbon tetrachloride	AST/ALT >1000 IU/L, rising bilirubin, INR >1.5
Acid-base status	Alcohols, salicylates, carbon monoxide, cyanide	pH <7.2 or >7.6, HCO_3 <15 mEq/L

Interpretation of blood pressure trends requires integration with other hemodynamic parameters and understanding of expected toxicant time course, as apparent "improvement" may reflect transition between phases of toxicity rather than genuine clinical resolution.

Temperature monitoring serves multiple purposes in toxicological assessment. Hyperthermia may indicate sympathomimetic excess, serotonin syndrome, anticholinergic toxicity, malignant hyperthermia, or neuroleptic malignant syndrome, with specific patterns of associated findings differentiating these toxidromes. Core temperature measurement provides greater accuracy than peripheral methods, particularly important when implementing cooling measures or assessing response to specific interventions for hyperthermic syndromes.

Hypothermia may reflect sedative-hypnotic effect, hypothalamic depression from various toxicants, environmental exposure during unconsciousness, or shock states with poor peripheral perfusion. Active external warming generally addresses toxicant-induced hypothermia, with core rewarming techniques reserved for profound temperature depression or cases with cardiovascular instability.

Respiratory monitoring encompasses both rate and quality assessments. Continuous pulse oximetry provides noninvasive oxygenation monitoring, though with important limitations in specific poisonings: carbon monoxide binding produces falsely normal saturations; methemoglobinemia typically causes saturation readings around 85% regardless of actual oxygenation; and dyes like methylene blue interfere with measurement accuracy. Capnography increasingly complements pulse oximetry by providing continuous assessment of ventilation adequacy, particularly valuable in opioid-induced respiratory depression where significant hypoventilation may precede oxygen desaturation. Respiratory pattern recognition aids toxidrome identification: Kussmaul breathing suggesting metabolic acidosis in toxic alcohol or salicylate poisoning; Cheyne-Stokes respiration indicating delayed neurological toxicity in various central nervous system depressants; and ataxic breathing patterns suggesting brainstem involvement in advanced central nervous system depression.

Laboratory Monitoring

Serial laboratory assessment monitors toxicant levels, detects complications, and evaluates treatment efficacy throughout the poisoning course. Toxicant-specific quantitative measurements guide management decisions when therapeutic windows are established: acetaminophen levels interpreted on the Rumack-Matthew nomogram determine need for N-acetylcysteine therapy; salicylate levels correlate with toxicity severity and need for enhanced elimination; digoxin concentrations guide Fab fragment dosing; and lithium, carbamazepine, phenytoin, and valproic acid levels inform both toxicity assessment and enhanced elimination decisions. Timing of measurements requires careful consideration relative to ingestion, with premature testing potentially missing peak levels for substances with delayed absorption. Interpretation considers both absolute values and trends, as rising levels despite supportive care may indicate ongoing absorption, sustained-release preparations, or developing complications affecting elimination.

Organ system function markers require systematic tracking to detect toxicant-induced damage or complications. Hepatic function monitoring includes transaminases, bilirubin, alkaline phosphatase, and synthetic function markers like albumin and prothrombin time. Transaminase elevation patterns provide diagnostic information: AST predominance suggesting muscle injury rather than primary hepatotoxicity; rapid extreme elevation (>10,000 IU/L) indicating severe acute injury as in acetaminophen toxicity; and delayed elevation emerging 24-72 hours after exposure with many hepatotoxic substances. Renal function assessment includes blood urea nitrogen, creatinine, electrolytes, and urinalysis, with attention to trends rather than single values to detect early injury. Urinalysis provides particularly valuable information regarding myoglobinuria (positive blood on dipstick without erythrocytes on microscopy), crystalluria (ethylene glycol, acyclovir, indinavir), and urinary pH relevant to ionizable toxicant elimination.

Metabolic and hematologic parameters require monitoring based on specific toxicant properties and clinical presentation. Serum glucose measurement addresses both hypoglycemia from insulin, sulfonylureas, and various natural toxins, and hyperglycemia from sympathomimetic excess, iron poisoning, or calcium channel blocker toxicity treated with high-dose insulin. Complete blood count monitors for toxicant-induced bone marrow suppression, hemolysis, methemoglobinemia, or developing infection. Coagulation studies identify both direct anticoagulant effects and developing hepatic dysfunction. Inflammatory markers including C-reactive protein and procalcitonin help distinguish infection from non-infectious inflammatory response to certain toxicants, particularly valuable when fever complicates the clinical picture. Serum lactate provides both prognostic information and treatment response assessment in numerous poisonings including carbon monoxide, cyanide, metformin, and various shock states.

Specialized laboratory monitoring addresses specific toxicological scenarios. Methemoglobin levels guide treatment decisions in oxidizing agent exposures, with values above 20-30% or symptomatic presentations warranting methylene blue administration. Carboxyhemoglobin measurements through co-oximetry (not standard pulse oximetry) assess carbon monoxide poisoning severity and treatment response. Cholinesterase activity quantifies organophosphate or carbamate poisoning severity, though interpretation requires understanding of significant inter-individual variation in baseline values. Anion gap and osmolal gap calculations provide screening tools for numerous toxicants—elevated anion gap suggesting toxic alcohols, salicylates, metformin, or certain anticonvulsants; osmolal gap elevation indicating alcohols, acetone, or certain glycols. The combination of both gaps with appropriate clinical context guides further specific testing and empiric management decisions when more definitive analyses remain unavailable or pending.

Toxicokinetic Monitoring

Toxicokinetic principles guide monitoring frequency and duration based on substance-specific absorption, distribution, metabolism, and elimination characteristics. Extended-release formulations necessitate prolonged observation even when initial presentations appear benign, as demonstrated by delayed cardiotoxicity from sustained-release calcium channel blockers or beta-blockers emerging 12-24 hours after ingestion. Medications with active metabolites require monitoring beyond expected parent compound elimination: tramadol produces the active metabolite O-desmethyltramadol with prolonged effect; carbamazepine forms the active epoxide metabolite contributing to toxicity; and some benzodiazepines generate long-acting active compounds exceeding parent drug duration. Substances undergoing enterohepatic circulation, including many natural toxins and certain pharmaceuticals, may demonstrate secondary peaks in concentration and clinical effect as the compound recirculates from biliary excretion back into intestinal absorption.

> **Remember**
>
> **Disposition decisions for poisoned patients must consider the specific toxin's time course, anticipated complications, required monitoring capabilities, and patient-specific factors including intentionality and comorbidities**

Tissue redistribution phenomena necessitate extended monitoring for lipophilic substances, which may demonstrate apparent clinical improvement as the toxicant redistributes from central nervous system to peripheral tissues, followed by recurrent toxicity as redistribution continues during elimination. This pattern appears classically with tricyclic antidepressants, where premature discontinuation of monitoring based on initial improvement may miss life-threatening recurrent cardiotoxicity. Similar concerns apply to numerous lipophilic agents including calcium channel blockers, antipsychotics, and local anesthetics. Recognition of these redistribution patterns guides appropriate monitoring duration, typically extending at least 24 hours after apparent clinical improvement for highly lipophilic toxicants with significant cardiovascular or neurological effects.

Elimination half-life considerations determine optimal monitoring intervals and necessary observation duration. For substances with short half-lives (1-3 hours) like morphine, meperedine, or salicylates, frequent assessments at 1-2 hour intervals capture rapidly changing clinical states. Intermediate half-life toxicants (8-24 hours) like phenobarbital, amitriptyline, or diazepam require assessments at 4-6 hour intervals to detect significant trends. Long half-life substances (>24 hours) like digoxin, methotrexate, or fluoxetine necessitate daily monitoring to assess gradual recovery. Expected duration of monitoring typically extends through at least 4-5 half-lives of the parent compound and significant metabolites, though this general rule requires modification based on toxicity severity, individual patient factors affecting elimination, and specific treatment interventions that may alter normal elimination patterns.

Therapeutic drug monitoring principles apply with important modifications in toxicological scenarios. Sampling timing requires adjustment for altered pharmacokinetics in overdose situations, where normal peak and trough patterns may not apply due to delayed or prolonged absorption, saturation of metabolic pathways, or impaired elimination. Reference ranges established for therapeutic use often have limited relevance in toxicity assessment, with correlation between concentration and clinical effect frequently following different patterns in overdose compared to normal use. Specimen selection considerations include potential interference effects in certain matrices; detection window differences between blood, urine, and other biological samples; and special handling requirements for unstable compounds. Interpretation of monitoring results requires integration with clinical assessment rather than standalone decision-making, as individual variations in receptor sensitivity, underlying health status, and coingestants significantly affect response to similar toxicant concentrations.

Special Monitoring

Pediatric poisonings present unique monitoring challenges reflecting developmental differences in physiology, body composition, and manifestation of toxicity. Weight-based calculations guide equipment selection, with appropriately sized blood pressure cuffs, pulse oximeter sensors, and vascular access devices essential for accurate monitoring. Vital sign interpretation requires age-specific reference ranges, as normal parameters vary substantially across developmental stages. Laboratory monitoring considers age-appropriate reference values and sampling limitations, with microtechniques employing minimal blood volumes particularly important for smaller children. Clinical assessment tools require developmental adaptation, with age-appropriate neurological examinations and pain assessment scales. Parental presence during monitoring provides both comfort to the child and valuable observational information, as parents often detect subtle behavioral changes not apparent to healthcare providers less familiar with the child's baseline.

Psychiatric monitoring complements physiological assessment in intentional overdoses, with structured evaluation of suicidal ideation, risk for self-harm, and underlying psychiatric conditions informing both acute management and discharge planning. Initial assessment occurs after medical stabilization but before potential discharge, with standardized screening tools complementing clinical interview techniques. Serial assessments monitor for emergence of suicidal thoughts during recovery, particularly relevant with substances causing dysphoria or agitation during resolution. Constant observation protocols with appropriately trained personnel prevent self-harm attempts during vulnerable periods. Consultation with mental health specialists establishes necessary follow-up arrangements, with direct transitions to psychiatric facilities when indicated rather than emergency department discharge. This integrated monitoring approach addresses the frequently intertwined medical and psychiatric aspects of intentional overdose, recognizing that attention to both components improves overall outcomes.

Withdrawal monitoring becomes essential when poisonings involve substances with dependence potential, as physiological dependence may emerge even after brief exposure to high doses of certain agents. Structured assessment tools guide monitoring and intervention: the Clinical Institute Withdrawal Assessment for Alcohol (CIWA-Ar) quantifies alcohol withdrawal severity; the Clinical Opiate Withdrawal Scale (COWS) measures opioid withdrawal manifestations; and the Benzodiazepine Withdrawal Scale tracks symptoms during benzodiazepine discontinuation. Recognition of less common withdrawal syndromes proves equally important, including gamma-hydroxybutyrate (GHB) withdrawal with autonomic instability and delirium, baclofen withdrawal with spasticity and seizures, and clonidine withdrawal with rebound hypertension.

Pregnancy presents specialized monitoring requirements when toxicological emergencies affect expectant mothers. Maternal monitoring follows standard principles with consideration of physiological changes of pregnancy affecting normal parameters: increased respiratory rate, elevated cardiac output, reduced blood pressure, and altered laboratory reference ranges. Fetal monitoring through electronic fetal heart rate assessment, contraction monitoring, and ultrasonography evaluates for toxicant effects on the fetus and potential pregnancy complications. Interpretation of fetal monitoring requires consultation with obstetrical specialists familiar with both normal patterns and toxicant-specific concerns. Pharmacokinetic changes during pregnancy, including increased volume of distribution, altered protein binding, enhanced renal clearance, and modified hepatic metabolism, may necessitate adjustment of expected toxicokinetic parameters. Multidisciplinary collaboration between toxicology, critical care, and maternal-fetal medicine specialists optimizes monitoring approaches for these complex scenarios where management decisions must consider both maternal and fetal wellbeing.

Summary

Emergency toxicology focuses on the time-sensitive management of acute poisonings, beginning with immediate stabilization followed by targeted interventions for specific toxins. Initial management follows the ABCDE approach, with particular attention to securing compromised airways in obtunded patients, supporting ventilation in respiratory depression, establishing vascular access for medication administration, addressing hypotension and dysrhythmias, and thoroughly examining for toxin-related findings. Simultaneous efforts focus on toxin identification through clinical assessment, toxidrome recognition, collateral history, and review of the exposure scene. Critical care management addresses organ-specific complications including hepatotoxicity (acetaminophen, amatoxin), nephrotoxicity (ethylene glycol, heavy metals), cardiotoxicity (calcium channel blockers, digoxin), and neurotoxicity (isoniazid, organophosphates). Specialized interventions include hyperinsulinemia-euglycemia therapy for calcium channel blocker toxicity, sodium bicarbonate for tricyclic antidepressant cardiotoxicity, and lipid emulsion therapy for local anesthetic toxicity. Continuous monitoring ranges from basic vital signs to advanced parameters including continuous ECG monitoring with focus on QRS and QT intervals, capnography for ventilation assessment, invasive hemodynamic monitoring in severe cardiotoxicity, and serial laboratory studies targeted to the specific toxin. Toxin-specific parameters include anion gap and osmolal gap in toxic alcohol ingestions, cholinesterase levels in organophosphate exposures, and methemoglobin levels with oxidizing agents. Documentation includes the clinical presentation, interventions performed, response to treatment, consultation with poison centers or toxicologists, laboratory findings, and disposition decisions, which range from brief observation to intensive care unit admission based on toxin characteristics, exposure severity, and anticipated clinical course.

Self-Assessment Questions

1. Describe the key airway management considerations in acutely poisoned patients, including indications for early intubation and special concerns with specific toxins.
2. Analyze how different toxins affect vital signs, creating patterns that aid in early recognition and management when the specific agent is unknown.
3. Explain the pathophysiology, recognition, and management approach to sodium channel blockade in tricyclic antidepressant overdose, including the role of sodium bicarbonate therapy.
4. Describe the approach to managing severe hypotension in calcium channel blocker overdose, including conventional therapies and high-dose insulin-euglycemia therapy.
5. Discuss the indications, contraindications, and implementation of extracorporeal membrane oxygenation (ECMO) in toxic cardiac arrest or severe cardiotoxicity.
6. Analyze the approach to seizure management in toxin-induced seizures, with specific considerations for isoniazid, tricyclic antidepressants, and withdrawal states.
7. Explain the significance and management of specific laboratory abnormalities in poisoned patients, including elevated anion gap, osmolal gap, and methemoglobinemia.
8. Describe the essential components of toxicology documentation in the emergency setting and how this documentation supports both ongoing clinical care and potential legal proceedings.
9. Discuss the approach to the undifferentiated poisoned patient, including initial diagnostic considerations, empiric therapies, and early management priorities.
10. Analyze the criteria for safe discharge, observation unit admission, general ward admission, or intensive care unit admission following toxic exposures, with specific examples of toxins in each category.

Bibliography

1. Nelson LS, Hoffman RS, Howland MA, Lewin NA, Goldfrank LR. Goldfrank's toxicologic emergencies. 11th ed. New York: McGraw Hill; 2019.
2. Howland MA, Smith SW, Lewin NA, Hoffman RS, Goldfrank LR, Flomenbaum NE. Antidotes in depth. In: Goldfrank's toxicologic emergencies. 10th ed. New York: McGraw-Hill Education; 2015. p. 457-1532.
3. Holstege CP, Eldridge DL, Rowden AK. ECG manifestations: the poisoned patient. Emerg Med Clin North Am. 2006;24(1):159-177.
4. Kirk MA, Baer AB. Toxicology secrets: questions and answers you need to succeed on the clinical rotations. Philadelphia, PA: Hanley & Belfus; 2001.
5. Cole JB, Stellpflug SJ, Ellsworth H, Harris CR. A blinded, randomized, controlled trial of three doses of high-dose insulin in poison-induced cardiogenic shock. Clin Toxicol (Phila). 2013;51(4):201-207.
6. Bebarta VS, Kao L, Froberg B, Clark RF, Lavonas E, Qi M, et al. A multicenter comparison of the safety of oral versus intravenous acetylcysteine for treatment of acetaminophen overdose. Clin Toxicol (Phila). 2010;48(5):424-430.
7. Betten DP, Vohra RB, Cook MD, Matteucci MJ, Clark RF. Antidote use in the critically ill poisoned patient. J Intensive Care Med. 2006;21(5):255-277.
8. Boyer EW, Shannon M. The serotonin syndrome. N Engl J Med. 2005;352(11):1112-1120.
9. Mokhlesi B, Leiken JB, Murray P, Corbridge TC. Adult toxicology in critical care: part I: general approach to the intoxicated patient. Chest. 2003;123(2):577-592.
10. Greene S, Harris C, Singer J. Gastrointestinal decontamination of the poisoned patient. Pediatr Emerg Care. 2008;24(3):176-186.

CHAPTER 7

PHARMACEUTICAL TOXICITY

Author

Mrs. Rohini Koratana, Assistant Professor, Department of Pharmacology, Sultan-ul-Uloom College of Pharmacy, Banjara Hills, Hyderabad, Telangana, India

Abstract

Pharmaceutical agents represent the most common causes of poisoning, with both intentional overdoses and therapeutic misadventures contributing significantly to morbidity and mortality. Analgesic toxicity varies widely by class, with acetaminophen causing delayed hepatotoxicity through toxic metabolite formation, while salicylates produce complex acid-base disturbances, hyperthermia, and multi-organ dysfunction. Opioid overdose presents with the classic triad of respiratory depression, miosis, and decreased consciousness, requiring prompt naloxone administration. Cardiovascular medication poisonings include beta-blocker and calcium channel blocker overdoses characterized by bradycardia, hypotension, and cardiogenic shock, often requiring high-dose insulin-euglycemia therapy or lipid emulsion treatment. Digoxin toxicity manifests with gastrointestinal symptoms, visual disturbances, and cardiac dysrhythmias responsive to specific antibody fragments. Among psychiatric medications, tricyclic antidepressant overdoses can cause life-threatening sodium channel blockade with QRS widening and seizures, while SSRI toxicity ranges from mild serotonin excess to life-threatening serotonin syndrome. Lithium's narrow therapeutic index leads to neurological toxicity with tremor, altered mental status, and seizures. Antimicrobial toxicities include aminoglycoside ototoxicity and nephrotoxicity, fluoroquinolone tendinopathies, and sulfonamide hypersensitivity reactions. Management principles emphasize toxin-specific interventions alongside supportive care tailored to the pharmaceutical agent's unique toxicokinetics and toxicodynamics

Keywords: *Acetaminophen, Opioids, Cardiovascular Medications, Antidepressants, Antipsychotics, Antimicrobial Toxicity*

Learning Objectives

After completion of the chapter, the learners should be able to:

- Identify the clinical manifestations of acetaminophen toxicity and implement appropriate N-acetylcysteine therapy based on ingestion time and serum levels.
- Recognize and manage salicylate poisoning with particular attention to acid-base disturbances, enhanced elimination, and indications for hemodialysis.
- Evaluate cardiovascular medication toxicity including beta-blockers, calcium channel blockers, and digoxin, and implement appropriate treatment including antidotes and advanced cardiovascular support.
- Differentiate between various psychiatric medication overdoses based on clinical presentation and ECG findings, with emphasis on managing life-threatening complications.
- Apply specific treatment approaches for tricyclic antidepressant toxicity including sodium bicarbonate therapy and benzodiazepines for seizures.
- Recognize antimicrobial toxicities including hypersensitivity reactions, organ-specific adverse effects, and drug interactions requiring monitoring or intervention.

ANALGESICS

Analgesic medications represent among the most common agents involved in pharmaceutical poisonings, with diverse mechanisms creating varied toxicological syndromes requiring specific management approaches.

Acetaminophen

Acetaminophen (paracetamol) toxicity represents one of the most common pharmaceutical poisonings worldwide, with its ubiquity, narrow therapeutic index, and potential for severe hepatotoxicity creating significant public health impact. Normal therapeutic metabolism occurs predominantly through glucuronidation (50-60%) and sulfation (25-35%), with a minor pathway (5-10%) involving cytochrome P450 2E1 oxidation to the reactive metabolite N-acetyl-p-benzoquinone imine (NAPQI). This toxic metabolite normally undergoes rapid glutathione conjugation and elimination. In overdose, however, saturation of primary metabolic pathways shunts more acetaminophen through the CYP2E1 system, depleting glutathione stores and allowing NAPQI to form covalent bonds with hepatocellular proteins, leading to cellular death and potential liver failure.

Table 7.1: Analgesic Toxicity - Clinical Presentation and Management

Analgesic Class	Laboratory Abnormalities	Treatment Approach	Antidote
Acetaminophen	↑AST/ALT, ↑PT/INR, ↑bilirubin	Based on Rumack-Matthew nomogram	N-acetylcysteine
Salicylates	Mixed acid-base disorder, ↑anion gap	Alkalinization, fluid resuscitation, HD in severe cases	None specific
NSAIDs	↑Cr, ↑BUN, prolonged bleeding time	Supportive care, H_2 blockers or PPI	None
Opioids	Hypoxemia, hypercarbia	Airway management, ventilatory support	Naloxone
TCAs (used for pain)	ECG abnormalities	Sodium bicarbonate for cardiotoxicity	None specific

Clinical manifestations evolve through four characteristic stages. Stage 1 (0-24 hours) presents with nonspecific symptoms including nausea, vomiting, diaphoresis, and malaise, though many patients remain asymptomatic despite potentially toxic ingestions. Stage 2 (24-72 hours) demonstrates apparent improvement in gastrointestinal symptoms while hepatic injury develops subclinically, with rising transaminases and right upper quadrant pain sometimes emerging. Stage 3 (72-96 hours) marks peak hepatotoxicity, with potential progression to fulminant hepatic failure manifesting as jaundice, coagulopathy, hypoglycemia, encephalopathy, and multiorgan dysfunction. Stage 4 (4-14 days) involves either resolution with gradual normalization of hepatic function or death from complications of hepatic failure.

Diagnostic evaluation centers on serum acetaminophen level measurement and correlation with time since ingestion using the Rumack-Matthew nomogram. Blood sampling should occur at least 4 hours post-ingestion to allow complete absorption, with earlier levels potentially misleading due to ongoing absorption. The nomogram plots acetaminophen concentration against time, with the standard treatment line beginning at 150 μg/mL at 4 hours and declining with a 4-hour half-life to 4.7 μg/mL at 24 hours. Levels above this line indicate potential hepatotoxicity warranting antidotal therapy. Modified nomograms with lower treatment thresholds apply to high-risk patients including those with induced CYP2E1 activity from alcohol use, those taking enzyme-inducing medications, and those with glutathione depletion from malnutrition or HIV. Extended-release formulations, massive ingestions (>30 g), and co-ingestants affecting gastrointestinal motility may require additional level measurements to capture peak concentration adequately.

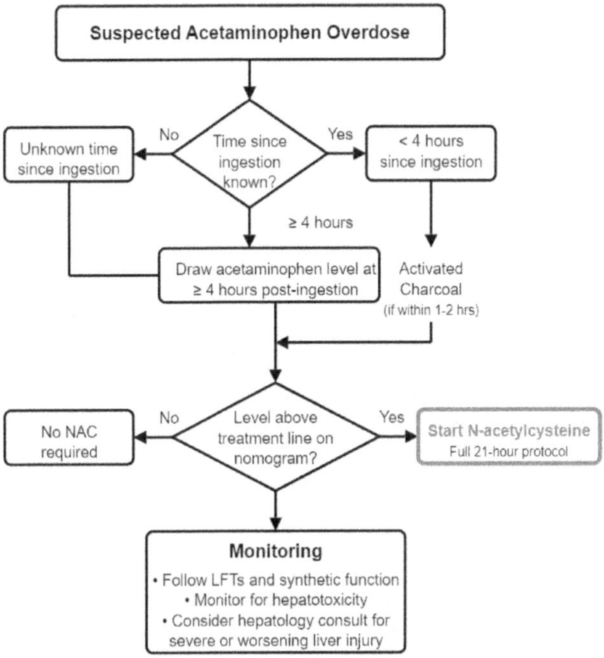

Figure 7.1: Acetaminophen Toxicity Management Algorithm

N-acetylcysteine (NAC) provides the definitive antidote for acetaminophen poisoning through multiple mechanisms: primarily replenishing glutathione stores, but also enhancing sulfation pathways, directly scavenging NAPQI, and providing anti-inflammatory and antioxidant effects that may reduce liver injury even after NAPQI formation. Oral administration follows a 72-hour protocol beginning with a loading dose of 140 mg/kg followed by 70 mg/kg every 4 hours for 17 additional doses. Intravenous administration employs a 21-hour protocol with 150 mg/kg over 60 minutes, followed by 50 mg/kg over 4 hours, and 100 mg/kg over 16 hours. Efficacy correlates strongly with early administration, approaching 100% hepatoprotection when initiated within 8 hours of ingestion but still providing benefit even in delayed presentations with established hepatotoxicity. Treatment indications include levels above the nomogram line, ingestions exceeding 150 mg/kg (or 7.5 g in adults) when levels cannot be obtained within 8 hours, evidence of hepatotoxicity, or concerning ingestions with unreliable history.

Remember

Acetaminophen toxicity causes predictable, dose-dependent hepatotoxicity through toxic metabolite formation, with N-acetylcysteine being highly effective when administered within 8-10 hours of ingestion but still beneficial even in delayed presentations

Management strategies beyond NAC administration include careful monitoring of hepatic synthetic function through serial prothrombin time/INR measurements, transaminases, bilirubin, albumin, and clinical assessments for encephalopathy development. Severe cases progressing to acute liver failure require intensive care management addressing potential complications including cerebral edema, coagulopathy, renal failure, hypoglycemia, and infection. Specific prognostic criteria including the King's College Criteria help identify patients who may benefit from liver transplantation evaluation, though decisions require careful consideration of intentionality assessment and psychiatric comorbidity when overdose was suicidal in nature. Prevention strategies include public education about acetaminophen presence in multiple over-the-counter preparations, blister packaging limiting quantity available, and placing antidotes in healthcare facilities serving remote locations with limited access to advanced care.

Nonsteroidal Anti-inflammatory Drugs

Nonsteroidal anti-inflammatory drugs (NSAIDs) includes a diverse medication class united by their inhibition of cyclooxygenase enzymes and resulting reduction in prostaglandin synthesis, with toxicological manifestations reflecting this mechanism alongside agent-specific effects. Most acute NSAID overdoses produce limited toxicity due to favorable safety profiles and relatively high therapeutic indices for most agents within this class. Significant exceptions include mefenamic acid, which can cause seizures in overdose, and phenylbutazone, associated with aplastic anemia and agranulocytosis even at therapeutic doses. Massive ingestions of even safer NSAIDs may produce serious toxicity, with ibuprofen ingestions exceeding 400 mg/kg sometimes causing severe metabolic acidosis, altered mental status, renal failure, and rarely cardiovascular collapse.

Gastrointestinal manifestations predominate in most NSAID toxicity presentations, reflecting both direct irritant effects and prostaglandin reduction impairing mucosal protective mechanisms. Symptoms typically include nausea, vomiting, epigastric pain, and occasionally gastrointestinal hemorrhage, particularly in patients with pre-existing ulcerative disease or concurrent anticoagulant use. Central nervous system effects remain generally limited to mild headache and dizziness at lower doses, though significant toxicity may produce lethargy, confusion, and rarely seizures, particularly with mefenamic acid or with severe acidosis complicating massive ibuprofen ingestions. Renal effects include acute kidney injury through multiple mechanisms: hemodynamically-mediated through prostaglandin inhibition reducing renal perfusion, acute interstitial nephritis representing hypersensitivity reactions, and rarely direct tubular toxicity.

Specific NSAID agents present unique toxicological considerations. Salicylates (discussed separately) create complex acid-base disturbances and multi-system toxicity distinct from other NSAIDs. Mefenamic acid demonstrates greater seizure risk in overdose, with convulsions sometimes occurring with ingestions just 3-5 times therapeutic doses. Phenylbutazone causes severe hematological toxicity including aplastic anemia, though rarely seen in contemporary practice due to limited clinical use. Ketorolac demonstrates particularly potent gastrointestinal toxicity, with bleeding risk substantially increased compared to most other NSAIDs. COX-2 selective inhibitors like celecoxib were initially developed to reduce gastrointestinal toxicity while maintaining anti-inflammatory efficacy, though subsequent recognition of cardiovascular risks has limited their use.

Management of NSAID overdoses generally employs supportive care addressing specific organ system effects without available antidotes. Gastrointestinal decontamination with activated charcoal may benefit patients presenting within 1-2 hours of significant ingestions, though generally unnecessary for minor overdoses. Intravenous fluid administration addresses potential dehydration from gastrointestinal losses while supporting renal perfusion. Acid-base monitoring identifies significant metabolic acidosis requiring intervention, most typically occurring with massive ibuprofen ingestions. Renal function requires monitoring with attention to fluid status, avoiding additional nephrotoxic agents, and occasionally temporary renal replacement therapy for significant acute kidney injury. Gastrointestinal bleeding management follows standard approaches including proton pump inhibitors, endoscopic intervention when indicated, and blood product support as needed.

Ibuprofen, the most commonly ingested NSAID, deserves specific consideration given its widespread availability and involvement in numerous overdoses. Acute toxicity severity correlates approximately with ingested amount: ingestions below 100 mg/kg typically produce minimal symptoms; doses between 100-400 mg/kg may cause significant gastrointestinal symptoms, mild central nervous system depression, and occasionally mild renal dysfunction; while ingestions exceeding 400 mg/kg risk severe toxicity with metabolic acidosis, seizures, coma, and cardiovascular depression. Anion gap metabolic acidosis represents a key marker of serious toxicity, with severe persistent acidosis despite appropriate bicarbonate therapy and fluid resuscitation indicating potential need for hemodialysis in extreme cases. Cardiovascular effects include myocardial depression and hypotension in severe overdoses, occasionally necessitating vasopressor support. Prognosis remains generally favorable even in significant overdoses when appropriate supportive care addresses complications.

Salicylates

Salicylate poisoning creates a distinctive toxidrome affecting multiple organ systems through mechanisms including direct cellular effects, uncoupling of oxidative phosphorylation, and complex acid-base disturbances. Sources include aspirin (acetylsalicylic acid) in various formulations, oil of wintergreen (methyl salicylate, with 1 teaspoon equivalent to approximately 7 g of aspirin), and various topical preparations. Toxicokinetics demonstrate notable complexities, including saturable protein binding causing disproportionate increases in free drug concentrations with rising levels, pH-dependent ionization affecting distribution (with decreased serum pH enhancing central nervous system penetration), and dose-dependent elimination kinetics leading to prolonged half-lives in severe toxicity.

Pathophysiology encompasses multiple mechanisms creating the characteristic clinical presentation. Direct stimulation of the medullary respiratory center produces respiratory alkalosis, typically the earliest acid-base disturbance. Uncoupling of oxidative phosphorylation increases metabolic demands while impairing ATP production, resulting in hyperthermia, hypoglycemia, and lactic acidosis. Enhanced lipolysis produces ketoacids contributing to the metabolic acidosis component. Direct irritant effects cause gastrointestinal symptoms and potential pulmonary injury. These combined processes create the classic mixed acid-base disturbance, with respiratory alkalosis predominating initially, followed by concurrent metabolic acidosis in moderate to severe poisonings as compensatory mechanisms become overwhelmed.

Clinical manifestations evolve from initial predominance of respiratory alkalosis with tachypnea, tinnitus, nausea, and vomiting, to more severe presentations including hyperthermia, altered mental status, non-cardiogenic pulmonary edema, coagulopathy, renal failure, and seizures. Chronic toxicity presents differently from acute poisoning, often with more insidious onset of confusion, delirium, and metabolic findings without prominent early respiratory alkalosis or tinnitus, creating diagnostic challenges. Special population considerations include children's vulnerability to rapid deterioration from relatively smaller ingestions and the entity of Reye's syndrome, a rare but potentially fatal hepatic encephalopathy historically associated with aspirin administration during viral illnesses in children.

Diagnostic evaluation centers on serum salicylate level measurement interpreted in clinical context, as correlation between levels and symptoms varies considerably between individuals and exposures. The Done nomogram, which correlates salicylate levels with time since ingestion and toxicity severity, provides general guidance but requires cautious application due to limitations including enteric-coated or sustained-release formulations causing delayed peak levels, chronic toxicity having poorer correlation with measured concentrations, and significant individual variation in susceptibility. Comprehensive assessment includes arterial blood gas analysis demonstrating the characteristic acid-base disturbances, electrolytes revealing potential abnormalities (including hypokalemia from renal potassium wasting), glucose measurement addressing hypoglycemia risk, and renal and hepatic function evaluation. Additional studies based on clinical presentation may include coagulation studies, complete blood count, chest radiography for non-cardiogenic pulmonary edema, and neuroimaging when altered mental status etiology remains uncertain.

Management strategies address the complex pathophysiology through multiple interventions. Gastrointestinal decontamination with activated charcoal benefits patients presenting within 1-2 hours of ingestion, with multiple-dose regimens potentially valuable for enteric-coated preparations. Enhanced elimination through urinary alkalinization represents a cornerstone of treatment, with intravenous sodium bicarbonate administration targeting urine pH above 7.5-8.0, increasing ionization of salicylate in tubular fluid and dramatically reducing reabsorption. Hemodialysis provides definitive management for severe poisonings, with indications including levels exceeding 100 mg/dL in acute toxicity (lower thresholds for chronic exposures), severe acid-base disturbances refractory to conventional management, progressive clinical deterioration despite appropriate therapy, significant end-organ damage including pulmonary edema or central nervous system effects, and patients with impaired elimination capacity due to renal or hepatic dysfunction. Supportive care addresses hyperthermia, coagulopathy, pulmonary edema, dehydration, and electrolyte abnormalities through standard approaches. Particular attention to potassium repletion remains essential during alkalinization therapy due to enhanced renal potassium wasting.

Special management considerations include careful fluid management balancing dehydration correction against pulmonary edema risk, glucose monitoring with supplementation as needed, avoidance of excessive mechanical ventilation that might eliminate compensatory respiratory alkalosis, and recognition of potential drug interactions with salicylate-displacing medications. Prognosis correlates with toxicity severity, time to appropriate intervention, and pre-existing comorbidities, with overall mortality between 5-10% in significant poisonings despite optimal management. Fatal outcomes typically result from cerebral edema, cardiopulmonary failure, or multisystem complications in severely poisoned patients, particularly those with delayed recognition or treatment.

Opioid Analgesics

Opioid analgesic toxicity has emerged as a leading cause of poisoning mortality worldwide, with changing patterns reflecting both pharmaceutical prescribing practices and illicit drug market dynamics. The diverse opioid class includes naturally derived agents (morphine, codeine), semi-synthetic compounds (hydrocodone, oxycodone, heroin), synthetic agents (fentanyl, methadone, tramadol), and mixed agonist-antagonists (buprenorphine, pentazocine). These compounds produce toxicity through agonist activity primarily at μ-opioid receptors, with individual agents demonstrating variable additional effects at δ and κ receptors or non-opioid targets like serotonin and norepinephrine transporters or NMDA receptors.

The classic opioid toxidrome presents with the triad of miosis, respiratory depression, and central nervous system depression, though considerable variation exists based on specific agent, co-ingestants, tolerance status, and individual factors. Respiratory depression represents the primary life-threatening effect, resulting from decreased responsiveness of brainstem respiratory centers to carbon dioxide. This manifests as decreased respiratory rate and tidal volume, potentially progressing to apnea. Pupillary constriction occurs through parasympathetic effects, though may be absent with certain synthetic opioids or in severe hypoxia. Additional manifestations include decreased gastrointestinal motility causing constipation or ileus, urinary retention, histamine-mediated pruritus and flushing (with certain agents), hypotension through both direct vasodilation and bradycardia, and occasionally pulmonary edema through mechanisms not fully elucidated but potentially involving neurogenic pulmonary vascular permeability changes.

Specific opioid agents present unique toxicological considerations beyond the classic toxidrome. Methadone demonstrates significantly prolonged respiratory depression (24-48 hours) compared to most other opioids, along with distinctive QT prolongation creating torsades de pointes risk. Tramadol produces seizures through non-opioid mechanisms, particularly serotonin and norepinephrine reuptake inhibition, with convulsions sometimes occurring independent of significant opioid effects. Buprenorphine creates complex scenarios due to its partial agonist properties, high receptor affinity, and ceiling effect on respiratory depression when used alone, though this ceiling effect diminishes substantially with concurrent benzodiazepine or alcohol use. Fentanyl and its analogs demonstrate extreme potency (50-10,000 times morphine), creating both rapid-onset toxicity and management challenges including potential exposure risks to first responders and healthcare personnel through dermal or inhalational routes.

Contemporary challenges include high-potency synthetic opioids, adulterated street drugs, and extended-release formulations. Illicitly manufactured fentanyl and its analogs (carfentanil, acrylfentanyl, furanyl fentanyl) have increasingly contaminated heroin, counterfeit prescription tablets, and other drugs, creating extreme overdose risk for users unaware of their presence. Toxicity management complexities include rapid onset leaving minimal intervention time, extended duration requiring prolonged naloxone administration, and extreme potency potentially overwhelming standard naloxone dosing regimens. Extended-release pharmaceutical formulations create prolonged absorption and toxicity duration, sometimes exceeding naloxone's effective period and necessitating extended monitoring and repeated antagonist administration. Adulterated products containing multiple substances, including benzodiazepines, cocaine, or novel psychoactive substances, create complex mixed toxidromes requiring broader management approaches beyond opioid antagonism.

Management centers on respiratory support and opioid antagonism, with naloxone providing competitive μ-receptor blockade that reverses respiratory and central nervous system depression. Initial naloxone dosing typically begins at 0.4 mg intravenously in adults, with subsequent dose escalation to 2 mg and then potentially to 10 mg if needed for partial response, particularly with potent synthetic opioids. Alternative administration routes include intramuscular, subcutaneous, intranasal, and endotracheal, with intranasal delivery (2-4 mg) increasingly employed in community settings through commercially available devices. Naloxone's short half-life (30-90 minutes) relative to many opioids necessitates repeated dosing or continuous infusion (starting at two-thirds the effective bolus dose per hour) to maintain reversal with longer-acting agents. Potential complications include precipitation of withdrawal in opioid-dependent individuals, cardiovascular stress responses including hypertension and dysrhythmias, and pulmonary edema, though the latter more likely represents underlying toxicity unmasked by reversal rather than direct antagonist effect.

Supportive care focuses on airway management and respiratory support, with bag-valve-mask ventilation providing temporizing oxygenation and ventilation while naloxone administration is prepared. Additional measures address hypothermia, aspiration risk, rhabdomyolysis from prolonged immobility, and associated injuries. Decontamination plays limited role in most cases, though activated charcoal may benefit patients presenting within 1-2 hours of substantial oral ingestion, particularly with extended-release formulations. Public health approaches include expanded naloxone distribution to at-risk individuals and community members, prescription monitoring programs addressing inappropriate prescribing, medication-assisted treatment expanding access to opioid use disorder therapy, and drug checking services identifying high-risk adulterants in street drugs.

CARDIOVASCULAR DRUGS

Cardiovascular medications represent a significant source of pharmaceutical toxicity, with their narrow therapeutic indices, complex pharmacodynamics, and widespread use creating potential for severe poisoning with limited physiological reserve.

Table 7.2: Cardiovascular Medication Toxicity

Drug Class	Clinical Manifestations	Management Priorities
Beta-blockers	Bradycardia, hypotension, hypoglycemia, bronchospasm	Glucagon, calcium, high-dose insulin-euglycemia therapy
Calcium channel blockers	Bradycardia, hypotension, hyperglycemia, ileus	Calcium, high-dose insulin-euglycemia, vasopressors
Digoxin	Nausea, visual disturbances, dysrhythmias	Digoxin-specific antibody fragments for severe toxicity
ACE inhibitors/ARBs	Hypotension, hyperkalemia, renal insufficiency	Fluid resuscitation, vasopressors, dialysis for severe cases
Antidysrhythmics	Depends on class: bradycardia, QT prolongation, hypotension	Class-specific interventions, magnesium for torsades

Beta-Adrenergic Blockers

Beta-adrenergic blocker toxicity presents distinctive management challenges due to antagonism of physiological compensatory mechanisms normally employed in shock states. These agents competitively block β-adrenergic receptors with varying selectivity for β_1 (cardiac) versus β_2 (bronchial, vascular) subtypes. Cardioselective agents including metoprolol, atenolol, and esmolol demonstrate relative β_1 selectivity at therapeutic doses, though this selectivity diminishes in overdose. Non-selective agents including propranolol, nadolol, and timolol block both receptor subtypes, potentially producing bronchospasm and peripheral vasodilation in addition to cardiac effects. Additional pharmacological properties creating clinically relevant differences include lipophilicity (affecting blood-brain barrier penetration, with propranolol exhibiting high CNS penetration), intrinsic sympathomimetic activity (partial agonist effects at β-receptors, potentially moderating toxicity), membrane-stabilizing activity (sodium channel blockade producing quinidine-like effects, particularly with propranolol), and extended-release formulations (creating prolonged toxicity duration and delayed peak effects).

> **Remember**
>
> **Beta-blocker and calcium channel blocker overdoses cause significant cardiovascular toxicity through different but synergistic mechanisms, often requiring aggressive intervention including high-dose insulin-euglycemia therapy for refractory cases**

Clinical manifestations predominantly affect cardiovascular function through negative chronotropic, dromotropic, and inotropic effects. Bradycardia represents the hallmark finding, often proportional to ingested dose and potentially severe (heart rates below 40 beats per minute not uncommon in significant overdoses). Hypotension results from both reduced cardiac output and vasodilation through β_2-blockade eliminating compensatory vasoconstriction. Cardiovascular collapse may occur rapidly with minimal prodrome, particularly with highly lipophilic agents like propranolol. Conduction disturbances including atrioventricular blocks, intraventricular conduction delays, and occasionally asystole can occur independent of simple bradycardia. Central nervous system manifestations range from mild lethargy to seizures and coma, particularly with lipophilic agents crossing the blood-brain barrier. Hypoglycemia may result from impaired glycogenolysis and gluconeogenesis through β_2-receptor blockade. Bronchospasm affects primarily patients with underlying reactive airway disease, though may occur in previously asymptomatic individuals with non-selective agents. Unique agent-specific toxicities include potential sotalol-induced QT prolongation through additional potassium channel blocking effects.

Diagnostic evaluation begins with electrocardiographic assessment demonstrating bradycardia, PR prolongation, QRS widening (particularly with agents possessing membrane-stabilizing activity), and occasionally QT prolongation. Hemodynamic evaluation through blood pressure monitoring, assessment of end-organ perfusion, and sometimes advanced parameters like central venous pressure or echocardiography guides both severity assessment and therapeutic intervention. Laboratory studies include electrolytes, renal function, glucose monitoring, and arterial blood gas analysis assessing for metabolic acidosis indicative of tissue hypoperfusion. Specific beta-blocker levels rarely provide clinical utility due to limited availability, long turnaround times, and poor correlation with toxicity severity. Toxicological screening may identify co-ingestants affecting management approaches, particularly calcium channel blockers or other cardioactive substances.

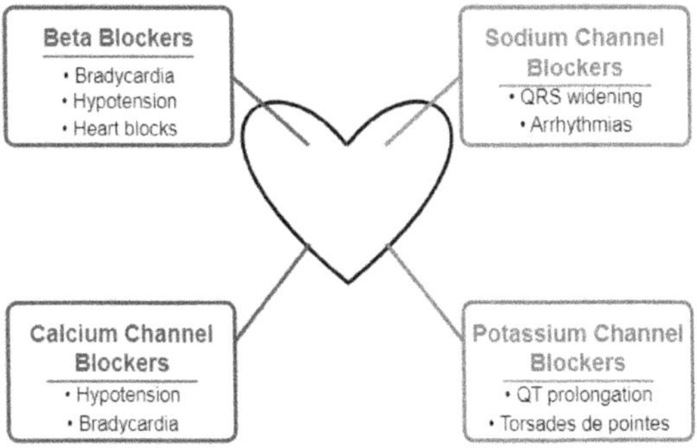

Management

Beta Blockers:	Glucagon, high-dose insulin-euglycemia
CCBs:	Calcium, high-dose insulin-euglycemia, lipid
Na+ Channel Blockers:	Sodium bicarbonate (target pH 7.45-7.55)
K+ Channel Blockers:	Magnesium, isoproterenol, overdrive pacing

Figure 7.2: Cardiotoxic Drug Effects and Management

Management strategies address the complex pathophysiology, with approaches extending beyond conventional resuscitation paradigms. Initial interventions include comprehensive supportive care with airway management, supplemental oxygen, and intravenous access. Gastrointestinal decontamination with activated charcoal may benefit patients presenting within 1-2 hours of ingestion, with extended windows sometimes appropriate for sustained-release formulations. Atropine addresses bradycardia through vagolytic effects but typically demonstrates limited efficacy in significant beta-blocker poisoning where direct cardiac effects predominate rather than vagally-mediated bradycardia. Glucagon, administered as 5-10 mg intravenous bolus followed by infusion at 1-5 mg/hour, activates adenylate cyclase through a non-beta-receptor-mediated pathway, increasing myocardial cAMP and potentially improving heart rate and contractility. This effect often proves transient due to tachyphylaxis, requiring dose escalation or additional therapies.

High-dose insulin euglycemia therapy (HIET) has emerged as a cornerstone of severe beta-blocker toxicity management, addressing the fundamental pathophysiology through multiple mechanisms: improved cardiac glucose utilization, positive inotropic effects, and peripheral vasodilation improving tissue perfusion. Protocol typically begins with regular insulin bolus of 1 unit/kg followed by infusion starting at 0.5-1 unit/kg/hour, titrated up to 10 units/kg/hour in severe cases, with concurrent dextrose administration maintaining euglycemia. Close monitoring includes frequent glucose measurements (every 30 minutes initially), potassium levels addressing potential hypokalemia, and hemodynamic parameters guiding dose titration. Clinical response may require 30-60 minutes to manifest, necessitating patience before concluding treatment failure. Additional pharmacological approaches include calcium administration (1-2 g calcium chloride or 2-4 g calcium gluconate) potentially opposing the negative inotropic effects, vasopressors (epinephrine, norepinephrine) providing chronotropic and inotropic support, phosphodiesterase inhibitors like milrinone increasing cardiac cAMP levels through reduced degradation rather than increased production, and sodium bicarbonate addressing QRS prolongation when present due to membrane-stabilizing activity.

Refractory cases may necessitate mechanical circulatory support, with intra-aortic balloon pumps providing afterload reduction and coronary perfusion enhancement, and venoarterial extracorporeal membrane oxygenation (VA-ECMO) offering complete cardiopulmonary support during profound cardiovascular collapse. Case series demonstrate impressive survival rates exceeding 80% with VA-ECMO implementation for severe beta-blocker poisonings unresponsive to maximal pharmacological intervention, emphasizing the importance of early consideration and consultation with centers capable of providing this resource. Enhanced elimination techniques including hemodialysis demonstrate limited utility for most beta-blockers due to large volumes of distribution and high protein binding, though may benefit specific agents like atenolol with more favorable elimination characteristics. Particular attention to extended observation periods remains essential with sustained-release formulations, which may demonstrate delayed toxicity onset and prolonged duration requiring extended supportive care and monitoring.

Calcium Channel Blockers

Calcium channel blocker poisoning represents among the most lethal pharmaceutical overdoses, with mortality rates approaching 10% despite optimal management. These agents inhibit voltage-dependent L-type calcium channels, reducing calcium influx during depolarization and subsequently decreasing intracellular calcium availability. Dihydropyridines (amlodipine, nifedipine, felodipine) predominantly affect vascular smooth muscle, producing vasodilation with limited cardiac effects at therapeutic doses, though this selectivity diminishes in overdose. Non-dihydropyridines including verapamil and diltiazem demonstrate greater cardiac effects, with significant negative chronotropy, dromotropy, and inotropy at both therapeutic and toxic doses. Toxicokinetic considerations include substantial first-pass metabolism for most agents, extensive protein binding, large volumes of distribution limiting extracorporeal removal, and sustained-release formulations creating prolonged absorption and delayed peak toxicity, sometimes exceeding 24 hours after ingestion.

Pathophysiological mechanisms extend beyond simple cardiovascular depression, incorporating complex metabolic derangements with substantial management implications. Direct cardiac effects include decreased sinoatrial node automaticity, atrioventricular conduction impairment, and reduced myocardial contractility through diminished excitation-contraction coupling. Vascular smooth muscle relaxation produces peripheral vasodilation and decreased systemic vascular resistance. Pancreatic calcium channel blockade inhibits insulin release, creating insulin resistance and hyperglycemia characteristic of significant poisonings. The combination of hypoinsulinemia, insulin resistance, and impaired myocardial glucose utilization creates an "energy crisis" where cardiomyocytes cannot access needed glucose despite hyperglycemia, explaining the apparent paradox of hyperglycemia in shock states that normally produce hypoglycemia through stress responses.

Clinical manifestations vary based on specific agent, dose, formulation, and individual factors. Hemodynamic effects include hypotension, which may be profound and refractory to conventional vasopressors, particularly with dihydropyridines where peripheral vasodilation predominates. Bradycardia and conduction disturbances occur more prominently with non-dihydropyridines like verapamil and diltiazem, though may develop with any agent in severe overdose. Cardiovascular collapse may evolve rapidly or develop insidiously over hours, especially with sustained-release preparations creating a false sense of security during early evaluation. Metabolic abnormalities include hyperglycemia resulting from impaired insulin release and metabolic acidosis reflecting tissue hypoperfusion. Neurological manifestations range from mild lethargy to seizures and coma in severe toxicity, reflecting both hypoperfusion and direct central nervous system effects of some agents. Pulmonary edema may develop through multiple mechanisms including myocardial dysfunction, altered capillary permeability, and precapillary vasodilation.

Diagnostic evaluation begins with electrocardiographic assessment demonstrating bradycardia, PR prolongation, various degrees of heart block, and occasionally junctional or idioventricular rhythms in severe poisoning. Hemodynamic monitoring includes continuous arterial pressure measurement when available, assessment of perfusion through mental status, urine output, and peripheral perfusion, and often central venous pressure monitoring guiding volume status management. Echocardiography provides valuable assessment of ventricular function, filling status, and response to interventions. Laboratory evaluation includes electrolytes, renal function, glucose (with hyperglycemia serving as both diagnostic clue and severity marker), arterial blood gas analysis assessing acid-base status, and calcium levels (though serum calcium typically remains normal despite functional deficiency at the cellular level). Specific calcium channel blocker levels rarely provide clinical utility due to limited availability and poor correlation with clinical severity.

Management approaches address the complex underlying pathophysiology rather than simply targeting presenting vital sign abnormalities. Initial stabilization includes airway management, oxygen supplementation, and establishment of reliable vascular access, ideally including central venous access in significant poisonings. Gastrointestinal decontamination with activated charcoal benefits patients presenting within 1-2 hours of ingestion, with whole bowel irrigation potentially valuable for sustained-release preparations when presenting within 4-6 hours. Calcium administration (calcium chloride 1 g or calcium gluconate 3 g intravenously, repeated every 15-20 minutes for 3-4 doses) attempts to overcome channel blockade by increasing the concentration gradient driving calcium entry, though clinical response often remains limited in significant poisonings. Atropine addresses bradycardia through vagolytic effects but typically demonstrates minimal efficacy when negative chronotropy results primarily from direct calcium channel blockade rather than vagal mechanisms.

High-dose insulin euglycemia therapy (HIET) has revolutionized calcium channel blocker poisoning management, addressing both cardiac dysfunction and peripheral vascular resistance through multiple mechanisms: improved cardiac glucose utilization overcoming the calcium-channel-blocker-induced energy failure, direct positive inotropic effects independent of calcium flux, and vasodilation improving microcirculation. Protocol typically begins with regular insulin bolus of 1 unit/kg followed by infusion starting at 0.5-1 unit/kg/hour, titrated up to 10 units/kg/hour based on hemodynamic response, with concurrent dextrose administration maintaining euglycemia. Response assessment includes hemodynamic parameters, vasopressor requirement reduction, and metabolic improvement including reduced lactate levels. Frequent glucose monitoring (every 20-30 minutes initially, then hourly when stable) and potassium assessment prevent hypoglycemia and hypokalemia complications.

Vasopressor and inotrope selection addresses the underlying pathophysiology, with epinephrine or norepinephrine typically preferred for initial support given their combined inotropic and vasopressor effects. Vasopressin (0.01-0.04 units/minute) provides additional benefit through non-catecholamine-dependent vasoconstriction that bypasses the calcium-dependent mechanisms blocked by the toxicant. Phosphodiesterase inhibitors like milrinone increase intracellular cAMP, potentially improving contractility through mechanisms less dependent on calcium channel function. Lipid emulsion therapy (1.5 mL/kg 20% lipid emulsion bolus followed by 0.25 mL/kg/minute infusion) may benefit selected patients through proposed mechanisms including lipid sink sequestration of lipophilic calcium channel blockers, enhanced cardiac energy substrate availability, and direct inotropic effects.

Refractory cases may require mechanical circulatory support, with venoarterial extracorporeal membrane oxygenation (VA-ECMO) providing definitive management for profound cardiovascular collapse unresponsive to pharmacological interventions. Case series demonstrate survival exceeding 75% with ECMO implementation despite initial refractory shock, emphasizing the importance of early consideration and transfer to capable centers when managing potentially severe calcium channel blocker poisonings. Continuous renal replacement therapy provides minimal enhancement of calcium channel blocker elimination due to large volumes of distribution and high protein binding but may address associated metabolic derangements and fluid management. Methylene blue (1-2 mg/kg) represents an investigational approach potentially addressing distributive components of shock through nitric oxide pathway modulation. Observation duration must account for sustained-release preparations, with monitoring typically continuing at least 24 hours after clinical stabilization and resolution of all toxicity manifestations.

Cardiac Glycosides

Cardiac glycoside poisoning creates distinctive toxicological challenges incorporating both direct cardiotoxicity and critical electrolyte derangements. These compounds, derived traditionally from plants including foxglove (Digitalis species), lily of the valley (Convallaria majalis), and oleander (Nerium oleander), share a core mechanism of sodium-potassium ATPase inhibition, though with varying potencies, pharmacokinetics, and additional properties. Digoxin represents the most commonly encountered pharmaceutical preparation, while acute poisonings increasingly involve botanicals used in traditional medicine, ornamental plants ingested accidentally, and intentional exposures to concentrated plant extracts. Toxicokinetic considerations include narrow therapeutic windows, extensive tissue distribution, variable protein binding, and elimination predominantly through renal excretion for digoxin compared to hepatic metabolism for many plant-derived glycosides.

Pathophysiological mechanisms involve complex cellular effects extending beyond simple enzyme inhibition. Sodium-potassium ATPase blockade increases intracellular sodium concentration, subsequently reducing the sodium gradient driving the sodium-calcium exchanger and ultimately increasing intracellular calcium. This calcium excess enhances myocardial contractility at therapeutic doses while potentially causing arrhythmogenesis and cellular injury in overdose. Additional mechanisms include enhanced vagal tone producing atrioventricular conduction slowing, altered baroreceptor function, and direct central nervous system effects through both central sodium-potassium ATPase inhibition and cerebral ischemia secondary to dysrhythmias. Electrolyte abnormalities, particularly hyperkalemia resulting from extracellular potassium shift as intracellular sodium rises, create additional complications independently increasing mortality risk.

Clinical manifestations encompass cardiovascular, neurological, gastrointestinal, and metabolic effects with considerable individual variation. Cardiac features represent the predominant life-threatening concerns, with dysrhythmias including sinus bradycardia, sinoatrial block, atrioventricular conduction disturbances, atrial tachyarrhythmias with block, junctional ectopy, ventricular ectopy, bidirectional ventricular tachycardia (a relatively specific finding), and ventricular fibrillation. The classic aphorism "digitalis creates every arrhythmia except rapid atrial fibrillation" captures this diversity while highlighting the paradoxical slowing of atrial fibrillation characteristic of therapeutic effect. Gastrointestinal symptoms including nausea, vomiting, and abdominal pain often precede cardiac manifestations, occasionally creating diagnostic confusion with primary gastrointestinal illnesses. Neurological effects encompass altered color perception with characteristic yellow-green distortion (xanthopsia), peripheral visual field disturbances, confusion, hallucinations, and seizures. Hyperkalemia represents both a marker of toxicity severity and an independent contributor to dysrhythmia risk and mortality.

Diagnostic evaluation integrates clinical assessment with laboratory and electrocardiographic findings. Serum digoxin concentration measurement, ideally collected at least 6 hours post-ingestion to allow distribution completion, provides important management guidance. Therapeutic concentrations typically range from 0.8-2.0 ng/mL, with toxicity risk increasing substantially above this range, though considerable overlap exists between therapeutic and toxic ranges in chronic therapy. Acute ingestions typically demonstrate higher concentration thresholds for toxicity, with levels exceeding 10 ng/mL generally indicating severe poisoning risk. Important caveats include certain immunoassays cross-reacting with endogenous digoxin-like immunoreactive substances in renal failure, pregnancy, or hepatic dysfunction, potentially creating false elevations. Electrocardiography reveals characteristic findings including PR prolongation, QT shortening, ST segment "scooping" depression, T wave inversion, and various dysrhythmias previously described. Comprehensive metabolic assessment includes electrolytes (with particular attention to potassium, calcium, and magnesium affecting cardiac stability), renal function, and acid-base status.

Management strategies address both direct cardiotoxicity and associated metabolic derangements. Initial approaches include discontinuation of the offending agent, continuous cardiac monitoring, and establishment of reliable vascular access. Gastrointestinal decontamination with activated charcoal benefits patients presenting within 1-2 hours of acute ingestion. Hyperkalemia management follows standard protocols with calcium administration, insulin-glucose therapy, sodium bicarbonate, and potassium-binding resins, though with recognition that correction may occur rapidly with specific antidote administration. Bradyarrhythmia management employs atropine, temporary pacing when necessary, and addressing hyperkalemia which often exacerbates conduction disturbances. Magnesium sulfate (2 g intravenously) may reduce ventricular ectopy, though with careful monitoring in renal insufficiency. Class Ib antiarrhythmics like lidocaine may address ventricular dysrhythmias with less proarrhythmic risk than many alternatives.

Digoxin-specific antibody fragments (Fab) provide definitive treatment through neutralizing circulating digoxin molecules, with indications including life-threatening dysrhythmias, progressive bradycardia unresponsive to atropine, serum potassium exceeding 5.5 mEq/L, and digoxin level above 10 ng/mL in acute overdose. Dosing employs either empiric administration based on clinical scenario (typically 5-10 vials in life-threatening cases) or calculated dosing based on serum concentration or estimated ingested amount. Each vial binds approximately 0.5 mg of digoxin, with 38 mg of plant-derived cardenolides equating to approximately 0.5 mg digoxin for calculation purposes. Response typically occurs within 30-60 minutes, with most patients demonstrating significant improvement within 4 hours. Potential complications include allergic reactions (less common with fragments than whole antibodies), hypokalemia from rapid intracellular potassium shift as sodium-potassium ATPase function restores, and returning digitalis toxicity as fragments are eliminated before the redistributed digoxin in severe poisonings. Cross-reactivity with non-digoxin cardiac glycosides varies, with better neutralization of structurally similar compounds like digitoxin compared to more distantly related plant glycosides.

Plant-derived cardiac glycoside poisonings present additional challenges including uncertain concentration in biological materials, potential presence of multiple active compounds with varying properties, limited cross-reactivity with digoxin-specific Fab for some compounds, and often delayed presentation after initial symptoms are attributed to other causes. Management follows similar principles as pharmaceutical digoxin poisoning, with Fab administration remaining appropriate despite variable cross-reactivity, as even partial neutralization may provide hemodynamic improvement. Supportive care often requires more prolonged implementation due to extended elimination of certain plant compounds compared to digoxin. Prognosis remains generally favorable with appropriate intervention, though mortality approaching 30% has been reported in severe untreated poisonings, particularly when complicated by significant hyperkalemia or delayed recognition.

Antiarrhythmics and Antihypertensives

Antiarrhythmic medications create complex toxicological scenarios through their intended effects on cardiac electrophysiology, with Vaughan Williams classification providing a framework for understanding toxicity mechanisms and management approaches. Class Ia agents (quinidine, procainamide, disopyramide) block fast sodium channels, prolonging depolarization and creating QRS widening in overdose, along with QT prolongation through potassium channel effects. Management parallels other sodium channel blockers, with sodium bicarbonate (1-2 mEq/kg boluses) narrowing QRS complex through both sodium load and alkalinization effects. Class Ib agents (lidocaine, mexiletine) demonstrate less significant QRS widening but produce seizures and myocardial depression in overdose. Class Ic medications (flecainide, propafenone) create pronounced sodium channel blockade with minimal compensatory potassium channel effects, resulting in severe conduction disturbances, QRS widening, and refractory ventricular arrhythmias in overdose. Management includes aggressive sodium bicarbonate administration, consideration of hypertonic sodium solutions in refractory cases, and potential lipid emulsion therapy given the high lipophilicity of these agents.

Class II antiarrhythmics (beta-blockers) produce toxicity profiles and management approaches discussed previously. Class III agents (amiodarone, sotalol, dofetilide) block potassium channels, prolonging repolarization and extending QT interval with risk for torsades de pointes. Amiodarone demonstrates additional sodium and calcium channel effects, creating complex mixed toxicity with both bradyarrhythmias and QT prolongation, while its extremely long half-life (up to 60 days with chronic use) necessitates extended monitoring. Sotalol combines potassium channel blockade with beta-blocking properties, creating risk for both bradycardia and torsades de pointes. Management includes magnesium sulfate administration for torsades risk, temporary overdrive pacing when indicated, aggressive electrolyte correction maintaining potassium and magnesium in high-normal ranges, and avoidance of other QT-prolonging medications. Class IV agents (calcium channel blockers) follow management principles previously discussed.

Antihypertensive medications beyond beta-blockers and calcium channel blockers include multiple classes with diverse toxicological implications. Angiotensin-converting enzyme (ACE) inhibitors and angiotensin receptor blockers (ARBs) typically produce limited acute toxicity, with hypotension representing the predominant concern through interference with the renin-angiotensin-aldosterone system. Management includes fluid resuscitation and vasopressors when necessary, preferably norepinephrine or vasopressin, which function through mechanisms independent of the blocked renin-angiotensin system. Significant hypotension typically resolves within 4-6 hours given the relatively short duration of effect for most agents in this class.

Alpha-adrenergic antagonists, including peripheral agents like prazosin and doxazosin and centrally acting agents like clonidine, create hypotension through vasodilation and decreased sympathetic outflow respectively. Clonidine and similar imidazoline agents produce a distinctive toxidrome mimicking opioid poisoning, with miosis, central nervous system depression, bradycardia, and hypotension, though without response to naloxone. Management includes fluid resuscitation and alpha-adrenergic agonists, with higher dosing requirements due to receptor blockade by the toxicant. Phenylephrine provides particular benefit for peripheral alpha-blockers due to its selective alpha-1 agonism counteracting the primary mechanism of toxicity.

Diuretic overdose creates fluid and electrolyte abnormalities with severity related to specific agent properties. Loop diuretics (furosemide, bumetanide) produce volume depletion, hypokalemia, hypomagnesemia, hypocalcemia, and metabolic alkalosis, with management focusing on fluid and electrolyte repletion. Thiazide diuretics demonstrate similar though typically less severe effects, with additional risk for hyperglycemia through pancreatic effects. Potassium-sparing diuretics, particularly spironolactone and eplerenone, may cause hyperkalemia, especially in patients with renal insufficiency or concurrent medications affecting potassium handling. Severe hyperkalemia management follows standard protocols including calcium administration, insulin-glucose therapy, sodium bicarbonate, potassium-binding resins, and hemodialysis when indicated.

Vasodilators including hydralazine, minoxidil, and nitrates produce hypotension through direct vascular smooth muscle relaxation. Nitrate toxicity additionally creates methemoglobinemia through oxidation of hemoglobin iron, presenting with cyanosis unresponsive to oxygen supplementation, chocolate-brown blood, and pulse oximetry readings around 85% regardless of actual oxygenation. Diagnosis relies on co-oximetry or blood gas analysis specifically measuring methemoglobin percentage, with management including methylene blue (1-2 mg/kg intravenously) for symptomatic patients or levels exceeding 20-30%. Hydralazine rarely produces a delayed lupus-like syndrome with chronic use, though this seldom accompanies acute overdose.

General management principles for cardiovascular medication poisonings include recognition of potential delayed toxicity with extended-release formulations, anticipatory preparation for clinical deterioration even when initial presentation appears benign, consideration of multiple-drug ingestions common in both intentional and therapeutic misadventure scenarios, and heightened vigilance for patients with limited cardiovascular reserve due to pre-existing conditions. Prognosis generally depends on time to appropriate intervention, specific agent properties, ingested quantity, patient comorbidities, and availability of advanced supportive care including mechanical circulatory support for refractory cases.

PSYCHIATRIC MEDICATIONS

Psychiatric medication toxicity creates distinctive management challenges related to their diverse pharmacological properties, frequency in intentional overdoses, and potential for delayed or prolonged effects requiring extended monitoring and intervention.

Antidepressants

Tricyclic antidepressants (TCAs) remain among the most dangerous medications in overdose despite declining prescribing frequency, with mortality rates approaching 3-5% even with optimal management. Their complex pharmacology produces toxicity through multiple mechanisms: anticholinergic effects (muscarinic receptor antagonism), cardiovascular toxicity (sodium channel blockade, alpha-adrenergic blockade, catecholamine reuptake inhibition), seizure generation (lowered seizure threshold through unclear mechanisms), and serotonin toxicity (serotonin reuptake inhibition). Specific agents demonstrate variable potencies for these different mechanisms, with amitriptyline and dothiepin among the most anticholinergic and cardiotoxic, while clomipramine demonstrates greater serotonergic properties. Toxicokinetics include high lipophilicity creating large volumes of distribution, extensive protein binding limiting enhanced elimination options, and enterohepatic recirculation potentially extending toxicity duration.

> **Remember**
>
> **Tricyclic antidepressant overdose presents with anticholinergic effects, seizures, and life-threatening sodium channel blockade causing QRS prolongation and ventricular dysrhythmias, with sodium bicarbonate as the cornerstone of cardiotoxicity management**

Clinical manifestations typically develop rapidly, with significant toxicity often apparent within 1-2 hours of ingestion. Cardiovascular effects represent the predominant life-threatening concerns, with conduction disturbances (prolonged QRS and QT intervals), ventricular dysrhythmias, and hypotension creating high mortality risk. The anticholinergic toxidrome includes hyperthermia, mydriasis, dry mucous membranes, urinary retention, reduced bowel sounds, and altered mental status ranging from agitation to delirium and coma. Seizures occur in approximately 10-30% of significant overdoses, often preceding cardiovascular collapse. Distinctive toxicokinetic patterns include apparent clinical improvement followed by sudden deterioration as the toxicant redistributes between central and peripheral compartments, necessitating extended monitoring even when initial stabilization occurs.

Diagnostic evaluation focuses on electrocardiographic abnormalities providing both diagnostic and prognostic information. QRS prolongation beyond 100 ms suggests sodium channel blockade, with durations exceeding 160 ms associated with significantly increased risk for ventricular dysrhythmias. Terminal 40 ms rightward axis deviation in aVR, manifesting as an R wave or R' deflection, represents a relatively specific finding for cyclic antidepressant toxicity. Additional electrocardiographic findings include sinus tachycardia, atrioventricular block, QT prolongation, and ventricular dysrhythmias. Laboratory assessment includes comprehensive metabolic profile, arterial blood gas analysis for acid-base disturbances potentiating cardiotoxicity, and consideration of co-ingestants through appropriate toxicological screening.

Management employs both supportive care and specific interventions addressing sodium channel blockade.

Table 7.3: Psychiatric Medication Toxicity Patterns

Medication Class	Toxic Manifestations	Interventions	Complications to Anticipate
SSRIs	Usually mild; nausea, sedation, tremor, serotonin syndrome in severe cases	Supportive care, benzodiazepines, cyproheptadine for serotonin syndrome	Serotonin syndrome with multiple serotonergic agents
TCAs	Anticholinergic effects, QRS prolongation, CNS depression, seizures	Sodium bicarbonate for QRS >100ms, benzodiazepines for seizures	Delayed cardiotoxicity up to 24 hours
Lithium	Tremor, ataxia, altered mental status, seizures	IV fluids, hemodialysis for severe toxicity	Chronic toxicity more neurotoxic than acute
Antipsychotics	QT prolongation, extrapyramidal symptoms, sedation, hypotension	Benzodiazepines for agitation, magnesium for QT prolongation	Temperature dysregulation, NMS risk
Benzodiazepines	CNS depression, respiratory depression, ataxia	Supportive care, flumazenil (with caution)	Withdrawal risk with chronic use
Bupropion	Seizures, tachycardia, agitation, hallucinations	Benzodiazepines, anticonvulsants	Delayed-release preparations may cause prolonged toxicity

Gastrointestinal decontamination with activated charcoal benefits patients presenting within 1-2 hours of ingestion, with some evidence suggesting extended benefit given the anticholinergic effects potentially delaying gastric emptying. Sodium bicarbonate administration represents the cornerstone of cardiotoxicity management, with 1-2 mEq/kg boluses followed by continuous infusion targeting serum pH 7.5-7.55. This intervention narrows QRS complex width through multiple proposed mechanisms: increased extracellular sodium gradient overcoming channel blockade, alkalinization altering toxicant-receptor interactions, increased protein binding of the toxicant, and altered drug distribution. Refractory cases may benefit from hypertonic sodium solutions, though with careful attention to volume status.

Hypotension management addresses the complex underlying mechanisms, with fluid resuscitation targeting preload reduction from alpha-blockade, followed by direct-acting vasopressors (norepinephrine, epinephrine) for persistent hypotension. Pure alpha-agonists like phenylephrine may prove less effective due to the mixed alpha-blocking and cardiac-depressant properties of the toxicant. Seizure management employs benzodiazepines as first-line therapy, with phenobarbital or propofol for refractory seizures, avoiding phenytoin which may worsen sodium channel blockade. Dysrhythmia management focuses on correcting underlying abnormalities (acidosis, hypoxemia, electrolyte derangements) while maintaining alkalinization, with standard antiarrhythmics generally avoided due to potential exacerbation of conduction abnormalities. Refractory ventricular dysrhythmias may necessitate overdrive pacing or magnesium administration. Mechanical circulatory support including venoarterial extracorporeal membrane oxygenation provides rescue therapy for refractory cardiovascular collapse, with case reports demonstrating successful outcomes despite initial cardiopulmonary resuscitation requirements.

Selective serotonin reuptake inhibitors (SSRIs) demonstrate significantly improved safety profiles compared to tricyclic antidepressants, though particular toxicological concerns remain. Serotonin syndrome represents the principal life-threatening complication, particularly with co-ingestants possessing serotonergic properties, manifesting with the triad of autonomic instability, neuromuscular abnormalities (hyperreflexia, clonus, rigidity), and altered mental status. QT prolongation occurs with certain agents, particularly citalopram and escitalopram, with risk for torsades de pointes in substantial overdoses. Seizures occur less frequently than with TCAs but remain possible, particularly with citalopram at higher doses. Management includes gastrointestinal decontamination when presenting within the appropriate timeframe, benzodiazepines for agitation and hyperadrenergic features, cyproheptadine (4-8 mg orally or via nasogastric tube, repeated every 4-6 hours) for moderate to severe serotonin syndrome, and supportive care addressing hyperthermia, rhabdomyolysis, and metabolic abnormalities.

Serotonin-norepinephrine reuptake inhibitors (SNRIs) including venlafaxine, desvenlafaxine, and duloxetine combine serotonergic toxicity risk with potential cardiovascular effects and seizure generation. Venlafaxine particularly demonstrates higher seizure risk in overdose compared to most SSRIs, along with QRS and QT prolongation at higher doses, necessitating electrocardiographic monitoring. Management follows principles similar to SSRIs, with additional attention to cardiovascular parameters and lower threshold for seizure prophylaxis with benzodiazepines in substantial ingestions.

Atypical antidepressants present diverse toxicological profiles reflecting their heterogeneous pharmacology. Bupropion demonstrates substantial seizure risk through dopamine and norepinephrine effects, with convulsions occurring in up to 40% of significant overdoses, often delayed 4-8 hours after ingestion with extended-release formulations. QRS and QT prolongation may occur at higher doses. Management emphasizes seizure prophylaxis with benzodiazepines for substantial ingestions, extended monitoring for delayed complications with sustained-release preparations, and supportive care. Mirtazapine typically produces sedation and minimal cardiac effects, with most cases managed through supportive care alone. Trazodone overdose frequently causes significant sedation, priapism in males, and potentially hypotension through alpha-adrenergic antagonism, with management addressing specific manifestations as they occur.

Monoamine oxidase inhibitors (MAOIs), though now rarely prescribed, create distinctive toxicological emergencies when taken in overdose. Delayed onset hypertensive crisis represents the classic complication, sometimes emerging 6-24 hours after ingestion, with potential for intracerebral hemorrhage, seizures, hyperthermia, and rhabdomyolysis. Additional complications include serotonin syndrome when combined with serotonergic agents and anticholinergic effects with certain compounds. Management includes intensive monitoring through the at-risk period, aggressive blood pressure control with short-acting titratable agents (nitroprusside, phentolamine) for hypertensive crisis, benzodiazepines for agitation and seizures, and active cooling for hyperthermia. Dietary tyramine restriction, critical during therapeutic use, becomes less relevant in acute overdose where the toxicant itself rather than dietary interaction creates the predominant toxicity.

Antipsychotics

Antipsychotic medications encompass diverse pharmacological

agents unified by dopamine receptor antagonism but demonstrating variable additional properties creating agent-specific toxicity profiles. First-generation (typical) antipsychotics, including phenothiazines (chlorpromazine, thioridazine), butyrophenones (haloperidol), and others, primarily block dopamine D_2 receptors while variably affecting cholinergic, histaminergic, and adrenergic receptors. Second-generation (atypical) agents, including olanzapine, quetiapine, risperidone, and aripiprazole, generally demonstrate broader receptor activity with relatively less D_2 antagonism, creating distinctive toxicological considerations. Clozapine occupies a unique position with minimal extrapyramidal effects but significant anticholinergic, antihistaminic, and anti-alpha-adrenergic properties contributing to its toxicity profile.

Cardiovascular toxicity represents a primary concern with many antipsychotics, manifesting through multiple mechanisms. QT prolongation occurs with numerous agents, most notably thioridazine, ziprasidone, iloperidone, and high-dose quetiapine, creating risk for torsades de pointes particularly with electrolyte abnormalities or co-ingestants. Sodium channel blockade resembling tricyclic antidepressant effects occurs with certain phenothiazines, producing QRS widening and ventricular dysrhythmias. Alpha-adrenergic blockade creates vasodilatory hypotension, particularly pronounced with low-potency first-generation agents like chlorpromazine and with quetiapine among atypicals. Direct myocardial depression occurs through unclear mechanisms with certain agents, potentially contributing to cardiovascular collapse in severe overdoses.

Neurological manifestations include sedation (through histamine H_1 antagonism and other mechanisms), extrapyramidal syndromes, seizures, and thermoregulatory disturbances. Extrapyramidal effects may present as dystonia, akathisia, or parkinsonism, reflecting dopamine blockade in the nigrostriatal pathway. Seizures occur more commonly with clozapine and low-potency phenothiazines, with incidence correlating with dose and specific agent properties. Neuroleptic malignant syndrome (NMS), characterized by muscular rigidity, hyperthermia, autonomic instability, and altered mental status, represents a life-threatening complication occurring with therapeutic use but also presenting in overdose scenarios. Temperature dysregulation results from hypothalamic dopamine blockade impairing thermoregulation, plus muscular hyperactivity generating excess heat in NMS.

Anticholinergic effects predominate with low-potency first-generation agents and certain atypicals, particularly clozapine and olanzapine, creating the classic toxidrome of hyperthermia, mydriasis, dry mucous membranes, reduced bowel sounds, urinary retention, and altered mental status. Antihistaminic properties contribute to sedation, which may become profound with agents possessing strong H_1 antagonism. Metabolic derangements include hyperglycemia through complex mechanisms potentially including pancreatic effects and insulin resistance, with olanzapine particularly associated with glucose abnormalities in both therapeutic use and overdose.

Toxicity management integrates supportive care with targeted interventions addressing specific manifestations. Airway protection remains paramount given the frequent occurrence of significant sedation and aspiration risk. Cardiovascular support includes fluid resuscitation addressing hypotension from alpha-blockade, followed by direct-acting vasopressors when necessary, with norepinephrine generally preferred due to combined alpha and beta effects. QT prolongation management includes avoidance of additional QT-prolonging medications, aggressive correction of electrolyte abnormalities (particularly potassium and magnesium), and consideration of magnesium sulfate (1-2 g intravenously) for torsades risk. Sodium bicarbonate administration (1-2 mEq/kg) addresses QRS prolongation when present, following principles similar to tricyclic antidepressant management.

Extrapyramidal manifestations respond to anticholinergic agents (benztropine 1-2 mg or diphenhydramine 25-50 mg intravenously) for dystonic reactions and akathisia. Benzodiazepines provide both seizure management and adjunctive treatment for extrapyramidal symptoms and agitation. Neuroleptic malignant syndrome requires intensive supportive care with aggressive cooling for hyperthermia, benzodiazepines for muscle rigidity, and consideration of specific agents including dantrolene for severe cases (though evidence remains limited), bromocriptine providing dopamine agonism potentially counteracting the fundamental pathophysiology, and amantadine through similar dopaminergic mechanisms.

Agent-specific considerations influence management approaches. Quetiapine frequently causes significant sedation, QT prolongation at higher doses, and anticholinergic effects, with management focusing on supportive care and monitoring for delayed cardiac complications. Olanzapine demonstrates prominent antihistaminic and anticholinergic properties creating severe sedation and occasionally delirium, along with metabolic derangements including hyperglycemia requiring monitoring. Clozapine overdose presents particularly high risk for seizures, anticholinergic toxicity, and respiratory depression, warranting lower thresholds for prophylactic anticonvulsant administration with substantial ingestions. Risperidone typically produces limited toxicity beyond extrapyramidal symptoms and sedation in most overdoses, though QT prolongation remains possible at higher doses.

Prognosis generally remains favorable with appropriate supportive care, with mortality rare except in massive ingestions, delayed presentation with complications like aspiration pneumonia, or cases involving vulnerable populations with limited physiological reserve. Most patients demonstrate resolution of acute toxicity within 24-48 hours, though extended-release formulations may require longer monitoring periods. Long-term neurological sequelae rarely occur with isolated antipsychotic overdoses, though persistent extrapyramidal symptoms occasionally require extended treatment. Neuroleptic malignant syndrome carries higher morbidity and mortality risk compared to simple overdose, with aggressive early intervention critical for optimizing outcomes.

Mood Stabilizers

Lithium toxicity presents distinctive management challenges related to its narrow therapeutic index, variable elimination kinetics, and potential for severe neurological sequelae. Three patterns of toxicity occur with different management implications: acute overdose in previously lithium-naïve individuals, acute-on-chronic toxicity in patients taking lithium therapeutically who then take an acute overdose, and chronic toxicity developing gradually from altered elimination or drug interactions in patients on stable therapy. Toxicokinetics include minimal protein binding, distribution primarily in total body water, limited tissue binding in acute exposure versus extensive tissue distribution in chronic therapy, and elimination almost exclusively through renal mechanisms with significant reabsorption in the proximal tubule.

Clinical manifestations evolve with rising serum concentrations, beginning with gastrointestinal symptoms (nausea, vomiting, diarrhea), fine tremor, and hyperreflexia at lower levels. Progressive toxicity produces neurological deterioration including confusion, dysarthria, ataxia, myoclonus, and altered consciousness. Severe toxicity may create seizures, coma, cardiovascular collapse, and permanent neurological sequelae. Chronic toxicity often presents insidiously with prominent neurological manifestations sometimes out of proportion to measured serum concentrations, reflecting equilibration between serum and brain tissue. Additional complications include nephrogenic diabetes insipidus, thyroid dysfunction with prolonged use, serotonin syndrome when combined with serotonergic agents, and cardiac conduction disturbances in severe cases.

Diagnostic evaluation centers on serum lithium concentration measurement, though interpretation requires consideration of exposure pattern and timing. Therapeutic concentrations typically range from 0.6-1.2 mEq/L, with acute toxicity generally developing above 1.5 mEq/L, though considerable individual variation exists. Serial measurements provide essential trending information, with rising levels despite supportive care suggesting ongoing absorption or declining renal function. Electrocardiographic assessment may reveal nonspecific T-wave changes or QT prolongation in significant toxicity. Comprehensive metabolic profile evaluates renal function and electrolytes, with particular attention to sodium levels as hyponatremia enhances lithium-induced neurotoxicity. Neuroimaging may be warranted in patients with focal findings or progressive deterioration despite decreasing lithium levels to exclude alternative or concurrent pathology.

Management strategies vary based on toxicity pattern and severity. Mild to moderate acute toxicity often responds to intravenous fluid administration enhancing renal elimination, with isotonic saline preferred to maintain euvolemia while avoiding hyponatremia that might exacerbate neurotoxicity. Gastrointestinal decontamination with activated charcoal provides no benefit due to minimal binding, though whole bowel irrigation may theoretically reduce absorption from sustained-release preparations. Enhanced elimination through hemodialysis represents definitive management for severe poisoning, with indications including lithium concentration exceeding 4 mEq/L in acute ingestion, levels above 2.5 mEq/L with significant symptoms, progressive clinical deterioration despite supportive care, and patients with impaired elimination capacity due to renal insufficiency or concurrent conditions. Continuous renal replacement therapy provides an alternative when conventional hemodialysis remains unavailable or patient instability precludes intermittent therapy.

Special management considerations include recognition of rebound elevation in lithium concentrations after hemodialysis discontinuation, often necessitating repeated or prolonged treatment due to redistribution from tissue stores. Sodium polystyrene sulfonate, while historically suggested, provides no meaningful enhancement of lithium elimination and should be avoided. Forced diuresis demonstrates limited efficacy while potentially creating fluid and electrolyte imbalances. Neurological sequelae, including persistent cerebellar dysfunction, extrapyramidal syndromes, and memory impairment, may develop despite appropriate intervention, particularly in chronic toxicity or delayed treatment initiation. These complications occasionally persist for months or become permanent, necessitating extended follow-up and rehabilitation. Prevention strategies include patient education regarding recognition of early toxicity signs, regular monitoring during therapeutic use, caution with potential interacting medications (especially NSAIDs, ACE inhibitors, and diuretics), and maintained euvolemia particularly during illness or environmental heat exposure.

Valproic acid toxicity creates multi-system effects through diverse mechanisms including GABA potentiation, mitochondrial dysfunction, and metabolic derangements. Therapeutic uses span epilepsy, bipolar disorder, and migraine prophylaxis, with toxicity occurring through both acute overdose and chronic accumulation. Toxicokinetics include extensive protein binding (90-95%) that becomes saturated in overdose, leading to disproportionate increases in free drug concentration with rising total levels, and hepatic metabolism with capacity for auto-induction with chronic therapy. Clinical manifestations include central nervous system depression ranging from mild somnolence to profound coma, occasionally with paradoxical agitation in early stages; cerebral edema in severe cases; hyperammonemia through carnitine depletion and urea cycle inhibition; metabolic abnormalities including hypoglycemia, hypernatremia, and anion gap metabolic acidosis; and hematological effects including thrombocytopenia, leukopenia, and rarely bone marrow suppression. Hepatotoxicity ranges from transient transaminase elevation to fulminant hepatic failure, with higher risk in pediatric patients, those with inborn errors of metabolism, and polytherapy scenarios.

Diagnostic evaluation includes serum valproic acid concentration, with therapeutic range typically 50-100 μg/mL and toxicity increasingly likely above 100 μg/mL, though clinical manifestations guide management more than absolute values. Significant central nervous system depression typically emerges at levels exceeding 450 μg/mL, with levels above 850-1000 μg/mL associated with profound coma and life-threatening complications. Additional laboratory assessment includes ammonia level (with hyperammonemia potentially causing encephalopathy independent of direct valproic acid effects), complete blood count, comprehensive metabolic profile, coagulation studies, and pancreatic enzymes given potential pancreatitis association. Electroencephalography may detect subclinical seizure activity in patients with unexplained altered consciousness, while neuroimaging evaluates for cerebral edema in severe toxicity.

Management approaches include gastrointestinal decontamination with activated charcoal for recent ingestions, supportive care addressing specific organ system effects, and consideration of antidotal therapy. L-carnitine supplementation (100 mg/kg up to 6 g/day intravenously or orally divided into 3-4 doses) addresses mitochondrial dysfunction and hyperammonemia through restoring fatty acid metabolism pathways, with particular benefit in chronic toxicity, pediatric patients, and cases with significant hyperammonemia or hepatotoxicity. Enhanced elimination through hemodialysis significantly increases valproic acid clearance despite high protein binding, as the free fraction increases substantially in severe overdose. Indications include levels exceeding 900-1000 μg/mL, profound coma unresponsive to supportive care, severe hyperammonemia, or significant acidosis. The lipid-soluble nature of valproic acid creates potential for lipid emulsion therapy in refractory cases, though evidence remains limited to case reports rather than controlled studies.

Carbamazepine toxicity affects primarily neurological and cardiovascular systems, with significant risk for delayed or prolonged effects due to erratic absorption, enterohepatic recirculation, and active metabolites. Therapeutic uses span epilepsy, trigeminal neuralgia, and bipolar disorder, with toxicity mechanisms including sodium channel blockade, anticholinergic effects, and GABA receptor modulation. Clinical manifestations typically begin with nystagmus, ataxia, and drowsiness, progressing to respiratory depression, coma, and seizures in severe cases. Cardiac effects include sinus tachycardia, QRS prolongation from sodium channel blockade, and hypotension through both myocardial depression and peripheral vasodilation. Distinctive toxicokinetic patterns include delayed peak toxicity with extended-release formulations, potential for secondary deterioration 24-48 hours after apparent improvement due to enterohepatic recirculation, and auto-induction of metabolism with chronic therapy potentially creating different toxicity patterns compared to naïve patients.

Management includes gastrointestinal decontamination with activated charcoal for patients presenting within 1-2 hours of ingestion, with multiple-dose regimens potentially beneficial given enterohepatic recirculation. Cardiovascular toxicity management parallels approaches for other sodium channel blockers, with sodium bicarbonate administration (1-2 mEq/kg) addressing QRS prolongation, though typically less dramatic than seen with tricyclic antidepressants. Hemodynamic support includes fluid resuscitation followed by vasopressors when necessary, with norepinephrine typically preferred given the mixed cardiovascular toxicity mechanisms. Enhanced elimination through multiple-dose activated charcoal demonstrates documented efficacy in reducing carbamazepine half-life, while hemodialysis or hemoperfusion may benefit severe cases with levels exceeding 60 mg/L, profound coma, refractory seizures, or significant QRS prolongation unresponsive to conventional management. Extended observation periods remain essential given the potential for delayed deterioration, particularly with sustained-release formulations or substantial ingestions.

Lamotrigine toxicity predominantly affects neurological and cardiac systems, with principal mechanisms including sodium channel modulation, glutamate release inhibition, and 5-HT3 receptor effects. Clinical manifestations include neurotoxicity ranging from tremor, ataxia, and nystagmus to seizures and altered mental status; cardiac conduction abnormalities including QRS and QT prolongation; and distinctive movement disorders including myoclonus, choreiform movements, and tic-like behaviors. Severe toxicity may produce brainstem dysfunction affecting respiratory drive, necessitating ventilatory support. Management primarily involves supportive care addressing specific manifestations, with sodium bicarbonate administration for QRS prolongation, benzodiazepines for seizures and movement disorders, and respiratory support as needed. Enhanced elimination techniques demonstrate limited efficacy due to high volume of distribution and moderate protein binding, making supportive care the mainstay of management while awaiting natural elimination.

Sedative-Hypnotics

Benzodiazepine toxicity predominantly manifests through central nervous system depression, reflecting their therapeutic mechanism of gamma-aminobutyric acid (GABA) potentiation at GABAA receptors. When taken alone, even substantial overdoses rarely produce life-threatening toxicity due to their wide therapeutic index and limited effects on cardiovascular and respiratory centers at standard doses. However, co-ingestion with other central nervous system depressants, particularly alcohol or opioids, creates synergistic toxicity with significantly increased risk for profound respiratory depression and airway compromise. Agent-specific properties creating clinically relevant differences include lipophilicity affecting onset and distribution (highly lipophilic agents like diazepam demonstrating rapid onset but shorter duration due to redistribution), metabolic pathways (oxidative metabolism through cytochrome P450 versus direct conjugation), presence of active metabolites (particularly desmethyldiazepam from numerous parent compounds), and elimination half-lives varying from 2-4 hours for midazolam to over 100 hours for diazepam when including active metabolites.

Clinical manifestations predominantly include central nervous system depression ranging from mild sedation and ataxia to profound unconsciousness. Respiratory depression severity correlates with sedation depth, though typically remains modest with isolated benzodiazepine ingestion at standard doses. Paradoxical reactions including agitation, aggression, and disinhibition occasionally occur, particularly in elderly patients, those with underlying brain pathology, or with certain agents like midazolam. Cardiovascular effects remain minimal in most cases, with preserved hemodynamic stability even in significant overdose. This toxicological profile creates the classic "normal vital signs except respiratory rate" presentation characteristic of isolated benzodiazepine overdose, contrasting with most other sedative-hypnotic classes which typically produce more significant hemodynamic effects.

Management begins with supportive care addressing airway

protection and respiratory support when necessary. Flumazenil, a competitive GABAA receptor antagonist, reverses benzodiazepine effects through direct receptor competition. Initial dosing begins at 0.2 mg intravenously, with titration up to a cumulative dose of 3-5 mg. Despite demonstrated efficacy, flumazenil use remains controversial and generally limited due to seizure risk, particularly in patients with benzodiazepine dependence, mixed overdoses involving proconvulsant agents (especially tricyclic antidepressants), or underlying seizure disorders. Additional concerns include the potentially short duration of action relative to the offending benzodiazepine and precipitation of benzodiazepine withdrawal, which may prove life-threatening. These risks generally confine appropriate use to iatrogenic oversedation scenarios and limited diagnostic applications rather than routine management of undifferentiated overdose.

Non-benzodiazepine sedative-hypnotics ("Z-drugs" including zolpidem, zaleplon, and zopiclone) act through similar GABAA receptor modulation but at different binding sites, creating somewhat different clinical profiles. While generally demonstrating similar toxicity patterns to benzodiazepines, these agents more frequently produce visual hallucinations, complex sleep behaviors (eating, driving, sexual activity without conscious awareness), and occasionally prolonged delirium, particularly in elderly patients. Management follows principles similar to benzodiazepine toxicity, with flumazenil demonstrating variable efficacy reflecting the modified binding site interactions of these compounds.

Barbiturate toxicity creates substantially greater risk than benzodiazepines due to steeper dose-response curves and significant cardiovascular depression in overdose. Although now rarely prescribed, these agents occasionally appear in overdose scenarios through remaining legitimate prescriptions for specific indications like epilepsy (phenobarbital), intentional procurement through veterinary sources, or international sources where prescribing restrictions differ. Toxicity mechanisms include GABAA receptor potentiation through binding sites distinct from benzodiazepines, direct inhibition of excitatory neurotransmission, and uncoupling of oxidative phosphorylation at higher doses. Clinical manifestations include dose-dependent central nervous system depression potentially progressing to coma, respiratory failure, hypotension through both myocardial depression and peripheral vasodilation, hypothermia, and characteristic cutaneous bullae at pressure points from immobility and tissue hypoperfusion.

Barbiturate management requires aggressive supportive care without available specific antidotes. Airway protection and ventilatory support address respiratory depression, while hypotension management includes fluid resuscitation followed by vasopressors when necessary. Enhanced elimination techniques demonstrate variable efficacy depending on specific agent properties. Multiple-dose activated charcoal significantly enhances phenobarbital elimination through interruption of enterohepatic circulation and potentially "gut dialysis" effects. Urinary alkalinization increases ionization and excretion of phenobarbital but provides minimal benefit for most other barbiturates. Hemodialysis effectively removes phenobarbital due to its relatively low protein binding and volume of distribution but demonstrates less utility for more lipophilic barbiturates. Prolonged supportive care often becomes necessary given extended elimination half-lives, particularly for phenobarbital which may require ventilatory support for several days in severe overdoses.

GHB (gamma-hydroxybutyrate) and its precursors (GBL, 1,4-butanediol) produce toxicity through GHB receptor agonism, GABAB receptor effects, and possibly additional mechanisms. Clinical presentation includes rapid onset central nervous system depression, often with abrupt transitions between normal consciousness and profound unresponsiveness, occasional seizure-like activity, emesis with aspiration risk, and bradycardia that typically remains hemodynamically stable. The characteristic toxidrome of essentially normal vital signs with profound but short-lived unconsciousness, often followed by abrupt awakening without residual sedation, provides important diagnostic clues in undifferentiated coma. Management focuses on supportive care addressing airway protection during the period of unconsciousness, typically lasting 2-4 hours with complete resolution without sequelae in uncomplicated cases. No specific antidote exists, with flumazenil and naloxone demonstrating no efficacy given the distinct receptor mechanisms. GHB withdrawal represents a separate clinical entity requiring specialized management, characterized by autonomic instability, agitation, delirium, and occasionally life-threatening complications when abrupt discontinuation follows regular use.

ANTIMICROBIALS

Antimicrobial agents represent a diverse pharmaceutical category with agent-specific toxicity profiles reflecting their varied chemical structures, mechanisms of action, and pharmacokinetic properties.

Beta-Lactam Antibiotics

Beta-lactam antibiotics, encompassing penicillins, cephalosporins, carbapenems, and monobactams, share the common structural beta-lactam ring but demonstrate significant differences in toxicity profiles and severity. Hypersensitivity reactions represent the predominant concern with this class, ranging from mild rashes to life-threatening anaphylaxis or severe cutaneous adverse reactions (SCARs) including Stevens-Johnson syndrome and toxic epidermal necrolysis. True IgE-mediated hypersensitivity occurs more frequently with penicillins compared to other beta-lactams, with approximate incidence of serious reactions between 0.01-0.05% of administrations. Cross-reactivity between penicillins and cephalosporins, historically overstated, actually occurs in approximately 2-10% of cases, with greatest risk for first-generation cephalosporins and those with similar side chains to the implicated penicillin. Carbapenems demonstrate approximately 1% cross-reactivity with penicillins, while monobactams (aztreonam) show negligible cross-reactivity except in patients with specific allergy to ceftazidime which shares an identical side chain.

Neurotoxicity occurs with various beta-lactams, particularly at high doses, in renal impairment, or with blood-brain barrier disruption. Clinical manifestations include seizures, myoclonus, altered mental status, and occasionally non-convulsive status epilepticus identified only through electroencephalography. Mechanism involves inhibition of GABA receptor function through structural similarities between beta-lactams and GABA inhibitory neurotransmitter. Specific agents demonstrating greater neurotoxic potential include cefepime, ceftazidime, and imipenem, with seizure risk for imipenem significantly reduced through the addition of cilastatin which prevents renal metabolism to a neurotoxic metabolite. Management involves drug discontinuation or dose reduction, anticonvulsants for seizure control (benzodiazepines generally most effective given the GABA-related mechanism), and occasional hemodialysis for severe symptoms in the context of renal failure with drug accumulation.

Hematological toxicity varies across the beta-lactam class. Hemolytic anemia occasionally accompanies high-dose penicillin therapy, particularly in patients with glucose-6-phosphate dehydrogenase deficiency. Neutropenia occurs with various beta-lactams, typically after prolonged administration and through immune-mediated mechanisms rather than direct bone marrow suppression. Platelet dysfunction with penicillins results from inhibition of ADP-induced platelet aggregation, occasionally causing clinical bleeding in patients with renal failure or other coexisting coagulation abnormalities. Ceftriaxone uniquely forms insoluble calcium complexes potentially causing biliary sludging and pseudolithiasis, with rare reports of fatal outcomes in neonates receiving both ceftriaxone and calcium-containing solutions, leading to contraindication of this combination.

> **Remember**
>
> **Antimicrobial toxicities range from dose-dependent effects requiring therapeutic drug monitoring (aminoglycosides, vancomycin) to idiosyncratic reactions that are unpredictable and potentially severe, necessitating prompt recognition and drug discontinuation**

Nephrotoxicity associated with certain beta-lactams occurs through various mechanisms. Interstitial nephritis represents an immunological reaction, typically developing after 7-10 days of therapy, with higher risk associated with specific agents including methicillin (now rarely used), nafcillin, and piperacillin. Acute tubular necrosis can occur with aminopenicillins in high doses. Carbapenems, particularly imipenem, may cause nephrotoxicity in rare cases. Management includes drug discontinuation, supportive care, and consideration of corticosteroids for severe interstitial nephritis, though evidence remains limited regarding steroid efficacy. Specific electrolyte disturbances include hypokalemia with ticarcillin and piperacillin (containing potassium-binding moieties) and sodium overload with high doses of sodium-containing preparations like nafcillin, potentially problematic in patients with heart failure or other sodium-sensitive conditions.

Management of beta-lactam toxicity primarily involves recognition and drug discontinuation, with additional supportive care and targeted interventions for specific complications. Hypersensitivity reactions follow standard approaches based on severity, from antihistamines and corticosteroids for mild to moderate reactions to epinephrine, airway management, and vasopressor support for anaphylaxis. Desensitization protocols enable administration in cases of absolute necessity despite prior hypersensitivity, though requiring specialized implementation under controlled conditions. Neurotoxicity management includes anticonvulsants for seizures, electroencephalographic monitoring for non-convulsive status, and occasionally hemodialysis for severe symptoms in the context of renal dysfunction with drug accumulation. Hemodialysis effectively removes most beta-lactams due to their low protein binding and predominantly renal elimination, providing both therapeutic drug removal and supportive renal function in appropriate cases.

Aminoglycosides

Aminoglycoside antibiotics, including gentamicin, tobramycin, amikacin, and streptomycin, create distinctive toxicity concerns predominating in renal and auditory systems. Nephrotoxicity occurs through direct proximal tubular cell injury following drug uptake via megalin-mediated endocytosis, with resulting phospholipidosis, mitochondrial dysfunction, and oxidative stress. Clinical manifestation typically involves non-oliguric acute kidney injury developing after 5-7 days of therapy, with urinalysis showing minimal abnormalities beyond occasional tubular epithelial cells and low-grade proteinuria. Risk factors include pre-existing renal impairment, concurrent nephrotoxic medications, advanced age, volume depletion, and extended therapy duration. Once-daily dosing strategies, compared to traditional multiple daily administrations, demonstrate equivalent efficacy with reduced nephrotoxicity risk due to saturable uptake mechanisms and concentration-dependent bacterial killing. Toxicity monitoring includes regular renal function assessment through serum creatinine measurement, with detection of rising trends prompting intervention before significant injury occurs.

Ototoxicity affects both vestibular and cochlear functions through similar mechanisms involving uptake into inner ear sensory cells, reactive oxygen species generation, and calcium dysregulation leading to apoptosis. Vestibular toxicity manifests as vertigo, ataxia, and nystagmus, while cochlear damage produces high-frequency hearing loss potentially progressing to broader frequency involvement and eventual deafness. Risk factors include genetic susceptibility (particularly mitochondrial DNA mutations at position 1555), concurrent ototoxic medications, pre-existing hearing impairment, advanced age, and extended treatment duration. Unlike nephrotoxicity, ototoxic effects often prove irreversible due to limited regenerative capacity of inner ear sensory cells. Monitoring approaches include audiometry before and during treatment for cochlear function assessment, though vestibular testing remains less standardized in routine practice.

Neuromuscular blockade represents a rare but potentially life-threatening complication of aminoglycoside therapy, manifesting as progressive muscle weakness occasionally culminating in respiratory failure. Mechanism involves presynaptic inhibition of acetylcholine release and postsynaptic competition at the neuromuscular junction, with risk factors including concurrent neuromuscular blocking agents, hypocalcemia, hypermagnesemia, and underlying neuromuscular disorders. This complication occurs most commonly with rapid administration of large doses, particularly in the perioperative setting or in patients with myasthenia gravis. Management includes drug discontinuation, respiratory support when necessary, and calcium gluconate administration (10 mL of 10% solution) potentially attenuating the blockade through increased acetylcholine release.

Management strategies for aminoglycoside toxicity focus on prevention through careful patient selection, appropriate dosing, therapeutic drug monitoring, and recognition of early toxicity signs. Therapeutic drug monitoring employs both peak and trough concentration measurements, with trough levels particularly correlating with toxicity risk. Target trough concentrations vary by specific agent, with gentamicin and tobramycin typically maintained below 2 μg/mL in multiple daily dosing regimens or below 1 μg/mL with once-daily administration. Peak concentrations ensure therapeutic efficacy while contributing less to toxicity risk assessment. Established toxicity management includes immediate drug discontinuation or dose adjustment, ensuring adequate hydration to support renal perfusion, and avoiding concurrent nephrotoxic agents. Ototoxicity requires audiological consultation, communication strategies for established hearing loss, and vestibular rehabilitation for balance disturbances. Enhanced elimination through hemodialysis effectively removes aminoglycosides due to their low protein binding and water solubility, potentially indicated in cases of inadvertent overdose, though rarely necessary in standard therapeutic toxicity.

Fluoroquinolones

Fluoroquinolone antibiotics, including ciprofloxacin, levofloxacin, moxifloxacin, and ofloxacin, demonstrate a broad toxicity profile resulting in significant prescribing restrictions by regulatory agencies worldwide. Central nervous system effects include a spectrum from mild headache and dizziness to severe reactions including seizures, psychosis, hallucinations, and altered mental status. Mechanism involves both GABA receptor antagonism and excitatory NMDA receptor activation, with seizure risk increasing with concurrent NSAIDs, advanced age, renal dysfunction, and prior seizure history. Management employs benzodiazepines as first-line therapy for seizures, addressing the GABA antagonism mechanism, with drug discontinuation and supportive care for other neurological manifestations.

Tendinopathy, particularly affecting the Achilles tendon, represents a distinctive fluoroquinolone toxicity occurring in approximately 0.1-0.4% of treated patients. Manifestations range from tendon pain and inflammation to complete rupture, sometimes occurring weeks after therapy completion. Pathophysiology involves disruption of tenocyte function through inhibition of mitochondrial function, altered gene expression, and enhanced matrix metalloproteinase activity. Risk factors include age over 60, concurrent corticosteroid therapy, renal dysfunction, previous tendon disorders, and strenuous physical activity during treatment. Management requires immediate drug discontinuation, rest, immobilization, orthopedic consultation for severe cases or rupture, and extended avoidance of fluoroquinolones in affected patients.

Cardiovascular toxicity primarily manifests as QT interval prolongation with associated risk for torsades de pointes, demonstrating variable risk across the class. Moxifloxacin shows the greatest effect, followed by levofloxacin, with ciprofloxacin demonstrating the least QT impact. Risk amplifies with concurrent QT-prolonging medications, electrolyte abnormalities (particularly hypokalemia and hypomagnesemia), structural heart disease, female gender, and advanced age. Monitoring includes baseline and follow-up electrocardiography for high-risk patients, with proactive electrolyte correction, dose adjustment in renal dysfunction, and avoidance of drug interactions. Management of established arrhythmias follows standard approaches including magnesium sulfate administration, avoidance of other QT-prolonging agents, overdrive pacing when necessary, and emergency defibrillation for hemodynamically unstable ventricular arrhythmias.

Photosensitivity reactions occur with variable frequency across different fluoroquinolones, manifesting as exaggerated sunburn-like reactions on sun-exposed areas. Mechanism involves both phototoxicity through reactive oxygen species generation and photoallergy through immunological hypersensitivity to light-altered drug molecules. Lomefloxacin and sparfloxacin (both now rarely used) demonstrate highest risk, with ciprofloxacin and levofloxacin showing intermediate potential, and moxifloxacin associated with lowest incidence. Management includes photoprotection through clothing and broad-spectrum sunscreens, scheduling outdoor activities outside peak ultraviolet exposure periods, and drug discontinuation for severe reactions. Hypersensitivity reactions ranging from maculopapular rash to life-threatening Stevens-Johnson syndrome occur with similar frequency to other antibiotics, requiring standard management approaches based on reaction severity.

Recent recognition of potentially permanent adverse effects has significantly altered fluoroquinolone prescribing patterns. Fluoroquinolone-associated disability (FQAD) encompasses a constellation of symptoms including peripheral neuropathy, tendinopathy, joint pain, psychiatric effects, and autonomic dysfunction persisting for months or years after drug discontinuation. Pathophysiology remains incompletely understood but likely involves mitochondrial dysfunction, oxidative stress, and altered gene expression in susceptible individuals. Management remains largely supportive, with no established interventions reliably reversing established damage. Regulatory agencies including the FDA have implemented increasingly restrictive boxed warnings and recommendations limiting fluoroquinolone use to situations where no alternative antibiotics exist, particularly for uncomplicated infections. Prevention focuses on appropriate antibiotic stewardship, avoiding fluoroquinolones for minor infections, and careful patient selection considering individual risk factors and alternative therapeutic options.

Antivirals and Antimycobacterials

Antiviral medications encompass diverse chemical classes with agent-specific toxicity profiles reflecting their mechanisms of action and pharmacological properties. Nucleoside reverse transcriptase inhibitors (NRTIs) including zidovudine, stavudine, and didanosine cause mitochondrial toxicity through polymerase gamma inhibition, manifesting as myopathy, peripheral neuropathy, pancreatitis, lactic acidosis, and hepatic steatosis. Lactic acidosis with hepatic steatosis represents a rare but potentially fatal complication, with risk factors including female gender, pregnancy, obesity, and prolonged therapy. Early recognition through monitoring of lactate levels, liver enzymes, and symptoms including unexplained nausea, abdominal pain, and dyspnea enables prompt intervention through drug discontinuation and supportive care addressing acidosis and organ dysfunction.

Protease inhibitors demonstrate complex metabolic effects including insulin resistance, dyslipidemia, and lipodystrophy. Ritonavir particularly causes significant gastrointestinal intolerance and demonstrates extensive drug interactions through potent cytochrome P450 inhibition. Non-nucleoside reverse transcriptase inhibitors (NNRTIs) like nevirapine and efavirenz produce distinctive toxicity profiles including rash, hepatotoxicity, and neuropsychiatric effects. Nevirapine-associated rash and hepatotoxicity occur more frequently in females with higher CD4 counts, while efavirenz causes vivid dreams, dizziness, and occasionally severe psychiatric disturbances necessitating administration at bedtime and consideration of alternative agents in patients with psychiatric comorbidities.

Integrase strand transfer inhibitors (INSTIs) including raltegravir, dolutegravir, and bictegravir generally demonstrate more favorable toxicity profiles, though neuropsychiatric effects including insomnia, depression, and anxiety occur with some agents, particularly dolutegravir. Newer antivirals for hepatitis C treatment, including direct-acting antivirals like sofosbuvir, ledipasvir, and glecaprevir, show substantially improved safety profiles compared to older interferon-based regimens, though drug interactions remain important considerations due to their effects on drug transporters including P-glycoprotein.

Ribavirin, used for various viral infections including hepatitis C and respiratory syncytial virus, causes dose-dependent hemolytic anemia through oxidative damage to erythrocytes. Management includes dose reduction for significant hemoglobin decreases, discontinuation for severe anemia, and consideration of erythropoietin in selected cases. Acyclovir and related antivirals (valacyclovir, famciclovir) occasionally cause nephrotoxicity through crystal deposition, particularly with rapid intravenous administration, dehydration, or pre-existing renal impairment. Prevention involves adequate hydration and appropriate dosing adjustments in renal dysfunction, with management of established toxicity including drug discontinuation, volume expansion, and rarely urinary alkalinization enhancing crystal solubility.

Antimycobacterial agents used for tuberculosis and related infections present significant toxicological challenges, often necessitating extended treatment durations increasing cumulative toxicity risk. Isoniazid (INH) causes hepatotoxicity through generation of toxic metabolites, with clinical presentation ranging from asymptomatic transaminase elevation to fulminant hepatic failure. Risk factors include age over 35, alcohol use, pre-existing liver disease, concurrent hepatotoxic medications, and specific genetic polymorphisms affecting acetylation rate. Management includes baseline and periodic liver enzyme monitoring, patient education regarding early symptoms, and immediate drug discontinuation if significant hepatotoxicity develops. Peripheral neuropathy represents another common isoniazid toxicity, resulting from pyridoxine (vitamin B6) depletion through formation of INH-pyridoxine complexes. Preventive pyridoxine supplementation (10-50 mg daily) during isoniazid therapy reduces neuropathy risk, with higher doses (100 mg daily) indicated for patients with additional risk factors including diabetes, alcohol use, malnutrition, or pregnancy.

Rifampin causes hepatotoxicity through both direct toxicity and enhancement of isoniazid toxic metabolite generation when used in combination. Additional toxicities include immunological reactions (flu-like syndrome typically occurring with intermittent dosing), orange discoloration of body fluids potentially staining contact lenses or soft tissues, and extensive drug interactions through potent cytochrome P450 induction. Ethambutol primarily causes optic neuritis through copper chelation interfering with mitochondrial function, manifesting as decreased visual acuity, altered color perception (particularly red-green discrimination), and central scotoma. Risk increases with higher doses, renal impairment, and treatment duration beyond two months. Monthly visual acuity and color discrimination testing enables early detection, with prompt drug discontinuation typically resulting in vision recovery if identified early, though irreversible damage may occur with delayed recognition.

Pyrazinamide demonstrates significant hepatotoxicity through uncertain mechanisms, potentially including formation of reactive metabolites and altered nicotinamide metabolism. Additional toxicities include hyperuricemia through inhibition of renal tubular urate secretion, rarely causing clinical gout, and occasionally hypersensitivity reactions. Second-line antimycobacterials used for resistant infections pose additional toxicological challenges: fluoroquinolones with toxicities previously discussed; aminoglycosides causing nephrotoxicity and irreversible ototoxicity necessitating regular audiometry during extended treatment; cycloserine producing neuropsychiatric effects including seizures, psychosis, and depression through NMDA receptor agonism; and bedaquiline causing QT prolongation requiring electrocardiographic monitoring throughout therapy.

Management of antimycobacterial toxicity presents particular challenges given the essential nature of these medications for treating potentially life-threatening infections and the requirement for multi-drug regimens to prevent resistance development. Strategies include careful baseline assessment identifying risk factors for specific toxicities, patient education regarding monitoring and early symptom recognition, regular clinical and laboratory surveillance throughout treatment, prompt intervention when toxicity develops, and regimen modification rather than complete treatment discontinuation when feasible. Liver toxicity management follows established protocols with definitions of significant injury warranting intervention: ALT greater than 3 times upper limit of normal with symptoms, greater than 5 times upper limit when asymptomatic, or any bilirubin elevation above 2 times upper limit. Rechallenge protocols allow cautious reintroduction of essential agents following toxicity resolution, typically employing sequential introduction with careful monitoring to identify the specific causative agent when multiple hepatotoxic medications were used concurrently

Summary

Pharmaceutical agents represent the most common causes of poisoning across all age groups, with both therapeutic misadventures and intentional overdoses contributing to significant morbidity and mortality. Analgesic toxicity presents distinct patterns based on drug class. Acetaminophen toxicity follows a predictable four-stage progression culminating in hepatic necrosis through toxic metabolite formation, with efficacy of N-acetylcysteine treatment highly time-dependent. Salicylate poisoning produces a complex mixed acid-base disturbance, hyperthermia, and multi-organ dysfunction requiring aggressive alkalization and potential hemodialysis. Opioid overdose manifests with the classic triad of respiratory depression, miosis, and decreased consciousness, requiring prompt naloxone administration and airway management. NSAIDs primarily cause gastrointestinal, renal, and platelet dysfunction through prostaglandin inhibition. Cardiovascular medication toxicity includes beta-blocker and calcium channel blocker overdoses characterized by bradycardia, hypotension, and cardiogenic shock, often requiring high-dose insulin-euglycemia therapy, vasopressors, and potentially lipid emulsion or extracorporeal support in severe cases. Digoxin toxicity presents with gastrointestinal symptoms, visual disturbances, and cardiac dysrhythmias responsive to specific antibody fragments when indicated. Psychiatric medication toxicity spans a spectrum from benzodiazepine-induced sedation to life-threatening tricyclic antidepressant cardiotoxicity with sodium channel blockade, seizures, and anticholinergic effects. Lithium's narrow therapeutic index leads to progressive neurotoxicity with tremor, altered mental status, seizures, and potential permanent neurological sequelae. Antimicrobial toxicities include concentration-dependent aminoglycoside ototoxicity and nephrotoxicity, fluoroquinolone neurotoxicity and tendinopathies, and idiosyncratic reactions with various agents. Management principles emphasize early recognition, toxin-specific interventions, and supportive care tailored to the pharmaceutical agent's unique toxicokinetics and mechanisms of toxicity.

Self-Assessment Questions

1. Describe the pathophysiology of acetaminophen hepatotoxicity, including the role of glutathione depletion, and explain how the Rumack-Matthew nomogram guides treatment decisions.
2. Analyze the acid-base disturbances characteristic of salicylate poisoning and explain the therapeutic rationale for urinary alkalinization in its management.
3. Compare and contrast the clinical presentations and management approaches for beta-blocker versus calcium channel blocker overdoses, including the role of high-dose insulin-euglycemia therapy.
4. Explain the mechanisms of cardiotoxicity in tricyclic antidepressant overdose and the physiological basis for sodium bicarbonate therapy in treating QRS prolongation.
5. Discuss the clinical manifestations of lithium toxicity at different serum levels and explain why hemodialysis might be indicated even at levels that would be therapeutic in other circumstances.
6. Describe the serotonin syndrome, including its distinguishing features from neuroleptic malignant syndrome, common precipitating medications, and management approach.
7. Analyze the toxicity concerns with newer anticoagulants (direct oral anticoagulants) compared to traditional agents like warfarin, including reversal strategies for life-threatening bleeding.
8. Explain the mechanisms, clinical presentation, and management of toxicity from antiepileptic medications, with particular attention to carbamazepine, valproic acid, and phenytoin.
9. Discuss the ototoxicity and nephrotoxicity associated with aminoglycoside antibiotics, including risk factors, monitoring approaches, and strategies for minimizing toxicity.
10. Compare and contrast the mechanisms, clinical features, and management of opioid overdose across different agents including full agonists, partial agonists, and synthetic opioids like fentanyl analogues.

Bibliography

1. Chiew AL, Gluud C, Brok J, Buckley NA. Interventions for paracetamol (acetaminophen) overdose. Cochrane Database Syst Rev. 2018;2(2):CD003328.
2. Juurlink DN. Antidepressants. In: Nelson LS, Hoffman RS, Howland MA, Lewin NA, Goldfrank LR, editors. Goldfrank's toxicologic emergencies. 11th ed. New York: McGraw-Hill Education; 2019. p. 896-907.
3. Hoegberg LCG, Gosselin S. Lipid resuscitation in acute poisoning: after a decade of experience, what have we learned? Curr Opin Crit Care. 2017;23(2):134-139.
4. Olson KR, Anderson IB, Benowitz NL, Blanc PD, Clark RF, Kearney TE, et al. Poisoning & drug overdose. 7th ed. New York: McGraw-Hill Education; 2018.
5. St-Onge M, Anseeuw K, Cantrell FL, Gilchrist IC, Hantson P, Bailey B, et al. Experts consensus recommendations for the management of calcium channel blocker poisoning in adults. Crit Care Med. 2017;45(3):e306-e315.
6. Lavergne V, Nolin TD, Hoffman RS, Roberts D, Gosselin S, Goldfarb DS, et al. The EXTRIP (EXtracorporeal TReatments In Poisoning) workgroup: guideline methodology. Clin Toxicol (Phila). 2012;50(5):403-413.
7. White CM. A review of potential cardiovascular uses of intravenous glucagon administration. J Clin Pharmacol. 1999;39(5):442-447.
8. Smilkstein MJ, Knapp GL, Kulig KW, Rumack BH. Efficacy of oral N-acetylcysteine in the treatment of acetaminophen overdose. Analysis of the national multicenter study (1976 to 1985). N Engl J Med. 1988;319(24):1557-1562.
9. Varpula T, Rapola J, Sallisalmi M, Kurola J. Treatment of serious calcium channel blocker overdose with levosimendan, a calcium sensitizer. Anesth Analg. 2009;108(3):790-792.
10. Konca C, Ertuğrul İ, Gül AE, Güllü UU, Atıcı SŞ, Yıldırım ZK. Torsades de pointes after overdose of escitalopram and propranolol: successful therapy with atrial pacing. J Emerg Med. 2015;48(5):e101-e104.

CHAPTER 8

ENVIRONMENTAL TOXINS

Author

Mrs. Bhagyasri Boyina, Assistant Professor,
Department of Pharmacy, Vikas Group of Institutions, Nunna,
Vijayawada Rural, Andhra Pradesh, India

Abstract

Environmental toxins represent a diverse category of hazardous substances encountered outside controlled pharmaceutical contexts, often producing distinctive toxicity patterns requiring specialized recognition and management. Heavy metal exposures include lead poisoning, with its neurodevelopmental effects in children and multisystem impacts in adults, requiring chelation therapy in severe cases. Arsenic toxicity presents with gastrointestinal, dermatological, and neurological manifestations alongside characteristic findings like Mees lines and garlic breath. Mercury exists in elemental, inorganic, and organic forms, each with unique toxicokinetics and target organ effects, particularly neurological and renal systems. Pesticide exposures vary by chemical class, with organophosphates and carbamates inhibiting acetylcholinesterase to produce cholinergic crisis requiring atropine and pralidoxime therapy. Pyrethroid insecticides primarily cause dermal and respiratory irritation, while organochlorine compounds produce CNS excitation and seizures. Industrial chemicals like cyanide rapidly inhibit cellular respiration, necessitating immediate hydroxocobalamin or sodium thiosulfate administration, while corrosives cause direct tissue damage requiring careful supportive care without neutralization attempts. Air pollutants include carbon monoxide, with its deceptive presentation and high mortality without prompt oxygen therapy, and irritant gases that produce progressive respiratory compromise potentially leading to delayed pulmonary edema. Management principles emphasize rapid identification, decontamination, specific antidotes where available, and supportive care addressing the unique pathophysiology of each environmental toxin.

Keywords: *Heavy Metals, Organophosphates, Carbon Monoxide, Chelation Therapy, Industrial Chemicals, Environmental Exposure*

Learning Objectives

After completion of the chapter, the learners should be able to:

- Identify clinical manifestations of common heavy metal poisonings including lead, arsenic, and mercury, and implement appropriate chelation therapies when indicated.
- Differentiate between various pesticide classes based on clinical presentation and cholinesterase activity, with emphasis on managing cholinergic crisis from organophosphate and carbamate exposures.
- Recognize and treat industrial chemical exposures including cyanide, hydrofluoric acid, and corrosives, with attention to specific antidotes and decontamination procedures.
- Evaluate carbon monoxide poisoning using appropriate diagnostic tests and determine indications for hyperbaric oxygen therapy versus normobaric oxygen treatment.
- Implement proper management of inhaled irritant gas exposures with attention to the risk of delayed-onset pulmonary edema and appropriate respiratory support.
- Develop surveillance and prevention strategies for environmental toxin exposures in occupational and community settings, including proper use of personal protective equipment.

HEAVY METALS

Heavy metals represent persistent environmental contaminants with significant human health effects through occupational, environmental, and occasionally deliberate exposures.

Lead

Lead toxicity remains a global public health challenge despite regulatory restrictions, with exposure sources including deteriorating lead-based paint in older housing, contaminated soil near industrial sites or roadways, lead-containing plumbing, certain occupations, contaminated folk remedies, and retained bullets or shrapnel. Toxicokinetics include gastrointestinal absorption significantly enhanced in children compared to adults (40-50% versus 10-15%), initial distribution in blood with approximately 95% bound to erythrocytes, subsequent redistribution to soft tissues and eventually to bone which serves as a long-term repository containing over 90% of total body burden in chronic exposure. This bone reservoir creates prolonged internal exposure through continuous mobilization, particularly during physiological states involving increased bone turnover including pregnancy, lactation, menopause, and immobilization. Elimination occurs predominantly through renal excretion, with biological half-life ranging from 30 days for blood lead to years or decades for bone lead stores.

> **Remember**
>
> **Lead toxicity affects multiple organ systems with particular concern for neurodevelopmental effects in children, requiring environmental intervention alongside medical management including chelation therapy at elevated blood levels.**

Pathophysiological mechanisms involve lead's strong affinity for sulfhydryl groups, resulting in inhibition of numerous enzymes, displacement of essential metals in metalloenzymes, disruption of calcium-dependent processes, and generation of oxidative stress. Specific enzyme targets include delta-aminolevulinic acid dehydratase and ferrochelatase in the heme synthesis pathway, contributing to anemia; sodium-potassium ATPase affecting cellular energy utilization; and various mitochondrial enzymes disrupting energy metabolism. Neurodevelopmental toxicity involves additional mechanisms including interference with neurotransmitter release, disruption of synaptic pruning, and impairment of cellular migration during critical developmental periods.

Clinical manifestations vary significantly with exposure intensity, duration, and patient age. Acute high-dose exposure, now rare in developed countries, produces lead encephalopathy with headache, confusion, seizures, coma, and potentially death through cerebral edema. More commonly encountered chronic toxicity presents with insidious multisystem effects: neurological manifestations include subtle neurocognitive deficits, peripheral neuropathy predominantly affecting motor function, and behavioral changes; hematological effects encompass microcytic anemia through both hemolysis and impaired hemoglobin synthesis; gastrointestinal symptoms include abdominal pain, constipation, and the classic but now rarely observed "lead line" (gingival hyperpigmentation); renal toxicity manifests as proximal tubular dysfunction and progressive nephropathy with chronic exposure. Children demonstrate enhanced susceptibility with neurodevelopmental effects occurring at substantially lower exposure levels than those causing symptomatic toxicity in adults, resulting in reduced intellectual function, attention deficits, behavioral problems, and diminished academic achievement without other obvious clinical signs.

Table 8.1: Heavy Metal Toxicity Profiles

Metal	Major Sources	Clinical Manifestations	Diagnostic Tests
Lead	Paint in older homes, contaminated water, industrial exposure	Abdominal pain, encephalopathy, peripheral neuropathy, anemia	Blood lead level, ZPP, CBC with peripheral smear
Mercury	Seafood, dental amalgams, industrial processes	Neurotoxicity, tremor, ataxia, sensory disturbances	Urine or blood mercury levels
Arsenic	Contaminated water, wood preservatives, pesticides	Garlic odor, GI symptoms, "rice milk" urine, peripheral neuropathy	24-hour urine arsenic, hair/nail analysis
Cadmium	Battery manufacturing, metal plating, cigarette smoke	Renal tubular damage, pulmonary irritation, bone effects	Urine cadmium, β_2-microglobulin
Chromium	Metal plating, leather tanning, welding	Skin/mucous membrane irritation, nasal septum perforation	Urine chromium, nasal examination

Diagnostic evaluation centers on blood lead level (BLL) measurement, which primarily reflects recent exposure rather than total body burden. Interpretation has evolved dramatically over decades, with current recognition that no safe threshold exists, particularly for neurodevelopmental effects. The CDC reference value for children, set at 3.5 μg/dL based on the 97.5th percentile of the population distribution, identifies children with exposures above most of the population, warranting investigation and intervention. Clinical toxicity becomes increasingly likely at higher levels: subtle neurocognitive effects begin below 5 μg/dL; hematological effects typically emerge above 20-25 μg/dL; frank symptomatic poisoning usually requires levels exceeding 60-70 μg/dL; and encephalopathy risk increases substantially above 100 μg/dL. Additional laboratory findings include basophilic stippling of erythrocytes, elevated zinc protoporphyrin reflecting impaired heme synthesis, hypochromic microcytic anemia, and elevated urinary delta-aminolevulinic acid. Radiographic findings in children may include metaphyseal lead lines representing increased metaphyseal density at long bone growth plates.

Management strategies encompass exposure identification and elimination, supportive care, chelation therapy when indicated, and long-term monitoring. Source identification requires detailed environmental and occupational history, home evaluation for lead hazards, and consideration of cultural practices or hobbies potentially involving lead exposure. Nutritional optimization, particularly ensuring adequate iron, calcium, and zinc intake, may reduce lead absorption and toxicity. Chelation therapy indications vary by blood lead level and clinical presentation: levels above 45 μg/dL generally warrant chelation in children, with lower thresholds for symptomatic patients; adult chelation typically begins at higher thresholds, often 70-100 μg/dL for asymptomatic cases. Specific chelating agents include succimer (2,3-dimercaptosuccinic acid, DMSA) for oral outpatient treatment at lower levels, calcium disodium ethylenediaminetetraacetic acid ($CaNa_2EDTA$) for parenteral therapy in more significant poisoning, and dimercaprol (British Anti-Lewisite, BAL) for severe toxicity, encephalopathy, or combined therapy with EDTA. Chelation endpoint typically targets blood lead reduction below chelation threshold levels, recognizing that bone lead stores will continue replenishing blood levels necessitating extended monitoring and potential repeated treatment courses.

Prevention strategies have evolved from treatment-focused approaches to primary prevention emphasizing exposure prevention before elevated levels occur. Public health interventions include elimination of lead from gasoline, residential paint, plumbing materials, and consumer products; remediation of contaminated housing through lead hazard control programs; enhanced surveillance systems identifying affected communities; and targeted screening programs for high-risk populations. Occupational protections include engineering controls minimizing workplace exposure, personal protective equipment, biological monitoring programs, and worker education regarding take-home exposure prevention. Clinical preventive services encompass anticipatory guidance regarding lead hazards, nutrition optimization, and selective screening based on risk assessment. Despite significant progress, ongoing challenges include legacy contamination from historical lead use, inadequate resources for housing remediation, and emerging exposure sources requiring continued vigilance and policy development.

Mercury

Mercury toxicity manifests in distinctive patterns determined by the specific chemical form, exposure route, and duration. Elemental mercury (Hg^0), found in thermometers, dental amalgams, certain religious practices, and artisanal gold mining, creates toxicity primarily through inhalation of mercury vapor. Inhaled elemental mercury readily crosses the blood-brain barrier and placenta due to its lipophilicity, subsequently oxidizing to inorganic forms that become trapped within tissues. Inorganic mercury compounds (Hg^+, Hg^{2+}), including mercurous and mercuric salts used in some batteries, explosives, and historically in medications, demonstrate limited gastrointestinal absorption (approximately 10-15%) and poor central nervous system penetration due to their charged nature. Organic mercury compounds, particularly methylmercury formed through microbial methylation in aquatic environments, show extensive gastrointestinal absorption (>90%), pronounced lipophilicity facilitating blood-brain barrier and placental transfer, and undergo extensive enterohepatic circulation creating prolonged half-life (approximately 50 days).

Pathophysiological mechanisms center on mercury's strong affinity for sulfhydryl groups, resulting in enzyme inhibition, protein structural alteration, and disruption of cellular transport mechanisms. Specific cellular targets include mitochondrial enzymes creating energy production impairment, glutathione depletion reducing antioxidant capacity, microtubule disruption affecting neuronal function and cellular division, and metalloprotein displacement altering essential enzyme functions. These effects manifest predominantly in tissues with limited regenerative capacity, particularly the central nervous system where both direct toxicity and inflammatory responses contribute to progressive damage, and the kidneys where proximal tubular concentration of mercury creates focal injury patterns.

Clinical manifestations differ substantially between mercury forms. Acute elemental mercury vapor inhalation produces respiratory irritation progressing to pneumonitis, with systemic absorption leading to tremor, neurobehavioral changes, and potentially renal failure with higher exposures. Chronic elemental mercury exposure classically causes the triad of tremor, neuropsychiatric disturbances (historically termed "erethism" and including irritability, shyness, memory loss, and depression), and gingivostomatitis. These features contributed to the phrases "mad as a hatter" and "hatter's shakes" reflecting occupational toxicity in felt hat manufacturing which utilized mercury compounds. Inorganic mercury ingestion produces predominant gastrointestinal and renal effects, with corrosive gastroenteritis, hemorrhagic colitis, and acute tubular necrosis potentially progressing to oliguric renal failure. Classic manifestations include metallic taste, gingival inflammation with distinctive blue-black "mercurial line," and chelosis (inflammation at mouth corners).

Methylmercury toxicity, most commonly resulting from contaminated seafood consumption, demonstrates pronounced neurological tropism with a latency period between exposure and symptom development sometimes extending weeks to months. Classic manifestations of significant exposure include paresthesias beginning peripherally and progressing in a centripetal pattern, concentrically constricted visual fields, ataxia, dysarthria, hearing impairment, and eventually neuromuscular weakness potentially progressing to paralysis. Prenatal methylmercury exposure from maternal seafood consumption creates particular concern due to the developing brain's enhanced vulnerability, with large-scale poisoning incidents demonstrating severe neurodevelopmental consequences including cerebral palsy, microcephaly, intellectual disability, and sensory impairments. Milder exposures may produce subtle neurodevelopmental effects detectable only through specialized neuropsychological testing.

Diagnostic confirmation requires appropriate specimen selection based on exposure pattern. Blood mercury measurement primarily reflects recent exposure to elemental or inorganic mercury but may remain elevated for extended periods with organic mercury due to its longer half-life. Urinary mercury provides the best assessment of inorganic and elemental mercury body burden and current exposure, with 24-hour collections preferred over spot samples due to significant excretion variability. Hair analysis effectively documents methylmercury exposure through longitudinal analysis allowing retrospective exposure timing assessment, though external contamination remains a potential confounder requiring careful interpretation. Neuroimaging typically demonstrates nonspecific findings in mercury toxicity, though magnetic resonance imaging may reveal characteristic patterns in severe methylmercury poisoning, particularly bilateral damage to the visual cortex and cerebellum.

Management strategies depend on mercury form, exposure timing, and symptom severity. For elemental mercury vapor exposure, immediate removal from the contamination source and respiratory support represent initial priorities, with chelation consideration for symptomatic patients or those with significantly elevated mercury levels. Acute inorganic mercury ingestion may benefit from gastric lavage if performed within one hour of exposure, followed by activated charcoal administration. Methylmercury poisoning management emphasizes supportive care with limited evidence for chelation efficacy due to the strong tissue binding and established cellular damage often present before diagnosis. Chelation agents include succimer (DMSA) for oral outpatient treatment of less severe cases, dimercaprol (BAL) for more significant poisoning requiring parenteral therapy, and occasionally penicillamine though with higher adverse effect profile. Specific chelation thresholds vary by mercury form: urinary mercury exceeding 50 μg/g creatinine or blood mercury above 50 μg/L for elemental/inorganic exposure; blood mercury above 100 μg/L for organic mercury exposure. Hemodialysis may provide adjunctive therapy for acute inorganic mercury poisoning with renal failure, both supporting renal function and enhancing mercury elimination.

Public health approaches emphasize exposure prevention through regulatory standards limiting industrial emissions, occupational exposure limits with biological monitoring programs, consumer product restrictions, and fish consumption advisories for vulnerable populations including pregnant women and young children. The Minamata Convention on Mercury, a global treaty effective since 2017, commits signatory nations to reducing mercury use and emissions through multiple strategies including phasing out certain mercury-containing products, implementing emission control technologies, regulating artisanal gold mining practices, and ensuring proper waste management for mercury-containing materials. Despite these measures, ongoing challenges include legacy contamination, atmospheric transport creating global distribution patterns, and socioeconomic factors limiting implementation of safer alternatives in certain industries and regions.

Arsenic

Arsenic toxicity presents complex clinical and diagnostic challenges due to its diverse chemical forms, exposure sources, and manifestation patterns. Environmental sources include naturally contaminated groundwater affecting millions globally, particularly in Bangladesh and parts of India, China, Taiwan, Argentina, Chile, and the United States; industrial contamination from mining, smelting, and wood preservation; agricultural sources including pesticides and animal feed additives; and certain foods naturally concentrating arsenic, particularly rice and some seafoods. Occupational exposures occur in metal refining, semiconductor manufacturing, wood treatment, and glass production. Intentional poisoning cases, though rare, continue occurring due to arsenic's availability, delayed symptom onset, and nonspecific initial presentation.

Toxicokinetics vary significantly between inorganic and organic arsenic compounds. Inorganic arsenic, the predominant form in contaminated water and most toxic species, demonstrates high gastrointestinal absorption (80-90%), undergoes hepatic methylation to monomethylarsonic acid (MMA) and dimethylarsinic acid (DMA), and eliminates primarily through urinary excretion with a typical half-life of

4 days. This methylation, once considered purely detoxification, now appears more complex, as certain methylated intermediates demonstrate significant toxicity. Organic arsenicals found naturally in seafood (primarily arsenobetaine and arsenocholine) show limited toxicity due to minimal biotransformation and rapid urinary elimination unchanged. Toxicokinetic variations including methylation efficiency demonstrate significant genetic polymorphism affecting individual susceptibility, with less efficient methylators showing higher toxicity risk at equivalent exposures.

Pathophysiological mechanisms reflect arsenic's thiol reactivity, leading to critical enzyme inhibition, cellular energy disruption, and oxidative stress generation. Specific mechanisms include pyruvate dehydrogenase inhibition disrupting cellular energy production, competitive substitution for phosphate in biochemical reactions including ATP formation, thiol binding inactivating over 200 enzymes, and DNA repair inhibition enhancing carcinogenic potential. Microvascular effects including endothelial damage and increased permeability contribute to characteristic skin manifestations and potentially to carcinogenesis through compromised tissue oxygenation. Recent evidence suggests epigenetic mechanisms, including DNA methylation alterations and histone modifications, may contribute to both immediate toxicity and long-term health effects including carcinogenesis.

Clinical manifestations demonstrate characteristic temporal patterns and organ system involvement. Acute poisoning classically presents with severe gastrointestinal symptoms including abdominal pain, violent vomiting, cholera-like diarrhea, and eventually cardiovascular collapse through both direct myocardial toxicity and capillary leak. Garlic odor on breath represents a classic though inconsistently present finding. Acute encephalopathy may develop with significant exposures, manifesting as confusion, seizures, and coma. Subacute presentations typically developing weeks after exposure include peripheral neuropathy predominantly affecting sensory functions in a stocking-glove distribution, though motor involvement may occur with higher exposures. This neuropathy results from axonal degeneration rather than demyelination, creating prolonged recovery periods often extending months to years.

Chronic arsenic toxicity produces pathognomonic dermatological manifestations including hyperpigmentation with characteristic "raindrops on a dusty road" appearance (guttate pattern of small hypopigmented macules on a hyperpigmented background), palmar-plantar hyperkeratosis, and ultimately potential development of Bowen's disease (squamous cell carcinoma in situ) and other skin malignancies. Mees' lines (transverse white bands on nails) may appear

4-6 weeks after acute exposure, reflecting disrupted nail matrix function. Peripheral vascular disease manifests as acrocyanosis potentially progressing to gangrene, historically termed "blackfoot disease" in endemic regions. Hepatic effects include non-cirrhotic portal hypertension, fibrosis, and occasionally cirrhosis with prolonged exposure. Hematological manifestations encompass anemia, leukopenia, and thrombocytopenia through bone marrow suppression. Long-term effects include significantly increased malignancy risk, particularly for skin, bladder, and lung cancers, with latency periods sometimes extending decades after exposure cessation.

Diagnostic evaluation requires appropriate specimen selection and testing methodology based on exposure timing. For recent acute exposure, blood arsenic measurement provides useful information, though levels decline rapidly limiting utility beyond 24-48 hours post-exposure. Urine arsenic represents the preferred biomarker for both acute and chronic exposure assessment, with 24-hour collections preferred over spot samples due to excretion variability. Critical interpretation factors include speciation analysis distinguishing toxic inorganic and methylated metabolites from relatively non-toxic organic arsenicals found in seafood, which otherwise create potential false elevations. Hair and nail analysis provide longer-term exposure assessment useful for historical exposure documentation, though external contamination remains a potential confounder requiring careful sample collection and preparation. Radiographic findings in chronic exposure may include characteristic punctate calcifications in soft tissues, particularly evident on chest radiography.

Treatment approaches include exposure elimination, supportive care, and chelation therapy when indicated. Gastrointestinal decontamination for acute oral exposure follows standard approaches with activated charcoal administration if presenting within 1-2 hours of ingestion. Fluid resuscitation addressing gastrointestinal losses and capillary leak represents a critical intervention in acute poisoning. Chelation therapy indications include symptomatic acute poisoning, confirmed significant exposure with elevated biological markers, and occasionally chronic high-level exposure with progressive symptoms. Chelating agents include dimercaprol (BAL) for severe acute poisoning requiring parenteral therapy, typically at 3-5 mg/kg intramuscularly every 4-6 hours; succimer (DMSA) for less severe cases amenable to oral therapy at 10 mg/kg three times daily for 5 days then twice daily for 14 days; and d-penicillamine as an alternative oral agent though with higher adverse effect profile. Supportive management of established complications includes pain control and gabapentinoids for neuropathic pain, physical therapy for neurological deficits, and enhanced skin cancer surveillance for patients with dermatological manifestations of chronic exposure.

Prevention encompasses both individual and population-level approaches. Water testing and treatment in affected regions represent primary interventions, with technologies including precipitation/coagulation with iron or aluminum compounds, ion exchange resins, reverse osmosis, and oxidation filtration systems. Public health measures include enhanced surveillance in high-risk regions, regulatory standards limiting arsenic in drinking water and food products, occupational exposure monitoring, and remediation of contaminated sites. Dietary modifications for individuals in affected regions include diversification beyond heavily reliant on arsenic-accumulating foods like rice, using water with confirmed safety for cooking as well as drinking, and awareness of potential dietary supplements or traditional medicines potentially containing arsenic. These multilevel approaches have successfully reduced exposure in many regions, though significant global challenges remain due to extensive natural contamination affecting impoverished areas with limited infrastructure and resources.

Cadmium

Cadmium toxicity represents a significant environmental health concern due to its accumulation in the environment, efficient biological uptake, extremely long biological half-life, and multiple target organ effects. Exposure sources include industrial emissions from metal refining, battery manufacturing, and pigment production; tobacco smoke containing cadmium concentrated by tobacco plants; contaminated foods particularly grains and vegetables grown in cadmium-rich soils; and occupational exposures in electroplating, welding, and pigment handling. Environmental background exposure occurs universally, with significantly enhanced levels in industrial regions and among smokers who may receive double the cadmium burden of non-smokers due to efficient pulmonary absorption and cadmium concentration in tobacco leaves.

Toxicokinetics involve relatively limited gastrointestinal absorption (approximately 5-10%) contrasting with efficient pulmonary uptake (40-60%), potentially enhanced gastrointestinal absorption with iron deficiency, and extremely prolonged biological half-life estimated at 10-30 years. This extended half-life reflects cadmium's binding to metallothionein, a cysteine-rich protein induced by cadmium exposure that both detoxifies by limiting free cadmium availability and inadvertently creates long-term storage facilitating accumulation. Renal cortical concentration reaches levels 20-fold higher than blood, creating pronounced nephrotoxic potential. Minimal biliary excretion and negligible transplacental transfer occur, though cadmium concentrates in the placenta potentially affecting placental function. Major body burden resides in liver and kidneys, with total accumulation continuing throughout life under typical environmental exposure conditions.

Pathophysiological mechanisms include displacement of essential metals (particularly zinc, iron, and calcium) from metalloenzymes and binding proteins, direct enzyme inhibition through sulfhydryl binding, cellular energy production disruption, enhanced oxidative stress, and interference with DNA repair mechanisms. Renal toxicity involves both glomerular and tubular damage, with initial manifestations of tubular dysfunction progressing to glomerular filtration impairment with continued exposure. Bone effects result from both direct osteotoxicity and secondary changes from altered calcium metabolism and vitamin D activation. Reproductive toxicity mechanisms include placental damage, disruption of steroid hormone synthesis, and direct effects on developing gametes, though placental barrier function limits direct fetal exposure.

Clinical manifestations reflect both acute high-dose and chronic low-level exposure patterns. Acute inhalational exposure primarily affects the respiratory system, producing chemical pneumonitis, pulmonary edema, and in severe cases, acute respiratory distress syndrome developing 24-48 hours post-exposure. Ingestion of highly concentrated cadmium creates severe gastroenteritis with vomiting, diarrhea, abdominal pain, and potential shock through third-spacing of fluids. Chronic exposure produces more insidious multisystem effects with renal manifestations predominating, initially presenting as tubular dysfunction with increased excretion of low molecular weight proteins (β2-microglobulin, retinol binding protein, α1-microglobulin) and eventually progressing to decreased glomerular filtration and chronic kidney disease.

Skeletal effects include osteomalacia and osteoporosis through both direct bone toxicity and secondary hyperparathyroidism from altered vitamin D metabolism, historically recognized in the "Itai-Itai" (ouch-ouch) disease affecting postmenopausal women in cadmium-polluted regions of Japan who developed painful bone deformities and fractures. Cardiovascular effects encompass hypertension through renal mechanisms and potentially direct vascular effects, with epidemiological evidence suggesting increased cardiovascular mortality with higher cadmium exposure. Reproductive consequences include decreased sperm parameters in males and potential effects on female reproductive function, though evidence remains less conclusive than for other target organs. Carcinogenic potential has been established through both animal studies and epidemiological evidence, with cadmium classified as a known human carcinogen particularly associated with lung cancer and possibly prostate, renal, and breast malignancies.

Diagnostic evaluation employs both exposure biomarkers and effect biomarkers providing complementary information. Blood cadmium primarily reflects recent exposure with typical levels below 1 μg/L in non-smokers from non-industrial regions, while urinary cadmium better represents total body burden due to its correlation with renal cortical concentration. Urinary β2-microglobulin and other low molecular weight proteins serve as early effect biomarkers indicating tubular dysfunction before clinical manifestations develop. Reference ranges require adjustment for smoking status, with smokers typically showing 2-3 fold higher cadmium biomarkers. Bone density measurement may reveal decreased mineralization in chronic high-level exposure, while pulmonary function testing assesses respiratory effects in occupational inhalational exposure.

Management strategies emphasize exposure cessation and supportive care, as no effective chelation therapy exists for chronic cadmium toxicity due to its tight metallothionein binding. For acute high-level exposure, particularly pulmonary exposure, early chelation with succimer (DMSA) or dimercaprol (BAL) may provide some benefit, though evidence remains limited. Calcium disodium EDTA demonstrates poor efficacy for cadmium and may paradoxically enhance nephrotoxicity by increasing renal tubular exposure to cadmium-EDTA complexes. Supportive management addresses specific manifestations including respiratory support for pulmonary injury, renal function monitoring with appropriate chronic kidney disease management for established nephropathy, and bone health optimization through calcium and vitamin D supplementation for skeletal effects. Nutritional interventions maintaining adequate iron, calcium, and zinc status may reduce cadmium absorption and potentially mitigate certain toxic effects through competitive interactions, though without significantly enhancing elimination of established body burden.

Prevention strategies encompass regulatory, occupational, and individual approaches. Environmental regulations limiting industrial emissions and establishing food content standards reduce population exposure, while occupational protections include engineering controls minimizing workplace dust and fume generation, respiratory protection programs, and biological monitoring for exposed workers. Individual measures include smoking cessation, dietary diversity rather than reliance on single potentially contaminated food sources, and maintenance of adequate iron status particularly in menstruating women who demonstrate enhanced cadmium absorption with iron deficiency. For contaminated regions, soil remediation and agricultural practices minimizing plant uptake, such as maintaining neutral soil pH and adequate zinc fertilization, may reduce dietary exposure. These multilevel approaches have successfully reduced cadmium exposure in some industrialized nations, though global challenges remain, particularly in rapidly industrializing regions with limited environmental regulation enforcement.

PESTICIDES

Pesticides encompass diverse chemical classes designed to control unwanted organisms, with human toxicity reflecting their mechanisms of action, exposure patterns, and physicochemical properties.

Organophosphates and Carbamates

Organophosphate and carbamate insecticides remain among the most toxicologically significant pesticides worldwide, causing thousands of annual fatalities through both unintentional exposures and deliberate ingestions. These compounds share the common mechanism of acetylcholinesterase (AChE) inhibition, though with distinctive chemical structures, toxicokinetic properties, and clinical features. Organophosphates include diverse compounds such as chlorpyrifos, parathion, malathion, and diazinon used across agricultural, residential, and public health applications. Carbamates include aldicarb, carbaryl, and propoxur, likewise employed across multiple settings. Military nerve agents including sarin, VX, and tabun represent organophosphate derivatives designed specifically for human toxicity, with chemical structures optimized for enhanced potency and distinctive physical properties facilitating weaponization.

The fundamental toxicological mechanism involves inhibition of acetylcholinesterase, the enzyme responsible for hydrolyzing acetylcholine at cholinergic synapses and neuromuscular junctions. This inhibition results in acetylcholine accumulation and consequent overstimulation of muscarinic and nicotinic receptors throughout the body. Important distinctions between compound classes affect clinical presentation and management: organophosphates form a covalent bond with AChE requiring days to weeks for new enzyme synthesis to restore function, while carbamates create a more readily reversible carbamylated enzyme complex typically resolving within hours. Organophosphates undergo bioactivation requiring conversion from thion (P=S) to oxon (P=O) forms through cytochrome P450 metabolism, creating potential for delayed onset and prolonged toxicity. Lipophilicity varies substantially between compounds, affecting distribution patterns, storage in adipose tissue, and potential for delayed recutting after apparent recovery.

Clinical manifestations reflect excessive cholinergic stimulation across multiple organ systems, classically categorized through receptor subtypes.

Table 8.2: Pesticide Classification and Toxicity

Pesticide Class	Mechanism of Toxicity	Clinical Features	Specific Antidotes
Organophosphates	Acetylcholinesterase inhibition	SLUDGEM syndrome, bradycardia, respiratory depression	Atropine, pralidoxime
Carbamates	Reversible acetylcholinesterase inhibition	Similar to organophosphates but shorter duration	Atropine (pralidoxime rarely needed)
Pyrethroids	Sodium channel modulation	Paresthesias, dizziness, GI symptoms, rarely seizures	None specific
Organochlorines	CNS stimulation, GABA antagonism	Seizures, headache, dizziness, paresthesias	None specific, benzodiazepines for seizures
Glyphosate	Surfactant toxicity more than active ingredient	GI irritation, pulmonary edema with surfactants	None specific

Muscarinic effects create the "SLUDGE" syndrome (Salivation, Lacrimation, Urination, Defecation, Gastric emesis, Emesis) reflecting secretory gland stimulation, along with bronchorrhea, bronchospasm, bradycardia, and miosis. Nicotinic manifestations include fasciculations, muscle weakness potentially progressing to paralysis, tachycardia (potentially masking muscarinic-induced bradycardia), hypertension, and in severe cases, respiratory failure through diaphragmatic weakness. Central nervous system effects encompass anxiety, restlessness, confusion, seizures, and respiratory center depression. Symptom onset typically occurs within minutes to hours of exposure, though certain highly lipophilic organophosphates with significant bioactivation requirements may demonstrate delayed toxicity onset up to 48 hours post-exposure.

Three distinctive temporal toxicity patterns require recognition. Acute cholinergic crisis represents the initial manifestation with symptom onset and severity proportional to the degree of AChE inhibition.

> **Remember**
>
> **Organophosphate and carbamate pesticides inhibit acetylcholinesterase producing the cholinergic toxidrome (SLUDGE: Salivation, Lacrimation, Urination, Defecation, Gastrointestinal distress, Emesis) and requiring treatment with atropine and pralidoxime.**

Intermediate syndrome develops 24-96 hours after acute cholinergic crisis resolution, manifesting as proximal muscle weakness predominantly affecting neck flexors, respiratory muscles, and proximal limbs, sometimes necessitating ventilatory support for 5-18 days. This syndrome likely results from receptor desensitization at the neuromuscular junction rather than cholinesterase inhibition. Organophosphate-induced delayed polyneuropathy (OPIDN) represents a rare complication developing 1-3 weeks after exposure to specific organophosphates, particularly those inhibiting neuropathy target esterase, presenting with distal symmetric sensorimotor polyneuropathy that may progress to irreversible deficits.

Diagnosis combines clinical assessment, exposure history, and laboratory confirmation when available. Cholinesterase measurement provides both diagnostic confirmation and severity assessment, with two complementary approaches: red blood cell (RBC) acetylcholinesterase more specifically reflects nervous system effects and recovers slowly, while plasma pseudocholinesterase (butyrylcholinesterase) shows greater sensitivity to exposure but less correlation with clinical severity and more rapid recovery. Depression below 50% of reference values typically produces clinical manifestations, with levels below 20% often associated with severe toxicity. Limitations include absence of pre-exposure baseline measurements, significant interpersonal variation in normal values, and various medical conditions affecting pseudocholinesterase independent of pesticide exposure. Specific compound identification through analytical toxicology provides valuable prognostic and management information, particularly regarding lipophilicity and aging rate affecting treatment duration requirements.

Management employs a structured approach addressing both inhibitor removal and cholinergic receptor antagonism. Initial stabilization focuses on airway protection and ventilatory support addressing profound secretions and potential respiratory muscle weakness. Decontamination includes clothing removal and thorough skin washing for dermal exposures, activated charcoal for recent oral ingestions, and careful attention to protective equipment for healthcare providers preventing secondary exposure, particularly with highly dermal-active compounds or nerve agents. Atropine provides competitive antagonism at muscarinic receptors, administered at initial doses of 1-5 mg intravenously (0.05 mg/kg in children) and doubled every 3-5 minutes until bronchial secretions diminish, with total requirements occasionally reaching hundreds of milligrams in severe cases. Importantly, atropine addresses only muscarinic manifestations without affecting nicotinic receptor overstimulation or directly restoring cholinesterase function.

Oximes, particularly pralidoxime (2-PAM), reactivate phosphorylated acetylcholinesterase through nucleophilic displacement of the phosphoryl group, but only before "aging" occurs—a time-dependent process where the phosphoryl-enzyme complex loses an alkyl group creating a permanently inhibited enzyme. Pralidoxime dosing typically involves 1-2 g intravenously followed by either intermittent dosing (1-2 g every 4-6 hours) or continuous infusion (500 mg/hour) until clinical improvement occurs and maintenance can be weaned. Efficacy varies between compounds based on aging rate, with soman having a half-time of aging of just minutes making oximes ineffective, while VX and many insecticidal organophosphates have aging half-times of hours to days allowing meaningful reactivation with prompt therapy. Carbamates generally do not require oxime therapy due to their spontaneous decarbamylation, with some evidence suggesting pralidoxime may potentially worsen carbamate toxicity through complex kinetic interactions.

Benzodiazepines play critical roles addressing both seizures and central nervous system cholinergic excess, with diazepam (5-10 mg intravenously in adults) representing the traditional agent, though alternative benzodiazepines demonstrate similar efficacy. Seizure management assumes particular importance as prolonged seizure activity substantially increases mortality and neurological sequelae. Additional therapies with limited evidence include sodium bicarbonate potentially enhancing organophosphate hydrolysis through alkalinization, and extracorporeal elimination for specific highly toxic compounds with favorable toxicokinetic properties, though evidence remains insufficient for routine recommendation.

Prevention strategies encompass regulatory, occupational, and public health approaches. Regulatory measures include registration requirements with toxicity testing, application restrictions for highly toxic compounds, certification requirements for applicators, and mandatory reentry intervals after application. Occupational protections incorporate engineering controls minimizing exposure, personal protective equipment appropriate to the specific compound and application method, and medical monitoring programs for workers with regular exposure. Public health measures include education regarding storage safety, proper application practices, recognition of exposure symptoms, and appropriate decontamination and medical care seeking behavior. Enhanced availability of atropine and pralidoxime in agricultural regions with high organophosphate usage has demonstrated mortality reduction in regions previously experiencing significant fatalities from delayed treatment access.

Organochlorines

Organochlorine pesticides represent a diverse chemical class characterized by chlorinated hydrocarbon structures, environmental persistence, lipophilicity, and shared neurotoxic mechanisms despite varying chemical configurations. While largely banned or severely restricted in developed nations due to ecological and human health concerns, these compounds persist in the environment decades after application cessation and continue being manufactured and utilized in certain developing regions due to their low cost and effectiveness against disease vectors including malaria-transmitting mosquitoes. Major compounds include dichlorodiphenyltrichloroethane (DDT) and its metabolites, chlordane, aldrin, dieldrin, endrin, heptachlor, toxaphene, and lindane (gamma-hexachlorocyclohexane). Their historical widespread application created global environmental contamination affecting virtually all human populations through dietary exposure, though at substantially lower levels than during peak usage periods.

Toxicokinetics reflect high lipophilicity creating distinctive patterns of distribution, storage, and elimination. Gastrointestinal absorption varies from 40-90% depending on specific compound and vehicle, with enhanced absorption in the presence of dietary lipids. Dermal absorption occurs significantlys, particularly with organic solvent vehicles increasing penetration. Distribution initially follows blood flow patterns but rapidly redistributes to adipose tissue creating long-term storage reservoirs, with half-lives ranging from 24 hours for less persistent compounds like lindane to years or decades for DDT and its metabolites. Enterohepatic circulation further extends biological persistence, while lipid mobilization during weight loss, pregnancy, or illness may release stored compounds causing elevated blood levels years after exposure cessation. Metabolism varies between compounds but generally involves cytochrome P450-mediated dehydrochlorination and oxidation, sometimes creating metabolites with greater toxicity or persistence than parent compounds, exemplified by DDT conversion to DDE (dichlorodiphenyldichloroethylene) which demonstrates greater stability and potential endocrine disruption.

Neurotoxic mechanisms primarily involve voltage-gated sodium channel modulation in neuronal membranes, with binding to the channel in its open state delaying repolarization and creating hyperexcitability through repetitive discharges after single stimuli. Additional mechanisms include antagonism of GABA-mediated inhibitory neurotransmission through interaction with GABA-A receptor chloride channels, inhibition of Na^+/K^+-ATPase and Ca^{2+}-ATPase disrupting ion gradients essential for normal neuronal function, and enhanced neurotransmitter release potentially contributing to excitotoxicity. These collective actions create neural hyperexcitability manifesting clinically as distinctive seizure patterns and movement disorders. Certain organochlorines additionally demonstrate endocrine disruption through estrogen receptor interactions (DDT and metabolites) or anti-androgenic effects (DDE), potentially affecting reproductive development and function at exposures below those causing obvious neurotoxicity.

Clinical manifestations vary with exposure intensity, specific compound, and individual susceptibility factors. Acute high-dose exposure typically produces progressively developing neurological symptoms beginning with hyperesthesia (particularly facial), headache, dizziness, nausea, and confusion, potentially progressing to myoclonic jerking, seizures, coma, and respiratory arrest in severe cases. Distinctive features differentiating organochlorine toxicity from other provulsant poisonings include early myoclonus often preceding frank seizures, seizures typically refractory to standard anticonvulsants but responsive to benzodiazepines, and prominent hyperreflexia. Cardiotoxicity manifests through myocardial sensitization to catecholamines, creating risk for malignant dysrhythmias particularly with physiological stress or exogenous sympathomimetic administration. Hepatotoxicity occurs with certain compounds, particularly chlordane and heptachlor, through mechanisms including microsomal enzyme induction and oxidative stress generation.

Chronic low-level exposure appears more toxicologically significant in contemporary contexts, with potential effects including subtle neurodevelopmental impacts from prenatal exposure, endocrine disruption affecting reproductive function and potentially contributing to disorders including polycystic ovary syndrome and altered gonadal development, immunomodulation with evidence suggesting potential autoimmune disorder links, and possible carcinogenicity with strongest evidence for compounds including DDT (classified as probable human carcinogen). These chronic effects typically occur without obvious clinical manifestations attributable to organochlorine exposure, but rather through epidemiological associations requiring careful interpretation due to numerous potential confounding factors.

Diagnostic evaluation for acute toxicity relies primarily on clinical presentation and exposure history, as rapid laboratory confirmation remains generally unavailable. Blood and adipose tissue measurements provide exposure documentation but correlate poorly with acute symptomatology due to rapid redistribution. Electroencephalography during acute toxicity typically demonstrates paroxysmal epileptiform activity corresponding to myoclonic jerking, though without pathognomonic patterns. For chronic exposure assessment, serum measurements of selected compounds and metabolites (particularly DDE) can document body burden, with interpretation requiring population-specific reference ranges reflecting background environmental exposure. Adipose tissue sampling provides more accurate total body burden assessment but involves invasive collection rarely justified in clinical contexts.

Management of acute organochlorine toxicity employs supportive care and seizure control without specific antidotes available. Gastrointestinal decontamination with activated charcoal benefits patients presenting within 1-2 hours of oral exposure, with consideration of multiple-dose regimens potentially interrupting enterohepatic circulation of certain compounds. Seizure management centers on benzodiazepines at aggressive dosing, with diazepam (0.2-0.5 mg/kg IV) traditionally preferred based on historical experience and lipophilicity potentially enhancing central nervous system penetration. Phenobarbital provides second-line therapy for seizures refractory to benzodiazepines, while propofol or general anesthesia may be required for status epilepticus unresponsive to conventional anticonvulsants. Critical management considerations include avoidance of epinephrine and other sympathomimetics due to myocardial sensitization creating malignant dysrhythmia risk, and recognition that recovery may require days with supportive care continuation throughout this period.

Enhanced elimination has demonstrated limited efficacy due to large volumes of distribution and adipose sequestration, though specific approaches may benefit selected scenarios. Cholestyramine binding interrupts enterohepatic circulation for compounds undergoing significant biliary excretion. Olestra, a non-absorbable fat substitute, enhances fecal elimination through solubilization in its lipid matrix, with evidence supporting modest acceleration of chlordecone (Kepone) elimination. Extracorporeal techniques including hemodialysis and hemoperfusion demonstrate minimal efficacy due to extensive tissue binding and large distribution volumes. Management of chronic exposure consequences remains largely supportive due to limited evidence for interventions affecting established endocrine, neurodevelopmental, or other systemic effects.

Prevention emphasizes reduced environmental release and

exposure mitigation where compounds remain in use. Alternative pest management strategies including integrated pest management and less persistent chemical classes have successfully replaced organochlorines in most agricultural applications. Vector control programs balancing malaria prevention against organochlorine exposure risks employ usage patterns minimizing human exposure while maintaining efficacy against disease vectors. Dietary exposure reduction includes consumption of lower-fat animal products (as organochlorines concentrate in animal fat), fatty fish consumption guidance balancing contaminant exposure against nutritional benefits, and agricultural practices minimizing uptake from historically contaminated soils. These approaches have successfully reduced human body burdens in many regions, with serum DDE levels in the United States declining approximately 90% since peak usage periods, though detectable levels remain nearly universal reflecting environmental persistence and continued low-level exposure.

Bipyridyl Herbicides

Bipyridyl herbicides, primarily paraquat and diquat, create distinctive toxicological challenges due to their unique mechanisms, specific organ tropisms, and absence of effective antidotes despite significant global usage. These compounds function agriculturally as non-selective contact herbicides disrupting photosynthesis through free radical generation, with applications including pre-planting weed control, crop desiccation before harvest, and aquatic weed management. Paraquat presents particular clinical significance due to its narrow therapeutic index, specific pulmonary concentration, and delayed progressive fibrosis mechanism creating mortality rates exceeding 50% despite intensive supportive care. Regulatory restrictions in many nations reflect these toxicity concerns, though agricultural advantages including rapid environmental degradation, soil inactivation preventing prolonged residual activity, and cost-effectiveness maintain widespread usage particularly in developing regions.

Toxicokinetics differ significantly between the principal bipyridyl compounds. Paraquat demonstrates limited gastrointestinal absorption (1-5%) but undergoes active uptake into pneumocytes through polyamine transporters, creating progressive pulmonary concentration up to 10 times plasma levels within 24 hours of systemic distribution. This active concentration mechanism explains both specific pulmonary toxicity and continued progression despite declining plasma levels. Minimal metabolism occurs, with elimination primarily through renal excretion of unchanged compound. Developing renal failure, common in significant poisoning, creates prolonged exposure through decreased elimination. Diquat shares similar gastrointestinal absorption characteristics but lacks the specific pulmonary transport mechanism, creating different distribution patterns with greater toxicity to the intestinal mucosa, liver, and kidneys rather than progressive pulmonary damage.

Pathophysiological mechanisms center on redox cycling generating reactive oxygen species. The paraquat dication (PQ^{2+}) undergoes single-electron reduction to form a free radical ($PQ^{+}\bullet$) which reacts with molecular oxygen producing superoxide radical and regenerating the parent compound. This cyclical process creates continuous free radical production until either the paraquat or reducing equivalents (primarily NADPH) become depleted. Resultant oxidative stress produces lipid peroxidation, mitochondrial dysfunction, DNA damage, and ultimately cellular apoptosis or necrosis depending on exposure intensity. The pulmonary tropism creates particular vulnerability in pneumocytes, with alveolar damage triggering inflammatory cascades and fibroblast activation leading to progressive fibrosis resembling accelerated acute respiratory distress syndrome. Additional mechanisms include NADPH depletion interrupting glutathione regeneration and nitric oxide synthase inhibition potentially contributing to pulmonary hypertension development.

Clinical manifestations evolve through characteristic phases following paraquat ingestion. Initial gastrointestinal effects include corrosive injury to oral mucosa, esophagus, and stomach due to direct caustic effects, creating painful ulcerations potentially progressing to perforation with larger volumes. The second phase, developing 24-48 hours post-ingestion, involves multiorgan dysfunction predominantly affecting kidneys, liver, and heart, with acute kidney injury particularly significant both as a direct toxicity manifestation and through its impact on paraquat elimination. The third and typically fatal phase involves progressive pulmonary damage evolving from initial chemical pneumonitis to fibroproliferative diffuse alveolar damage and eventually pulmonary fibrosis with respiratory failure developing 3-14 days post-exposure. Distinctive clinical features include painful oral ulcerations with blue-black discoloration developing after approximately 24 hours, reflecting local paraquat reduction to a colored radical species, and progressive worsening of respiratory function despite declining plasma concentrations, reflecting the continuing damage cascade initiated during early exposure.

Diagnostic confirmation integrates clinical presentation, exposure history, and laboratory testing when available. Qualitative screening employs the sodium dithionite test applied to urine, with development of blue coloration indicating paraquat presence at concentrations above approximately 1 mg/L. More precise quantification through spectrophotometric or chromatographic methods provides prognostic information, with plasma concentrations exceeding 2-3 mg/L at 24 hours or 0.1-0.2 mg/L at 48 hours generally associated with fatal outcomes. Pulmonary function assessment through both spirometry and diffusion capacity measurement documents functional impairment progression, while radiographic evaluation demonstrates evolving infiltrates typically beginning with peripheral distribution and progressing to confluent opacities with eventual fibrotic changes in survivors. Renal and hepatic function monitoring guides both prognostication and supportive care decisions.

Management strategies address toxin removal, reactive oxygen species mitigation, antifibrotic interventions, and supportive care, though with limited evidence for mortality reduction beyond early decontamination efforts. Gastrointestinal decontamination includes activated charcoal administration for patients presenting within 1-2 hours of ingestion, with additional benefit from Fuller's earth or bentonite clay which bind paraquat through cation exchange capacity rather than simple adsorption. Enhanced elimination employs hemoperfusion, ideally initiated within 4 hours of ingestion, though limited by rapid tissue distribution and specific pulmonary uptake creating ongoing damage despite plasma concentration reduction. Additional enhanced elimination approaches include hemodialysis and continuous renal replacement therapy, which may provide supportive benefit for renal failure while offering modest toxin removal.

Antioxidant interventions target the fundamental oxidative stress mechanism with numerous agents investigated, though none demonstrating consistent mortality reduction. Approaches studied include N-acetylcysteine providing glutathione precursors, vitamin E and C as direct antioxidants, superoxide dismutase and catalase analogs, spin-trapping agents, and iron chelators reducing Fenton reaction contribution to hydroxyl radical formation. Immunosuppressive and anti-inflammatory regimens, including cyclophosphamide combined with methylprednisolone or dexamethasone, demonstrate potential benefit through interruption of inflammatory cascades leading to fibrosis, though evidence quality remains limited with inconsistent results across studies. Supportive care emphasizes oxygen restriction to the minimum required for adequate saturation, as higher concentrations potentially enhance pulmonary toxicity through increased superoxide generation, along with standard respiratory, renal, and cardiovascular support.

Prevention strategies include regulatory restrictions limiting access to highly concentrated formulations, development of alternative formulations incorporating deterrent additives such as emetics, stenching agents, blue coloration, and alerting agents creating immediate recognition of potential ingestion. Product stewardship programs promoting secure storage, certified applicator restrictions, and rapid spill response procedures reduce accidental exposure risk. Public health interventions include education regarding toxicity recognition and immediate management, with emphasis on the importance of immediate decontamination and medical evaluation even for apparently minor exposures given the potential for progressive toxicity despite initial minimal symptoms.

Rodenticides

Rodenticide toxicity presents diverse clinical scenarios reflecting the multiple chemical classes employed for vertebrate pest control, with anticoagulants representing the most commonly encountered agents in human exposures but several alternative classes creating distinctive toxicological concerns. Superwarfarins, including brodifacoum, difethialone, and bromadiolone, function as vitamin K antagonists with significantly greater potency and duration compared to traditional warfarin, creating potential for severe coagulopathy persisting weeks to months after exposure. Metal phosphides, particularly aluminum and zinc phosphide, release phosphine gas upon contact with moisture or acid, producing cytotoxic effects through mitochondrial dysfunction and oxidative stress. Strychnine induces generalized muscle contractions through glycine receptor antagonism, while bromethalin produces cerebral edema and spongiform myelinopathy through uncoupling oxidative phosphorylation. Sodium monofluoroacetate (compound 1080) and fluoroacetamide metabolize to fluorocitrate blocking the tricarboxylic acid cycle with resultant energy failure and cardiotoxicity. Each class demonstrates distinctive clinical presentation, diagnostic approach, and management considerations.

Anticoagulant rodenticides create human toxicity through vitamin K antagonism, inhibiting vitamin K epoxide reductase and consequently blocking activation of clotting factors II, VII, IX, and X plus regulatory proteins C and S. First-generation compounds including warfarin demonstrate relatively short half-lives (15-20 hours) and duration of action (2-3 days), while second-generation "superwarfarins" show substantially enhanced potency (up to 100-fold) and markedly prolonged half-lives (16-69 days or longer) creating extended toxicity potential. Clinical manifestations typically develop gradually as functional clotting factors deplete through normal consumption without adequate replacement, with factor VII (shortest half-life at 6 hours) declining first, followed by factors IX, X, and II. Initial presentation may include mucosal bleeding, particularly epistaxis or gingival bleeding, gastrointestinal hemorrhage manifesting as hematemesis or melena, hematuria, or excessive menstrual bleeding, potentially progressing to life-threatening hemorrhage including intracranial bleeding. Important clinical distinctions from therapeutic anticoagulation include the prolonged duration requiring extended treatment and monitoring, the lack of anticoagulant dose titration data potentially leading to unpredictable response to typical reversal protocols, and the potential for delayed presentation weeks after exposure.

Diagnostic evaluation for anticoagulant rodenticides centers on coagulation studies and specific compound identification when possible. Prothrombin time (PT/INR) elevation typically occurs earlier than activated partial thromboplastin time (aPTT) prolongation due to the shorter half-life of factor VII affecting the extrinsic pathway first. Mixing studies help distinguish between factor deficiency and inhibitor presence, with correction suggesting factor deficiency consistent with anticoagulant exposure. Specific anticoagulant identification through high-performance liquid chromatography or mass spectrometry provides valuable management guidance, particularly regarding treatment duration requirements, though clinical decisions regarding initial intervention should not await these results when significant coagulopathy exists. Normal coagulation studies effectively exclude clinically significant anticoagulant rodenticide toxicity, providing reassurance in cases of suspected pediatric exposures with uncertain ingestion amount.

Management strategies for anticoagulant rodenticide poisoning balance hemorrhage risk against treatment costs and complications. For patients with confirmed significant exposure but normal coagulation studies, management options include observation with serial coagulation studies, empiric low-dose vitamin K_1 (phytonadione) prophylaxis, or discharge with scheduled laboratory follow-up based on specific compound, exposure circumstances, and patient reliability. For established coagulopathy without active bleeding, oral vitamin K_1 (typically 15-25 mg daily in adults, adjusted based on response) provides effective reversal, though with treatment duration potentially extending weeks to months with superwarfarin exposure. Active hemorrhage or critical coagulopathy (INR >20) necessitates immediate factor replacement through fresh frozen plasma or prothrombin complex concentrate administration, alongside intravenous vitamin K_1 (typically 10 mg slow infusion, avoiding rapid administration which may cause anaphylactoid reactions). Treatment monitoring includes regular coagulation studies with frequency determined by clinical stability, exposure characteristics, and treatment response, recognizing that premature discontinuation commonly results in coagulopathy recurrence due to the long half-life of second-generation compounds.

Metal phosphides, particularly aluminum and zinc phosphide used as grain fumigants and rodenticides, create toxicity through phosphine gas generation upon exposure to moisture or gastric acid. Phosphine produces cellular toxicity through multiple mechanisms including inhibition of cytochrome c oxidase disrupting mitochondrial respiration, catalase inhibition increasing oxidative stress, and direct membrane lipid peroxidation. Clinical manifestations develop rapidly, typically within hours of exposure, with initial gastrointestinal symptoms including vomiting, abdominal pain, and diarrhea progressing to multiorgan dysfunction predominantly affecting cardiovascular system (hypotension, dysrhythmias, myocardial depression), lungs (pulmonary edema, acute respiratory distress syndrome), and central nervous system (altered consciousness, seizures). Distinctive features include garlic-like breath odor reflecting phosphine elimination, severe metabolic acidosis disproportionate to hemodynamic status, and fulminant cardiovascular collapse resistant to conventional resuscitation measures. Diagnosis relies primarily on exposure history and clinical presentation, with positive silver nitrate paper testing of gastric contents or breath providing confirmation when available, though treatment should not be delayed awaiting confirmation.

Management for metal phosphide poisoning focuses on supportive care without effective specific antidotes available. Gastrointestinal decontamination has limited evidence with theoretical concerns about lavage fluid accelerating phosphine release, though some protocols employ potassium permanganate (1:10,000) gastric lavage attempting to oxidize phosphine to less toxic phosphate. Vegetable oils or liquid paraffin administration has been suggested to reduce phosphine formation and absorption based on limited evidence. Hemodynamic support often requires aggressive fluid resuscitation and vasopressor therapy, occasionally with intra-aortic balloon pump or extracorporeal support for refractory shock. Additional supportive measures include mechanical ventilation for respiratory failure, continuous renal replacement therapy for acute kidney injury, sodium bicarbonate for severe metabolic acidosis, and antioxidant therapy with N-acetylcysteine, though with limited evidence for outcome improvement. Mortality remains high (approximately 30-70%) even with intensive supportive care, with prognosis correlating with exposure amount, time to treatment initiation, and development of multiorgan failure.

Bromethalin produces distinctive neurotoxicity through uncoupling of oxidative phosphorylation in the central nervous system, creating energy failure with resultant cerebral edema and spongy degeneration of white matter. Clinical presentations include two distinct syndromes: acute cerebral edema manifesting with altered mental status, seizures, cerebral herniation, and potentially death within 24-36 hours of significant exposure; and subacute spongiform myelinopathy presenting with progressive hindlimb weakness, paresthesias, tremors, and eventually paralysis developing 1-5 days post-exposure. No specific antidote exists, with management centering on supportive care including cerebral edema control through osmotic diuretics, seizure management, and respiratory support when necessary. Gastrointestinal decontamination with activated charcoal benefits patients presenting within 1-2 hours of ingestion, with potential consideration of multiple-dose regimens interrupting enterohepatic circulation.

Strychnine creates excitotoxicity through competitive antagonism at post-synaptic glycine receptors in the spinal cord and brainstem, blocking inhibitory neurotransmission and resulting in unmodulated excitatory stimulation manifesting as generalized muscle contractions. Clinical presentation includes heightened sensitivity to stimuli, muscle rigidity, painful tetanic seizures classically described as "awake seizures" due to preserved consciousness during episodes, trismus, opisthotonos, and eventual respiratory arrest from respiratory muscle spasm or exhaustion. Characteristic features differentiating strychnine from other seizure etiologies include precipitation by minimal stimuli, preservation of consciousness during episodes, and the distinctive opisthotonic posture with generalized extension. Management employs aggressive benzodiazepine administration controlling muscle hyperactivity, with addition of barbiturates, propofol, or neuromuscular blockade with mechanical ventilation for refractory cases. Supportive care addresses metabolic acidosis from muscle activity, hyperthermia, and rhabdomyolysis with potential acute kidney injury. Gastrointestinal decontamination with activated charcoal benefits patients presenting within 1-2 hours of ingestion, with recovery typically complete without sequelae when adequate supportive care prevents hypoxic injury during the acute toxicity phase.

Prevention strategies for rodenticide exposures integrate regulatory, product design, and educational approaches. Regulatory measures include restricted usage patterns for highly toxic compounds like strychnine and sodium fluoroacetate, bait station requirements minimizing non-target exposure, and obligatory bittering agents making accidental ingestion less likely. Product design modifications include distinctive colorants aiding recognition, pellet sizes reducing ingestion risk, and packaging improvements with child-resistant containers. Educational interventions focus on proper storage practices, recognition of potential exposure symptoms, appropriate decontamination and healthcare-seeking behaviors, and alternatives to chemical rodent control in settings with high pediatric exposure risk. These multilevel approaches have successfully reduced severe poisoning incidence while maintaining effective pest control options, though ongoing vigilance remains necessary particularly regarding emerging resistance patterns potentially driving development of new rodenticide classes with uncertain human toxicity profiles

INDUSTRIAL CHEMICALS

Industrial chemicals create human toxicity exposure scenarios through occupational settings, environmental releases, and consumer product applications, with diverse mechanisms and exposure patterns necessitating specialized assessment and management approaches.

Table 8.3: Industrial Chemical Exposure - Acute Effects and Management

Chemical	Route of Exposure	Initial Management	Delayed Effects to Monitor
Hydrogen sulfide	Inhalation	100% oxygen, supportive care, consider hydroxocobalamin	Pulmonary edema, neurological sequelae
Chlorine	Inhalation	Remove from exposure, humidified oxygen, bronchodilators	Reactive airways dysfunction syndrome
Carbon monoxide	Inhalation	100% oxygen, hyperbaric oxygen in severe cases	Delayed neuropsychiatric syndrome
Cyanide	Inhalation, ingestion, dermal	Hydroxocobalamin or sodium thiosulfate	Rare delayed neurological effects
Hydrofluoric acid	Dermal, inhalation	Calcium gluconate (topical, infiltration, or IV)	Hypocalcemia, cardiac effects

Hydrocarbons

Hydrocarbon toxicity encompasses effects from a diverse chemical category united by hydrogen and carbon composition but demonstrating variable toxicological properties based on structural characteristics and additives. Aliphatic hydrocarbons (straight or branched chain structures) include compounds like gasoline, kerosene, mineral oil, and petroleum distillates, while aromatic hydrocarbons (containing benzene rings) include benzene, toluene, xylene, and naphthalene. Halogenated hydrocarbons incorporate chlorine, fluorine, bromine or other halogens, creating compounds with distinctive toxicity profiles including carbon tetrachloride, trichloroethylene, and methylene chloride. Exposure routes include inhalation (particularly for volatile compounds), ingestion (especially in pediatric exposures to household products), and dermal contact, with toxicokinetics and target organ effects varying substantially between specific agents and exposure patterns.

Pulmonary aspiration represents the principal concern with ingested aliphatic hydrocarbons, particularly those with low viscosity, low surface tension, and high volatility like gasoline, kerosene, and lamp oil. These physical properties facilitate distal airway penetration creating chemical pneumonitis, with clinical manifestations developing within minutes to hours after aspiration and including cough, tachypnea, hypoxemia, and characteristic radiographic findings of perihilar infiltrates often in right-sided predominance reflecting common aspiration anatomy. Progression may include pneumatocele formation, pneumothorax, bacterial superinfection, and acute respiratory distress syndrome in severe cases. Management emphasizes supportive respiratory care without established benefit from prophylactic antibiotics or corticosteroids. Controversially, gastrointestinal decontamination including induced emesis or gastric lavage is generally avoided due to aspiration risk potentially exceeding benefits, though activated charcoal administration may be considered for specific hydrocarbon types with significant systemic toxicity potential when airway protection is ensured.

Systemic toxicity varies substantially between hydrocarbon classes. Aliphatic compounds generally demonstrate limited systemic effects except with massive exposure, where central nervous system depression and occasionally dysrhythmias from myocardial sensitization to catecholamines may occur. Aromatic hydrocarbons produce greater systemic toxicity, with acute effects including central nervous system depression, hepatorenal injury, and cardiac dysrhythmias. Benzene specifically demonstrates hematological toxicity through metabolite binding to cellular macromolecules, creating acute myelosuppression with high-level exposure and chronic effects including aplastic anemia, myelodysplastic syndrome, and acute myelogenous leukemia with long-term exposure. Halogenated hydrocarbons typically produce the most significant systemic toxicity, with carbon tetrachloride creating severe hepatotoxicity through CYP2E1-mediated formation of trichloromethyl free radicals, while chlorinated solvents like trichloroethylene produce central nervous system effects, hepatotoxicity, nephrotoxicity, and cardiotoxicity with specific patterns varying between compounds.

Intentional inhalation for euphoric effects, termed "huffing," "sniffing," or "bagging" depending on the specific technique employed, creates distinctive toxicological concerns. Acute effects include initial excitation followed by central nervous system depression, with progression to respiratory arrest possible with continued exposure or substances stored in confined spaces creating oxygen displacement. "Sudden sniffing death syndrome" refers to dysrhythmic cardiac arrest, particularly ventricular fibrillation, occurring when sensitized myocardium encounters endogenous or exogenous catecholamines, such as during physical exertion or emotional stress following hydrocarbon inhalation. Chronic inhalation produces progressive multisystem effects including neurocognitive dysfunction with cerebral and cerebellar atrophy, peripheral neuropathy, hepatorenal toxicity, bone marrow suppression, and cardiomyopathy, with specific patterns reflecting particular agents and exposure characteristics.

Occupational exposure to hydrocarbons creates potential for both acute and chronic toxicity, with petroleum refineries, chemical manufacturing, painting, degreasing operations, and vehicle repair representing high-risk settings. Acute high-level exposure typically occurs during spills, confined space work, or equipment failure, while chronic lower-level exposure may occur through everyday operations with inadequate ventilation or protective equipment. Long-term health effects include neurobehavioral changes, peripheral neuropathy, hepatic enzyme elevation, nephrotoxicity including specific glomerulopathies with certain compounds, hematological abnormalities, and carcinogenicity, with benzene (leukemia), vinyl chloride (angiosarcoma), and trichloroethylene (renal cell carcinoma) representing established human carcinogens. Biological monitoring programs measuring either parent compounds or metabolites in blood or urine provide exposure assessment complementing environmental monitoring, with specific markers including hippuric acid for toluene exposure, mandelic acid for styrene, and trans,trans-muconic acid for benzene.

Management strategies address specific toxicity manifestations without available antidotes for most hydrocarbon exposures. Pulmonary aspiration management includes supportive care with supplemental oxygen, bronchodilators for bronchospasm, mechanical ventilation when necessary, and vigilance for secondary bacterial pneumonia developing 3-5 days after initial chemical pneumonitis. Systemic toxicity management follows organ-specific supportive protocols, with particular attention to cardiac monitoring for dysrhythmias, liver and renal function assessment, and neurological evaluation. Specific interventions based on metabolic activation patterns include N-acetylcysteine administration for carbon tetrachloride hepatotoxicity, resembling protocols used for acetaminophen poisoning, though with limited evidence basis. Chronic exposure consequences require specialized evaluation and management approaches, including occupational medicine consultation, neuropsychological assessment for cognitive effects, and enhanced surveillance for potential malignancies associated with specific exposures.

Prevention emphasizes both primary exposure reduction and secondary measures limiting toxicity when exposure occurs. Engineering controls including closed systems, local exhaust ventilation, and substitution with less hazardous alternatives represent the primary occupational exposure prevention hierarchy. Administrative controls encompass worker education, standard operating procedures minimizing exposure, and biological monitoring programs detecting excessive exposure before clinical toxicity develops. Personal protective equipment provides a final protection layer when other controls prove insufficient, with respirator selection requiring specific consideration of the particular hydrocarbons involved, as certain compounds may penetrate standard activated carbon cartridges. Consumer product safety measures include child-resistant packaging, product reformulation replacing highly toxic hydrocarbons with safer alternatives when feasible, adequate labeling regarding hazards and emergency procedures, and public education regarding proper storage preventing both pediatric and intentional misuse exposures.

Corrosives

Corrosive chemicals produce tissue destruction through direct chemical reactions, with toxicity dependent on substance properties, concentration, duration of contact, and exposed tissue vulnerability. Acids cause coagulation necrosis through protein denaturation, creating a coagulum that may limit further penetration except with highly concentrated exposures. Alkalis produce liquefaction necrosis through saponification of fats, protein dissolution, and cellular disruption, typically resulting in deeper tissue penetration and more extensive injury compared to equivalent acid exposures. Exposure scenarios encompass occupational settings including manufacturing, cleaning operations, and laboratory work; household exposures to cleaning products, drain cleaners, and batteries; and intentional exposures in suicide attempts or assaults. The most commonly encountered corrosives include sulfuric acid (battery acid, certain drain cleaners), hydrochloric acid (metal cleaners, pool chemicals), hydrofluoric acid (glass etching, rust removal), sodium hydroxide (lye, drain cleaners), and bleach (sodium hypochlorite, which forms hypochlorous acid in water).

Dermal corrosive exposures produce distinctive injury patterns varying with specific agent properties. Acid burns typically create well-demarcated areas of necrosis with eschar formation, while alkali burns demonstrate more diffuse boundaries with deeper tissue involvement. Hydrofluoric acid creates particularly concerning injuries through dual mechanisms: direct corrosive action from the hydrogen ion and specific fluoride ion toxicity through calcium binding, creating progressive deeper tissue destruction potentially out of proportion to initial appearance. Clinical evaluation includes assessment of injury depth using standard burn classification (superficial, partial thickness, full thickness), extent using percent body surface area calculation, and location with particular concern for areas overlying major vessels, joints, or functional structures. Distinctive features suggesting specific agents include the gray-white appearance of hydrofluoric acid burns, often with disproportionate pain; yellow discoloration with nitric acid; and brownish discoloration with sulfuric acid burns.

Ocular corrosive exposures represent ophthalmic emergencies with potential for permanent vision impairment. Alkalis demonstrate particular ophthalmologic concern due to rapid penetration through the cornea potentially damaging intraocular structures before decontamination can be completed. Clinical assessment focuses on visual acuity measurement, conjunctival and scleral evaluation for hyperemia and ischemia, corneal examination for epithelial defects, opacification or haze, and anterior chamber assessment for inflammatory response. The pH of tears provides critical diagnostic and therapeutic guidance, with continued irrigation necessary until normalization occurs. Complications include corneal scarring, symblepharon (adhesion between bulbar and palpebral conjunctivae), chronic dry eye syndrome, glaucoma, cataract formation, and potentially blindness, with prognosis dependent on involved agent, exposure duration, decontamination speed, and subsequent medical management.

Ingestion of corrosive substances creates complex management scenarios due to potential injury throughout the upper gastrointestinal tract. Clinical manifestations include oropharyngeal pain, drooling, vomiting (sometimes with blood), chest or abdominal pain, and respiratory symptoms when laryngeal or epiglottic injury occurs. Important clinical findings include circumoral burns, oropharyngeal erythema or ulceration, stridor suggesting airway compromise, subcutaneous emphysema indicating esophageal perforation, and peritoneal signs suggesting gastric perforation. The absence of oropharyngeal injury does not reliably exclude significant esophageal damage, particularly with liquid corrosives which may rapidly transit the mouth. Complications include acute perforation, stricture formation, gastric outlet obstruction, and long-term increased risk for esophageal carcinoma following significant caustic injury, necessitating endoscopic evaluation and long-term surveillance in significant exposures.

Management of corrosive exposures begins with immediate decontamination appropriate to the specific scenario. For dermal exposure, clothing removal and copious water irrigation represents the universal initial approach, with irrigation duration of at least 15-20 minutes and much longer for concentrated exposures. Hydrofluoric acid exposures require specific management with calcium gluconate gel (2.5-10%) application to affected areas, sometimes requiring calcium gluconate injections for deeper burns or higher concentration exposures. Ocular exposures necessitate immediate and prolonged irrigation, ideally with isotonic saline but with plain water acceptable when specialized solutions are unavailable, continued until tear pH normalizes with verification at least 15-30 minutes after irrigation cessation to detect rebounding acidosis from deep tissue stores.

Ingestion management includes several key principles: first, contraindication of neutralization attempts due to potential exothermic reactions causing additional thermal injury; second, avoidance of emetics or gastric lavage which may re-expose tissue to the corrosive; third, careful consideration of endoscopic evaluation timing and technique; and fourth, proactive management of anticipated complications. Endoscopic grading systems guide subsequent management: Grade 0 (normal appearance) typically requires no specific intervention; Grade 1 (edema and erythema) warrants observation and supportive care; Grade 2 (ulcerations and pseudomembrane formation) indicates significant injury requiring close monitoring and potential intervention; and Grade 3 (deep ulceration, necrosis, or perforation) represents severe injury potentially requiring surgical management. Specific interventions may include proton pump inhibitors reducing acid reflux exacerbation of injuries, early enteral nutrition support when feasible, and consideration of corticosteroids for Grade 2 injuries though evidence remains contradictory regarding stricture prevention efficacy.

Prevention strategies incorporate regulatory, engineering, and educational approaches. Regulatory measures include packaging requirements with child-resistant features for consumer products, concentration limitations in household formulations, and workplace standards specifying handling protocols and personal protective equipment requirements. Engineering controls encompass closed systems preventing direct contact, substitution with less hazardous alternatives when feasible, and improved container design reducing spill and splash risk. Educational initiatives include hazard communication programs in workplaces, residential safety education emphasizing proper storage and hazard recognition, and first aid training regarding appropriate initial management of corrosive exposures including immediate irrigation principles and rapid medical evaluation. These multilevel approaches have reduced incidence of serious exposures despite widespread corrosive chemical availability in both industrial and consumer settings.

Metals and Solvents

Metallic compounds beyond the heavy metals previously discussed create distinctive occupational and environmental toxicity concerns through diverse mechanisms and exposure patterns. Chromium toxicity varies with oxidation state, with hexavalent chromium [Cr(VI)] demonstrating significantly greater toxicity than trivalent [Cr(III)] forms due to enhanced cellular penetration through anion channels and subsequent intracellular reduction generating reactive intermediates and oxidative stress. Occupational exposures occur in chrome plating, stainless steel welding, pigment production, and leather tanning, with health effects including irritant and allergic contact dermatitis, chronic ulceration (historically termed "chrome holes"), respiratory manifestations ranging from irritation to occupational asthma, nasal septum perforation with chronic exposure, and lung cancer with sufficient exposure duration and intensity. Biological monitoring employs urinary chromium measurement, with industrial hygiene surveillance critical due to carcinogenic potential.

Manganese neurotoxicity manifests through accumulation in basal ganglia and other brain regions with high metabolic activity, creating a parkinsonian syndrome with distinctive features including prominent gait disturbance with less pronounced tremor compared to idiopathic Parkinson's disease, frequent psychiatric manifestations including hallucinations and personality changes, and limited response to traditional dopaminergic therapies. Occupational settings creating exposure risk include welding, steel production, battery manufacturing, and fossil fuel combustion, with absorption occurring primarily through inhalation. Management emphasizes exposure cessation, with chelation generally ineffective for established neurotoxicity, though recent research suggests potential benefit from specific chelators binding manganese with greater affinity than traditional agents.

Nickel compounds create multiple toxicological concerns depending on specific solubility and composition characteristics. Soluble nickel salts commonly cause allergic sensitization manifesting as contact dermatitis, particularly from jewelry and other skin-contact items. Occupational inhalation exposures to nickel compounds, especially in refining operations, create respiratory effects including irritation, chronic bronchitis, reduced pulmonary function, and increased lung and nasal cancer risk with certain nickel species. Biological monitoring typically employs urinary nickel measurement, though with careful interpretation required due to significant influence of recent exposure and dietary sources. Prevention focuses on engineering controls minimizing aerosol generation, appropriate respiratory protection, and skin contact avoidance through protective equipment and hygiene practices.

Industrial solvents represent a diverse chemical category united by their ability to dissolve other substances, with widespread applications including degreasing, painting, printing, pharmaceutical manufacturing, and chemical synthesis. Solvent neurotoxicity represents a principal concern, with both acute and chronic manifestations. Acute effects reflect CNS depression proportional to solvent concentration, progressing from headache, dizziness, and incoordination to confusion, impaired judgment, and eventually unconsciousness with sufficient exposure. Chronic neurotoxicity presents more insidiously with subtle neurocognitive dysfunction affecting memory, attention, processing speed, and executive function, sometimes termed "chronic solvent encephalopathy" or "painters' syndrome" reflecting common occupational associations. Diagnosis requires integration of exposure history, neuropsychological testing, and exclusion of alternative etiologies, with management focusing on exposure cessation which may result in partial improvement, though established deficits often remain permanent.

Non-neurological solvent effects vary by specific agent characteristics. Hepatotoxicity occurs with several chlorinated solvents including carbon tetrachloride, chloroform, and trichloroethylene through metabolic activation generating free radicals and subsequent lipid peroxidation. Nephrotoxicity manifests particularly with certain halogenated compounds through both direct tubular toxicity and immunologically-mediated glomerular injury, with trichloroethylene-associated membranous nephropathy representing a classic example. Reproductive toxicity has been documented with several solvents including glycol ethers reducing sperm parameters and certain chlorinated solvents associated with increased spontaneous abortion risk. Hematopoietic effects include benzene-induced bone marrow suppression and leukemogenicity through genotoxic metabolites. Appropriate biological monitoring programs vary by specific solvent, including urinary metabolites (hippuric acid for toluene, mandelic acid for styrene), unchanged solvent in expired air, or blood solvent levels, typically obtained at end-of-shift sampling to capture workday exposure.

Management of acute high-level solvent exposure addresses both immediate toxicity and prevention of delayed effects. Removal from exposure source represents the initial priority, with particular attention to confined space scenarios where rescuer protection remains essential. Supportive care follows principles for other causes of CNS depression, with careful attention to potential cardiac dysrhythmias from myocardial sensitization, particularly with halogenated solvents. Specific antidotal approaches exist for selected solvents, including ethanol or fomepizole for methanol and ethylene glycol preventing toxic metabolite formation, N-acetylcysteine for carbon tetrachloride potentially reducing free radical-mediated hepatotoxicity, and oxygen for carbon monoxide displacing the toxicant from hemoglobin and enhancing elimination. Chronic solvent toxicity management emphasizes exposure cessation, with established neurological deficits typically managed through compensatory strategies rather than direct treatment of the underlying pathology.

Solvent exposure reduction incorporates substitution, engineering controls, and appropriate personal protective equipment. Substitution with water-based or less toxic alternatives has successfully reduced exposure in many applications, including paint formulations, cleaning processes, and extraction procedures. Engineering controls encompass closed systems preventing vapor release, local exhaust ventilation capturing emissions at their source, and scheduling modifications reducing exposure frequency and duration. Personal protective equipment selection requires specific solvent consideration, as breakthrough times vary substantially between glove materials and solvent types, while respiratory protection necessitates appropriate cartridge selection with recognition of limitations including breakthrough, saturation, and inadequate protection against certain compounds. Biological monitoring programs provide objective exposure assessment verifying control effectiveness, with action levels triggering investigation and intervention before clinical toxicity develops.

Prevention of both metal and solvent toxicity requires integration of regulatory standards, workplace controls, medical surveillance, and worker education. Regulatory frameworks establish permissible exposure limits, monitoring requirements, and medical surveillance protocols for substances with established toxicity. Workplace implementations include engineering controls as the primary prevention strategy, administrative controls including exposure rotation and scheduling modifications, and personal protective equipment as the final control level. Medical surveillance programs combine exposure monitoring, biological monitoring where appropriate biomarkers exist, and targeted clinical evaluation addressing specific toxicity concerns for particular agents. Worker hazard communication includes training regarding recognition of overexposure symptoms, appropriate work practices minimizing exposure, and proper use of control measures. These comprehensive approaches have substantially reduced occupational metal and solvent toxicity incidence in regulated settings, though significant challenges remain in small businesses, developing nations, and nontraditional work arrangements where regulatory oversight and resource availability may be limited.

Gases and Vapors

Toxic gases and vapors present distinctive hazards through their physical properties allowing rapid distribution, potentially imperceptible presence, and efficient exposure through inhalation directly accessing the bloodstream without first-pass metabolism. Carbon monoxide (CO) represents the most common lethal inhaled toxicant, producing hypoxic injury through multiple mechanisms: tight binding to hemoglobin with affinity 200-250 times greater than oxygen, shifting the oxyhemoglobin dissociation curve leftward reducing oxygen offloading at tissues, and direct inhibition of mitochondrial cytochrome oxidase disrupting cellular respiration even when adequate oxygen delivery occurs. Exposure sources include incomplete combustion from heating systems, engines, fires, and tobacco smoke, with distinctive risk scenarios including poorly ventilated heating appliances, indoor use of gasoline-powered equipment, vehicle exhaust in enclosed spaces, and structure fires creating both acute poisoning and potential long-term neurological sequelae.

> **Remember**
>
> **Carbon monoxide poisoning presents with nonspecific symptoms and normal pulse oximetry, requiring high clinical suspicion, carboxyhemoglobin measurement, and prompt oxygen therapy with consideration of hyperbaric treatment for severe cases**

Clinical manifestations of carbon monoxide poisoning reflect tissue hypoxia, with severity proportional to exposure concentration, duration, and individual susceptibility factors including age, underlying cardiovascular disease, and baseline anemia. Initial symptoms include headache, dizziness, nausea, and visual disturbances, potentially progressing to confusion, syncope, seizures, coma, and death in severe exposures. Characteristic findings include bright red venous blood from carboxyhemoglobin formation, though cyanosis may develop with severe tissue hypoxia despite normal appearing blood. Cherry red skin coloration historically described occurs rarely and typically only post-mortem. Cardiovascular manifestations include myocardial ischemia, dysrhythmias, and hypotension, with particular vulnerability in patients with pre-existing coronary disease. Delayed neurological sequelae, developing days to weeks after apparent recovery from acute poisoning, affect 10-30% of significantly poisoned patients with manifestations including cognitive impairment, personality changes, parkinsonian features, focal neurological deficits, and rarely persistent vegetative state.

Diagnosis combines exposure history, clinical presentation, and carboxyhemoglobin measurement, though limitations in each element necessitate integrated assessment. Standard pulse oximetry proves unreliable due to inability to distinguish oxyhemoglobin from carboxyhemoglobin, both absorbing similarly at measured wavelengths, creating falsely normal readings despite significant hypoxemia. Co-oximetry specifically measuring multiple hemoglobin species provides accurate carboxyhemoglobin quantification, with levels typically below 3% in non-smokers, 5-10% in smokers, and potentially exceeding 50% in severe poisonings, though correlation between levels and symptoms remains imperfect due to variable exposure timing and individual susceptibility factors. Arterial blood gas analysis typically demonstrates normal PaO_2 despite tissue hypoxia, with metabolic acidosis developing in severe cases reflecting anaerobic metabolism from cellular hypoxia.

Management centers on oxygen administration displacing carbon monoxide from hemoglobin and enhancing elimination, with concentration and delivery method determined by poisoning severity. Normobaric oxygen (100% via non-rebreather mask or endotracheal tube) reduces carboxyhemoglobin half-life from approximately 4-6 hours breathing room air to 40-80 minutes. Hyperbaric oxygen therapy, providing 100% oxygen at pressures typically 2.5-3 atmospheres absolute, further reduces half-life to approximately 20-30 minutes while potentially providing additional benefit through enhanced oxygen dissolution in plasma independent of hemoglobin binding. Indications for hyperbaric treatment remain somewhat controversial, with various protocols considering factors including carboxyhemoglobin level (typically >25%), pregnancy (lower thresholds, often >15-20%), presence of neurological symptoms, cardiac ischemia or significant dysrhythmias, severe metabolic acidosis, and age extremes. Treatment efficacy for preventing delayed neurological sequelae remains incompletely established, with some studies suggesting benefit while others show no significant difference compared to normobaric oxygen, potentially reflecting treatment timing variations with greater benefit for earlier intervention.

Prevention strategies incorporate engineering controls, detection technology, public education, and targeted interventions for high-risk scenarios. Engineering approaches include improved combustion efficiency in heating appliances and vehicles, ventilation requirements for spaces containing combustion sources, and catalytic converters reducing carbon monoxide emission. Detection technology encompasses carbon monoxide alarms with mandatory installation in residential settings in many jurisdictions, featuring electrochemical sensors detecting carbon monoxide at levels below those causing symptoms and providing warning before significant exposure occurs. Public education focuses on recognition of poisoning symptoms, proper installation and maintenance of fuel-burning appliances, appropriate ventilation practices, and understanding situations creating elevated risk including operation of gas-powered equipment in enclosed spaces. Targeted interventions for high-risk populations, particularly elderly individuals during heating seasons, include home safety assessments and heating system inspection programs that have demonstrated reduced poisoning incidence in implemented areas.

Hydrogen cyanide and related cyanide compounds create cellular asphyxiation through inhibition of cytochrome c oxidase in the mitochondrial electron transport chain, blocking oxygen utilization at the cellular level despite adequate delivery. Exposure sources include industrial processes utilizing cyanide compounds (electroplating, metallurgy, chemical synthesis), combustion of nitrogen-containing materials particularly synthetic polymers during structure fires, certain foods containing cyanogenic glycosides (bitter almonds, cassava, apricot kernels), and specific industrial chemicals releasing cyanide upon metabolism, notably nitriles and certain fumigants. Clinical manifestations develop rapidly with significant exposure, including headache, dizziness, tachypnea, nausea, vomiting, altered consciousness, seizures, and cardiovascular collapse. Distinctive findings include bright red venous blood despite metabolic acidosis (reflecting decreased oxygen extraction), bitter almond odor detectable by approximately 60% of the population with genetic olfactory ability, and initial respiratory stimulation followed by respiratory depression with progressive toxicity.

Diagnosis relies predominantly on clinical recognition in appropriate exposure contexts, as rapid laboratory confirmation remains generally unavailable in emergency settings. Blood cyanide levels correlate with toxicity severity, with concentrations below 0.5 mg/L typically asymptomatic, 0.5-1.0 mg/L causing minor symptoms, 1.0-2.5 mg/L creating moderate to severe toxicity, and levels above 2.5-3.0 mg/L frequently fatal without treatment. Elevated lactate levels (typically >8-10 mmol/L) provide an important surrogate marker reflecting blocked aerobic metabolism, with correlation between lactate elevation and cyanide level established in several studies. Additional laboratory findings include metabolic acidosis with elevated anion gap, frequently normal PaO_2 contrasting with significantly decreased central or mixed venous oxygen saturation reflecting decreased extraction, and occasionally elevated carboxyhemoglobin in fire-related cases with combined toxic exposures.

Management employs both supportive measures and specific

antidotes, with treatment initiation based on clinical suspicion rather than awaiting confirmation given the rapidly lethal potential. Supportive care includes high-flow oxygen administration which may partially overcome cytochrome c oxidase inhibition through mass action, ventilatory support when necessary, and hemodynamic stabilization addressing hypotension through fluid resuscitation and vasopressors. Specific antidotal approaches include hydroxocobalamin (vitamin B12a), which directly binds cyanide forming cyanocobalamin (vitamin B12), with adult dosing typically 5 g intravenously (70 mg/kg in children) administered over 15 minutes, with potential repeat dosing for persistent toxicity. Alternative approaches include sodium nitrite followed by sodium thiosulfate (the traditional "cyanide kit"), with nitrite converting hemoglobin to methemoglobin which preferentially binds cyanide, and thiosulfate enhancing conversion to thiocyanate through rhodanese enzyme activity. Hydroxocobalamin demonstrates advantages through lack of methemoglobin formation, particular benefit in smoke inhalation victims with potential concurrent carbon monoxide poisoning, and favorable safety profile, though with higher acquisition cost and limited shelf stability compared to sodium nitrite and thiosulfate.

Chemical asphyxiants beyond carbon monoxide and cyanide include hydrogen sulfide, presenting similar cellular toxicity through cytochrome c oxidase inhibition but with distinctive "rotten egg" odor at low concentrations, though olfactory fatigue occurs rapidly potentially eliminating this warning property with continued exposure. Occupational settings including petroleum refining, sewer maintenance, manure pit operations, and certain industrial processes create exposure risk, with management following similar principles to cyanide though with less established antidotal efficacy. Simple asphyxiants including nitrogen, methane, helium, and carbon dioxide produce hypoxia through oxygen displacement without direct cellular toxicity, creating rapidly developing central nervous system manifestations progressing from cognitive impairment to unconsciousness and death when inspired oxygen concentration falls sufficiently, typically below 10-12%. These scenarios require immediate removal from the exposure environment, respiratory support, and recognition of potential confined space hazards creating risk to rescuers without appropriate respiratory protection.

Irritant and corrosive gases create direct tissue damage upon contact, primarily affecting respiratory mucosa but potentially causing systemic effects with sufficient absorption. Chlorine, commonly used in water treatment, household bleach products, and industrial processes, reacts with mucosal moisture forming hydrochloric and hypochlorous acids creating direct chemical injury. Clinical manifestations range from mild mucous membrane irritation at lower concentrations (1-3 ppm) to severe bronchospasm, pulmonary edema, and acute respiratory distress syndrome at higher levels (>40-60 ppm). Ammonia, utilized in fertilizer production, refrigeration systems, and cleaning products, creates direct alkaline injury through formation of ammonium hydroxide upon contact with moist mucosa, with water solubility resulting in predominant upper airway effects except at very high concentrations where lower respiratory injury may occur. Management principles for irritant gas exposures include immediate removal from the contaminated environment, supportive respiratory care including supplemental oxygen and bronchodilators for bronchospasm, careful fluid management addressing potential pulmonary edema development, and vigilance for delayed manifestations including bronchiolitis obliterans developing days to weeks after the initial exposure.

Prevention strategies for gas and vapor exposures incorporate environmental monitoring, respiratory protection programs, confined space protocols, and emergency response planning. Continuous monitoring systems detecting specific gases at concentrations below those causing health effects provide early warning of leaks or accumulation. Respiratory protection selection requires careful matching to specific contaminants, with air-purifying respirators suitable for certain scenarios but supplied air systems necessary for oxygen-deficient environments or extremely toxic substances exceeding cartridge capabilities. Confined space entry protocols including atmospheric testing, ventilation, and standby rescue capability address the particular hazards created when gases accumulate in enclosed areas. Emergency response planning includes evacuation procedures, sheltering guidance when appropriate, and community notification systems for facilities using or producing hazardous gases that might affect surrounding populations through accidental release. These comprehensive approaches have substantially reduced fatalities from industrial gas exposures, though significant challenges remain particularly in emergency response to transportation accidents and in developing regions where regulatory frameworks and resources for implementation may be limited.

AIR POLLUTANTS

Air pollutants create complex toxicological scenarios through diverse chemical species, variable concentration and duration exposure patterns, and population-wide impact potential affecting vulnerable subgroups disproportionately.

Particulate Matter

Particulate matter (PM) represents a complex mixture of solid particles and liquid droplets suspended in air, with composition varying by source, region, and meteorological conditions. Size-based classification provides the principal regulatory and toxicological framework: coarse particles (PM_{10}, aerodynamic diameter 2.5-10 μm) primarily originate from mechanical processes including road dust, construction activities, and agricultural operations; fine particles ($PM_{2.5}$, diameter <2.5 μm) derive predominantly from combustion sources and atmospheric chemical reactions; and ultrafine particles ($PM_{0.1}$, diameter <0.1 μm) form primarily through high-temperature combustion and photochemical reactions. This size distribution determines deposition patterns within the respiratory tract, with coarse particles predominantly impacting in the nasopharyngeal and tracheobronchial regions, fine particles reaching the bronchioles and alveoli, and ultrafine particles demonstrating efficient alveolar deposition with potential translocation across the respiratory epithelium into systemic circulation.

Compositional diversity creates varied toxicological mechanisms. Transition metals including iron, copper, vanadium, and nickel participate in Fenton reactions generating reactive oxygen species. Organic compounds including polycyclic aromatic hydrocarbons (PAHs) and quinones induce oxidative stress through redox cycling, aryl hydrocarbon receptor activation, and electrophilic reactions with cellular macromolecules. Biologic components including endotoxin from bacterial cell walls stimulate inflammatory responses through toll-like receptor activation. Surface characteristics including charge, shape, and reactive groups influence particle-cell interactions determining uptake and processing. This complex composition creates multiple pathophysiological pathways leading to pulmonary and systemic effects, with oxidative stress, inflammation, autonomic nervous system modulation, and direct particle translocation representing primary mechanisms connecting exposure to health outcomes.

Cardiovascular effects have emerged as the predominant mortality driver for particulate air pollution, with both acute exposure episodes and chronic lower-level exposure contributing to adverse outcomes. Short-term exposure increases risk for acute myocardial infarction, decompensated heart failure, stroke, and cardiac arrhythmias, with initial mechanisms including enhanced thrombogenicity, endothelial dysfunction, autonomic modulation shifting toward sympathetic predominance, and direct effects of translocated ultrafine particles on vascular function. Long-term exposure accelerates atherosclerosis development and progression through sustained inflammatory processes, oxidative modification of lipoproteins, and impaired vascular repair mechanisms. Hypertension development and exacerbation occurs through vascular endothelial dysfunction, increased arterial stiffness, and altered renal sodium handling. These diverse pathways create population-level cardiovascular risk reflected in epidemiological associations between PM exposure and cardiovascular mortality, with meta-analyses suggesting approximately 0.5-1% increased cardiac mortality risk per 10 μg/m^3 increase in $PM_{2.5}$ concentration.

Respiratory effects include both acute exacerbation of existing conditions and chronic pathology development or progression. Asthma exacerbations increase with short-term PM exposure through mechanisms including enhanced airway inflammation, oxidative epithelial injury, increased bronchial hyperreactivity, and potential altered response to pathogens. Chronic obstructive pulmonary disease (COPD) exacerbations similarly demonstrate exposure-response relationships, with increased hospitalization rates during pollution episodes. Long-term exposure contributes to accelerated lung function decline exceeding age-related changes, impaired lung development in children with potential lifelong consequences, and increased risk for adult-onset asthma development. Emerging evidence suggests potential associations with idiopathic pulmonary fibrosis progression and bronchiectasis exacerbation. Lung cancer risk increases with chronic PM exposure, with the International Agency for Research on Cancer classifying outdoor air pollution and particulate matter as Group 1 carcinogens based on sufficient evidence from both epidemiological and experimental studies.

Vulnerable populations demonstrate enhanced susceptibility through both increased exposure patterns and heightened biological sensitivity. Children experience higher exposure doses relative to body size due to increased minute ventilation, greater physical activity, more time spent outdoors, and proportionally greater pulmonary deposition. Their developing respiratory and immune systems create biological vulnerability, with exposure during critical developmental windows potentially programming lifelong susceptibility. Elderly individuals demonstrate reduced physiological reserve, age-related changes in respiratory clearance mechanisms, and higher prevalence of underlying cardiopulmonary conditions creating enhanced vulnerability to additional stressors. Pre-existing cardiopulmonary disease, particularly heart failure, coronary artery disease, COPD, and asthma, substantially increases risk from particulate exposure. Socioeconomic factors often amplify vulnerability through increased baseline exposure in disadvantaged communities, limited healthcare access, higher prevalence of comorbidities, nutritional factors affecting antioxidant status, and housing characteristics that may increase indoor penetration of outdoor pollutants.

Exposure assessment employs both population-level monitoring and individual exposure estimation approaches. Regulatory monitoring networks provide spatiotemporal concentration data for major metropolitan areas, though with limitations including incomplete spatial coverage and focus on regulated particle size fractions without detailed compositional analysis. Satellite remote sensing using aerosol optical depth measurements increasingly supplements ground-level monitoring, providing greater spatial coverage though with reduced accuracy for individual exposure assessment. Land-use regression models incorporate geographical indicators including road proximity, population density, and industrial sources to estimate exposure at unmonitored locations. Personal monitoring using portable sensors provides individual exposure assessment accounting for microenvironments and activity patterns, though typically limited to research settings rather than clinical application due to cost and complexity. These complementary approaches enable both population-level health impact assessment and identification of high-exposure settings warranting targeted intervention.

Preventive strategies incorporate regulatory standards, technological interventions, urban planning, personal measures, and clinical approaches addressing susceptible populations. Regulatory frameworks establish ambient air quality standards with specific particulate matter limits, though with substantial international variation in both stringency and enforcement. Technological interventions include improved combustion efficiency, advanced emission control technologies for vehicles and stationary sources, and transition toward cleaner energy sources. Urban planning approaches incorporate transportation system design minimizing high-density traffic near residential areas, creation of green spaces providing both filtration and buffer zones, and building codes requiring enhanced filtration for structures in high-exposure settings. Personal measures include awareness of air quality forecasts with activity modification during pollution episodes, use of high-efficiency particulate air (HEPA) filtration in homes and vehicles, and route selection for active transportation minimizing major roadway proximity. Clinical interventions for susceptible individuals include optimization of underlying condition management, potential prophylactic medication adjustment during anticipated high-pollution periods, and enhanced monitoring for early detection of pollution-related exacerbations.

The future research agenda addresses several critical knowledge gaps. Identification of specific particulate components driving health effects would enable more targeted regulatory and technological interventions focusing on the most harmful constituents rather than simple mass concentration. Elucidation of ultrafine particle health impacts, currently unregulated despite increasing evidence of toxicity, could inform future regulatory approaches. Determination of biological mechanisms linking exposure to specific health outcomes would facilitate development of targeted preventive and therapeutic interventions. Integration of emerging sensor technologies with healthcare systems could enable personalized risk assessment and intervention matching individual exposure profiles and susceptibility factors. These advances would significantly enhance both population-level protection through refined regulatory approaches and individual risk management through targeted clinical interventions.

Ozone and Nitrogen Oxides

Tropospheric ozone (O_3) represents a secondary air pollutant formed through photochemical reactions between nitrogen oxides (NO_x) and volatile organic compounds (VOCs) in the presence of sunlight, distinct from stratospheric ozone providing ultraviolet radiation protection. This formation process creates characteristic temporal patterns with peak concentrations typically occurring during afternoon hours of summer months when sunlight intensity maximizes photochemical reactions. Spatial distribution demonstrates complex patterns influenced by precursor emission sources, meteorological conditions, and atmospheric chemistry, with potential for both urban centers and downwind suburban or rural areas to experience elevated concentrations depending on specific conditions. Major precursor sources include vehicle emissions, industrial processes, power generation, and natural sources including certain plants emitting VOCs like isoprene and terpenes which react with anthropogenic nitrogen oxides.

Pathophysiological mechanisms for ozone toxicity primarily involve direct oxidative damage to airway epithelial cells through reaction with cellular components creating reactive oxygen species, lipid peroxidation products, and protein adducts. This initial injury triggers inflammatory cascades with neutrophil recruitment, cytokine release, and epithelial permeability increases. Neural activation through bronchial C-fibers and irritant receptors contributes to symptomatology and physiological responses including bronchoconstriction. Adaptation phenomena occur with repeated exposure, though this likely represents adjustment of antioxidant defenses and inflammatory pathways rather than absence of continuing injury with potential cumulative effects despite symptomatic accommodation. Significant individual susceptibility variation exists, partially explained by genetic polymorphisms affecting antioxidant enzyme capacity, inflammatory response regulation, and neural reaction to irritant stimulation.

Clinical manifestations predominantly affect the respiratory system, with symptoms including cough, throat irritation, chest tightness, shortness of breath, and decreased exercise capacity. Objective physiological changes include decreased lung function parameters, particularly forced expiratory volume in one second (FEV_1) and forced vital capacity (FVC), increased airway hyperresponsiveness, and enhanced allergic inflammation in sensitized individuals. Controlled human exposure studies demonstrate measurable FEV_1 decrements beginning at concentrations around 60-70 ppb with 6-8 hours exposure, with greater effects at higher concentrations or with exercise increasing minute ventilation. Population studies show increased emergency department visits and hospitalizations for respiratory conditions including asthma and COPD during high ozone episodes, with a typical lag period of 0-3 days between exposure and healthcare utilization. Long-term exposure associations include accelerated lung function decline, increased asthma development risk, and potentially enhanced susceptibility to respiratory infections through epithelial barrier disruption and altered immune response.

Cardiovascular effects, while less established than respiratory impacts, appear to involve both direct and indirect mechanisms. Short-term exposure demonstrates associations with myocardial infarction, heart failure exacerbation, and cardiac arrhythmias in epidemiological studies, though with less consistency than particulate matter associations. Proposed mechanisms include systemic inflammation following pulmonary oxidative stress, autonomic nervous system modulation through irritant receptor stimulation, and potentially direct effects of oxidant molecules or inflammatory mediators entering circulation. Long-term exposure shows associations with increased cardiovascular mortality in some cohort studies, though distinguishing independent effects from co-pollutants presents methodological challenges. Metabolic effects including insulin resistance and type 2 diabetes exacerbation represent emerging concerns, with initial evidence suggesting potential impacts on glucose homeostasis through inflammatory pathways and mitochondrial dysfunction.

Nitrogen oxides, particularly nitrogen dioxide (NO_2), represent both primary pollutants directly emitted from combustion processes and precursors for secondary pollutant formation including ozone and certain particulate components. Major sources include vehicle emissions (especially diesel engines), power plants, industrial boilers, and home heating systems. Indoor sources including gas stoves and unvented heating appliances can create indoor concentrations exceeding outdoor levels, particularly in poorly ventilated spaces. Toxicological mechanisms include direct oxidative damage to respiratory epithelium, increased susceptibility to respiratory infections through impaired mucociliary clearance and macrophage function, enhanced allergic inflammation, and contribution to secondary pollutant formation through atmospheric chemical reactions.

Clinical effects of nitrogen dioxide exposure include increased respiratory symptoms, enhanced response to allergen challenge in sensitized individuals, and modest lung function decrements at higher concentrations. Epidemiological evidence associates short-term exposure with increased respiratory emergency department visits and hospitalizations, particularly for asthma exacerbations. Long-term exposure demonstrates associations with reduced lung function growth in children, increased asthma and respiratory infection incidence, and potential cardiovascular effects, though disentangling independent effects from traffic-related co-pollutants presents significant challenges. Susceptible populations include individuals with pre-existing respiratory conditions, children with developing respiratory systems, and residents of high-traffic areas who may experience both higher outdoor levels and enhanced indoor penetration.

Preventive strategies require integrated approaches addressing both individual pollutant exposures and their common sources and interactions. Regulatory frameworks establish ambient air quality standards for both ozone and nitrogen dioxide, though with recognized challenges in simultaneously controlling these pollutants due to complex atmospheric chemistry where NO_x reduction can sometimes increase ozone formation depending on specific VOC/NO_x ratios. Technological interventions include advanced emission control technologies for vehicles and stationary sources, transition toward cleaner energy sources, and improved efficiency reducing overall combustion requirements. Urban planning approaches incorporate transportation system design reducing high-density traffic areas, creation of green spaces providing both psychological benefits and potential pollution mitigation, and building codes requiring enhanced ventilation and filtration especially near major roadways or in areas with poor air quality.

Personal and clinical interventions address both exposure reduction and enhanced management of susceptible individuals. Exposure reduction strategies include awareness of air quality forecasts with activity modification during high pollution episodes, scheduling outdoor activities during lower ozone periods (typically mornings rather than afternoons), and indoor air quality management through ventilation practices coordinated with outdoor pollution levels. Clinical approaches for susceptible populations include optimization of underlying condition management, potential prophylactic medication adjustment during anticipated high-pollution periods, and enhanced symptom monitoring enabling early intervention for pollution-related exacerbations. Educational initiatives targeting healthcare providers, susceptible populations, and the general public increase awareness of both risks and mitigation strategies, with particular emphasis on vulnerable groups including children, elderly individuals, and those with pre-existing respiratory or cardiovascular conditions.

Research priorities include better understanding of combined pollutant effects reflecting real-world exposure scenarios rather than single-pollutant approaches, improved personal exposure assessment techniques accounting for microenvironmental factors and activity patterns, identification of specific biological mechanisms creating susceptibility variation, and development of targeted interventions addressing physiological pathways linking exposure to health outcomes. The complex interactions between climate change and air pollution present particular challenges, as warming temperatures may accelerate photochemical reactions, alter atmospheric circulation patterns affecting pollutant dispersion, and potentially create feedback loops through wildfire increase and ecosystem changes affecting natural VOC emissions. These interconnected challenges necessitate integrated research and policy approaches addressing both immediate health impacts and longer-term sustainability considerations.

Volatile Organic Compounds

Volatile organic compounds (VOCs) encompass a diverse chemical category defined by their carbon-containing structure and tendency to evaporate at normal temperature and pressure, creating vapors that may contribute to both outdoor and indoor air pollution. Outdoor sources include vehicle emissions, industrial processes, solvent usage, and natural emissions from vegetation; indoor sources encompass building materials, furnishings, consumer products, and occupant activities. The complex mixture varies substantially across environments, with outdoor VOCs typically dominated by components like benzene, toluene, ethylbenzene, and xylenes from traffic and industrial sources, while indoor environments often contain additional compounds including formaldehyde, acetaldehyde, limonene, and a-pinene from sources such as pressed wood products, cleaning agents, air fresheners, and personal care products. This diversity creates toxicological complexity through varying mechanisms, potencies, and potential interactions.

Formaldehyde represents one of the most extensively studied VOCs due to its ubiquity and established health effects. Sources include pressed wood products containing urea-formaldehyde resins, certain insulation materials, combustion processes including tobacco smoking, and natural emissions from some building materials and consumer products. Its high-water solubility results in efficient upper respiratory tract absorption, creating predominantly local effects at typical environmental concentrations. Acute effects include eye, nose, and throat irritation through direct reaction with mucosal proteins, with sensitive individuals reporting symptoms at concentrations as low as 0.1 ppm. Objective effects include decreased nasal mucociliary clearance, increased nasal resistance, and enhanced neurogenic inflammation. Sensitization in susceptible individuals may produce allergic contact dermatitis through dermal exposure and potentially contribute to asthma through respiratory sensitization, though mechanisms and exposure thresholds remain incompletely characterized. Carcinogenicity has been established through both epidemiological studies in occupational settings and experimental evidence, with nasopharyngeal cancer and leukemia representing the primary concerns, leading to classification as a known human carcinogen by the International Agency for Research on Cancer.

BTEX compounds (benzene, toluene, ethylbenzene, and xylenes) represent aromatic hydrocarbons commonly found in outdoor air pollution, primarily from vehicular emissions, fuel evaporation, and industrial processes. Benzene creates particular concern due to established hematotoxicity and leukemogenicity through metabolic activation producing compounds that directly damage bone marrow progenitor cells and induce chromosomal aberrations. Chronic environmental exposure at concentrations well below occupational limits shows associations with reduced blood cell counts in epidemiological studies, suggesting potential health impacts even at relatively low concentrations. Toluene, ethylbenzene, and xylenes demonstrate neurotoxicity as their primary effect at higher concentrations, with symptoms including headache, dizziness, and fatigue, though typical environmental levels generally remain below those causing overt neurological manifestations in most individuals.

Terpenes and their reaction products represent an emerging indoor air quality concern due to their increasing use in consumer products and potential secondary pollutant formation. Compounds like limonene (citrus scent), a-pinene (pine scent), and other terpenoids increasingly appear in cleaning products, air fresheners, and personal care items marketed as "natural" alternatives. While generally demonstrating low toxicity in their primary form, these compounds readily react with oxidants like ozone and nitrogen oxides present in indoor environments, creating secondary products including formaldehyde, acetaldehyde, and ultrafine particles. This indoor atmospheric chemistry creates potential for enhanced exposure to irritant compounds even in settings without traditional pollution sources, particularly when consumer product use coincides with elevated outdoor oxidant penetration creating ideal conditions for secondary pollutant formation.

Health effects from VOC mixtures extend beyond individual compound toxicity, with combined exposures potentially creating enhanced or novel effects through various mechanisms. Additive effects occur when compounds share similar mechanisms, with total irritant potential potentially exceeding that predicted from individual components. Synergistic interactions may develop through metabolic interference, as occurs when certain VOCs inhibit cytochrome P450 enzymes metabolizing other compounds, potentially enhancing toxicity of compounds requiring detoxification. Sensory effects demonstrate particular complexity, with evidence suggesting that certain mixtures may trigger symptoms at concentrations below individual thresholds through combined stimulation of multiple irritant receptors or amplification of neural signaling. These mixture complexities create significant challenges for both exposure assessment and development of health-protective standards traditionally based on single-compound toxicology.

Sick building syndrome (SBS) represents a constellation of non-specific symptoms associated with time spent in particular buildings, with VOCs among numerous potential contributing factors. Characteristic symptoms include irritation of eyes, nose, and throat; headache and fatigue; difficulty concentrating; nausea; and occasionally skin irritation, typically improving upon leaving the building. While multiple factors likely contribute, including ventilation inadequacy, particulate matter, bioaerosols, and psychosocial factors, VOC mixtures demonstrate associations with symptom prevalence in several studies. Proposed mechanisms include direct mucosal irritation, neurogenic inflammation, autonomic nervous system modulation, and potential central nervous system effects particularly for more lipophilic compounds capable of crossing the blood-brain barrier. Diagnostic approaches integrate building investigation, environmental sampling, occupant symptom documentation, and elimination of alternative medical explanations, with management typically employing enhanced ventilation, source removal or containment, and air cleaning technologies rather than specific medical interventions.

Multiple chemical sensitivity (MCS), also termed idiopathic environmental intolerance, describes a controversial condition involving reported multisystem symptoms triggered by exposure to diverse chemicals at concentrations well below those causing effects in the general population. While traditional toxicological mechanisms cannot fully explain the reported sensitivity levels, proposed pathophysiological models include neurogenic inflammation with sensitization of chemosensory pathways, limbic kindling altering central processing of sensory information, and altered xenobiotic metabolism creating enhanced susceptibility to certain compounds. Management approaches focus on exposure avoidance based on individual trigger identification, symptomatic treatment, and occasionally cognitive-behavioral approaches addressing the significant life disruption often accompanying the condition. The complex etiology likely involves interactions between biological vulnerability, psychological factors, and environmental exposures, necessitating integrated assessment and management approaches.

Monitoring and mitigation strategies address both outdoor and indoor VOC exposures through complementary approaches. Outdoor monitoring typically employs canister sampling or automated gas chromatography systems measuring specific compounds, while total VOC measurements using photoionization detectors provide screening capability with limited specificity. Indoor assessment commonly uses passive samplers collecting compounds over days to weeks, providing time-integrated exposure estimation, though with limited temporal resolution for identifying specific emission patterns. Mitigation approaches for outdoor sources emphasize regulatory emission controls for vehicles and industry, substitution with lower-VOC alternatives in industrial and commercial processes, and urban planning approaches reducing high-density traffic near residential areas. Indoor strategies prioritize source control through product selection, ventilation optimization balancing fresh air introduction against energy consumption and outdoor pollution infiltration, and in some cases air cleaning technologies including activated carbon filtration specifically targeting VOCs through adsorption mechanisms.

The future research agenda addresses several critical knowledge gaps regarding VOC health effects and exposure mitigation. Enhanced understanding of low-concentration, long-term exposure effects represents a priority, as most toxicological data derives from higher occupational exposures with uncertain relevance to environmental levels. Mixture toxicology development would provide more realistic health risk assessment compared to single-compound approaches typically employed in regulatory frameworks. Improved understanding of interpersonal susceptibility variation would enable identification of high-risk populations warranting enhanced protection. Development of advanced sensor technologies for real-time, specific VOC monitoring would facilitate both exposure assessment and mitigation effectiveness evaluation. Integration of emissions testing into product development and certification would enable informed consumer choices reducing unnecessary exposure. These advances would collectively enhance both regulatory approaches protecting general populations and targeted interventions addressing specific high-risk settings or susceptible individuals.

Indoor Air Quality

Indoor air quality represents a critical public health domain considering that people typically spend over 90% of their time in indoor environments where pollutant concentrations often exceed outdoor levels despite lower public awareness compared to ambient air pollution. Multiple factors influence indoor air quality including outdoor air penetration, building characteristics affecting ventilation and pollutant accumulation, indoor sources from building materials and occupant activities, and dynamic interactions between occupants and their environment. This complexity creates diverse exposure scenarios requiring integrated assessment and management approaches addressing physical, chemical, and biological contaminants while considering energy efficiency, comfort, and practicality considerations.

Combustion sources create significant indoor air quality challenges through diverse pollutant generation. Gas stoves, particularly when improperly vented or operated without exhaust ventilation, produce nitrogen dioxide, carbon monoxide, particulate matter, and formaldehyde, with concentration spikes during cooking activities often exceeding health-based guidelines. Environmental tobacco smoke, despite declining prevalence in many regions due to smoking restrictions, continues creating complex exposure mixtures including fine and ultrafine particles, numerous VOCs, and semi-volatile compounds persisting in dust and surface residues (third-hand smoke) even after visible smoke dissipates. Solid fuel combustion in cookstoves and heating appliances, affecting an estimated 3 billion people globally, produces substantial particulate emissions with strong associations with respiratory and cardiovascular disease, particularly affecting women and children with greater exposure duration. Unvented combustion appliances including certain space heaters create carbon monoxide exposure risk with potential for acute poisoning alongside chronic exposure effects.

Building materials and furnishings emit various pollutants through initial off-gassing, secondary emissions from material degradation, and compound migration from products to indoor air. Formaldehyde emissions from pressed wood products using urea-formaldehyde resins create sustained exposure conditions as these materials slowly release the compound over years. Plasticizers including phthalates and alternative agents used in vinyl flooring, wall coverings, and furnishings migrate into indoor air and dust, creating exposure through multiple pathways including inhalation, ingestion, and dermal contact. Flame retardants incorporated into furniture, electronics, and insulation materials similarly migrate into the indoor environment, with some classes demonstrating particular persistence. Flooring materials including certain carpets, vinyl products, and laminate flooring may emit various VOCs with composition depending on specific formulation and manufacturing processes. These emissions collectively contribute to background VOC concentrations while creating potential for higher exposures in recently constructed or renovated spaces where multiple new materials simultaneously emit compounds.

Consumer products represent significant pollutant sources through both intentional compound release (air fresheners, scented products) and unintentional emissions during product use. Cleaning products often contain solvents, fragrances, and reactive compounds that become airborne during application. Personal care products including perfumes, colognes, hair products, and cosmetics contribute to indoor VOC and semi-volatile organic compound (SVOC) levels, with potential for occupant exposure through both inhalation and dermal pathways. Electronic equipment emits various compounds including flame retardants from plastic components and VOCs from electronic components, particularly during initial use periods and when equipment heats during operation. Activities including cooking, cleaning, and hobby pursuits create episodic emission patterns that may generate substantial concentration spikes superimposed on background levels from more consistent sources.

Biological contaminants introduce additional complexity through their ability to grow, reproduce, and produce secondary compounds affecting indoor environments. Mold and fungal growth occurs when moisture enables spore germination on susceptible building materials, with subsequent colonization potentially producing spores, fragments, allergens, mycotoxins, and microbial VOCs. House dust mites thrive in humidity above approximately 50%, feeding on skin cells and producing allergenic proteins in their fecal particles. Bacterial growth in HVAC systems, humidifiers, and water-damaged materials may release endotoxin and other biologically active components. Pollen penetrates from outdoor sources through ventilation systems and building openings, while pet dander and other animal allergens accumulate in homes with pets. These biological pollutants create particular health concerns for sensitized individuals, with exposure potentially triggering allergic responses, asthma exacerbations, hypersensitivity pneumonitis, and various respiratory and dermatological symptoms depending on specific agents and individual susceptibility.

Health effects associated with indoor air quality problems demonstrate diverse manifestations reflecting the multiple potential exposures and varying individual susceptibility. Acute effects include irritation of eyes, nose, throat, and respiratory tract; headache; fatigue; dizziness; and cognitive effects including difficulty concentrating and reduced productivity. Specific constituents may trigger asthma exacerbations in sensitized individuals, with indoor allergens, irritants, and particulate matter all potentially contributing. Chemical sensitivities may develop in susceptible individuals, with symptoms triggered by levels well below those affecting most people. Chronic effects with stronger evidence include increased risk for respiratory infections, sustained inflammation potentially contributing to chronic respiratory conditions, and specific disease associations including lung cancer (radon, environmental tobacco smoke), cardiovascular disease (particulate matter), and allergic sensitization (certain biological contaminants). Emerging concerns include potential endocrine disruption from certain semi-volatile compounds, neurodevelopmental impacts from specific pesticides and flame retardants, and immunological effects from various indoor contaminants, though with currently limited evidence bases compared to more established respiratory outcomes.

Assessment methods include building investigation, environmental sampling, occupant symptom evaluation, and consideration of temporal patterns linking exposures with effects. Building investigation examines ventilation systems, potential moisture sources, visible mold or water damage, potential emission sources, and occupant activities potentially affecting air quality. Environmental sampling may include continuous monitoring of parameters like carbon dioxide (as ventilation indicator), particulate matter, temperature, and humidity; integrated sampling for specific compounds using various collection media; and targeted investigation of specific concerns like mold spore identification or radon measurement. Occupant symptom evaluation documents type, timing, and spatial distribution of complaints, with patterns sometimes suggesting specific sources or causative agents. Temporal associations between activities or occupancy patterns and symptom development provide valuable diagnostic information, particularly when building vacation periods consistently alleviate symptoms that recur upon return.

Mitigation strategies include source control as the primary intervention when feasible. Source elimination removes problematic materials or appliances creating ongoing emissions. Source substitution replaces high-emitting products with lower-emission alternatives maintaining functional equivalence. Source manipulation modifies usage patterns to reduce exposure, such as operating combustion appliances only with ventilation activated or conducting high-emission activities when buildings are unoccupied or can be thoroughly ventilated afterward. Ventilation enhancement addresses multiple contaminants simultaneously by diluting indoor pollutants with cleaner outdoor air, though with consideration of energy implications, outdoor air quality, and potential comfort effects. Filtration and air cleaning technologies provide targeted removal of specific pollutants, with particulate filtration through mechanical filters demonstrating strongest evidence base, while technologies addressing gaseous pollutants show more variable efficacy depending on specific compounds and operational parameters.

Summary

Environmental toxins encompass a diverse category of hazardous substances encountered outside controlled pharmaceutical contexts, often producing distinctive toxicity patterns requiring specialized recognition and management. Heavy metal exposures include lead poisoning, which primarily affects the nervous system, hematopoietic system, kidneys, and reproductive organs. Children show particular vulnerability to neurodevelopmental effects, while adults often present with abdominal pain, peripheral neuropathy, and cognitive changes. Chelation therapy with agents like succimer, EDTA, or dimercaprol is indicated at elevated blood levels. Arsenic toxicity presents with gastrointestinal, dermatological, and neurological manifestations alongside characteristic findings like Mees lines and garlic breath, requiring chelation with dimercaprol or succimer. Mercury exists in elemental, inorganic, and organic forms, each with unique toxicokinetics and target organ effects, particularly affecting the nervous system and kidneys. Pesticide exposures vary by chemical class, with organophosphates and carbamates inhibiting acetylcholinesterase to produce cholinergic crisis requiring atropine and pralidoxime therapy. Pyrethroid insecticides primarily cause dermal and respiratory irritation, while organochlorine compounds produce CNS excitation and seizures. Herbicides like paraquat cause progressive pulmonary fibrosis through redox cycling and oxidative stress. Industrial chemicals include cyanide, which rapidly inhibits cellular respiration by binding to cytochrome oxidase, necessitating immediate hydroxocobalamin or sodium thiosulfate administration. Corrosives cause direct tissue damage requiring careful supportive care without neutralization attempts. Air pollutants include carbon monoxide, with its deceptive presentation and high mortality without prompt oxygen therapy, and irritant gases like chlorine, ammonia, and nitrogen oxides that produce progressive respiratory compromise potentially leading to delayed pulmonary edema. Management principles emphasize rapid identification, decontamination, specific antidotes where available, and supportive care addressing the unique pathophysiology of each environmental toxin.

Self-Assessment Questions

1. Describe the clinical manifestations of lead poisoning in children versus adults, and explain the different management approaches for acute versus chronic exposures.
2. Analyze the mechanisms and clinical features of arsenic toxicity, including acute and chronic effects, and discuss appropriate diagnostic testing and treatment approaches.
3. Compare and contrast the toxicological properties of elemental, inorganic, and organic mercury compounds, including differences in absorption, distribution, target organs, and clinical manifestations.
4. Explain the pathophysiology of organophosphate poisoning, including the aging phenomenon, and discuss the roles of atropine and oximes in management.
5. Describe the mechanism of toxicity, clinical presentation, and management challenges associated with paraquat ingestion, including factors that influence prognosis.
6. Analyze the pathophysiology of cyanide toxicity and compare the advantages and limitations of different antidote regimens including hydroxocobalamin and the cyanide antidote kit.
7. Discuss the management of corrosive ingestions, including assessment of injury severity, role of endoscopy, contraindications to specific interventions, and potential long-term complications.
8. Explain the toxic mechanisms, clinical features, and management principles for carbon monoxide poisoning, including indications for hyperbaric oxygen therapy.
9. Describe the pathophysiology of pulmonary injury from irritant gas exposures (chlorine, ammonia, phosgene), including delayed effects and appropriate management strategies.
10. Analyze the occupational and environmental sources of toxic metal exposures in contemporary settings, and discuss approaches to prevention, surveillance, and early detection.

Bibliography

1. Kosnett MJ. Heavy metal intoxication and chelators. In: Katzung BG, Trevor AJ, editors. Basic and clinical pharmacology. 14th ed. New York: McGraw-Hill Education; 2018. p. 998-1011.
2. Flora SJS, Pachauri V. Chelation in metal intoxication. Int J Environ Res Public Health. 2010;7(7):2745-2788.
3. Bradberry S, Cage S, Proudfoot A, Vale JA. Poisoning due to pyrethroids. Toxicol Rev. 2005;24(2):93-106.
4. Eddleston M, Buckley NA, Eyer P, Dawson AH. Management of acute organophosphorus pesticide poisoning. Lancet. 2008;371(9612):597-607.
5. Hampson NB, Piantadosi CA, Thom SR, Weaver LK. Practice recommendations in the diagnosis, management, and prevention of carbon monoxide poisoning. Am J Respir Crit Care Med. 2012;186(11):1095-1101.
6. Brent J, Burkhart K, Dargan P, Hatten B, Megarbane B, Palmer R, et al. Critical care toxicology: diagnosis and management of the critically poisoned patient. 2nd ed. Cham: Springer International Publishing; 2017.
7. Tchounwou PB, Yedjou CG, Patlolla AK, Sutton DJ. Heavy metal toxicity and the environment. Exp Suppl. 2012;101:133-164.
8. Narahashi T. Neuronal ion channels as the target sites of insecticides. Pharmacol Toxicol. 1996;79(1):1-14.
9. Bjørling-Poulsen M, Andersen HR, Grandjean P. Potential developmental neurotoxicity of pesticides used in Europe. Environ Health. 2008;7:50.
10. Beasley DMG, Glass WI. Cyanide poisoning: pathophysiology and treatment recommendations. Occup Med (Lond). 1998;48(7):427-431..

CHAPTER 9

NATURAL TOXINS

Author

Mrs. Sreedevi Kudaravalli, Associate Professor,
Department of Pharmaceutical Biotechnology, Sultan-ul-Uloom College of Pharmacy, Banjara Hills, Hyderabad, Telangana, India

Abstract

Natural toxins represent a diverse array of biologically active substances produced by plants, animals, fungi, and marine organisms that can cause significant morbidity and mortality. Plant toxins include cardiac glycosides found in oleander and foxglove that inhibit Na+/K+-ATPase, causing hyperkalemia and potentially lethal cardiac dysrhythmias. Anticholinergic plants like jimsonweed produce the classic toxidrome of hyperthermia, dry skin, urinary retention, and delirium. Ricinogenic plants contain potent cytotoxins causing severe gastrointestinal symptoms and potential organ failure. Animal venoms vary widely, with snake envenomations producing local tissue damage, coagulopathy, neurotoxicity, or cytotoxicity depending on species. Scorpion stings may cause intense pain or life-threatening cardiopulmonary effects, while spider bites range from local necrosis with recluse spiders to neurotoxicity with widow spiders. Mycotoxins demonstrate important timing distinctions, with early-onset mushroom poisonings typically causing gastrointestinal or neurological effects, while delayed-onset amatoxin poisoning leads to potentially fatal hepatorenal failure. Marine toxins include paralytic shellfish poisoning, ciguatera from reef fish, scombroid from improperly stored fish, and tetrodotoxin from pufferfish. Management emphasizes identification, symptom-specific supportive care, and administration of specific antidotes or antivenoms when available, with recognition that conventional toxicology screening rarely detects these diverse compounds.

Keywords: *Phytotoxins, Envenomation, Mushroom Poisoning, Antivenom, Cardiac Glycosides, Marine Biotoxins*

Learning Objectives

After completion of the chapter, the learners should be able to:

- Identify major toxic plants by their characteristic appearances, toxic components, and clinical effects, with emphasis on cardiac glycosides, anticholinergics, and cytotoxic compounds.
- Differentiate between various snake envenomation syndromes and implement appropriate management including antivenom therapy, wound care, and supportive measures.
- Recognize the clinical presentations of amatoxin-containing mushrooms and implement time-sensitive interventions to mitigate hepatotoxicity.
- Compare and contrast the mechanisms and clinical manifestations of various marine toxins including ciguatera, scombroid, tetrodotoxin, and paralytic shellfish poisoning.
- Develop management strategies for arthropod envenomations including scorpions, spiders, and hymenopterans based on species-specific toxicity patterns.
- Evaluate the role of specific antidotes, antivenoms, and supportive care in the treatment of natural toxin exposures across different biological sources.

PLANT TOXINS

The plant kingdom produces diverse toxins resulting from evolutionary selection pressures favoring defensive compounds protecting against herbivory, microbial infection, and interspecies competition.

Cardioactive Glycosides

Cardiac glycosides represent a structurally related group of compounds characterized by a steroid nucleus linked to sugar moieties and a lactone ring, produced by numerous plant families including Apocynaceae (oleander, foxglove), Ranunculaceae (hellebore), Scrophulariaceae (digitalis), and Convallariaceae (lily of the valley). These compounds share a common mechanism of sodium-potassium ATPase inhibition, though with varying potencies, pharmacokinetics, and additional properties. This enzyme inhibition increases intracellular sodium concentration, subsequently reducing the sodium gradient driving the sodium-calcium exchanger and ultimately increasing intracellular calcium. This calcium excess enhances myocardial contractility at therapeutic doses while potentially causing arrhythmogenesis and cellular injury in overdose. Additional mechanisms include enhanced vagal tone producing atrioventricular conduction slowing, altered baroreceptor function, and direct central nervous system effects.

Table 9.1: Plant Toxin Categories and Clinical Effects

Toxin Category	Representative Plants	Major Toxic Effects	Treatment Priorities
Cardiac glycosides	Foxglove, oleander, lily of the valley	Nausea, visual changes, dysrhythmias, hyperkalemia	Digoxin-specific antibody fragments for severe toxicity
Anticholinergics	Jimsonweed, deadly nightshade	Hyperthermia, tachycardia, mydriasis, hallucinations	Benzodiazepines, physostigmine (with caution)
Sodium channel activators	Monkshood (aconite)	Paresthesias, dysrhythmias, hypotension	Supportive care, antiarrhythmics
Convulsants	Water hemlock	Rapid onset seizures, gastrointestinal irritation	Aggressive seizure control with benzodiazepines
Hepatotoxins	Certain mushrooms, comfrey	Delayed hepatic failure (1-3 days)	Supportive care, transplant evaluation

Oleander (*Nerium oleander*) contains numerous cardiac glycosides including oleandrin, digitoxigenin, and neriin, distributed throughout all plant parts with highest concentrations in seeds and sap. This ornamental evergreen shrub with distinctive pink, white, or red flowers grows widely in Mediterranean climates, creating exposure risk through accidental ingestion (particularly in children attracted to the flowers), intentional ingestion in suicide attempts, consumption of honey from bees feeding on oleander nectar, and occasionally through medicinal use in traditional healing systems. Yellow oleander (*Thevetia peruviana*), despite its common name, belongs to a different genus but contains similar cardiac glycosides including thevetin A and B, with particularly high concentrations in seeds. Foxglove (Digitalis species) produces principally digoxin and digitoxin, with medicinal derivatives representing among the earliest documented botanical medicines specifically targeting heart conditions.

> **Remember**
>
> **Plant toxins produce distinctive toxidromes including cardiac glycoside effects (digitalis-like plants), anticholinergic syndrome (Datura, Atropa), nicotinic stimulation (tobacco, poison hemlock), and cyanogenic potential (certain fruit pits, cassava).**

Clinical manifestations of cardiac glycoside plant poisoning reflect their pharmacological effects on cardiac conduction, contractility, and autonomic tone. Initial symptoms typically include gastrointestinal effects (nausea, vomiting, abdominal pain) often preceding cardiac manifestations. Cardiac features include bradycardia, various degrees of atrioventricular block, atrial tachyarrhythmias with block, ventricular ectopy and bigeminy, and occasionally bidirectional ventricular tachycardia representing a relatively specific finding. Hyperkalemia develops through inhibition of the sodium-potassium ATPase, creating both a marker of toxicity severity and an independent contributor to dysrhythmia risk. Central nervous system effects include altered color vision (particularly yellow-green visual disturbances with "halos" around lights), headache, delirium, and seizures in severe poisoning. The clinical course often demonstrates progression from predominantly gastrointestinal symptoms to cardiac conduction disturbances and finally to potentially lethal ventricular arrhythmias without appropriate intervention.

Management employs both supportive measures and specific antidotal therapy. Initial approaches include activated charcoal administration for recent ingestions, continuous cardiac monitoring, and establishment of reliable intravenous access. Hyperkalemia management follows standard protocols with calcium administration, insulin-glucose therapy, sodium bicarbonate, and potassium-binding resins, though with recognition that correction may occur rapidly with digoxin-specific antibody fragment (Fab) administration. Bradyarrhythmia management employs atropine, temporary pacing when necessary, and addressing hyperkalemia which often exacerbates conduction disturbances. Magnesium sulfate (2 g intravenously) may reduce ventricular ectopy, while phenytoin has demonstrated efficacy for ventricular arrhythmias associated with digitalis toxicity through membrane-stabilizing effects.

Digoxin-specific antibody fragments (Fab) provide definitive treatment through neutralizing circulating cardiac glycosides, with indications including life-threatening dysrhythmias, progressive bradycardia unresponsive to atropine, serum potassium exceeding 5.5 mEq/L, and significant ingestions predicted to produce severe toxicity. Cross-reactivity with non-digoxin cardiac glycosides varies between plant compounds, with dosing typically based on estimated digitalis equivalents when known, or empirically based on clinical severity when ingested amount remains uncertain. Response typically occurs within 30-60 minutes, with most patients demonstrating significant improvement within 4 hours. Potential complications include allergic reactions (less common with fragments than whole antibodies), hypokalemia from rapid intracellular potassium shift as sodium-potassium ATPase function restores, and returning toxicity as fragments are eliminated before the redistributed glycosides in severe poisonings.

Solanaceous Alkaloids

Solanaceous alkaloids, particularly tropane alkaloids including atropine, scopolamine, and hyoscyamine, occur in numerous plants within the Solanaceae family including *Atropa belladonna* (deadly nightshade), Datura species (jimsonweed, angel's trumpet), *Hyoscyamus niger* (henbane), and *Mandragora officinarum* (mandrake). These compounds act primarily as competitive antagonists at muscarinic acetylcholine receptors, blocking parasympathetic nervous system effects and creating the characteristic anticholinergic toxidrome. Structural similarities between these compounds result in qualitatively similar effects, though with variations in potency, specific receptor affinity, blood-brain barrier penetration, and duration of action creating somewhat different clinical pictures depending on the specific plant involved.

Exposure scenarios include accidental ingestion of berries or plant parts, particularly by children attracted to the sometimes appealing fruit; deliberate ingestion for hallucinogenic effects, especially with Datura species containing higher concentrations of the more hallucinogenic scopolamine; medicinal use in traditional healing practices; and occasional inadvertent exposures through contamination of food crops, exemplified by documented incidents of Datura contamination in commercially harvested grain. Jimsonweed (*Datura stramonium*) creates particular concern due to its worldwide distribution as a weed, distinctive seedpods containing hundreds of highly potent seeds, and reputation in folkloric knowledge and internet resources as a "natural high," contributing to its relatively frequent involvement in toxicological emergencies among adolescents and young adults seeking hallucinogenic experiences.

The anticholinergic toxidrome presents with characteristic features captured in the traditional mnemonic "hot as a hare, blind as a bat, dry as a bone, red as a beet, mad as a hatter." Specific manifestations include hyperthermia through impaired sweating and increased muscle activity; mydriasis with blurred vision and photophobia; dry mucous membranes and decreased secretions; flushed skin from cutaneous vasodilation; altered mental status ranging from agitation and hallucinations to frank delirium; urinary retention; decreased bowel sounds; and tachycardia. Central nervous system effects predominate with scopolamine-rich species due to its greater blood-brain barrier penetration, while peripheral effects may be more prominent with atropine or hyoscyamine predominance. Hallucinations frequently demonstrate distinctive characteristics with anticholinergic toxicity, often described as vivid, complex, occasionally lilliputian (seeing small people or animals), and typically experienced as real rather than recognized as hallucinatory, contributing to potentially dangerous behavior during the intoxication.

Diagnosis relies predominantly on clinical recognition of the characteristic toxidrome in the appropriate exposure context, as specific alkaloid levels typically remain unavailable in emergency settings. Anticholinergic poisoning differential diagnosis includes sympathomimetic toxicity, serotonin syndrome, neuroleptic malignant syndrome, and central nervous system infections, with distinguishing features including skin moisture (dry in anticholinergic toxicity versus diaphoretic in sympathomimetic and serotonergic states), pupillary response (mydriatic but still somewhat responsive to light in anticholinergic states versus fixed in certain CNS infections), bowel sounds (decreased or absent in anticholinergic poisoning versus normal or hyperactive in sympathomimetic states), and urinary retention (characteristic of anticholinergic effects). Specific plant identification, when available, may provide insight into the particular alkaloid profile, though treatment decisions typically proceed based on clinical presentation rather than botanical identification.

Management addresses both symptomatic support and specific antidotal therapy when indicated by severity. Supportive care includes external cooling for hyperthermia, intravenous fluids addressing dehydration from decreased fluid intake and increased losses, bladder catheterization for urinary retention, and cardiac monitoring for dysrhythmias. Benzodiazepines provide safer control of agitation and seizures compared to antipsychotics, which may exacerbate anticholinergic effects, lower seizure threshold, and potentiate hyperthermia. Gastrointestinal decontamination with activated charcoal benefits patients presenting within 1-2 hours of ingestion, with consideration for multiple-dose regimens in substantial ingestions given the anticholinergic effect of delayed gastric emptying potentially extending the absorption window.

Physostigmine, a reversible acetylcholinesterase inhibitor crossing the blood-brain barrier, provides specific antidotal therapy by increasing acetylcholine availability at receptor sites, addressing both central and peripheral anticholinergic manifestations. Indications include severe anticholinergic toxicity with dangerous hyperthermia, extreme agitation endangering patient or staff, or life-threatening tachyarrhythmias, with contraindications including known or suspected simultaneous ingestion of tricyclic antidepressants or other sodium channel blocking agents due to potential precipitation of seizures and arrhythmias. Administration typically employs 1-2 mg in adults (0.02 mg/kg in children) by slow intravenous push, with careful monitoring and availability of cardiac resuscitation equipment. Effects typically begin within minutes and last 30-60 minutes, occasionally requiring repeated dosing, though establishment of a continuous infusion generally remains avoided due to cholinergic crisis risk with excessive dosing.

Taxine Alkaloids

Taxine alkaloids occur in various species of yew (Taxus spp.), particularly English yew (*Taxus baccata*), Pacific yew (*Taxus brevifolia*), and Japanese yew (*Taxus cuspidata*), representing among the most rapidly lethal plant toxins. These evergreen trees and shrubs feature distinctive red arils (fleshy coverings surrounding seeds) contrasting with dark green needles, creating visual appeal contributing to their common use in ornamental landscaping. The seeds, needles, and bark contain taxine A and B alongside several related compounds, with only the aril lacking significant toxin content. These plants have historical significance in various cultures, with documented suicide cases dating to ancient Greek and Roman literature, continuing into the present as evidenced by contemporary forensic case series demonstrating yew's persistent role in both suicidal and accidental poisonings.

The principal cardiotoxic mechanism involves antagonism of calcium and sodium movement in myocardial cells, with functional effects resembling those of class I antiarrhythmic agents like quinidine. Specific effects include prolonged cardiac action potential, decreased atrioventricular and intraventricular conduction velocity, depression of sino-atrial node automaticity, and reduced contractility. Additional proposed mechanisms include antagonism at β-adrenergic receptors and disruption of mitochondrial function, contributing to the potent cardiotoxic effects observed clinically. While taxoids from these plants, particularly paclitaxel, demonstrate significant anticancer properties through microtubule stabilization and have been developed into important chemotherapeutic agents, these compounds differ from the cardiotoxic taxine alkaloids responsible for acute poisoning effects.

Clinical manifestations develop rapidly following ingestion, with initial gastrointestinal symptoms including nausea, vomiting, and abdominal pain frequently followed by cardiovascular collapse within hours. Cardiotoxic effects include initial tachycardia potentially progressing to bradycardia, atrioventricular conduction disturbances, ventricular arrhythmias (particularly wide-complex tachycardias), and ultimately electromechanical dissociation and asystole. The QRS complex widening on electrocardiography reflects the sodium channel blocking properties, while QT prolongation may occur through calcium current effects. Neurotoxicity occasionally manifests with seizures and altered consciousness, though cardiovascular effects typically predominate and may cause death before significant neurological manifestations develop. The rapid progression from ingestion to life-threatening toxicity creates particular management challenges, with documented cases of death occurring within 2-5 hours after consumption of relatively small amounts of plant material.

Diagnosis relies predominantly on exposure history and characteristic cardiotoxicity presentation, as specific taxine measurements remain unavailable in most clinical settings. Plant material identification through botanical expertise or, increasingly, digital image transmission to poison centers or botanical specialists may confirm exposure when history remains uncertain. Specific features suggesting taxine poisoning include rapid onset of cardiotoxicity, prominent QRS widening, and progressive conduction disturbances, particularly in contexts with potential exposure to ornamental landscaping or natural areas containing yew species. Differential diagnosis includes other cardiotoxic xenobiotics, particularly those with sodium channel blocking effects like tricyclic antidepressants, though the rapid progression and absence of significant anticholinergic effects typically distinguishes taxine toxicity.

Management employs aggressive supportive care without available specific antidotes. Gastrointestinal decontamination with activated charcoal benefits patients presenting within 1-2 hours of ingestion, with multiple-dose regimens potentially providing additional benefit through interruption of enterohepatic circulation documented with certain taxines. Cardiovascular support represents the management cornerstone, with interventions addressing specific manifestations: sodium bicarbonate (1-2 mEq/kg intravenously) for QRS prolongation reflecting sodium channel blockade; magnesium sulfate (2 g intravenously) for QT prolongation and torsades de pointes risk;

atropine, isoproterenol, or temporary pacing for symptomatic bradyarrhythmias; and electrical cardioversion or defibrillation for unstable tachyarrhythmias following standard advanced cardiac life support protocols.

Refractory cases may require aggressive interventions including high-dose insulin euglycemia therapy following protocols similar to calcium channel blocker overdose management, lipid emulsion therapy potentially binding lipophilic taxines, and mechanical circulatory support including extracorporeal membrane oxygenation (ECMO) maintaining perfusion until the toxins can be eliminated. Case reports document successful outcomes even in initially dire presentations when aggressive supportive care bridges the period of greatest toxicity. Prevention strategies include proper plant identification before consumption of any foraged materials, appropriate education of landscape professionals and homeowners regarding the extreme toxicity of these commonly planted ornamentals, and maintenance of landscape design standards minimizing use of highly toxic species in locations readily accessible to children or individuals with altered decision-making capacity.

Toxic Alkaloids and Glycosides

Cyanogenic glycosides occur in numerous plant species across diverse families, creating potential for hydrogen cyanide release upon hydrolysis through endogenous plant enzymes activated by crushing, grinding, or chewing plant material. Significant sources include fruit seeds from the Rosaceae family (apricot, cherry, peach, apple), with amygdalin representing the principal compound; cassava (Manihot esculenta) containing linamarin, creating potential for toxicity when inadequately processed; lima beans with varying linamarin content depending on cultivar; and several species within the Prunus genus including bitter almonds. The biochemical basis involves sequential enzymatic reactions: β-glucosidase first hydrolyzes the glycoside liberating a cyanohydrin, which subsequently decomposes either spontaneously or through hydroxynitrile lyase action to release hydrogen cyanide. This mechanism creates variable toxicity depending on processing methods, as cooking typically denatures the activating enzymes, reducing cyanide liberation.

Clinical manifestations reflect cellular hypoxia through cytochrome c oxidase inhibition in the mitochondrial electron transport chain, blocking oxygen utilization at the cellular level. Initial symptoms typically include headache, dizziness, nausea, vomiting, and anxiety, potentially progressing to altered mental status, seizures, cardiovascular collapse, and metabolic acidosis with significant exposures. Distinctive findings include bright red venous blood despite metabolic acidosis, reflecting decreased oxygen extraction, and bitter almond odor detectable by approximately 60% of individuals with genetic ability to smell cyanide. Management follows protocols established for cyanide poisoning, with oxygen administration, supportive care addressing specific manifestations, and antidotal therapy for significant toxicity. Specific antidotes include hydroxocobalamin (Cyanokit), which directly binds cyanide forming cyanocobalamin, and the traditional cyanide antidote kit containing sodium nitrite creating methemoglobin that preferentially binds cyanide, followed by sodium thiosulfate providing substrate for rhodanese-mediated detoxification.

Ricin, a potent protein toxin found in castor beans (*Ricinus communis*), demonstrates extreme toxicity through irreversible inhibition of protein synthesis. The seeds contain approximately 1-5% ricin by weight, with the protective outer coat limiting absorption unless damaged through chewing or crushing. Once absorbed, the toxin enters cells through endocytosis, with the catalytically active A chain inactivating ribosomes through removal of a specific adenine from ribosomal RNA, preventing protein synthesis and ultimately causing cell death. Clinical presentation varies by exposure route: ingestion typically causes severe gastroenteritis with vomiting, diarrhea, abdominal pain, and potential progression to hepatorenal failure, coagulopathy, and shock with large exposures; inhalation creates respiratory symptoms including chest tightness, cough, dyspnea, and potential acute respiratory distress syndrome; and injection (documented in assassination attempts) produces local tissue necrosis followed by systemic manifestations.

Diagnosis relies on clinical features in appropriate exposure context, with specific ricin testing available through specialized laboratories though rarely impacting acute management decisions due to result delays. Management remains predominantly supportive, addressing specific organ system effects without available antidotes. For recent oral ingestion, gastrointestinal decontamination with activated charcoal may provide benefit, though with caution regarding timing given the rapid onset of gastrointestinal symptoms potentially creating aspiration risk. Fluid management addressing significant gastrointestinal losses represents a management cornerstone, with additional supportive care directed toward specific manifestations including respiratory support for pulmonary involvement, renal replacement therapy for established kidney failure, and management of coagulopathy when present. Prevention emphasizes education regarding this common ornamental plant's toxicity, appropriate processing for castor oil production (which removes the water-soluble ricin from the lipid fraction), and security measures given ricin's potential use as a biological weapon.

Abrin, structurally and functionally similar to ricin, occurs in rosary peas (*Abrus precatorius*), distinctive red and black seeds used in jewelry making and ornamental objects. Like ricin, this toxalbumin inhibits protein synthesis through ribosomal inactivation, with comparable clinical effects including severe gastroenteritis following ingestion, potentially progressing to multiorgan failure with significant exposures. The seeds' hard coat provides some protection against absorption unless damaged, creating variable clinical presentations depending on whether seeds were chewed, crushed, drilled (for jewelry making), or swallowed intact. Management follows principles similar to ricin poisoning, with predominantly supportive care addressing specific manifestations without available antidotes.

Colchicine, an alkaloid from autumn crocus (*Colchicum autumnale*) and related species, disrupts cellular division through microtubule binding preventing spindle formation. This antimitotic effect creates particular toxicity for rapidly dividing cells, including gastrointestinal mucosa, bone marrow, and hair follicles. Exposures occur through accidental ingestion of the plant (sometimes mistaken for wild garlic), medicinal use (both appropriate for conditions like gout and inappropriate through dosing errors), and intentional ingestion in suicide attempts. Clinical progression typically involves three phases: initial gastrointestinal symptoms (vomiting, diarrhea, abdominal pain) developing within hours of ingestion; temporary apparent improvement potentially creating false reassurance; and multiorgan failure phase with bone marrow suppression, hepatorenal dysfunction, respiratory failure, cardiovascular collapse, and neuropathy developing 24-72 hours post-ingestion.

Diagnosis combines exposure history with characteristic clinical progression, as specific colchicine levels typically remain unavailable during the critical management timeframe. Laboratory abnormalities include leukocytosis potentially followed by leukopenia, thrombocytopenia, elevated transaminases, renal function impairment, and elevated creatine kinase from rhabdomyolysis. Management remains predominantly supportive, with activated charcoal administration for recent ingestions, aggressive fluid resuscitation addressing gastrointestinal losses, and specific supportive measures for organ systems affected during the third phase. Particular attention to infection risk during the bone marrow suppression period remains essential, with broad-spectrum antibiotics typically initiated for febrile episodes. While Fab fragments against colchicine have been developed experimentally, they remain unavailable for clinical use, leaving aggressive supportive care as the management cornerstone with mortality reaching 10-30% in significant poisonings.

ANIMAL VENOMS

Animal venoms represent complex bioactive mixtures specifically evolved for prey acquisition, defense, or competitor deterrence, with human envenomation typically representing defensive responses to perceived threats.

Snake Venoms

Snake venoms demonstrate remarkable compositional complexity and diversity reflecting evolutionary adaptations to specific predatory strategies and ecological niches. Fundamentally, these venoms comprise various proteins and peptides including enzymes, non-enzymatic toxins, and other bioactive components, with specific composition varying significantly between species and even within species based on geographical distribution, individual variation, and ontogenetic changes during development. While traditional classification broadly categorized venoms as predominantly hemotoxic, neurotoxic, or cytotoxic, contemporary understanding recognizes the significant overlap and complementary effects between these categories, with most venoms containing components affecting multiple physiological systems simultaneously.

Viperid venoms (family Viperidae, including rattlesnakes, cottonmouths, copperheads, and true vipers) typically contain high concentrations of enzymes producing prominent local tissue effects and coagulopathy. Metalloproteinases degrade extracellular matrix components and vascular basement membranes, contributing to local tissue destruction, hemorrhage, and edema. Phospholipases A_2 hydrolyze phospholipids in cell membranes, creating both direct cellular damage and releasing precursors for inflammatory mediators. Serine proteases affect the coagulation cascade through multiple mechanisms, potentially producing both procoagulant effects through direct activation of coagulation factors and anticoagulant effects through consumption coagulopathy. This complex interaction with the coagulation system creates diverse clinical presentations ranging from hypercoagulable states with thrombosis risk to severe hemorrhagic diathesis. Additional venom components include hyaluronidase facilitating venom spread through tissue planes, L-amino acid oxidases generating hydrogen peroxide contributing to tissue damage, and various other enzymes and toxins with specific pharmacological effects.

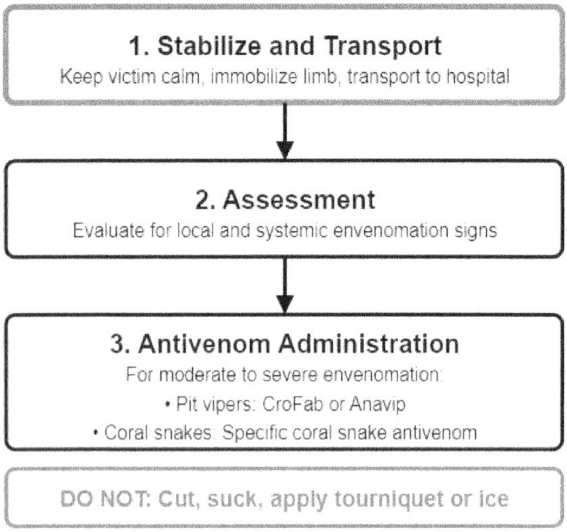

Figure 9.1: Venomous Snake Bite Management

Elapid venoms (family Elapidae, including coral snakes, cobras, mambas, and kraits) typically contain higher concentrations of low molecular weight neurotoxins producing systemic effects with less prominent local tissue damage. Alpha-neurotoxins bind postsynaptically to nicotinic acetylcholine receptors at the neuromuscular junction, preventing acetylcholine binding and creating a non-depolarizing neuromuscular blockade clinically resembling that produced by curare-like medications. Beta-neurotoxins act presynaptically, initially causing acetylcholine release but subsequently preventing neurotransmitter release, creating progressive weakness resistant to reversal with anticholinesterases. Certain elapids, particularly Australian species, additionally contain procoagulant toxins, myotoxins affecting skeletal muscle, and cardiotoxins producing direct myocardial effects. This diversity creates significant variation in clinical presentations depending on specific envenomation, from predominantly neurotoxic effects with minimal local reaction to complex syndromes involving multiple organ systems.

Clinical manifestations following snake envenomation vary substantially based on factors including specific species, venom quantity delivered, anatomical location of the bite, patient characteristics (age, size, comorbidities), and time to treatment. Local effects typically develop within minutes to hours, including pain, progressive edema, ecchymosis, and in severe cases, tissue necrosis. Systemic manifestations may include coagulopathy (detectable through prolonged clotting times, thrombocytopenia, hypofibrinogenemia, and elevated fibrin degradation products), neurotoxicity (progressive descending paralysis typically beginning with cranial nerve dysfunction manifesting as ptosis, ophthalmoplegia, and dysarthria), cardiovascular effects (hypotension through vasodilation and direct myocardial toxicity), and renal dysfunction (through direct nephrotoxicity, renal hypoperfusion, rhabdomyolysis effects, and microthrombi formation).

Table 9.2: Venomous Animal Exposures

Animal	**Venom Components**	**Clinical Manifestations**	**Treatment**
Pit vipers (rattlesnakes, copperheads)	Hemotoxins, myotoxins, cytotoxins	Local pain, swelling, ecchymosis, coagulopathy	Antivenom (CroFab or Anavip), supportive care
Coral snakes	Neurotoxins	Minimal local effects, delayed neurotoxicity	Antivenom if available, supportive care, airway management
Black widow spiders	Alpha-latrotoxin	Painful muscle cramping, autonomic effects	Calcium, benzodiazepines, antivenom for severe cases
Brown recluse spiders	Sphingomyelinase D	Local necrosis, rarely systemic hemolysis	Wound care, rarely dapsone or hyperbaric oxygen
Scorpions (Arizona bark)	Neurotoxins	Pain, paresthesias, neuromuscular effects	Antivenom for severe cases, benzodiazepines

Diagnosis relies primarily on clinical assessment integrated with knowledge of local snake species, as laboratory confirmation of specific venom components typically remains unavailable in emergency settings. Identification of the offending snake, when possible, provides valuable management guidance, though definitive species determination often proves challenging due to misidentification, incomplete observation, and similar appearance between venomous and non-venomous species in many regions. Laboratory evaluation includes complete blood count, coagulation studies, basic metabolic profile, urinalysis, and creatine kinase measurement, with specific testing based on clinical manifestations and local snake species. Serial assessments remain essential due to potentially progressive envenomation effects, particularly coagulopathy which may worsen over 24-48 hours even after antivenom administration in certain cases.

Management begins with appropriate first aid emphasizing victim immobilization, minimizing physical activity that could increase systemic venom absorption, and rapid transport to medical care. Historically recommended interventions including tourniquets, incision and suction, cryotherapy, and electrical shock have been abandoned due to evidence demonstrating either ineffectiveness or potential harm exceeding benefits. Australian pressure-immobilization technique, involving firm wrapping of the entire affected limb combined with splinting, may delay systemic absorption of certain neurotoxic venoms but requires specific training for proper application and remains inappropriate for venoms producing significant local tissue damage where increased local venom concentration could worsen tissue destruction.

> **Remember**
>
> **Snake envenomations require species-specific management, with antivenom administration guided by progressive symptoms rather than prophylactically, and careful monitoring for coagulopathy, neurotoxicity, and compartment syndrome.**

Antivenom administration represents the definitive treatment for clinically significant envenomations, with specific product selection based on regional snake species and observed clinical effects. These biological products contain antibodies (either whole immunoglobulin or Fab fragments) raised against specific venoms or venom mixtures, capable of binding and neutralizing venom components before they interact with target tissues. Indications for administration include progressive local effects beyond minor swelling, any systemic manifestations including coagulopathy even without bleeding, neurotoxicity, significant cardiovascular effects, or rhabdomyolysis with risk for renal injury. Potential adverse effects include acute hypersensitivity reactions ranging from mild urticaria to anaphylaxis, cytokine-mediated reactions with fever and rigors, and delayed serum sickness developing 7-14 days after administration. These risks necessitate appropriate risk-benefit assessment, with generally lower thresholds for administration in more severe envenomations, pediatric patients, bites involving anatomically critical locations, and patients with significant comorbidities increasing complication risks.

Supportive care addresses specific manifestations, with measures including airway management for progressive neurotoxicity affecting respiratory muscles, ventilatory support when necessary, intravenous fluid administration addressing hypotension, tetanus prophylaxis, and pain management. Coagulopathy management requires careful consideration, with blood product administration generally reserved for active hemorrhage rather than prophylactic correction of laboratory abnormalities, as the ongoing venom effects may rapidly consume transfused factors. Compartment syndrome evaluation requires vigilance, though with recognition that actual compartment syndrome occurs less frequently than the dramatic local swelling might suggest, with measurement of compartment pressures recommended when clinical suspicion exists rather than empiric fasciotomy which may worsen outcomes when performed unnecessarily. Wound management includes elevation of the affected extremity, regular reassessment of progression, and conservative debridement approaches allowing clear demarcation of nonviable tissue before extensive debridement.

Arthropod Venoms

Hymenoptera venoms from bees, wasps, and ants create significant medical concerns through both direct toxic effects and hypersensitivity reactions, with the latter responsible for most serious outcomes in humans. Honey bees (*Apis mellifera*) deliver approximately 50-100 μg of venom per sting, with the barbed stinger remaining embedded in the victim's skin along with the venom sac, which continues delivering venom until removed. Principal venom components include melittin (a membrane-active peptide creating direct cytotoxicity), phospholipase A_2 (enzymatically degrading phospholipids in cell membranes), hyaluronidase (facilitating tissue penetration), and various other peptides and enzymes with specific activities. Vespid venoms from wasps, hornets, and yellow jackets contain similar enzymatic components but different primary cytotoxic peptides, including mastoparans and kinins producing pain, vasodilation, and increased vascular permeability.

Clinical manifestations of Hymenoptera stings typically include localized pain, erythema, and swelling reflecting the direct cytotoxic and enzymatic effects of venom components. Large local reactions, exceeding 10 cm in diameter and persisting beyond 24 hours, represent IgE-mediated late-phase hypersensitivity responses, affecting approximately 5-10% of those stung. Systemic reactions range from mild, generalized cutaneous reactions (urticaria, pruritus, flushing) to life-threatening anaphylaxis involving respiratory compromise, cardiovascular collapse, and potentially death, occurring in approximately 3% of adults and 1% of children following stings. Mass envenomation involving numerous simultaneous stings (typically exceeding 50-100) may produce direct venom toxicity independent of allergic mechanisms, with manifestations including hemolysis, rhabdomyolysis, hepatorenal dysfunction, and coagulopathy.

Management strategies address both direct venom effects and hypersensitivity reactions. Initial measures include stinger removal (for honey bees) using scraping rather than grasping techniques to avoid additional venom expression, wound cleansing, cold pack application reducing pain and swelling, and oral analgesics. Local reactions typically resolve spontaneously within hours to days, occasionally benefiting from oral antihistamines and topical corticosteroids for symptomatic relief. Systemic reactions require treatment based on severity, with mild symptoms managed through oral or intramuscular antihistamines, while anaphylaxis necessitates immediate epinephrine administration (0.3-0.5 mg intramuscularly for adults, 0.01 mg/kg up to 0.3 mg for children), intravenous fluids, oxygen supplementation, and additional measures including antihistamines, corticosteroids, and bronchodilators as adjunctive therapy. Patients experiencing systemic reactions should receive allergy referral for venom immunotherapy consideration, which reduces future systemic reaction risk from approximately 60% to less than 5% with subsequent stings.

Spider venoms demonstrate remarkable diversity reflecting their predatory evolution across approximately 48,000 described species, though very few produce clinically significant effects in humans. Latrodectus species (widow spiders) produce α-latrotoxin, a high-molecular-weight protein binding to presynaptic neuronal receptors and creating calcium channels resulting in massive neurotransmitter release, particularly norepinephrine and acetylcholine. Clinical manifestations, termed latrodectism, include painful muscle contractions and cramping initially at the bite site and subsequently progressing to generalized involvement, occasionally with autonomic effects including hypertension, tachycardia, diaphoresis, and anxiety. The characteristic migratory, cramping pain, particularly involving large muscle groups and the abdomen, often leads to misdiagnosis as acute abdomen, renal colic, or other medical conditions when the bite history remains unrecognized.

Loxosceles species (recluse spiders) produce sphingomyelinase D, a phospholipase enzyme activating complement, platelets, and polymorphonuclear leukocytes, resulting in local ischemia, thrombosis, and potential tissue necrosis. Clinical presentations range from minor erythema and pruritus resolving spontaneously to characteristic dermonecrosis with the "red, white, and blue sign" (erythema, ischemia, and thrombosis) potentially progressing to eschar formation and ulceration. Systemic effects, occurring in a small percentage of cases, include intravascular hemolysis, rhabdomyolysis, coagulopathy, and acute kidney injury, collectively termed systemic loxoscelism. Factors influencing severity include specific species involved, venom quantity, anatomical location (with more adipose tissue potentially associated with greater necrosis), individual susceptibility, and potentially climatic conditions affecting venom potency.

Australian funnel-web spiders (Atrax and Hadronyche genera) produce complex venoms containing δ-hexatoxins that prevent sodium channel inactivation, leading to spontaneous repetitive firing and autonomic neurotoxicity. Envenomation creates a distinctive syndrome with rapidly developing symptoms including local pain, piloerection, facial paresthesias, muscle fasciculations, autonomic effects (salivation, lacrimation, diaphoresis), and in severe cases, pulmonary edema and progression to cardiovascular collapse. The development of specific antivenom has dramatically reduced mortality from these previously lethal envenomations.

Management approaches for spider bites vary based on specific species, envenomation severity, and available treatments. For Latrodectus envenomations, mild cases may respond to analgesics, muscle relaxants, and supportive care, while more severe presentations benefit from specific antivenom administration, which typically produces rapid pain relief. Loxosceles bites remain controversial regarding optimal management, with approaches including conservative wound care, early surgical excision (of questionable benefit and potentially harmful), dapsone (theoretical benefit through neutrophil inhibition though with limited supporting evidence and potential adverse effects), and various other treatments with minimal evidence basis. The cornerstone remains appropriate wound care, tetanus prophylaxis, and careful monitoring for systemic complications. Funnel-web spider envenomation represents a medical emergency requiring pressure-immobilization first aid, rapid transport to medical care, and prompt antivenom administration for moderate to severe envenomations.

Scorpion venoms contain complex mixtures of neurotoxic peptides, with clinical severity varying dramatically between species. Medically significant envenomations predominantly involve species from the Buthidae family, including Centruroides species in North America, Tityus in South America, Androctonus and Leiurus in North Africa and the Middle East, and Mesobuthus in Asia. These venoms primarily affect voltage-gated sodium channels, causing sustained membrane depolarization and massive release of neurotransmitters including acetylcholine, catecholamines, and glutamate. Clinical manifestations range from localized pain, which may be intense and radiating, to severe systemic effects including cranial nerve dysfunction, neuromuscular abnormalities, autonomic storm with hypertension and tachycardia, hypersalivation, bronchospasm, and pulmonary edema. Children demonstrate particular vulnerability to severe effects due to higher venom-to-body mass ratios and potentially less robust physiological compensatory mechanisms.

Management strategies for scorpion stings include both supportive care and specific antivenom therapy when available and indicated. Pain control employs local anesthetic infiltration, which may provide more effective relief than systemic analgesics for the intense neurogenic pain. Autonomic manifestations occasionally require specific interventions including alpha-blockers for severe hypertension or benzodiazepines for agitation and neuromuscular hyperactivity. Antivenom administration, where species-specific products exist, provides rapid symptom resolution for severe envenomations, with particular benefit in pediatric patients and those with significant systemic manifestations. Regional variations in available antivenoms and envenomation characteristics necessitate familiarity with local scorpion species, clinical presentations, and established treatment protocols, as management approaches demonstrating efficacy in one region may not translate to areas with different predominant species.

Marine Venoms

Marine envenomations encompass diverse taxonomic groups employing venom for both defensive and predatory purposes, with human exposures predominantly involving defensive responses to inadvertent contact. Cnidarians (jellyfish, anemones, corals) represent the most frequently encountered venomous marine creatures, utilizing specialized penetrant structures called nematocysts containing complex protein mixtures. Upon contact, these pressurized capsules discharge coiled threads penetrating the victim's skin and injecting venom through a combination of mechanical force and enzymatic activity. Different species produce vastly different clinical effects, from minor local irritation to potentially lethal systemic toxicity.

Box jellyfish (*Chironex fleckeri*) found in Indo-Pacific waters produce among the most potent known animal venoms, containing proteins with cardiotoxic, dermatonecrotic, and porogenic (pore-forming) activities. Envenomation produces immediate excruciating pain, distinctive linear wheals reflecting tentacle contact patterns, and potential rapid progression to cardiovascular collapse with documented fatalities occurring within minutes of severe stings. Physalia species (Portuguese man-of-war, bluebottle jellyfish) comprise colonies of specialized organisms rather than true jellyfish, with painful stings producing characteristic linear urticarial lesions, occasionally with systemic effects including nausea, vomiting, headache, muscle spasms, and rarely cardiovascular or respiratory compromise. Irukandji syndrome, initially described with *Carukia barnesi* but now recognized with several small carybdeid jellyfish species, produces minimal initial sting pain followed by delayed systemic effects including severe headache, back and abdominal pain, diaphoresis, hypertension, tachycardia, and potentially life-threatening cardiovascular complications—a dramatic example of severe systemic effects from seemingly minor initial envenomation.

Management of cnidarian stings begins with tentacle removal and nematocyst inactivation, with approach varying by specific species involved. Vinegar application (5% acetic acid) inactivates undischarged nematocysts from many species, particularly box jellyfish and other cubozoans, while potentially increasing venom discharge from certain others including some Physalia species, highlighting the importance of region-specific protocols based on predominant local species. After appropriate inactivation, tentacle removal using gloved hands, forceps, or splashed seawater (avoiding freshwater which may trigger additional nematocyst discharge through osmotic effects) completes initial decontamination. Pain management employs both topical (lidocaine, calamine) and systemic approaches. Specific antivenom exists for *Chironex fleckeri,* with administration indicated for severe envenomations involving extensive skin surface, significant pain unresponsive to conventional measures, or any systemic manifestations. Irukandji syndrome management focuses on pain control, often requiring high-dose opioids, and cardiovascular monitoring with intervention for hypertensive complications.

Venomous fish employ specialized venom apparatus typically associated with spines used defensively rather than for prey acquisition. Stingrays possess serrated spines with venom glands along the tail base, creating wounds through both mechanical trauma and venom effects. Principal venom components include serotonin, phosphodiesterase, and various peptides producing intense vasoconstriction, tissue necrosis, and extreme pain described as immediately incapacitating. Stonefish (Synanceia species) possess among the most potent fish venoms, delivered through 13 dorsal spines causing profound local pain, edema, and occasionally systemic effects including hypotension, arrhythmias, respiratory distress, and rarely cardiovascular collapse. Other notable venomous fish include scorpionfish, lionfish, and various catfish species, all employing specialized spines with associated venom glands producing predominantly localized effects of variable severity.

Management principles for fish envenomations emphasize wound irrigation, foreign body removal, heat therapy, and appropriate pain control. Heat immersion (water as hot as tolerable without burning, typically 42-45°C) provides both pain relief through possible venom protein denaturation and vasodilation counteracting the vasoconstrictive venom effects. This simple intervention often provides dramatic pain reduction when implemented promptly and maintained for 30-90 minutes, occasionally requiring repeated application for recurrent pain. Wound management includes careful irrigation, debridement of necrotic tissue, and appropriate tetanus prophylaxis. Pain control frequently requires systemic analgesics including opioids for moderate to severe envenomations. Specific antivenoms exist for certain species, particularly stonefish, with administration indicated for severe local effects unresponsive to conventional measures, multiple spine punctures, or systemic manifestations. Retained foreign bodies, particularly stingray barbs or spine fragments, may require surgical exploration and removal, with wound closure typically delayed due to infection risk.

Sea urchins possess numerous fragile spines and specialized triple-jawed pedicellariae containing various toxins. Spine punctures create mechanical trauma and potential for secondary infection, with certain species including toxin-containing sheaths around spines producing enhanced local effects. The unique concern involves spine fragmentation, with retained fragments potentially causing granulomatous inflammation, secondary infection, and in rare cases, systemic effects through delayed toxin release. Management emphasizes careful removal of visible spines, recognition that dark pigmentation may actually represent spine fragments rather than simple "tattoo" effect, and appropriate follow-up for potential development of granulomatous reactions requiring surgical intervention. Hot water immersion provides symptomatic relief similarly to fish envenomations, while topical or oral corticosteroids may benefit granulomatous reactions to retained fragments.

Cone snails (Conus species) employ specialized harpoon-like modified radulae to inject venom containing highly specific neurotoxic peptides (conotoxins) evolved for rapid prey immobilization. These compounds demonstrate remarkable pharmacological specificity for particular ion channels and receptors, creating research interest for novel drug development while simultaneously producing potentially lethal human envenomations. Clinical manifestations begin with local pain and paresthesias, potentially progressing to generalized paresthesias, flaccid paralysis, visual disturbances, and in severe cases, respiratory arrest through neuromuscular blockade. Management remains predominantly supportive, including respiratory support for significant neuromuscular effects, with full recovery typically occurring within 24 hours for non-fatal envenomations, though prolonged mechanical ventilation may be required in severe cases.

Vertebrate Venoms

Mammalian venoms, though rare across the approximately 5,500 mammalian species, occur in several taxa including certain shrews, solenodons, slow lorises, vampire bats, and most notably, the platypus (*Ornithorhynchus anatinus*). Male platypuses possess specialized crural spurs on their hind limbs containing venom glands activated during breeding season, predominantly serving male-male competition rather than predatory functions. The complex venom contains C-type natriuretic peptides, hyaluronidase, and defensin-like peptides, producing intense, prolonged pain poorly responsive to conventional analgesics, localized edema, and occasionally systemic effects including hyperalgesia and muscle wasting in human envenomations. Management focuses on pain control, often requiring high-dose opioids or regional nerve blocks, wound care, and monitoring for rarely reported systemic complications or secondary infection.

The slow loris (Nycticebus species), a nocturnal primate found in Southeast Asia, produces a distinctive venom through combination of a brachial gland exudate mixed with saliva, creating a toxic bite previously underappreciated in medical literature. The venom contains a protein (loris slow toxin) bearing structural similarity to the allergen Fel-d1 found in cat dander, potentially explaining the occasionally severe hypersensitivity reactions observed in human bites. Clinical manifestations include significant pain, edema, local tissue necrosis, and in sensitized individuals, potential anaphylactic reactions. Management follows principles for other mammalian bites, with particular attention to potential allergic complications and careful wound care addressing the relatively high infection rate associated with primate bites generally.

Several lizard species possess venom systems, most notably the Gila monster (*Heloderma suspectum*) and Mexican beaded lizard (*Heloderma horridum*), utilizing specialized grooved teeth connected to submandibular venom glands. These venoms contain various bioactive compounds including gilatoxin, hyaluronidase, serotonin, and helodermatine, a kallikrein-like serine protease activating kinin pathways. Clinical manifestations include intense local pain, progressive edema, lymphangitis, and occasionally systemic effects including hypotension, nausea, vomiting, and diaphoresis. The bite mechanism involves a tenacious grip with gradual venom introduction through capillary action along the grooved teeth, occasionally requiring careful mechanical disengagement to prevent additional envenomation. Management focuses on wound care, pain control, and supportive measures addressing specific manifestations, with most cases resolving without long-term sequelae though occasionally requiring hospitalization for pain management and monitoring for systemic effects.

Recent evidence has identified venom systems in previously unrecognized taxa, including certain species within Varanidae (monitor lizards), challenging traditional understandings of venom evolution. The Komodo dragon (*Varanus komodoensis*), previously thought to rely primarily on bacterial infection for prey acquisition, has been demonstrated to possess complex oral secretions with anticoagulant and hypotensive properties. While human envenomation reports remain limited, bites from large monitors including Komodo dragons produce significant bleeding, hypotension, and occasionally prolonged wound healing challenges. Management emphasizes wound care, infection prevention, bleeding control, and monitoring for systemic effects, with broader recognition of potential envenomation contributing to updated treatment protocols for these bites.

Amphibian venoms, particularly those from certain frog species, represent highly diverse chemical mixtures involving both defensive compounds secreted through specialized skin glands and occasionally true venom delivered through specialized structures. Dendrobatid frogs (poison dart frogs) produce various alkaloids including batrachotoxin, epibatidine, and numerous others, creating potential for significant toxicity through handling or consumption rather than envenomation in the traditional sense. These toxins predominantly affect sodium channels and nicotinic acetylcholine receptors, with potential cardiac, neuromuscular, and central nervous system effects. South American Rhinella toads (formerly Bufo) produce bufotoxins including bufadienolides with digoxin-like effects on the sodium-potassium ATPase, creating potential for clinically significant cardiotoxicity. Management for both scenarios focuses on decontamination through meticulous skin washing, supportive care addressing specific manifestations, and for bufotoxin exposure with significant cardiac effects, consideration of digoxin-specific antibody fragments which may neutralize the cardioactive effects through structural similarities between bufadienolides and cardiac glycosides.

The evolutionary convergence of venom systems across diverse vertebrate lineages highlights the adaptive value of these complex biochemical weapons, while simultaneously creating management challenges due to the mechanistic diversity and occasional unexpectedness of these exposures. Clinical approach emphasizes recognition of potential envenomation based on geographical location and animal identification when possible, appropriate first aid focused on victim stabilization and rapid medical evaluation, and management tailored to the specific manifestations and available treatments for the particular exposure. The expanding recognition of previously unappreciated venom systems across the animal kingdom suggests continued evolution of both biological understanding and clinical management approaches as additional information emerges regarding these fascinating yet potentially dangerous biochemical adaptations

MYCOTOXINS

Mycotoxins represent secondary metabolites produced by various fungi, primarily molds, with diverse chemical structures and biological activities creating significant human and animal health concerns through food contamination, agricultural impacts, and occasionally direct mushroom consumption.

Aflatoxins

Aflatoxins comprise a group of related difuranocoumarin compounds produced primarily by *Aspergillus flavus* and *Aspergillus parasiticus*, with aflatoxin B_1 representing the most toxic and prevalent variant. These fungi contaminate various food commodities including maize, peanuts, tree nuts, cottonseed, and spices, particularly in tropical and subtropical regions with high temperature and humidity conditions favoring fungal growth. Contamination may occur both pre-harvest, when crops experience drought stress increasing susceptibility, and post-harvest during improper storage with inadequate drying or pest damage creating favorable conditions for fungal proliferation. Global distribution demonstrates significant variation, with highest levels typically occurring in Sub-Saharan Africa and parts of Asia where regulatory oversight may be limited and environmental conditions favor fungal growth.

The principal toxicological mechanism involves metabolic activation through cytochrome P450 enzymes, particularly CYP3A4 and CYP1A2, converting aflatoxin B_1 to the highly reactive aflatoxin B_1-8,9-epoxide. This electrophilic metabolite forms covalent adducts with DNA, predominantly at the N7 position of guanine, creating mutagenic lesions with particular significance at the p53 tumor suppressor gene. The characteristic mutation involves G→T transversion at codon 249, creating a specific molecular signature strongly associated with hepatocellular carcinoma in high-exposure regions. Additional mechanisms involve protein adduct formation disrupting cellular function, oxidative stress induction, and immunomodulatory effects potentially contributing to both acute and chronic toxicity manifestations.

Acute aflatoxicosis, though relatively rare, presents with severe hepatotoxicity following high-dose exposure, typically through consumption of heavily contaminated food during shortage periods when quality controls may be compromised. Clinical manifestations include abdominal pain, vomiting, hepatomegaly, jaundice, and potential progression to fulminant hepatic failure with coagulopathy, encephalopathy, and ascites.

Table 9.3: Mushroom Toxicity by Onset Time

Toxin/Syndrome	**Examples**	**Clinical Features**	**Critical Interventions**
Muscarinic	Inocybe, Clitocybe	SLUDGE syndrome, bradycardia	Atropine for severe symptoms
Hallucinogenic	Psilocybe	Visual hallucinations, euphoria	Supportive care, benzodiazepines
Disulfiram-like	Coprinopsis atramentaria	Alcohol intolerance reaction	Avoid alcohol, supportive care
Amatoxins	*Amanita phalloides,* Galerina	Initial GI symptoms, delayed hepatorenal failure	Multi-dose activated charcoal, N-acetylcysteine, silibinin, transplant evaluation
Gyromitrin	Gyromitra species	GI symptoms, hepatorenal failure, seizures	Pyridoxine, supportive care
Orellanine	Cortinarius species	Delayed renal failure (2-14 days)	Supportive care, dialysis, transplant evaluation

Laboratory findings demonstrate markedly elevated transaminases, hyperbilirubinemia, hypoalbuminemia, and coagulopathy reflecting severe hepatocellular injury. Mortality rates in documented outbreaks have ranged from 25-40%, with children potentially demonstrating enhanced susceptibility. Diagnosis relies on exposure history, characteristic clinical presentation, and when available, toxin detection in food samples or measurement of aflatoxin-albumin adducts in serum providing biomarkers of recent exposure.

Chronic exposure effects predominantly involve hepatocellular carcinoma development, with aflatoxin established as a Group 1 human carcinogen by the International Agency for Research on Cancer. Epidemiological evidence from high-exposure regions demonstrates synergistic interactions between aflatoxin exposure and hepatitis B virus infection, with combined risk substantially exceeding the sum of individual risk factors. Additional chronic effects include growth impairment in children, with studies from multiple regions demonstrating associations between aflatoxin exposure biomarkers and stunting, though causal relationships remain incompletely established due to potential confounding factors. Immunomodulatory effects may include both humoral and cell-mediated immunity alteration, potentially contributing to infectious disease susceptibility in chronically exposed populations.

> Remember
>
> **Mushroom poisonings follow important temporal patterns: early-onset symptoms (within 2 hours) typically indicate less serious toxicity, while delayed onset (>6 hours) strongly suggests potentially lethal amatoxin-containing species requiring intensive intervention**

Management strategies for acute aflatoxicosis remain predominantly supportive without specific antidotes, following general approaches for acute liver failure including careful fluid management, correction of hypoglycemia, monitoring for and addressing complications including encephalopathy and bleeding diathesis, and consideration of liver transplantation in appropriate candidates with irreversible injury. Prevention represents the primary intervention approach, with strategies encompassing pre-harvest agricultural practices reducing crop susceptibility, proper drying and storage conditions minimizing post-harvest contamination, regular monitoring systems detecting contaminated products before consumption, and regulatory standards establishing maximum allowable concentrations in various food commodities.

Innovative approaches addressing aflatoxin exposure include biocontrol strategies utilizing non-toxigenic Aspergillus strains competitively excluding toxin-producing variants, development of molecular markers enabling breeding of resistant crop varieties, improved storage technologies including hermetic bags reducing fungal growth, chemical and physical decontamination methods reducing toxin levels in already contaminated products, and clay-based enterosorbents potentially binding aflatoxins in the gastrointestinal tract reducing absorption. Public health initiatives further include hepatitis B vaccination potentially reducing the synergistic liver cancer risk, educational programs improving food handling and storage practices, and market-based initiatives creating economic incentives for production of lower-contamination commodities.

Ochratoxins

Ochratoxins comprise a family of related pentaketide compounds produced by various Aspergillus and Penicillium species, with ochratoxin A (OTA) representing the most prevalent and toxicologically significant member. These mycotoxins contaminate diverse food commodities including cereals, coffee, wine, beer, dried fruits, and animal-derived products from livestock consuming contaminated feed. Their chemical stability during most food processing operations, including baking, roasting, and fermentation, creates potential for widespread human exposure through typical dietary patterns. Geographic distribution demonstrates variation, with higher levels typically occurring in regions with climates favoring specific producer species, though global food trade results in potential worldwide exposure regardless of local production conditions.

Toxicokinetics reveal distinctive features including high plasma protein binding (>99% to serum albumin), contributing to the exceptionally long half-life in humans (approximately 35 days) and creating potential for bioaccumulation with chronic low-level exposure. Distribution demonstrates particular concentration in kidney, liver, and adipose tissue, with minimal metabolism creating prolonged tissue exposure to the parent compound. Elimination occurs predominantly through renal mechanisms, with significant biliary excretion and enterohepatic circulation further extending systemic exposure duration.

Nephrotoxicity represents the principal toxicological concern, with ochratoxin A demonstrating particular affinity for proximal tubular cells through organic anion transporters. Mechanisms include inhibition of protein synthesis through competition with phenylalanine in phenylalanyl-tRNA synthetase reaction, mitochondrial dysfunction through effects on respiratory chain components, enhanced oxidative stress, and disruption of calcium homeostasis. These effects collectively result in tubular cell degeneration, interstitial fibrosis, and potentially progressive renal impairment with chronic exposure. Epidemiological evidence suggests potential association with Balkan endemic nephropathy, a chronic tubulointerstitial disease occurring in specific Balkan Peninsula regions, though causal relationships remain incompletely established due to potential confounding factors including other environmental exposures.

Carcinogenicity concerns arise from both animal studies demonstrating renal and hepatic tumor formation with chronic exposure and mechanistic evidence suggesting genotoxic potential through direct DNA adduct formation and indirect mechanisms including oxidative DNA damage. The International Agency for Research on Cancer classifies ochratoxin A as a Group 2B carcinogen (possibly carcinogenic to humans) based on sufficient evidence in experimental animals with limited human evidence. Additional toxicological effects include immunosuppression through both humoral and cell-mediated immunity impairment, teratogenicity in animal models, and potential neurotoxicity through mechanisms not fully elucidated but possibly involving oxidative stress and disruption of neurotransmitter systems. exposure assessment employs both food contamination surveillance and biomarkers reflecting individual exposure levels. Serum ochratoxin A measurement provides the most commonly employed biomarker, reflecting recent and ongoing exposure due to the toxin's long half-life, with detection in a high percentage of sampled populations worldwide indicating widespread low-level exposure. Urinary ochratoxin A and various metabolites offer alternative biomarkers, though with generally lower sensitivity due to limited renal clearance of the parent compound. Risk assessment approaches incorporate these exposure data alongside toxicological information establishing tolerable weekly intake levels, generally ranging from 100-120 ng/kg body weight across various regulatory authorities, though with some disagreement reflecting uncertainties in the dose-response relationship for chronic effects.

Prevention strategies predominantly focus on agricultural practices and food processing approaches reducing initial contamination or removing existing toxins. Pre-harvest interventions include appropriate crop rotation, fungicide application when warranted, and prompt harvesting reducing field exposure to producer fungi. Post-harvest approaches emphasize proper drying techniques achieving moisture content below fungal growth thresholds, appropriate storage conditions minimizing humidity and temperature fluctuations, and regular monitoring systems detecting contamination before distribution. Processing interventions include physical methods (sorting, milling), chemical approaches (ammoniation, ozonation), and binding agents potentially reducing bioavailability when added to animal feed. Regulatory standards establish maximum allowable concentrations in various food commodities, though with international variation creating potential trade implications and differential protection levels across populations.

Mushroom Toxins

Amatoxins represent a group of bicyclic octapeptides produced by several mushroom genera including Amanita, Galerina, and Lepiota, with α-amanitin and β-amanitin demonstrating greatest toxicological significance. *Amanita phalloides* (death cap) contains the highest concentrations, with a single specimen potentially delivering lethal doses, while creating particular risk through its resemblance to several edible species and occurrence in areas where mushroom foraging remains cultural practice. These thermostable toxins resist degradation during cooking or other food preparation processes, maintaining potency even in improperly preserved specimens. Toxicokinetics involve rapid gastrointestinal absorption, enterohepatic recirculation extending systemic exposure, and predominant renal elimination of unchanged compound, with hepatocytes and renal tubular cells demonstrating particular susceptibility through active transport uptake mechanisms.

The primary toxicological mechanism involves RNA polymerase II inhibition, preventing messenger RNA synthesis and subsequently blocking protein production, with particular impact on cells requiring high protein synthesis rates. This mechanism creates a characteristic clinical progression with delayed symptom onset (typically 6-24 hours post-ingestion) as existing cellular proteins become depleted, creating an asymptomatic latent period often falsely reassuring victims and potentially delaying medical evaluation. Clinical presentation evolves through phases: initial gastrointestinal symptoms including severe vomiting, diarrhea, and abdominal pain; apparent improvement during a transient latent phase; and subsequent hepatorenal phase with progressive hepatocellular injury potentially culminating in fulminant liver failure. Laboratory findings demonstrate marked transaminase elevation, coagulopathy, hyperbilirubinemia, and often renal function impairment reflecting both direct nephrotoxicity and hepatorenal syndrome mechanisms.

Management employs multiple approaches attempting to interrupt the progressive injury cascade. Gastrointestinal decontamination with activated charcoal may provide benefit even with relatively delayed presentation due to the enterohepatic circulation potentially creating ongoing absorption. Aggressive intravenous fluid resuscitation addresses significant gastrointestinal losses while supporting renal perfusion. Specific interventions with theoretical benefit include high-dose penicillin G potentially competing for the same hepatocyte uptake transporters as amatoxins, N-acetylcysteine providing generalized hepatoprotective effects through antioxidant mechanisms, and silibinin (from milk thistle) potentially inhibiting hepatocyte toxin uptake while providing antioxidant protection. Extracorporeal elimination techniques including hemodialysis and hemoperfusion demonstrate limited toxin removal due to rapid tissue distribution but may provide supportive benefit addressing metabolic complications of hepatorenal failure. Liver transplantation consideration becomes necessary for patients developing progressive hepatic failure despite maximal supportive care, with specific prognostic criteria including King's College Criteria guiding evaluation for this definitive intervention. Prognosis without transplantation for severe cases historically approached 10-30% survival, though modern intensive care and potential earlier intervention with transplantation have improved outcomes in centers with appropriate resources.

Gyromitrin and related hydrazones occur in false morel mushrooms (Gyromitra species), converting to monomethylhydrazine upon hydrolysis in the gastrointestinal tract. This compound interferes with pyridoxal phosphate (vitamin B6) dependent reactions, particularly affecting gamma-aminobutyric acid (GABA) production and potentially creating both hepatotoxicity and neurotoxicity. Clinical manifestations typically begin with gastrointestinal symptoms 5-12 hours post-ingestion, potentially progressing to headache, dizziness, ataxia, altered mental status, seizures, methemoglobinemia, and in severe cases, hepatic injury. Significant individual susceptibility variation exists, potentially reflecting differences in hydrazone hydrolysis rate, methylhydrazine metabolism, and baseline pyridoxine status. Management includes gastrointestinal decontamination for recent ingestions, pyridoxine administration (25 mg/kg, up to 15-20 g total) addressing the functional vitamin B6 deficiency, methylene blue for significant methemoglobinemia, anticonvulsants for seizure activity, and supportive care for specific manifestations.

Orellanine, a nephrotoxic bipyridine compound found in Cortinarius species (particularly *Cortinarius orellanus* and related species), creates distinctive delayed-onset renal failure sometimes termed "Orellanus syndrome." This toxin demonstrates particular affinity for proximal tubular cells, creating injury through oxidative stress generation, inhibition of cellular respiration, and disruption of RNA synthesis. The characteristic clinical presentation involves an exceptionally long latent period ranging from 2-20 days between ingestion and symptom onset, creating particular diagnostic challenges as the association with mushroom consumption may not be initially recognized. Manifestations begin with nonspecific symptoms including nausea, headache, myalgias, and chills, followed by evidence of renal injury including oliguria, flank pain, and progressive azotemia. Histopathology demonstrates interstitial nephritis and tubular necrosis, with recovery ranging from complete to permanent end-stage renal disease requiring dialysis or transplantation. Management remains predominantly supportive, with no established specific antidote, focusing on appropriate renal replacement therapy when indicated and monitoring for potential partial recovery which may continue for several months after the initial injury.

Muscarine, found in Inocybe and Clitocybe species, acts as a direct muscarinic acetylcholine receptor agonist creating a cholinergic toxidrome. Clinical manifestations typically begin within 30-60 minutes of ingestion, including hypersecretion (salivation, lacrimation, urination, diarrhea), bradycardia, miosis, bronchospasm, and potential hypotension through vasodilation. The rapid onset distinguishes muscarine toxicity from amatoxin poisoning, though co-ingestion remains possible necessitating appropriate monitoring periods. Management includes atropine administration (1-2 mg intravenously, repeated as needed) providing competitive antagonism at muscarinic receptors, with dosing guided by resolution of bronchial secretions rather than pupillary response or heart rate. Gastrointestinal decontamination with activated charcoal benefits patients presenting within 1-2 hours of ingestion. Most cases resolve without sequelae within 24 hours with appropriate supportive care and specific antidotal therapy when indicated.

Psilocybin and psilocin, structurally similar to serotonin, occur in numerous mushroom species within the Psilocybe, Panaeolus, and other genera, creating hallucinogenic effects through serotonin receptor agonism, particularly at 5-HT2A receptors. Clinical effects typically begin within 20-60 minutes of ingestion, including perceptual alterations (visual distortions, synesthesia), emotional lability, altered time perception, and occasionally more severe manifestations including panic reactions, psychosis-like symptoms, and rarely, self-injurious behavior. Physiological effects remain generally mild, including pupillary dilation, mild tachycardia and hypertension, and occasionally nausea or vomiting. Management emphasizes supportive care creating a calm environment reducing sensory stimulation, benzodiazepines for severe agitation or anxiety, and rarely antipsychotics for extreme behavioral disturbances, though generally avoided due to potential lowering of seizure threshold. Most cases resolve without sequelae within 6-12 hours as the compounds undergo hepatic metabolism and renal elimination.

Trichothecenes and Fumonisins

Trichothecenes represent a diverse family of sesquiterpenoid compounds produced by various Fusarium, Myrothecium, Trichoderma, and other fungal genera contaminating cereal grains including wheat, barley, oats, and maize. These mycotoxins share a common tetracyclic 12,13-epoxytrichothec-9-ene structure with varying side groups creating different type A (T-2 toxin, HT-2 toxin, diacetoxyscirpenol) and type B (deoxynivalenol, nivalenol) variants with somewhat different toxicity profiles. Fungal production increases under specific environmental conditions including temperature fluctuations, high humidity, and plant stress, with particular concern in temperate grain-producing regions experiencing wet harvest conditions or improper storage allowing post-harvest contamination.

The primary toxicological mechanism involves inhibition of protein synthesis through binding to the 60S ribosomal subunit, preventing peptidyl transferase activity and elongation of peptide chains. This fundamental cellular process disruption creates multiple downstream effects including ribotoxic stress response activation, mitogen-activated protein kinase signaling pathway alterations, apoptosis induction, and oxidative stress generation. Additional mechanisms include direct cellular membrane damage through interaction with lipid components and disruption of mitochondrial function. These processes collectively affect rapidly dividing cells particularly severely, explaining the prominent gastrointestinal, hematopoietic, and lymphoid tissue effects observed clinically.

Clinical manifestations vary with exposure route, specific trichothecene involved, and dose. Gastrointestinal effects predominate with oral exposure, including nausea, vomiting, abdominal pain, and diarrhea, occasionally progressing to hemorrhagic gastroenteritis with higher doses. Dermal contact produces irritation, pain, redness, and potential vesicle formation when concentrated material contacts skin. Inhalational exposure creates respiratory tract irritation, coughing, dyspnea, and potential airway inflammatory responses. Systemic effects with significant exposure may include leukopenia through bone marrow suppression, altered immune function through lymphoid tissue damage, and cardiovascular effects including hypotension and tachycardia. Historical incidents including "Alimentary Toxic Aleukia" affecting Soviet populations during World War II have demonstrated the potential severity of high-dose exposure, with mortality resulting from combined effects of gastrointestinal damage, bone marrow suppression with subsequent infection, and cardiovascular compromise.

Deoxynivalenol (DON, vomitoxin) represents the most commonly detected trichothecene in food supplies, with particular significance due to its stability during food processing and documented immunomodulatory effects at concentrations below those causing overt toxicity. Acute effects predominantly involve feed refusal and emesis mediated through both central mechanisms involving serotonergic and dopaminergic pathways and local effects on gastrointestinal enterochromaffin cells. Chronic exposure at lower concentrations produces more subtle effects including altered nutrient absorption, modified immune function potentially enhancing susceptibility to infections, and possible growth impairment reported in some animal studies. Biomarker development employing urinary deoxynivalenol and glucuronide metabolites allows population exposure assessment, with detection in a high percentage of sampled individuals worldwide indicating widespread low-level exposure through typical dietary patterns.

Regulatory approaches addressing trichothecene exposure include maximum allowable concentration standards for various foods, though with international variation creating potential trade implications. Decontamination technologies under investigation include physical methods (sorting, milling), chemical approaches (oxidizing agents, alkaline treatments), biological strategies utilizing specific bacterial strains capable of detoxification, and binding agents potentially reducing gastrointestinal absorption. Agricultural interventions focus on resistant crop variety development, appropriate fungicide application when warranted, harvest timing optimization reducing field exposure during susceptible growth stages, and proper drying and storage conditions minimizing post-harvest fungal proliferation.

Fumonisins, primarily produced by *Fusarium verticillioides* and Fusarium proliferatum, contaminate maize and maize-based products worldwide, with fumonisin B_1 representing the most abundant and toxicologically significant variant. These compounds structurally resemble sphingoid bases but lack the 1-hydroxyl group required for conversion to complex sphingolipids, creating their primary toxicological mechanism through competitive inhibition of ceramide synthase, a key enzyme in sphingolipid metabolism. This inhibition results in accumulation of sphinganine and sphingosine while reducing complex sphingolipid formation, disrupting critical cellular functions including membrane integrity, cell signaling pathways, and apoptosis regulation. Species demonstrate remarkable susceptibility variation, with horses particularly vulnerable to leukoencephalomalacia, pigs developing pulmonary edema, and rodent studies demonstrating hepatotoxicity and carcinogenic potential.

Human health effects remain less definitively established than animal toxicity, though epidemiological evidence suggests potential associations with several conditions. Esophageal cancer shows geographical correlation with high fumonisin exposure regions in certain parts of South Africa and China, though confounding factors including nutritional deficiencies and other concurrent exposures complicate causal attribution. Neural tube defects demonstrate potential association in some population studies, consistent with the mechanism of disrupted sphingolipid metabolism which plays critical roles in neural development. Limited evidence suggests possible growth impairment with chronic exposure, particularly in populations consuming maize as a dietary staple with limited dietary diversity. The International Agency for Research on Cancer classifies fumonisin B_1 as a Group 2B carcinogen (possibly carcinogenic to humans) based on sufficient evidence in experimental animals with inadequate human evidence.

Prevention strategies emphasize agricultural practices and

processing approaches reducing initial contamination or removing existing toxins. Pre-harvest interventions include resistant variety cultivation, irrigation management reducing drought stress which enhances susceptibility, appropriate insect control minimizing plant damage creating fungal entry points, and fungicide application when warranted. Post-harvest approaches emphasize proper drying techniques achieving moisture content below fungal growth thresholds, appropriate storage conditions minimizing humidity and temperature fluctuations, and regular monitoring systems detecting contamination before distribution. Processing interventions include physical methods (sorting, milling with removal of outer grain portions containing higher concentrations), alkaline treatments employed in traditional nixtamalization processes which hydrolyze the toxin, and potential dietary approaches including supplementation with substances that may reduce toxin effects, though with limited evidence basis for efficacy

MARINE TOXINS

Marine toxins encompass diverse compounds produced by various organisms including dinoflagellates, diatoms, cyanobacteria, and certain fish species, creating human health risks through seafood consumption, water exposure, and occasionally inhalation of aerosolized toxins.

Paralytic Shellfish Poisoning

Paralytic shellfish poisoning (PSP) results from consumption of shellfish contaminated with saxitoxins and related compounds produced primarily by dinoflagellates including Alexandrium, Gymnodinium, and Pyrodinium species during harmful algal blooms (HABs). These water-soluble, heat-stable neurotoxins accumulate in filter-feeding shellfish including mussels, clams, oysters, and scallops, which concentrate the toxins from large water volumes with minimal self-toxicity. Approximately 57 saxitoxin analogs have been identified, with varying potencies based on specific chemical structures, creating complex toxicity profiles in naturally contaminated shellfish. Global distribution demonstrates widespread occurrence, with particular concerns in temperate coastal regions experiencing seasonal temperature and nutrient conditions favoring dinoflagellate blooms, though climate change appears to be altering traditional geographical and seasonal patterns.

The fundamental toxicological mechanism involves highly specific binding to voltage-gated sodium channels in neuronal membranes, blocking ion conductance through the pore without affecting the voltage sensor function. This blockade prevents action potential generation and propagation, effectively interrupting neural signal transmission in both peripheral and central nervous systems. The molecular structure, particularly the positively charged guanidinium groups, creates an exceptionally tight binding configuration explaining both the high potency and the absence of effective antidotal approaches. Additional mechanisms potentially contributing to toxicity include calcium channel effects and glutamate receptor interactions, though sodium channel blockade represents the predominant pathophysiological pathway.

Remember

Marine toxins often involve heat-stable compounds unaffected by cooking, with distinct syndromes including ciguatera, scombroid, paralytic shellfish poisoning, and tetrodotoxin poisoning, each requiring specific supportive management.

Clinical manifestations typically begin rapidly, within minutes to hours of consumption, reflecting the toxins' immediate action without requiring metabolic activation. Initial perioral paresthesias create characteristic tingling and numbness of lips, tongue, and face, progressing to extremities in ascending fashion. This sensory disturbance may be accompanied or followed by gastrointestinal symptoms including nausea, vomiting, and diarrhea, though their prominence varies among individual cases. Progressive neuromuscular involvement produces weakness, incoordination, dysphagia, dysarthria, and in severe cases, respiratory muscle paralysis necessitating mechanical ventilation. Cardiovascular effects may include hypotension through peripheral vasodilation and occasionally dysrhythmias, though consciousness typically remains preserved even with significant neuromuscular paralysis, creating a particularly distressing experience for victims maintaining awareness despite inability to move or communicate effectively.

Diagnosis relies predominantly on exposure history and characteristic clinical presentation, as rapid laboratory confirmation of specific toxins typically remains unavailable in emergency settings. The distinctive progression beginning with perioral paresthesias followed by ascending neurological manifestations, particularly in a context of recent shellfish consumption from areas with known or suspected harmful algal blooms, should prompt consideration of PSP. Differential diagnosis includes similar marine toxin exposures (particularly tetrodotoxin), botulism (distinguished by its descending rather than ascending pattern and prominent anticholinergic features), and various neurotoxic snake envenomations. Detection of saxitoxins in remnant food samples using mouse bioassay or chemical analytical methods provides retrospective confirmation but rarely influences acute management decisions.

Treatment remains predominantly supportive without specific antidotes, focusing on respiratory support as the critical intervention preventing mortality in severe cases. Airway monitoring and management represent priorities, with mechanical ventilation implementation for patients demonstrating significant respiratory muscle involvement or inability to protect airway due to bulbar weakness. Gastrointestinal decontamination with activated charcoal may theoretically benefit patients presenting within 1-2 hours of consumption, though the rapid onset of symptoms often means presentation occurs after significant absorption has already occurred. Fluid management addresses potential hypotension and replaces gastrointestinal losses. Other supportive measures include nutrition support for prolonged cases, prophylaxis against complications of immobility, and respiratory therapy preventing atelectasis and pneumonia during mechanical ventilation.

Prognosis depends primarily on exposure severity and access to appropriate supportive care, particularly mechanical ventilation when required. With modern intensive care capabilities, mortality remains low despite the absence of specific antidotes, though in resource-limited settings without ventilatory support capability, severe cases may still prove fatal. Recovery typically occurs within days as the toxin undergoes renal elimination and sodium channel function restores, though occasionally prolonged weakness may persist for weeks in severe cases. Prevention relies on monitoring programs testing shellfish for saxitoxin content before commercial harvesting, public health closures of recreational harvesting during identified harmful algal blooms, and education regarding risks of consuming shellfish from unmonitored sources, particularly during red tide events which provide visible evidence of potential dinoflagellate proliferation.

Ciguatera Fish Poisoning

Ciguatera fish poisoning (CFP) represents the most common non-bacterial seafood poisoning worldwide, resulting from consumption of tropical and subtropical reef fish contaminated with ciguatoxins. These lipid-soluble, heat-stable polyether compounds originate in benthic dinoflagellates (primarily *Gambierdiscus toxicus*) growing on macroalgae, coral, and other surfaces in reef ecosystems. The toxins undergo bioaccumulation and biotransformation through the marine food chain, with herbivorous fish consuming toxin-producing dinoflagellates, followed by carnivorous fish preying upon the herbivores, creating highest concentrations in larger predatory species including barracuda, grouper, snapper, amberjack, and others commonly consumed by humans. This biomagnification process, combined with the extraordinary potency of ciguatoxins (active at sub-parts-per-billion concentrations), creates significant exposure risk despite the absence of reliable detection methods applicable to commercial fish monitoring.

The primary toxicological mechanism involves binding to voltage-gated sodium channels at site 5, causing the channel to remain open at resting membrane potential. This action creates excessive sodium influx leading to cellular depolarization, spontaneous firing, and eventually inactivation through depolarization block. The distinctive lipid solubility enables both gastrointestinal absorption and penetration of the blood-brain barrier, explaining the diverse neurological and systemic manifestations. Additionally, the compounds demonstrate remarkable stability, resisting degradation during cooking or freezing and persisting in affected fish tissue indefinitely, creating risk regardless of food preparation method.

Clinical manifestations typically begin within 1-24 hours of consumption, with initial gastrointestinal symptoms including nausea, vomiting, abdominal pain, and diarrhea frequently preceding neurological effects. The characteristic neurological presentation includes distinctive dysesthesias with reversal of temperature sensation (cold objects producing burning sensations and vice versa), perioral and extremity paresthesias, pruritus, myalgias, arthralgias, headache, and occasionally ataxia, vertigo, or muscle weakness. Cardiovascular effects may include bradycardia, hypotension, and rarely more complex dysrhythmias, particularly in patients with pre-existing cardiovascular disease. A pathognomonic finding, though not present in all cases, involves exacerbation of neurological symptoms following consumption of alcohol, certain fish products, nuts, or exercise, sometimes occurring months after the initial poisoning has apparently resolved.

Chronic and recurrent symptoms represent a distinctive and problematic aspect of ciguatera poisoning, with approximately 20-40% of patients experiencing persistence or episodic recurrence of neurological manifestations for months or occasionally years after initial exposure. These protracted courses may involve sensory disturbances, fatigue, cognitive complaints including memory and concentration difficulties, and mood disturbances including depression and anxiety. Recurrence triggers include not only the previously mentioned dietary factors but occasionally non-specific stressors, creating significant lifestyle limitations and psychological impact for affected individuals. The pathophysiological basis remains incompletely understood but may involve persistent sodium channel dysfunction, immunological mechanisms, or autonomic nervous system dysregulation.

Diagnosis relies predominantly on exposure history and clinical presentation, as commercially available tests for ciguatoxins in human specimens remain unavailable, and even specialized research laboratory methods demonstrate limited sensitivity given the extraordinarily low concentrations producing clinical effects. The combination of gastrointestinal symptoms followed by distinctive neurological manifestations, particularly temperature sensation reversal and pruritus, in a context of recent reef fish consumption should prompt consideration of ciguatera poisoning. Various bioassays and analytical methods including liquid chromatography with mass spectrometry can detect ciguatoxins in fish samples, though rarely available in routine clinical settings and generally employed for public health investigations rather than individual diagnosis.

Management remains predominantly supportive, addressing specific manifestations without established specific antidotes, though several approaches demonstrate potential benefit. Intravenous mannitol (1 g/kg of 20% solution) administered within 48-72 hours of symptom onset has shown benefit in some clinical reports, potentially acting through osmotic reduction of neuronal edema, free radical scavenging, or enhanced sodium channel competition, though evidence quality remains limited with conflicting results between studies. Symptomatic treatments include antiemetics for gastrointestinal manifestations, non-sedating antihistamines for pruritus, neuropathic pain medications (gabapentin, pregabalin) for dysesthesias, and amitriptyline for broader symptom management in chronic presentations. Supportive care addresses specific complications including fluid resuscitation for significant gastrointestinal losses or hypotension, and rarely cardiac monitoring and antiarrhythmic therapy for significant cardiovascular manifestations.

Prevention strategies emphasize both individual decision-making and public health approaches. Personal risk reduction includes avoiding larger reef predatory fish (particularly barracuda, which demonstrates highest risk), avoiding consumption of fish viscera where toxins concentrate, and recognizing that conventional food preparation methods neither inactivate the toxins nor produce reliable warning signs in affected fish, which typically appear, smell, and taste normal. Public health approaches include developing and implementing improved detection methods allowing commercial screening, enhancing surveillance systems documenting affected areas and species, and education of both healthcare providers regarding appropriate recognition and management and consumers regarding risk reduction strategies. Climate change impacts, including ocean warming and coral reef ecosystem alterations, appear to be expanding the geographical range of ciguatera risk, necessitating adapting monitoring and education efforts to address emerging threat areas previously considered low risk.

Scombroid Poisoning

Scombroid poisoning results from consumption of improperly handled or stored fish containing high levels of histamine and potentially other biogenic amines, creating a syndrome clinically resembling allergic reaction despite its non-immunological mechanism. While the name references scombroid fish family members including tuna, mackerel, and bonito which demonstrate higher risk due to naturally elevated free histidine content in their muscle tissue, non-scombroid species including mahi-mahi, sardines, anchovies, and others may also cause this poisoning under appropriate conditions. The fundamental process involves bacterial decarboxylation of histidine to histamine through histidine decarboxylase enzyme activity, occurring when fish experience temperature abuse allowing bacterial proliferation, typically above 20°C (68°F) for several hours. The resulting histamine, a heat-stable compound resistant to cooking or freezing once formed, creates the characteristic toxic effects when ingested.

Pathophysiological mechanisms center on histamine's pharmacological activity at H_1 and H_2 receptors, producing effects similar to those seen in allergic reactions, though without involving immunoglobulin E or other immune mechanisms. Additional biogenic amines including putrescine and cadaverine may potentiate histamine's effects by inhibiting intestinal histamine-metabolizing enzymes (diamine oxidase and histamine N-methyltransferase), enhancing absorption and prolonging activity. These non-immunological mechanisms explain several distinctive features of scombroid poisoning: the potential for all consumers of a contaminated fish to develop symptoms rather than only those with specific allergies; the occasional response to antihistamines in individuals who typically show limited benefit from these medications during true allergic reactions; and the possibility of symptoms despite negative allergy testing to fish proteins.

Clinical manifestations typically begin rapidly, within minutes to hours of consumption, with prominent cutaneous effects including flushing (particularly of the face, neck, and upper chest), sensation of warmth, urticaria, and occasionally angioedema. Gastrointestinal symptoms including nausea, vomiting, abdominal cramping, and diarrhea frequently accompany the cutaneous presentation. Additional manifestations may include headache, dizziness, palpitations, tachycardia, and occasionally bronchospasm or hypotension in severe cases, particularly in individuals with underlying cardiovascular disease or those taking medications affecting histamine metabolism including monoamine oxidase inhibitors or isoniazid. The condition typically remains self-limited, resolving within 12-48 hours even without specific treatment, though occasionally symptoms may persist longer with significant exposures.

Diagnosis relies predominantly on clinical presentation and exposure history, with the characteristic rapid onset of allergy-like symptoms following fish consumption, particularly when multiple individuals consuming the same fish develop similar manifestations. Laboratory confirmation through measurement of histamine levels in remaining fish samples provides retrospective evidence, with concentrations exceeding 50 mg/100 g generally considered indicative of spoilage and potential toxicity, though rarely influencing acute management decisions. Elevated urinary histamine or its metabolite N-methylhistamine may provide additional evidence but similarly seldom affects immediate treatment approaches. Differential diagnosis predominantly includes true IgE-mediated fish allergy, distinguished by typical history of consistent reactions to specific fish species regardless of storage conditions and potential confirmation through specific IgE testing, though this distinction may not alter initial management when presentations remain clinically indistinguishable.

Management primarily involves antihistamine administration addressing the fundamental pathophysiological mechanism. H_1 receptor antagonists including diphenhydramine (25-50 mg orally or intravenously) provide symptomatic relief for cutaneous and upper respiratory manifestations, while H_2 receptor antagonists including ranitidine or famotidine may provide additional benefit through complementary receptor blockade, particularly for gastrointestinal symptoms. Bronchodilators may benefit patients developing bronchospasm, though this manifestation occurs less frequently than in true allergic reactions. Fluid resuscitation addresses potential dehydration from gastrointestinal losses, while rarely, vasopressors may be required for significant hypotension unresponsive to fluid administration. Unlike true anaphylaxis, epinephrine administration is generally reserved for severe cases with bronchospasm or hypotension, as the non-immunological mechanism typically produces less dramatic cardiovascular and respiratory compromise than true allergic reactions.

Prevention focuses on proper fish handling and storage practices maintaining temperatures below 4°C (39°F) throughout the distribution chain from harvest to preparation, minimizing time periods allowing bacterial proliferation and consequent histamine formation. Commercial regulations in many jurisdictions establish maximum allowable histamine levels in marketed fish, though enforcement challenges and the invisible, odorless nature of the contamination (affected fish often appearing, smelling, and tasting normal) create ongoing risk despite regulatory frameworks. Consumer education regarding proper storage practices, recognition of potential warning signs including metallic or peppery taste sometimes associated with affected fish, and appropriate medical care seeking behavior represents an additional preventive approach. Healthcare provider education emphasizing distinction from true fish allergy in both acute management and subsequent dietary recommendations remains important, as inappropriate labeling of scombroid poisoning as fish allergy may create unnecessary long-term dietary restrictions for affected individuals.

Tetrodotoxin and Brevetoxins

Tetrodotoxin (TTX) represents a potent neurotoxin occurring in numerous marine and some terrestrial species, most notably pufferfish (family Tetraodontidae) but also found in certain gobies, blueringed octopuses, gastropods, newts, and frogs. This non-protein, heat-stable toxin demonstrates remarkable specificity for voltage-gated sodium channels, binding to site 1 and blocking ion conductance through the pore, creating functional effects similar to saxitoxin despite different chemical structures. Unlike many marine toxins produced by microorganisms, tetrodotoxin appears endogenously synthesized by certain bacteria, with some evidence suggesting symbiotic relationships between these bacteria and the animals accumulating the toxin. Pufferfish accumulate tetrodotoxin predominantly in liver, ovaries, intestines, and skin, with concentration in these non-muscle tissues creating particular risk from improper preparation removing these organs before consumption.

Clinical manifestations typically begin within 10-45 minutes of ingestion, though occasionally delayed up to several hours depending on consumed quantity and individual susceptibility. Initial symptoms include perioral paresthesias, rapidly progressing to involve the tongue, face, and distal extremities. Gastrointestinal effects including nausea, vomiting, and diarrhea frequently accompany or follow sensory disturbances. Progressive neurological involvement produces ataxia, aphonia, dysphagia, ascending motor paralysis potentially culminating in respiratory failure, hypotension, and occasionally fixed dilated pupils mimicking brainstem death, though with consciousness typically preserved until terminal stages. This preserved consciousness despite profound neuromuscular paralysis creates a particularly distressing experience described in surviving victims as terrifying awareness of inability to move or communicate.

Diagnosis relies predominantly on exposure history and characteristic clinical presentation, as laboratory confirmation of tetrodotoxin typically remains unavailable in emergency settings. The combination of rapid onset perioral paresthesias progressing to ascending paralysis following consumption of known tetrodotoxin-containing species, particularly pufferfish (fugu), should prompt immediate consideration of this diagnosis. Differential diagnostic considerations include similar marine toxin exposures (particularly paralytic shellfish poisoning), certain neurotoxic snake envenomations, and botulism, though the latter typically demonstrates slower onset with prominent anticholinergic features and descending rather than ascending paralysis pattern. Various analytical methods including liquid chromatography with mass spectrometry can detect tetrodotoxin in clinical and food samples, though generally available only in specialized research or reference laboratories rather than routine clinical settings.

Management remains predominantly supportive without specific antidotes, focusing on respiratory support as the critical intervention preventing mortality. Aggressive airway monitoring and management represent priorities, with mechanical ventilation implementation for patients demonstrating significant respiratory muscle involvement or inability to protect airway due to bulbar weakness. Gastrointestinal decontamination with activated charcoal may theoretically benefit patients presenting within 1-2 hours of consumption, though the rapid onset of symptoms often means presentation occurs after significant absorption has already occurred. Cardiovascular support addresses hypotension through fluid resuscitation and occasionally vasopressors for refractory cases. Traditional remedies including tea from Coptis japonica rhizome, containing berberine alkaloids that may theoretically compete with tetrodotoxin at receptor binding sites, lack robust evidence basis but remain culturally important in some regions with endemic exposure.

Prognosis correlates predominantly with exposure severity and access to appropriate supportive care, particularly mechanical ventilation when required. With modern intensive care capabilities, mortality has declined substantially compared to historical rates, though in resource-limited settings without ventilatory support capability, severe cases may still prove fatal. Recovery typically occurs within 2-3 days as the toxin undergoes renal elimination and sodium channel function restores, creating a considerably shorter clinical course than would be expected from the profound nature of the neuromuscular blockade. Prevention relies primarily on strict regulation of pufferfish preparation by specifically licensed and trained chefs in countries where fugu consumption remains cultural practice, proper identification of hazardous species by recreational and subsistence fishers, and education regarding risks of consuming potentially tetrodotoxin-containing organisms, particularly as climate change alters traditional species distributions potentially introducing toxic species to new regions.

Brevetoxins represent a group of lipid-soluble, heat-stable polyether compounds produced by the dinoflagellate Karenia brevis during harmful algal blooms commonly termed "red tides," particularly in the Gulf of Mexico and along Florida coastlines. These toxins create human health effects through multiple exposure routes: ingestion via contaminated shellfish causing neurotoxic shellfish poisoning (NSP); inhalation of aerosolized toxins in sea spray causing respiratory and ocular irritation; and direct skin contact during swimming or beach activities causing dermatological effects. The primary toxicological mechanism involves binding to voltage-gated sodium channels at site 5 (similar to ciguatoxin but different specific binding configuration), causing the channels to remain open and producing membrane depolarization, spontaneous firing, and eventually depolarization block.

Clinical manifestations vary by exposure route. Neurotoxic shellfish poisoning from ingestion typically produces combined gastrointestinal and neurological effects, including nausea, vomiting, diarrhea, paresthesias, reversal of temperature sensation similar to ciguatera poisoning, ataxia, and rarely more severe neuromuscular dysfunction. Symptom onset usually occurs within minutes to hours of consumption, with resolution typically within 2-3 days. Respiratory exposure through aerosolized toxins predominantly affects the upper respiratory tract and eyes, causing cough, bronchospasm, rhinorrhea, sneezing, tearing, and conjunctival irritation. These effects typically resolve quickly upon leaving the exposure area, though individuals with pre-existing respiratory conditions including asthma may experience more prolonged symptoms sometimes persisting 3-5 days. Dermal contact may produce localized irritation and occasionally pruritic rashes, particularly in areas of skin covered by swimwear where toxins may become concentrated.

Management remains predominantly supportive for all exposure routes, addressing specific manifestations without available specific antidotes. For neurotoxic shellfish poisoning, approach follows principles similar to ciguatera poisoning management, including antiemetics for gastrointestinal symptoms, analgesics for pain, and potentially neuropathic pain medications for dysesthesias. Respiratory exposures benefit from removal from the exposure source (leaving affected beach areas), bronchodilators for bronchospasm, and nasal saline irrigation or antihistamines for upper respiratory and ocular symptoms. Dermal manifestations typically respond to thorough washing removing residual toxins, with topical corticosteroids occasionally beneficial for pronounced inflammatory responses. Prevention relies on monitoring programs detecting Karenia brevis blooms, public health closures of shellfish harvesting during identified red tide events, beach advisories during active blooms, and education regarding risk reduction strategies including wearing masks near affected shorelines during active bloom periods to reduce respiratory exposure.

The expanding threats from marine toxins reflect multiple interacting factors including increased global seafood consumption, international trade expanding distribution of potentially contaminated products, climate change altering traditional patterns of harmful algal blooms, and improved detection and reporting systems identifying previously underrecognized exposures. Management challenges include limited laboratory testing availability in many clinical settings, absence of specific antidotes for most marine toxins, and insufficient healthcare provider familiarity with these relatively uncommon but potentially severe poisonings. These factors collectively emphasize the importance of preventive approaches, including robust monitoring programs, appropriate regulatory frameworks, and education of both healthcare providers and consumers regarding recognition, management, and risk reduction strategies for these distinctive and evolving toxicological threats.

Summary

Natural toxins represent a diverse array of biologically active substances produced by plants, animals, fungi, and marine organisms that can cause significant morbidity and mortality through various mechanisms. Plant toxins include cardiac glycosides found in oleander, foxglove, and lily of the valley that inhibit Na+/K+-ATPase, causing hyperkalemia and potentially lethal cardiac dysrhythmias treatable with digoxin-specific antibody fragments in severe cases. Anticholinergic plants like jimsonweed (Datura) produce the classic toxidrome of hyperthermia, dry skin, urinary retention, delirium, and mydriasis through muscarinic receptor antagonism. Ricinogenic plants contain potent cytotoxins causing severe gastrointestinal symptoms and potential organ failure. Animal venoms vary widely in composition and effects, with snake envenomations producing local tissue damage, coagulopathy, neurotoxicity, or cytotoxicity depending on species. North American pit vipers primarily cause local tissue destruction and coagulopathy, while coral snakes and many non-native species produce neurotoxicity. Antivenom administration requires careful consideration of indications, timing, and potential adverse reactions. Scorpion stings may cause intense pain or life-threatening cardiopulmonary effects, while spider bites range from local necrosis with recluse spiders to neurotoxicity with widow spiders. Mycotoxins demonstrate important timing distinctions, with early-onset mushroom poisonings (1-2 hours) typically causing gastrointestinal or neurological effects with good outcomes, while delayed-onset Amanita phalloides poisoning (>6 hours) leads to potentially fatal hepatorenal failure through RNA polymerase inhibition. Marine toxins include paralytic shellfish poisoning with sodium channel blockade, ciguatera from reef fish affecting sodium and potassium channels, tetrodotoxin from pufferfish blocking sodium channels, and scombroid from histamine formation in improperly stored fish. Management emphasizes identification, symptom-specific supportive care, and administration of specific antidotes or antivenoms when available, with recognition that conventional toxicology screening rarely detects these diverse compounds.

Self-Assessment Questions

1. Describe the mechanism of toxicity, clinical manifestations, and management approach for cardiac glycoside-containing plants, including the role of digoxin-specific antibody fragments.
2. Compare and contrast the clinical presentations and management approaches for North American pit viper envenomations versus coral snake envenomations.
3. Analyze the pathophysiology of amatoxin-containing mushroom poisoning, including the clinical phases, diagnostic approach, and current treatment modalities.
4. Explain the mechanism, clinical features, and management principles for ciguatera fish poisoning, including distinguishing characteristics from other seafood-related illnesses.
5. Describe the evaluation and management of brown recluse spider bites, including indications for various treatment approaches and management of local necrosis.
6. Discuss the toxic principles in common household plants, focusing on plants with highest morbidity and mortality potential and appropriate triage of exposures.
7. Analyze the neurotoxic mechanisms and management approaches for various animal venoms and plant toxins that affect the nervous system.
8. Explain how to differentiate between anticholinergic plant poisoning and other causes of delirium based on clinical presentation and response to physostigmine.
9. Describe the toxic principles, clinical presentation, and management of exposure to plants containing oxalates, including both soluble and insoluble forms.
10. Discuss the approach to management of unknown mushroom ingestions, including key history elements, laboratory testing, and determining which patients require aggressive intervention.

Bibliography

1. Diaz JH. Syndromic diagnosis and management of confirmed mushroom poisonings. Crit Care Med. 2005;33(2):427-436.
2. White J, Warrell D, Eddleston M, Currie BJ, Whyte IM, Isbister GK. Clinical toxinology—where are we now? J Toxicol Clin Toxicol. 2003;41(3):263-276.
3. Schep LJ, Slaughter RJ, Vale JA, Beasley DM. The clinical toxicology of plant cardiotoxins. Part I: Glycosides. Clin Toxicol (Phila). 2019;57(10):891-902.
4. Gummin DD, Mowry JB, Spyker DA, Brooks DE, Beuhler MC, Rivers LJ, et al. 2018 Annual Report of the American Association of Poison Control Centers' National Poison Data System (NPDS): 36th Annual Report. Clin Toxicol (Phila). 2019;57(12):1220-1413.
5. Lavonas EJ, Ruha AM, Banner W, Bebarta V, Bernstein JN, Bush SP, et al. Unified treatment algorithm for the management of crotaline snakebite in the United States: results of an evidence-informed consensus workshop. BMC Emerg Med. 2011;11:2.
6. Friedman MA, Fernandez M, Backer LC, Dickey RW, Bernstein J, Schrank K, et al. An updated review of ciguatera fish poisoning: clinical, epidemiological, environmental, and public health management. Mar Drugs. 2017;15(3):72.
7. Pinillos MA, Gómez J, Elizalde J, Dueñas A. Intoxication by amatoxin-containing mushrooms: report of 13 cases. Eur J Emerg Med. 2007;14(6):330-333.
8. Isbister GK, Fan HW. Spider bite. Lancet. 2011;378(9808):2039-2047.
9. Gummin DD, Mowry JB, Beuhler MC, Spyker DA, Bronstein AC, Rivers LJ, et al. 2020 Annual Report of the American Association of Poison Control Centers' National Poison Data System (NPDS): 38th Annual Report. Clin Toxicol (Phila). 2021;59(12):1282-1501.
10. Karlson-Stiber C, Persson H. Cytotoxic fungi—an overview. Toxicon. 2003;42(4):339-349..

CHAPTER 10

PEDIATRIC TOXICOLOGY

Author

Mr. Sanat Mahendra Dhoke, PharmD Scholar, Department of Pharmacy Practice, Parul Institute of Pharmacy & Research, Faculty of Pharmacy, Parul University, Vadodara, Gujarat, India

Abstract

Pediatric toxicology addresses the unique physiological, developmental, and exposure characteristics that differentiate children from adults in toxic emergencies. Age-specific concerns include altered toxicokinetics with greater absorption through immature gastrointestinal tracts and skin, different distribution patterns due to higher body water proportions, underdeveloped hepatic enzyme systems affecting metabolism, and variable elimination capabilities. These factors often increase vulnerability to toxins while producing different clinical manifestations than seen in adults. Exposure patterns change dramatically with development: infants primarily experience caregiver medication errors; toddlers and preschoolers suffer exploratory ingestions of household products, medications, and plants; school-age children face increasing risk from recreational substances and intentional misuse; and adolescents demonstrate adult-pattern exposures including self-harm attempts. Treatment modifications necessitate weight-based dosing calculations, careful fluid management, adjusted decontamination approaches, and antidote adaptations. Children's smaller airways, decreased glycogen reserves, and immature thermoregulation require special consideration during supportive care. Prevention strategies target developmental stage-specific risks through proper storage practices, child-resistant packaging, supervision appropriate to developmental capabilities, and age-appropriate education. Effective management requires understanding these distinctive aspects while recognizing red flags suggesting non-accidental poisoning requiring child protection involvement.

Keywords: *Pediatric Poisoning, Developmental Toxicology, Accidental Ingestion, Weight-Based Dosing, Child-Resistant Packaging, Toxicokinetic Differences*

Learning Objectives

After completion of the chapter, the learners should be able to:

- Explain how developmental differences in absorption, distribution, metabolism, and excretion affect toxic responses in pediatric patients across different age groups.
- Identify common toxic exposures specific to different developmental stages from infancy through adolescence.
- Calculate appropriate pediatric doses for decontamination methods, antidotes, and supportive medications based on weight, body surface area, and age-specific factors.
- Modify treatment approaches for pediatric toxic exposures with consideration for airway differences, fluid requirements, glucose homeostasis, and thermoregulation.
- Implement age-appropriate prevention strategies including safe storage practices, caregiver education, and recognition of household hazards.
- Differentiate between accidental and non-accidental poisonings using history, clinical presentation, and exposure patterns, and initiate appropriate interventions when malicious intent is suspected

AGE-SPECIFIC CONCERNS

Pediatric toxicology involves distinct developmental, physiological, and behavioral factors creating unique challenges in exposure assessment, management, and prevention.

Developmental Toxicodynamics

Developmental toxicodynamics addresses how age-related differences in physiological systems affect responses to toxic exposures across pediatric developmental stages. The immature blood-brain barrier, particularly in neonates and young infants, demonstrates increased permeability to numerous compounds that would be excluded in mature systems. This heightened central nervous system vulnerability results from both incomplete tight junction formation between capillary endothelial cells and reduced expression of efflux transporters including P-glycoprotein that actively remove potentially toxic substances. Specific agents demonstrating enhanced central nervous system effects in young children due to this mechanism include certain antibiotics, opioids, and antihistamines, which may produce unexpected neurological manifestations at doses well-tolerated by older children and adults.

Receptor expression and sensitivity fluctuate throughout development, creating variable responses to receptor-mediated toxicants across age groups. Alpha-adrenergic receptors demonstrate both decreased density and reduced coupling efficiency to downstream signaling pathways in neonates and infants, potentially diminishing responses to both therapeutic and toxic sympathomimetic effects. Conversely, gamma-aminobutyric acid (GABA) receptors show enhanced sensitivity in young children, particularly to benzodiazepines and other GABA-potentiating agents, explaining the increased risk for respiratory depression with these medications compared to older age groups. Cholinergic systems undergo significant maturation during early development, with variable muscarinic and nicotinic receptor expression across brain regions creating potentially unpredictable responses to both anticholinergic and cholinergic toxicants.

Metabolic enzyme ontogeny significantly affects both activation and detoxification pathways for numerous toxic substances. Cytochrome P450 isoforms demonstrate distinct developmental trajectories: CYP3A7 predominates in fetal liver but rapidly declines after birth as CYP3A4 expression increases; CYP2D6 and CYP2C9 remain significantly below adult activity until several months of age; while CYP1A2 may not reach mature activity until early childhood. These patterns create specific vulnerabilities, such as reduced capacity to metabolize caffeine (a CYP1A2 substrate) in infants, explaining their prolonged half-life for this common dietary constituent. Phase II conjugation pathways similarly show developmental patterns, with glucuronidation particularly deficient in neonates due to immature uridine diphosphate glucuronosyltransferase expression, creating risk for both reduced clearance of certain toxicants and potential alternative metabolism through more toxic pathways.

Organ system maturation affects functional reserve capacity and compensatory responses to toxic insults. The developing kidney demonstrates both reduced glomerular filtration rate and incomplete tubular function in neonates and young infants, limiting toxicant elimination and potentially enhancing nephrotoxicity from agents excreted through renal mechanisms. Cardiovascular compensatory mechanisms, including baroreceptor sensitivity and adrenergic responsiveness, develop progressively throughout infancy and early childhood, creating potential for more rapid decompensation in young children exposed to cardiotoxic substances. Thermoregulatory capacity remains limited in infants due to both physiological factors (higher surface area to volume ratio, reduced subcutaneous fat, immature sweating mechanisms) and behavioral limitations restricting autonomous temperature regulation responses, creating enhanced vulnerability to toxicants affecting thermoregulatory processes.

Long-term developmental consequences may result from exposures during critical windows of susceptibility, particularly affecting brain development, reproductive system maturation, and immune function. The concept of the developmental origins of health and disease recognizes that exposures during these sensitive periods may program lifelong alterations in physiological systems through epigenetic modifications, altered cell differentiation pathways, or permanent structural changes.

Table 10.1: Developmental Factors Affecting Toxicity in Pediatric Patients

Age Group	Physiological Differences	Toxicokinetic Impact
Neonates (0-1 month)	Immature blood-brain barrier, reduced GFR, higher body water %	Enhanced CNS penetration, reduced elimination, larger Vd for water-soluble drugs
Infants (1-12 months)	Higher gastric pH, developing CYP450 enzymes, reduced plasma protein	Enhanced absorption of basic compounds, altered metabolism, higher free drug fraction
Toddlers (1-3 years)	Higher metabolic rate, ongoing organ development, higher BSA:weight ratio	Faster metabolism of some toxins, target organ sensitivity, increased absorption/elimination rates
Children (4-12 years)	Maturing enzyme systems, smaller fat stores than adults	Approach adult patterns but with quantitative differences
Adolescents (13-18 years)	Hormonal changes, approaching adult physiology	Similar to adults for most toxicokinetic parameters

Neurodevelopmental toxicants, including lead, methylmercury, and certain pesticides, may produce subtle cognitive or behavioral effects at exposure levels below those causing obvious acute toxicity, with manifestations potentially delayed until developmental demands reveal functional deficits years after the exposure. This temporal disconnect between exposure and manifest effects creates particular assessment challenges, as causative relationships may remain unrecognized without specific investigation.

Pediatric Toxicokinetics

Pediatric toxicokinetics addresses how developmental differences in absorption, distribution, metabolism, and elimination processes affect the disposition of toxic substances across age groups. Gastrointestinal absorption demonstrates several age-dependent variations potentially affecting toxic exposures. Gastric pH remains relatively neutral (compared to adult acidic environments) until approximately 2 years of age, enhancing absorption of basic compounds while potentially reducing acidic substance uptake. Gastrointestinal transit time shows greater variability in infants and young children, creating unpredictable absorption patterns, particularly for extended-release formulations designed assuming adult physiology. Enhanced permeability of the immature intestinal mucosa potentially increases absorption of compounds normally limited by the mature intestinal barrier, though this effect generally resolves within the first months of life as tight junction formation completes.

> **Remember**
>
> **Children differ from adults toxicologically due to developmental variations in absorption, distribution, metabolism, and excretion, with factors including higher body surface-to-weight ratio, lower plasma protein levels, immature hepatic enzymes, and variable renal function.**

Distribution patterns reflect significant body composition differences across pediatric age groups. Total body water constitutes approximately 75-80% of body weight in neonates compared to 55-60% in adults, with particularly expanded extracellular compartments creating larger distribution volumes for water-soluble compounds and potentially lower peak plasma concentrations after fixed mg/kg dosing. Adipose tissue percentage increases during infancy, then fluctuates throughout childhood with characteristic patterns including the adiposity rebound during early childhood, affecting distribution of lipophilic compounds. Plasma protein binding capacity demonstrates quantitative and qualitative differences, with reduced albumin concentrations and altered binding characteristics in neonates and young infants, potentially increasing free fractions of highly protein-bound toxicants. Additionally, endogenous substances including bilirubin and free fatty acids may compete for binding sites, further displacing toxicants from protein binding in neonates.

Hepatic metabolism undergoes profound maturation throughout pediatric development, affecting both detoxification and bioactivation processes for numerous xenobiotics. Phase I oxidative metabolism through cytochrome P450 enzymes follows isoform-specific developmental trajectories, creating age-dependent vulnerability or resistance to specific toxicants based on their metabolic pathways. Phase II conjugation demonstrates similar developmental patterns with clinical significance: glucuronidation, catalyzed by uridine diphosphate glucuronosyltransferases, remains markedly reduced in neonates and young infants, necessitating alternative metabolic pathways for certain compounds and potentially creating increased toxicity risk when these alternative pathways generate reactive metabolites. Paradoxically, some metabolic pathways may actually show enhanced activity during certain developmental windows, creating potential for increased toxicity from metabolite-mediated mechanisms compared to adults exposed to the same xenobiotics.

Renal elimination capacity demonstrates substantial postnatal development affecting toxicant clearance. Glomerular filtration rate approaches adult values (when adjusted for body surface area) by approximately 6-12 months of age, though remains significantly reduced in neonates, creating prolonged elimination of renally excreted toxicants during this period. Tubular secretion and reabsorption processes mature more gradually, with some transport mechanisms not reaching adult capacity until later childhood. This differential maturation of filtration versus tubular functions potentially alters the clearance patterns of toxicants compared to adult predictions, particularly for compounds where tubular secretion represents a significant elimination mechanism. For toxicants undergoing enterohepatic circulation, age-related differences in biliary transport and intestinal microbiota composition potentially affect reabsorption patterns and overall elimination kinetics.

Collectively, these toxicokinetic factors necessitate specific consideration when evaluating potential toxicity and determining appropriate interventions across pediatric age groups. Dosage calculations based solely on weight or body surface area may inadequately account for developmental differences in absorption, distribution, metabolism, and elimination processes. Age-appropriate pharmacokinetic models incorporating these developmental changes provide more accurate predictions of toxicant disposition, though remain incompletely developed for many substances. Clinical vigilance regarding potentially unexpected toxicokinetic patterns remains essential when managing pediatric exposures, particularly for substances whose properties have been primarily characterized in adult populations.

Behavioral Development

Behavioral development profoundly influences exposure risk patterns throughout childhood, with characteristic age-specific behaviors creating distinctive vulnerability periods for particular toxicants. Oral exploration represents a fundamental developmental behavior beginning in early infancy, intensifying during the 6-24 month period when hand-to-mouth activity peaks as part of normal sensory development and object exploration. This natural exploratory behavior creates significant ingestion risk for accessible household substances, medications, and small objects, particularly as mobility develops allowing access to previously unreachable areas. Compounding this risk, genuine taste discrimination remains undeveloped in young children, who may willingly consume bitter or unpleasant substances that would trigger rejection in adults, including harmful chemicals in attractive containers or medications designed without consideration of taste aversion as a protective factor.

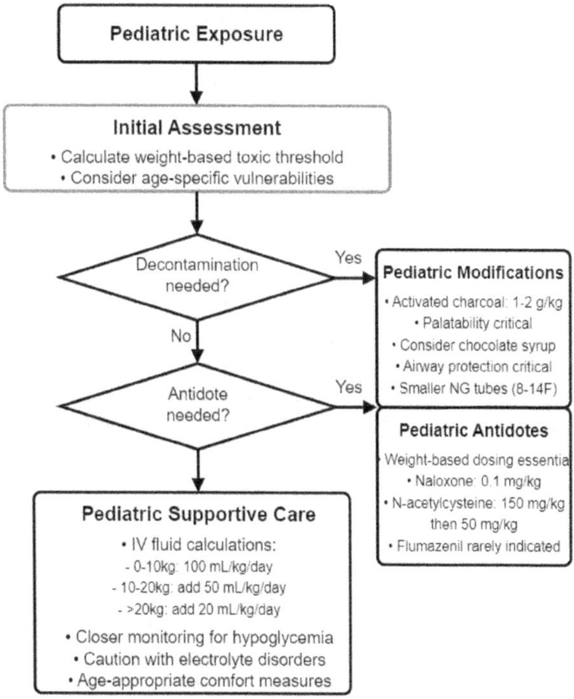

Figure 10.1 Modifications in Pediatric Treatment

Expanding environmental interaction characterizes the developmental progression from infancy through early childhood. Crawling emergence (typically 7-10 months) dramatically expands the accessible environment, providing access to low-lying hazards including houseplants, pest control products, fallen medications, and spilled household chemicals. Walking development further extends this environmental exploration, with vertical reach progressively increasing through climbing behaviors emerging around 12-18 months. These mobility developments occur before corresponding cognitive abilities to recognize and avoid hazards, creating a high-risk period where physical capabilities outpace safety awareness. This developmental mismatch necessitates environmental modification rather than reliance on educational approaches during this stage.

> **Remember**
>
> **Developmental stage significantly influences exposure risk, with exploratory ingestions peaking in toddlers (especially household products and medications), while adolescents exhibit intentional exposures including recreational substance use and self-harm attempts**

Cognitive development follows predictable patterns affecting risk recognition and safety behavior implementation throughout childhood. Preoperational thinking (approximately 2-7 years) includes several characteristics increasing poisoning vulnerability: egocentrism limiting perspective-taking and understanding of others' safety warnings; magical thinking potentially creating misconceptions about substance properties; concrete interpretation of information without abstract understanding of harm concepts; and limited cause-effect reasoning affecting comprehension of delayed toxicity. During this period, safety rules may be followed concretely without underlying comprehension, requiring consistent external monitoring rather than reliance on independent judgment. School-age children (approximately 7-11 years) develop increased capacity for logical operations and cause-effect reasoning, enabling more effective safety education, though still benefit from environmental protections for high-risk substances.

Adolescent development introduces distinct risk patterns reflecting both neurodevelopmental changes and social-environmental factors. Risk-taking behaviors increase during adolescence, influenced by normative neurodevelopmental processes including heightened reward sensitivity, sensation-seeking tendencies, and still-developing executive function capabilities affecting impulse control and consequence evaluation. These developmental characteristics, combined with increased independence from adult supervision and peer influence significance, create vulnerability to intentional misuse of substances for recreational purposes or through nonsuicidal self-harm behaviors. Approximately 85-90% of substance misuse begins during the adolescent period, highlighting the critical importance of prevention efforts during this developmental window. Additionally, role experimentation including identity formation through appearance-focused behaviors may increase exposure to potentially harmful consumer products including cosmetics, weight control substances, and performance-enhancing compounds.

Digital media influence on exposure risk represents an emerging consideration across pediatric age groups. Online challenges promoting potentially harmful behaviors have resulted in documented toxic exposures, including the "cinnamon challenge" causing respiratory irritation from inhaled spice, laundry pod consumption promoted through social influence, and various ethnobotanical exposures popularized through online forums. These digital influences evolve rapidly, creating challenges for traditional toxicovigilance systems and necessitating engagement with contemporary media platforms to identify emerging exposure trends. Concurrently, online information access may provide both benefits through readily available poisoning prevention information and risks through misinformation about home remedies or potentially harmful substances misrepresented as safe or beneficial through unregulated platforms.

COMMON EXPOSURES

Pediatric poisoning epidemiology demonstrates distinctive patterns reflecting developmental behaviors, environmental access, and caregiver practices across different age groups.

Pharmaceutical Agents

Analgesics consistently rank among the most common pharmaceutical exposures in children, with acetaminophen representing the single most frequently reported medication in pediatric poisoning surveillance data. Exploratory ingestions typically involve liquid formulations accessible to young children, created in appealing flavors to facilitate therapeutic administration but consequently reducing taste aversion as a protective factor against accidental consumption. Dosing confusion represents another significant exposure mechanism, particularly with liquid preparations where caregivers may misinterpret dosing instructions, confuse milliliter with teaspoon measurements, or use inappropriate measuring devices creating substantial overdose potential. Toxicity risk assessment must consider both acute single ingestions and repeated supratherapeutic dosing, as the latter may create cumulative hepatotoxicity despite individual doses below acute toxic thresholds. Management follows principles similar to adult protocols, with N-acetylcysteine administration based on serum acetaminophen levels plotted on the Rumack-Matthew nomogram, though with consideration that the traditional treatment line assumes normal glutathione stores which may not apply to malnourished or chronically ill children.

Table 10.2: Common Pediatric Toxic Exposures by Age Group

Age Group	**Most Common Exposures**	**Unique Considerations**	**Management Priorities**
<6 months	Medications given in error, plant exposures	Limited mobility means exposures often iatrogenic	Careful weight-based calculations
6-12 months	Household cleaners, personal care products, medications	Crawling/cruising enables access to low-lying hazards	Home safety assessment, cabinet locks, proper storage
1-3 years	Medications, cleaning products, foreign bodies, button batteries	Hand-to-mouth behavior, climbing ability, inability to assess danger	Immediate intervention for high-risk ingestions (button batteries, caustics)
4-6 years	Medications, arts/crafts supplies, plants	Curious about adult behaviors, can access higher locations	Distinguish between exploratory ingestion and potential self-harm
7-12 years	Medications, household products	May ingest on dares or from peer pressure	Consider social context of exposure
13-18 years	Alcohol, recreational drugs, intentional medication overdoses	Intentional exposures predominate	Mental health assessment, substance use evaluation

Cardiovascular medications create significant pediatric toxicity concerns despite relatively fewer exposure numbers, as minimal dosing (often a single tablet) of certain agents can produce profound effects in small children. Calcium channel blockers, particularly immediate-release nifedipine and extended-release formulations of various agents, produce disproportionate toxicity in children through both vasodilation and cardiac depression mechanisms. Beta-blockers similarly create substantial risk, with lipophilic agents like propranolol demonstrating particular concern due to additional central nervous system effects alongside the expected cardiac manifestations. Clonidine and related centrally-acting antihypertensives demonstrate distinctive pediatric significance, as their small tablet size and clinical use for attention-deficit/hyperactivity disorder place them in many households with children. The characteristic toxidrome includes miosis, bradycardia, hypotension, and central nervous system depression potentially mimicking opioid toxicity, though without response to naloxone. These cardiovascular medication exposures require intensive monitoring, aggressive supportive care, and consideration of specific interventions including high-dose insulin therapy for calcium channel blocker and beta-blocker toxicity, with pediatric-specific dosing protocols tailored to developmental physiology.

Psychotropic medications present increasing exposure concerns reflecting changing prescription patterns, with rising pediatric exposures correlating with increased presence in households. Selective serotonin reuptake inhibitors generally demonstrate wider therapeutic margins compared to earlier antidepressant classes, though still produce significant toxicity in overdose, particularly serotonin syndrome risk with its characteristic triad of neuromuscular abnormalities, autonomic instability, and mental status changes. Atypical antipsychotics produce predominantly sedation and miosis in small ingestions, with larger exposures creating risk for QT prolongation, extrapyramidal symptoms, and anticholinergic effects varying by specific agent profiles. Stimulant medications prescribed for attention-deficit/hyperactivity disorder create exposure risk through both exploratory ingestion and therapeutic misuse, with manifestations including tachycardia, hypertension, hyperthermia, agitation, and seizure potential with significant overdoses. Management approaches emphasize supportive care addressing specific manifestations, with particular attention to serotonin syndrome recognition requiring cyproheptadine consideration and cardiac monitoring for agents with potential QT effects.

Cough and cold preparations, though widely available in pediatric formulations despite limited efficacy evidence, create substantial toxicity risk through multiple mechanisms. Many combination products contain diphenhydramine or dextromethorphan alongside decongestants, creating complex toxidromes with concurrent anticholinergic and serotonergic or NMDA antagonist effects in overdose. Pediatric-specific concerns include paradoxical excitation sometimes observed with antihistamines in young children rather than the expected sedation and enhanced susceptibility to the dysrhythmogenic effects of sympathomimetic decongestants. Historical formulation changes removing pseudoephedrine from many over-the-counter preparations reduced sympathomimetic toxicity potential but created substitution with phenylephrine, which demonstrates different adverse effect profiles. Codeine-containing preparations, though less common following regulatory restrictions, create risk through both direct opioid effects and unpredictable metabolism to morphine through CYP2D6, with ultrarapid metabolizers potentially experiencing toxicity at standard doses.

Oral hypoglycemic agents deserve specific consideration due to their increasing presence in households related to rising diabetes prevalence and their potential for prolonged, profound hypoglycemia in pediatric exposures. Sulfonylureas stimulate pancreatic insulin release independent of serum glucose levels, creating potential for refractory hypoglycemia persisting beyond the expected duration based on the parent drug's pharmacokinetics. This prolonged effect reflects both the potent insulin secretion stimulus that may continue after drug levels decline and the limited glycogen reserves in children that reduce their ability to mount sustained counter-regulatory responses. Management requires extended observation periods, continuous glucose monitoring, frequent small feedings when tolerated, and intravenous dextrose administration titrated to maintain euglycemia. Octreotide, a somatostatin analog inhibiting insulin release, may benefit cases with recurrent or refractory hypoglycemia despite conventional dextrose administration, though with careful monitoring for potential adverse effects including gastrointestinal symptoms and gallbladder sludging.

Household Products

Cleaning products consistently rank among the most frequently reported pediatric exposures, reflecting their ubiquitous household presence and common storage in accessible locations. Toxicity potential varies dramatically within this category, from relatively benign dilute surfactant-based cleaners to highly caustic drain openers capable of producing full-thickness tissue injury upon contact. Bleach (sodium hypochlorite) represents the single most common cleaning product exposure, with household concentrations (typically 3-6%) generally producing limited toxicity beyond mild gastrointestinal irritation, though concentrated products available for pool maintenance may create more significant caustic injuries. Quaternary ammonium compounds ("quats") found in many disinfectants demonstrate greater toxicity potential, with ingestion causing both corrosive effects and systemic toxicity including central nervous system depression and hypotension in significant exposures. Toilet bowl cleaners containing acids create particular concern due to both their corrosive properties and common storage within reach of toddlers exploring bathroom environments. Risk assessment must consider both product concentration and formulation characteristics, as many modern products contain bittering agents, thickeners to reduce splashing, or distinctive colors aiding recognition—features that may reduce exposure severity compared to historical patterns.

Laundry products have gained increased toxicological significance with the introduction of highly concentrated "pod" or "packet" formulations containing detergents, enzymes, surfactants, and brighteners in premeasured dissolvable packaging. These products create distinctive exposure patterns compared to traditional liquid or powder detergents, with higher rates of significant toxicity including respiratory distress from aspiration, profound central nervous system depression of unclear mechanism, caustic injury to oral and esophageal tissues, and metabolic derangements. The colorful, soft-textured packaging resembling candy or toys creates particular appeal to young children, while the concentrated contents and rapid dissolution upon contact with mucous membranes or saliva allows ingestion of substantial quantities before taste aversion or caregiver intervention. Management approaches include careful airway assessment and protection given aspiration risk, supportive care addressing specific manifestations, and consideration of endoscopic evaluation for patients with significant oropharyngeal involvement or persistent symptoms. Prevention strategies targeting both product design (less appealing appearances, more resilient packaging) and consumer education have demonstrated partial success in reducing these exposures.

Button battery ingestions represent a pediatric toxicological emergency with distinctive mechanisms and management considerations. These small, disc-shaped power sources, increasingly common in household devices including remote controls, toys, watches, and hearing aids, create severe tissue injury through several mechanisms: electrolysis generating hydroxide at the negative pole, direct electrical current causing tissue liquefaction, and pressure necrosis between mucosal surfaces and the rigid battery. The resulting alkaline environment can produce full-thickness esophageal damage within 2 hours of impaction, with potential progression to catastrophic complications including aortoesophageal fistula formation, vertebral erosion, and mediastinitis. Risk assessment considers battery size (20-25 mm diameter batteries pose greatest esophageal impaction risk), location (esophageal impaction creates highest urgency), and time since ingestion. Management protocols emphasize immediate radiographic localization followed by emergent endoscopic removal for esophageal batteries, with subsequent surveillance for delayed perforation or stricture formation. Ingestions confirmed in the stomach may permit observation without immediate removal for smaller batteries in older children, though with close monitoring and follow-up imaging ensuring passage beyond the pylorus.

Hydrocarbons encompass a diverse product category including fuels, solvents, lubricants, and lamp oils, with varying toxicity profiles based on specific chemical properties. Aspiration risk represents the primary concern with many aliphatic hydrocarbons, as their low viscosity and surface tension facilitate distal airway penetration if even small amounts enter the respiratory tract during ingestion or subsequent vomiting. The resulting chemical pneumonitis typically presents with cough, respiratory distress, and characteristic radiographic findings developing within hours of exposure. Management emphasizes respiratory support, with gastrointestinal decontamination generally avoided due to concerns that induced emesis or lavage may increase aspiration risk. Certain hydrocarbons create additional concerns beyond respiratory effects: halogenated compounds may produce hepatotoxicity; aromatic compounds may cause central nervous system effects and bone marrow toxicity with significant absorption; and compounds containing additives such as camphor, metals, or pesticides may create specific systemic toxicity requiring targeted interventions. Prevention strategies include appropriate storage in original child-resistant containers, avoiding transfer to food or beverage containers where children might misidentify contents.

Cosmetics and personal care products consistently rank among the most frequently reported pediatric exposures due to their widespread household presence, often in easily accessible locations including bathrooms, bedrooms, and purses. Most exposures involve products with limited toxicity potential, including shampoos, lotions, and makeups, though exceptions exist requiring specific risk assessment. Mouthwash containing ethanol may create significant intoxication risk in small children due to the relatively high alcohol concentrations in some formulations. Essential oils, increasingly popular for various applications, demonstrate significant toxicity potential including seizures with certain compounds (camphor, eucalyptus, clove), chemical pneumonitis with aspiration, and dermal irritation or sensitization with topical exposure. Hair care products including relaxers and permanents contain various caustics or oxidizers capable of producing significant mucosal injury. Personal care product exposures require individualized risk assessment considering specific ingredients, concentration, quantity, and route of exposure, with management ranging from simple observation for minimally toxic exposures to specific interventions for products containing alcohols, caustics, or other potentially harmful components.

Environmental Toxins

Lead exposure remains a persistent pediatric public health concern despite significant regulatory reductions over recent decades, with children under 6 years demonstrating particular vulnerability due to developmental neurotoxic effects, enhanced absorption compared to adults, and characteristic behaviors including hand-to-mouth activity and pica that increase exposure risk. Primary sources include deteriorating lead-based paint in older housing, contaminated dust and soil, certain consumer products including imported toys or ceramics, and occasionally water contamination through lead-containing plumbing materials. Clinical presentation varies with exposure level: overt symptomatic lead poisoning, while now rare in developed nations, presents with nonspecific symptoms including abdominal pain, irritability, anorexia, and constipation; subclinical toxicity affects neurodevelopment without obvious immediate manifestations, potentially reducing cognitive function, altering behavior, and impairing academic achievement. Management follows tiered intervention protocols based on blood lead levels, including environmental investigation identifying and remediating exposure sources, nutritional optimization focusing on adequate iron, calcium and vitamin C intake, developmental monitoring for affected children, and chelation therapy for levels exceeding intervention thresholds (typically 45 μg/dL for asymptomatic children). Prevention emphasizes screening programs identifying at-risk populations, housing remediation eliminating lead hazards, and regulatory standards reducing lead in consumer products and environmental media.

Carbon monoxide represents a leading cause of unintentional poisoning death, with children demonstrating both physiological vulnerability and exposure risk through malfunctioning heating systems, improperly ventilated fuel-burning appliances, and generator use during power outages. Developmental factors affecting pediatric susceptibility include higher metabolic rates creating increased relative carbon monoxide production from the same percentage of hemoglobin binding, more rapid onset of cellular hypoxia due to higher baseline oxygen utilization, and limited capacity to verbalize early symptoms in young children. Clinical presentation often includes nonspecific symptoms making diagnosis challenging without specific consideration: headache, nausea, vomiting, dizziness, and fatigue may be misattributed to viral illnesses; more severe toxicity produces confusion, syncope, seizures, and coma potentially misconstrued as primary neurological emergencies. Management includes immediate removal from the exposure source, high-flow oxygen administration accelerating carboxyhemoglobin dissociation, and consideration of hyperbaric oxygen therapy for severe poisonings based on both carboxyhemoglobin levels and clinical presentation. Prevention strategies include carbon monoxide detector installation, regular maintenance of fuel-burning appliances, appropriate ventilation practices, and education regarding proper generator placement during emergency scenarios.

Pesticide exposures demonstrate both acute toxicity concerns and potential long-term developmental effects in pediatric populations. Organophosphate and carbamate insecticides, though increasingly restricted in residential settings, create particular concern through acetylcholinesterase inhibition producing the characteristic cholinergic toxidrome with muscarinic (salivation, lacrimation, urination, defecation, emesis, bronchospasm, bradycardia) and nicotinic (muscle fasciculations, weakness, tachycardia) manifestations. Pyrethroids, commonly replacing organophosphates in many residential applications, generally demonstrate lower mammalian toxicity but may produce paresthesias, salivation, nausea, and seizures with significant exposures. Exposure sources include agricultural applications with drift or take-home contamination on worker clothing, residential pest control treatments, pet products including flea and tick preventatives, and improperly stored containers. Management approaches address both decontamination through thorough skin washing for dermal exposures and specific antidotes including atropine for symptomatic cholinergic excess and pralidoxime for organophosphate-induced acetylcholinesterase inhibition. Emerging evidence suggests potential neurodevelopmental effects from chronic low-level exposures, particularly for organophosphates, though regulatory frameworks increasingly incorporate these concerns through application restrictions in settings where children may experience exposure.

Recreational drugs and substances of abuse create evolving pediatric exposure concerns through both accidental ingestion of substances present in the household and, in older children and adolescents, intentional experimentation or misuse. Cannabis exposures have increased significantly in regions implementing legalization or decriminalization, with edible products including gummies, brownies, and candies creating particular pediatric appeal and potentially containing highly concentrated forms resulting in significant toxicity. Clinical effects include altered mental status ranging from mild agitation to obtundation, conjunctival injection, tachycardia, and occasionally respiratory depression with substantial exposures, particularly with synthetic cannabinoids. Opioid exposures, reflecting the broader public health crisis, create critical pediatric concerns due to the extreme potency of synthetic opioids like fentanyl, where even minimal exploratory contact may produce severe respiratory depression in small children. Management approaches include appropriate respiratory support, naloxone administration for opioid-induced respiratory depression, and benzodiazepines for sympathomimetic-induced agitation or seizures, with specific interventions guided by the particular substance involved. Prevention strategies require adaptation to evolving substance use patterns, with particular attention to safe storage practices for both prescribed medications and recreational substances legally available in some jurisdictions.

Environmental envenomations and exposures to naturally occurring toxins demonstrate significant regional variation in pediatric populations. Snake envenomations affect children disproportionately due to both curiosity-driven interaction with potentially dangerous species and greater toxin effects per body weight from the same venom volume. Management follows principles established for adults, including appropriate immobilization, prompt transport to medical care, and specific antivenom administration when indicated, though with pediatric-specific considerations regarding fluid volumes, antivenom dosing, and monitoring parameters. Plant exposures represent frequent pediatric poison center calls, with most involving non-toxic or minimally toxic species, though important exceptions include cardiac glycoside-containing plants (foxglove, oleander, lily of the valley), highly nephrotoxic species (certain lilies in cats but minimally toxic to children), and plants containing solanaceous alkaloids (jimsonweed, deadly nightshade) producing anticholinergic toxicity. Management approach depends on specific identification and quantity, ranging from simple observation for non-toxic species to gastrointestinal decontamination, enhanced elimination, and specific antidotes for highly toxic plant ingestions.

Nonaccidental Poisoning

Münchhausen syndrome by proxy (factitious disorder imposed on another) represents a form of child abuse where a caregiver, typically a parent, fabricates, exaggerates, or induces illness in a child to fulfill psychological needs for attention and the caregiver role. Poisoning represents one manifestation, with documented cases involving administration of various substances including insulin causing hypoglycemia, salt causing hypernatremia, ipecac causing chronic emesis, and medications including sedatives, laxatives, or anticoagulants producing diverse clinical presentations. Several features suggest potential factitious poisoning: symptoms that occur only in the presence of a particular caregiver; recurrent unexplained illness defying conventional diagnostic approaches; clinical presentations inconsistent with the reported history; symptoms that do not respond to appropriate treatment but resolve in structured settings like hospitals; caregivers with unusual medical knowledge or apparent comfort in the healthcare environment; and caregivers who seem inappropriately calm or even satisfied with the child's illness or hospitalization.

Diagnosis requires comprehensive evaluation integrating medical, psychological, and social assessments. Medical investigation may include comprehensive toxicological screening beyond routine panels, with specific testing directed by clinical suspicion; careful chain of custody procedures ensuring sample integrity; and occasionally covert observation or restriction of caregiver access to determine whether symptoms persist without potential for medication administration. Psychological assessment evaluates both the child's adjustment to chronic illness and the caregiver's psychological functioning, while social investigation examines family dynamics, potential secondary gains, and historical patterns across multiple healthcare encounters, often requiring medical record review from various treatment facilities. Management necessitates multidisciplinary collaboration including medical providers, child protection services, mental health professionals, and often legal authorities, with primary focus on ensuring child safety while developing appropriate intervention strategies addressing the underlying psychological issues driving the abuse pattern.

Chemical submission or facilitated assault involves intentional administration of substances to impair a victim's consciousness, judgment, or resistance, typically for purposes of sexual assault or other crimes. While most commonly affecting older adolescents, documented cases involve children across age ranges, with perpetrators typically being caregivers or other trusted individuals. Substances employed include benzodiazepines, particularly flunitrazepam (Rohypnol) and similar potent sedatives; gamma-hydroxybutyrate (GHB) and related compounds; antihistamines with sedative properties; and ethanol, either alone or potentiating other agents. Clinical presentations typically involve sudden, unexplained alterations in consciousness, amnesia for specific time periods, and occasionally physical evidence of assault discovered during medical evaluation. Diagnostic challenges include the often-delayed presentation after symptoms resolve, rapid elimination of many implicated substances from conventional testing matrices, and potential misattribution of symptoms to recreational substance use in adolescent victims.

Toxicological investigation requires specific consideration of detection windows and appropriate specimens. Hair analysis may identify certain substances weeks to months after exposure, while conventional urine or serum testing typically detects substances for only hours to days, necessitating prompt specimen collection when chemical submission is suspected. Specialized reference laboratories can perform targeted testing for specific agents like GHB or flunitrazepam that may be missed on standard toxicology screens. Management involves both medical care addressing any injuries or exposures and appropriate psychosocial support, including trauma-informed approaches recognizing the profound psychological impact of such victimization. Forensic considerations require chain of custody documentation, appropriate evidence collection following jurisdiction-specific protocols, and collaboration with law enforcement when crimes are suspected.

Intentional pediatric poisoning encompasses scenarios where caregivers deliberately administer harmful substances with intent to cause injury or death rather than the attention-seeking motivation characteristic of factitious disorder. While rare compared to other forms of child maltreatment, these cases present particular diagnostic and management challenges. Clinical presentations raising concern include symptoms inconsistent with the reported history, exposure to substances not typically accessible to children, simultaneous illness in multiple siblings, or previous unexplained deaths in the family. Management priorities include ensuring immediate child safety through appropriate protective measures, comprehensive medical evaluation identifying and addressing all potential exposures, toxicological testing with proper chain of custody, and mandatory reporting to child protective services and law enforcement agencies according to jurisdictional requirements. These cases necessitate careful documentation meeting legal evidentiary standards, as criminal prosecution often follows confirmed intentional poisoning.

Suicide attempts and nonsuicidal self-injury using poisoning or overdose demonstrate increasing prevalence in pediatric populations, particularly among adolescents, with concerning upward trends over recent decades. Risk factors include previous suicide attempts, mental health conditions (particularly depression, anxiety, and borderline personality traits), substance use disorders, history of trauma or abuse, LGBTQ+ identity in non-supportive environments, and exposure to suicidal behavior among peers including through social media. Clinical assessment must address both the immediate toxicological concerns and the underlying psychological factors, with particular attention to distinguishing between nonsuicidal self-injury (self-harm without genuine death intent) and true suicide attempts, as management approaches differ significantly. Hospitalization decisions integrate medical necessity based on the specific overdose with psychiatric safety considerations including ongoing suicidal ideation, plan, and protective factors. Discharge planning must include safety measures addressing means restriction, appropriate mental health referrals with confirmed follow-up appointments, crisis response planning, and family education regarding supervision and support strategies

TREATMENT MODIFICATIONS

Pediatric toxicology necessitates specific treatment modifications addressing developmental physiology, practical implementation challenges, and unique risk-benefit considerations.

Gastrointestinal Decontamination

Gastric lavage has undergone substantial reevaluation in pediatric toxicology, with contemporary practice substantially restricting its use compared to historical approaches. Procedural modifications required for pediatric implementation include appropriate tube selection based on age and size (typically 16-28 French catheters for children compared to 36-40 French in adults), reduced lavage fluid volumes (5-10 mL/kg per aliquot rather than fixed 200-300 mL volumes), and particular attention to thermoregulation as the substantial fluid volumes may contribute to hypothermia in small children. Indications have narrowed significantly to rare circumstances involving life-threatening ingestions presenting within 60 minutes with substances not adsorbed by activated charcoal, and only when performed by experienced personnel with appropriate airway protection capability. Contraindications include unprotected airway without endotracheal intubation in obtunded patients, ingestion of hydrocarbons or caustics where the procedure may increase aspiration or perforation risk, and hemodynamic instability or respiratory compromise where the procedure may worsen the clinical status. Complications including aspiration, laryngospasm, and fluid/electrolyte imbalances occur more frequently in pediatric populations, contributing to the general shift away from this intervention in contemporary practice.

Activated charcoal administration represents the most widely employed gastrointestinal decontamination method in pediatric poisonings, though with important implementation modifications. Dosing follows weight-based guidelines (typically 1 g/kg) rather than standardized adult doses, with maximum recommendations typically not exceeding 50-100 g regardless of size. Administration challenges in children include palatability concerns limiting voluntary consumption and potential aspiration risk in uncooperative patients. Strategies addressing these challenges include commercial preparations with improved flavor profiles, mixing with small amounts of food substances compatible with binding efficacy (chocolate syrup, fruit purees), and occasionally administration via nasogastric tube when oral acceptance proves impossible but the risk-benefit assessment supports proceeding. Contraindications require particularly careful consideration in pediatric practice, as the risk of aspiration may outweigh decontamination benefits in situations involving uncooperative patients without definitive airway protection, especially young children with limited understanding and cooperation capacity.

Table 10.3: Pediatric Treatment Modifications for Common Toxicological Interventions

Intervention	Pediatric Modifications	Contraindications
Activated charcoal	1-2 g/kg (max 50-100g), palatability crucial	Same as adults, more concern for aspiration
Antidotes	Weight-based dosing essential Naloxone: 0.1 mg/kg N-acetylcysteine: 150 mg/kg load, then 50 mg/kg Flumazenil: 0.01 mg/kg	Flumazenil rarely indicated in pediatrics
IV fluid therapy	Careful calculation based on weight: 0-10kg: 100 mL/kg/day 10-20kg: add 50 mL/kg/day >20kg: add 20 mL/kg/day	Fluid overload risk in renal/cardiac impairment
Enhanced elimination	Lower threshold for dialysis in specific toxins (salicylates, lithium)	Equipment limitations for very small patients
Decontamination	Smaller equipment sizes (NG tubes 8-14F based on age)	Same as adults, higher risk of complications

Multiple-dose activated charcoal regimens demonstrate potentially enhanced efficacy for specific toxicants undergoing enterohepatic circulation or demonstrating prolonged gastrointestinal transit, though with pediatric-specific considerations affecting implementation. Compared to adult protocols, pediatric regimens typically employ reduced per-dose charcoal amounts (0.5 g/kg rather than fixed 25-50 g doses) administered at 4-6 hour intervals, with total treatment duration determined by clinical response and specific toxicant properties. Complications requiring specific monitoring include electrolyte abnormalities from intestinal losses, particularly hypokalemia with prolonged therapy; constipation or intestinal obstruction, especially with inadequate fluid intake; pulmonary aspiration with repeated administration attempts in uncooperative patients; and potential interaction with other essential medications administered during the treatment course. These concerns necessitate careful patient selection, considering both specific toxicant properties justifying the approach and the individual child's ability to tolerate the regimen safely.

Whole bowel irrigation employs large volumes of polyethylene glycol electrolyte solution to physically remove toxicants from the gastrointestinal tract, with pediatric applications requiring specific protocol modifications. Dosing follows age-based guidelines rather than standardized adult rates: 500 mL/hour for children 9 months to 6 years, 1000 mL/hour for ages 6-12 years, and adult doses (1500-2000 mL/hour) only for adolescents with adult size parameters. Administration typically requires nasogastric tube placement in younger children, as voluntary consumption of the necessary volumes proves impractical, with careful attention to tube position confirmation before initiating the procedure. Monitoring during the procedure must address potential fluid and electrolyte shifts, especially in smaller children where improperly formulated solutions might create significant imbalances; thermoregulation concerns with room-temperature solutions potentially contributing to hypothermia in extended procedures; and abdominal distention or vomiting indicating intolerance and potentially necessitating rate reduction or temporary discontinuation. Indications primarily include substances not effectively bound by activated charcoal, sustained-release pharmaceutical preparations, drug packets in body packers, and toxic metals or other foreign bodies requiring physical removal, with careful consideration of whether the anticipated benefits justify the procedural challenges in pediatric patients.

Cathartics, historically administered concurrently with activated charcoal under the premise of accelerating gastrointestinal transit and reducing toxicant absorption, demonstrate particularly problematic risk-benefit profiles in children and are generally discouraged in contemporary pediatric practice. Significant concerns include fluid and electrolyte disturbances occurring more readily in children's smaller fluid compartments with reduced regulatory capacity, potential for excessive fluid losses creating dehydration, and limited evidence supporting efficacy beyond that provided by the concurrently administered adsorptive agent. When deemed necessary in specific circumstances, single-dose cathartic administration using sorbitol (0.5 g/kg in children, maximum 25 g) demonstrates the most favorable profile, with particular caution in children under 1 year where regulatory mechanisms remain less developed. Multiple-dose cathartic regimens are specifically contraindicated in pediatric patients due to the substantial fluid and electrolyte disturbance risks without demonstrated additional benefit.

Remember

Treatment modifications for pediatric poisonings include precise weight-based dosing, careful fluid management, consideration of hypoglycemia risk, equipment size adjustments, and special attention to airway management given anatomical differences.

Enhanced elimination considerations including urinary alkalinization and extracorporeal techniques require pediatric-specific approaches addressing both practical implementation and developmental physiology. Urinary alkalinization for weakly acidic toxicants like salicylates employs sodium bicarbonate administration with pediatric dosing of 1-2 mEq/kg IV bolus followed by continuous infusion titrated to maintain urinary pH between 7.5-8.0, with careful attention to fluid volume status, potassium levels requiring concurrent replacement, and monitoring parameters appropriate to developmental stage. Hemodialysis indications follow principles similar to adult parameters but with recognition that smaller body fluid compartments and potentially enhanced end-organ susceptibility may justify intervention at different relative toxicant levels compared to adult guidelines. Technical aspects of extracorporeal procedures require pediatric expertise ensuring appropriate vascular access selection, circuit parameters, and anticoagulation protocols reflecting developmental hemodynamics and coagulation system maturation.

Antidotal Therapy

Antidotal therapy in pediatric toxicology requires specific considerations regarding dosing, administration routes, potential adverse effects, and efficacy assessment across developmental stages. N-acetylcysteine (NAC) for acetaminophen toxicity follows weight-based protocols with identical target doses to adults but requiring volume adjustments for both oral administration (loading dose of 140 mg/kg followed by 70 mg/kg every 4 hours, typically diluted to 5% concentration for palatability) and intravenous regimens (same three-step protocol but with careful attention to sodium load and fluid volumes in smaller children). Efficacy assessment employs the same Rumack-Matthew nomogram with identical treatment thresholds, though some experts advocate for more conservative approaches in infants under 1 year where glutathione metabolism demonstrates developmental variations potentially affecting detoxification capacity. Adverse effect monitoring requires recognition that children demonstrate higher rates of vomiting with oral administration and may exhibit anaphylactoid reactions to intravenous formulations, occasionally necessitating administration rate adjustments or temporary discontinuation with rechallenge at slower rates when reactions subside.

Naloxone administration for opioid toxicity involves crucial pediatric modifications addressing both appropriate dosing for developmental body weight and implementation considerations for various clinical scenarios. Initial dosing follows weight-based guidelines of 0.1 mg/kg for most clinical situations, though with adjustments based on individual exposure characteristics—suspected fentanyl or other high-potency synthetic opioid exposures may warrant higher initial doses given their relative naloxone resistance. Administration routes provide particular flexibility in pediatric scenarios: intravenous delivery offers most rapid effect when access exists; intramuscular or subcutaneous administration provides alternatives when intravenous access proves challenging; intranasal delivery through commercially available devices or improvised atomizers creates non-invasive options particularly valuable in community settings; and intraosseous administration using established pediatric emergency vascular access protocols provides additional options in critical scenarios. Dosing intervals require careful consideration of naloxone's relatively short half-life (30-90 minutes) compared to many opioids, particularly extended-release formulations, creating potential for recurrent toxicity as antagonist effects wane before the opioid eliminates. Continuous infusions, when indicated for persistent or recurrent effects, typically employ hourly rates of two-thirds the effective reversal dose.

Flumazenil, a competitive benzodiazepine antagonist, demonstrates particularly controversial applications in pediatric toxicology due to seizure risk concerns similar to those in adult populations but potentially magnified by children's enhanced seizure susceptibility. When deemed appropriate after careful risk-benefit assessment, pediatric dosing employs 0.01 mg/kg (maximum 0.2 mg) administered intravenously over 30 seconds, with repeat dosing at one-minute intervals to maximum cumulative dose of 1 mg. Absolute contraindications include known or suspected co-ingestion of proconvulsant agents (particularly tricyclic antidepressants), history of seizure disorder, known benzodiazepine dependence, and evidence of cyclic antidepressant toxicity on electrocardiogram (QRS prolongation), as antagonism in these scenarios may precipitate refractory seizures. Limited appropriate indications include iatrogenic benzodiazepine oversedation during procedural sedation and diagnostic evaluation of altered mental status in specific circumstances where the risk-benefit assessment supports administration. The relatively short duration of action (typically 30-60 minutes) compared to most benzodiazepines necessitates extended monitoring after administration, as recurrent sedation may occur as antagonist effects wane while the benzodiazepine remains present.

Heavy metal chelation therapy requires particularly careful pediatric considerations due to both the enhanced vulnerability of developing organ systems to metal toxicity and potential adverse effects from the chelating agents themselves. Lead chelation employs tiered approaches based on blood lead levels, with current guidelines typically recommending oral succimer (dimercaptosuccinic acid, DMSA) for levels exceeding 45 μg/dL without encephalopathy at doses of 10 mg/kg every 8 hours for 5 days, followed by the same dose every 12 hours for 14 days. More severe toxicity with higher levels or encephalopathic manifestations typically warrants parenteral therapy with dimercapril (BAL) at 4-5 mg/kg/dose deep intramuscularly combined with calcium disodium EDTA (25 mg/kg/dose intravenously or intramuscularly). Mercury chelation similarly employs succimer for most non-emergent cases, with dimercaprol reserved for more severe acute toxicity or manifestations suggesting central nervous system involvement. Arsenic chelation follows similar protocols, though with recognition of different relative efficacies for various arsenic species. Common implementation challenges include the unpleasant sulfur odor of many chelating agents affecting palatability, painful injection sites with parenteral dimercaprol administration, and coordination of chelation therapy with environmental intervention addressing ongoing exposure sources.

Digoxin-specific antibody fragments (Fab) represent a critical antidote in pediatric toxicology given both accidental ingestions of cardiac glycoside-containing plants and medications and the extreme sensitivity of the pediatric myocardium to these agents. Dosing calculations employ either direct approaches based on serum digoxin level and weight (dose in vials = [serum digoxin concentration × weight in kg] ÷ 100) or empiric regimens (typically 10-20 vials for severe acute overdose in adolescents, with proportionately adjusted doses for smaller children). For plant-derived cardiac glycosides, dosing estimates convert the approximate plant content to digoxin equivalents, though often with significant uncertainty necessitating symptom-based titration.

Administration requires attention to potential allergic reactions, though less common with fragments than whole antibodies, and monitoring for hypokalemia resulting from rapid reversal of the hyperkalemia characteristic of cardiac glycoside toxicity. Early utilization receives particular emphasis in pediatric patients given their limited cardiovascular reserve and potential for rapid decompensation with these exposures.

Fomepizole (4-methylpyrazole) for toxic alcohol poisoning has largely replaced ethanol in pediatric practice due to its more favorable adverse effect profile, predictable pharmacokinetics, and absence of central nervous system depression. Pediatric dosing follows the standard protocol of 15 mg/kg loading dose followed by 10 mg/kg every 12 hours for 4 doses, then 15 mg/kg every 12 hours until methanol or ethylene glycol levels decrease below 20 mg/dL, with adjustments to 4-hour intervals during hemodialysis. The absence of hypoglycemia risk, sedation, and complex monitoring requirements that complicate ethanol therapy creates particular advantages in children, where these adverse effects may prove more problematic than in adults. Implementation typically involves administration in 100 mL of normal saline or 5% dextrose infused over 30 minutes, with attention to potential infusion site irritation. Combined therapy approaches employing both alcohol dehydrogenase inhibition through fomepizole and enhanced elimination through hemodialysis receive particular consideration in pediatric patients with significant toxic alcohol levels, where rapid toxicant removal may prevent irreversible end-organ damage to developing systems.

Supportive Care

Fluid management in pediatric toxicology necessitates specific approaches reflecting developmental physiology, with both volume requirements and composition requiring careful consideration. Maintenance fluid calculations follow either weight-based approaches (100 mL/kg/day for the first 10 kg, plus 50 mL/kg/day for 10-20 kg, plus 20 mL/kg/day for weight exceeding 20 kg) or body surface area methods (1500-2000 mL/m^2/day), with adjustments based on specific toxicant properties and clinical manifestations. Composition selection requires consideration of potential electrolyte abnormalities associated with specific poisonings, with particular attention to sodium content in scenarios involving potential cerebral edema where hypertonic solutions may provide benefit, and dextrose concentration addressing hypoglycemia risk with certain toxicants including insulin secretagogues, beta-blockers, and alcohols. Dehydration correction employs deficit calculations typically estimated through clinical assessment with degree-based replacement strategies (mild dehydration calculated as 50 mL/kg deficit, moderate as 100 mL/kg, severe as 150 mL/kg), with rehydration rates determined by hemodynamic stability and specific toxicant characteristics. Monitoring parameters must address both overhydration and underhydration risks, with children demonstrating more rapid decompensation with volume depletion but also enhanced vulnerability to fluid overload complications including pulmonary edema.

Airway management incorporates developmental anatomy considerations substantially affecting both assessment and intervention. The relatively larger occiput of infants and young children creates natural neck flexion in the supine position, potentially exacerbating airway obstruction and necessitating towel placement under the shoulders rather than the neck typically positioned in adult patients. The proportionally larger tongue relative to oropharyngeal dimensions increases soft tissue obstruction risk, particularly in obtunded patients, while the shorter neck and anterior laryngeal position create more challenging direct visualization during intubation attempts. Equipment selection follows age-adjusted guidelines, with endotracheal tube size estimated through various methods including age-based formulas (size = [age in years + 4] ÷ 4) or comparison with anatomical structures like the patient's little finger diameter. Rapid sequence induction medication selection addresses the vulnerability of the pediatric cardiovascular system to certain induction agents, with etomidate or ketamine typically providing more stable hemodynamic profiles compared to propofol or barbiturates in critically ill poisoned children. Definitive airway management thresholds may differ somewhat from adult guidelines, as children demonstrate both more rapid oxygen desaturation due to higher metabolic rates and smaller functional residual capacity, and increased risk for hypercapnia-induced acidosis exacerbating certain toxicities.

Cardiovascular support requires pediatric-specific approaches addressing both normal developmental physiological differences and toxicant-induced alterations. Hemodynamic parameter targets follow age-adjusted normal ranges rather than standardized adult values, with particular attention to heart rate as a primary determinant of cardiac output in infants and young children whose limited stroke volume reserve creates reliance on chronotropic mechanisms. Fluid resuscitation for hypotension typically begins with 10-20 mL/kg crystalloid boluses, with reassessment after each administration to prevent overload, as children may transition rapidly from inadequate organ perfusion to pulmonary edema with excessive fluid. Vasopressor and inotrope selection addresses the shifting adrenergic receptor density and responsiveness throughout childhood development, with dopamine historically employed as first-line therapy in younger children due to its combined inotropic and chronotropic effects at moderate doses, though contemporary critical care practice increasingly favors epinephrine or norepinephrine with more predictable effects. Toxicant-specific cardiovascular support follows principles similar to adult management but with pediatric dosing adjustments, exemplified by high-dose insulin euglycemia therapy for calcium channel blocker or beta-blocker toxicity employing 1 unit/kg regular insulin bolus followed by infusion starting at 0.5-1 unit/kg/hour, with concomitant glucose administration and monitoring proportional to size.

Neurological management addresses the distinctive features of central nervous system toxicity in children, including their enhanced susceptibility to certain neurotoxic effects and different manifestations compared to adult populations. Seizure management employs weight-based benzodiazepine dosing (typically lorazepam 0.05-0.1 mg/kg IV or midazolam 0.1-0.2 mg/kg IV/IM), with lower thresholds for intervention given the potential for more rapid progression to status epilepticus in pediatric patients and the enhanced neurological vulnerability to prolonged seizure activity in developing brains. Second-line anticonvulsant selection for refractory seizures typically favors phenobarbital (15-20 mg/kg IV) or levetiracetam (20-60 mg/kg IV) over phenytoin due to the latter's potential exacerbation of cardiotoxicity with certain poisonings and its variable efficacy against toxicant-induced seizures. Increased intracranial pressure management, when indicated for specific poisonings including severe salicylate toxicity or certain hydrocarbon exposures, employs both standard approaches including head elevation, normocapneic ventilation, and osmotic agents at pediatric doses (mannitol 0.25-1 g/kg or 3% saline 2-5 mL/kg) and careful evaluation of potential endotracheal intubation effects, as the transient hypercarbia during the procedure may transiently worsen cerebral edema.

Thermoregulation support addresses the enhanced vulnerability of pediatric patients to temperature dysregulation from both direct toxicant effects and environmental factors during prolonged evaluations or procedures. Hyperthermia management for toxicological causes including sympathomimetics, anticholinergics, salicylates, or serotonergic agents employs active external cooling measures (mist and fan techniques, ice packs to groin and axillae, cooling blankets) with careful temperature monitoring preventing overcorrection. Severe hyperthermia (>40-41°C) may require more aggressive approaches including cold intravenous fluid administration or rarely endovascular cooling devices in larger children and adolescents. Pharmacological approaches address underlying mechanisms when possible: benzodiazepines for sympathomimetic excess and certain serotonin syndrome presentations; anticholinergics like physostigmine in carefully selected cases of anticholinergic toxicity without contraindications; and specific agents like dantrolene for malignant hyperthermia or cyproheptadine for serotonin syndrome. Hypothermia prevention receives particular attention during prolonged procedures like gastrointestinal decontamination or extended observation periods, where children's higher surface area to volume ratio and limited physiological compensatory mechanisms create enhanced vulnerability. Active warming through pre-warmed intravenous fluids, appropriate environmental temperature control, and external warming devices maintains normothermia and prevents the additional physiological stress hypothermia would place on already compromised systems.

PREVENTIVE MEASURES

Poisoning prevention in pediatric populations requires multilevel approaches addressing developmental vulnerability, environmental modifications, caregiver education, and regulatory frameworks.

Product Engineering

Child-resistant packaging represents among the most successful injury prevention interventions in public health history, with U.S. implementation through the Poison Prevention Packaging Act of 1970 estimated to prevent approximately 200,000 childhood poisonings annually. These packaging mechanisms incorporate designs requiring coordinated actions exceeding typical developmental capabilities of young children, while remaining accessible to adults including those with physical limitations. Standard testing protocols require that at least 80% of children under five years cannot open the container within 10 minutes, while at least 90% of adults can properly close and open the package. Designs include push-and-turn mechanisms requiring simultaneous pressure and rotation, alignment systems necessitating precise positioning before opening, and locking blisters requiring multiple steps for medication access. Contemporary approaches increasingly incorporate adaptability features allowing consumers to select between child-resistant and easy-open configurations based on household composition and storage practices.

Despite demonstrated effectiveness, this engineering control presents several important limitations necessitating complementary approaches. Proper functioning requires consistent re-securing after each use, with observational studies demonstrating significant rates of improper closure in everyday household use. Effectiveness diminishes as children approach 5 years of age, with some developmentally advanced younger children demonstrating capability to defeat these mechanisms. Transfer of products from original containers to non-child-resistant storage frequently occurs for convenience, particularly with medications taken regularly or products used in multiple household locations. These limitations highlight the need for comprehensive prevention approaches rather than reliance solely on packaging interventions, though continuous improvement efforts address identified shortcomings through innovative design modifications including single-use packaging, enhanced visual and tactile feedback for proper closure, and designs addressing common defeat methods identified through ongoing research.

Unit-dose packaging represents an evolution beyond traditional child-resistant approaches, limiting potential exposure quantities through individually wrapped single doses rather than relying solely on container access restriction. This approach creates multiple protective barriers, as children would need to defeat both the outer container mechanism and individual dose wrappings to access harmful quantities. Additionally, the time required to open multiple individual packages may increase the likelihood of caregiver discovery before significant quantities are consumed. Pharmaceutical applications include blister packs for solid oral medications and single-use containers for liquid formulations, while household product adaptations include dissolvable packets for laundry and dishwasher detergents and single-use cleaning product capsules. Demonstrated benefits include reduced severity of exposures when they occur, as children typically access fewer doses before discovery compared to traditional bulk-container products. Implementation challenges include increased manufacturing costs potentially affecting consumer acceptance, environmental concerns regarding additional packaging materials, and occasionally reduced accessibility for individuals with disabilities requiring alternative designs balancing safety with usability.

Active dispensing systems incorporate technological approaches limiting medication access to appropriate timing and dosing, with particular value for households with both young children and individuals requiring complex medication regimens. Simple mechanical timer devices prevent reopening of containers until scheduled dose times, while more sophisticated electronic systems incorporate features including biometric identification, remote monitoring capabilities allowing caregiver alerts when doses are accessed, and automated dispensing of only the appropriate medication quantity. These systems demonstrate particular benefit in households with children where high-risk medications including opioid analgesics or cardiovascular agents necessitate regular use by adults, creating ongoing exposure risk despite traditional safety measures. Limitations include cost barriers affecting widespread implementation, potential technical failures requiring backup access methods, and the observation that partial protection may still allow determined adolescents to defeat these mechanisms for intentional misuse. Future development directions include integration with smartphone technology for enhanced monitoring and alert capabilities, reduced cost implementations for broader accessibility, and designs specifically addressing adolescent misuse patterns while maintaining appropriate therapeutic access.

Formulation modifications address inherent product properties creating specific toxicity risks, with approaches including addition of bittering agents creating taste aversion, emetics inducing vomiting upon overdose, or antagonists activated only when consumed in excessive quantities. Denatonium benzoate, an extremely bitter substance detectable at minute concentrations, has been incorporated into various products including antifreeze, nail polish removers, and certain medications, though with mixed evidence regarding effectiveness in preventing pediatric ingestions. While some studies demonstrate reduced consumption volumes in simulated exposure scenarios, others indicate that young children may continue ingesting despite the unpleasant taste, particularly with sweet vehicles partially masking the bitterness. More sophisticated approaches include abuse-deterrent opioid formulations incorporating naloxone that remains inactive with normal oral administration but activates upon crushing for misuse, and acetaminophen preparations containing methionine providing glutathione precursors activated during overdose. Consumer product adaptations include reduced-concentration formulations of household chemicals balancing cleaning efficacy with improved safety profile when accidental exposures occur, such as automatic dishwasher detergents reformulated with reduced alkalinity and oxidizing potential following recognition of significant esophageal injury risk from the original high-concentration products.

Enhanced warning systems incorporate visual, auditory, or electronic alerts identifying potential exposure risks before injury occurs. Applications include carbon monoxide and natural gas detectors providing early warning of these otherwise imperceptible toxic gases; medication reminder systems that also track potential excessive consumption through electronic monitoring; and emerging "smart home" technologies capable of recognizing unusual patterns suggesting potential poisoning scenarios. Pediatric-specific adaptations include lower placement of monitoring devices reflecting children's breathing zone closer to the floor where heavier-than-air gases concentrate, and visual warning systems using symbols and colors recognizable to preliterate children rather than text warnings requiring reading ability. Implementation challenges include cost barriers limiting widespread adoption, potential for alarm fatigue with frequent non-emergency activations, and the need for regular maintenance ensuring continued proper functioning. Future development directions include integration with broader home safety systems, reduced cost implementations for underserved communities demonstrating higher poisoning rates, and designs specifically addressing developmental characteristics of the highest risk pediatric populations.

Educational Programs

Caregiver education represents a cornerstone of pediatric poisoning prevention, with approaches tailored to specific developmental stages and corresponding risk patterns. Anticipatory guidance delivered through healthcare visits provides developmentally timed information addressing emerging mobility and exploratory behaviors before they create exposure risks. This preventive counseling typically begins during prenatal care and early infancy, establishing safe medication and household chemical storage practices before the infant develops mobility. Content expands as developmental capabilities increase, addressing crawling-stage hazards around 6 months, walking and climbing capabilities around 12 months, and progressive environmental access through early childhood. Educational materials employ multiple formats accommodating diverse learning styles and preferences, including written handouts, visual demonstrations, video content, and interactive teaching methods, with evidence suggesting that multimodal approaches combining various instructional methods demonstrate superior knowledge retention and behavior implementation compared to single-methodology education.

The universal precautions concept has evolved from infectious disease applications to poisoning prevention, advancing the principle that all medications and household chemicals should be considered potentially harmful and stored securely regardless of specific toxicity levels. This approach addresses several confirmed limitations of selective protection strategies: caregiver uncertainty regarding which specific products require restricted access; changing household composition when visitors including grandchildren or other young guests create unanticipated exposure risks; and the observation that children's capability to access ostensibly secure locations increases rapidly and often unexpectedly throughout development. Implementation emphasizes consistent application of prevention strategies across all potential toxicants, with specific recommendations including storage at heights exceeding 5 feet (above typical climbing reach), use of locked cabinets or containers for all medications and household chemicals, and prompt proper disposal of unused medications and chemicals rather than long-term storage creating ongoing exposure opportunity.

Child education approaches must address developmental limitations affecting comprehension and implementation of safety information. For children under 3 years, education targets caregivers exclusively, as developmental capabilities preclude effective direct child education at this stage. Preschool children (approximately 3-5 years) benefit from concrete safety rules like "ask a grown-up" before touching or consuming any potential toxicant, though with recognition that their developmental egocentrism and limited cause-effect reasoning create inconsistent application requiring continued environmental protections rather than reliance on educational approaches alone. School-age children demonstrate increased capability for safety education, with programming focused on specific substance identification, understanding of basic poison concepts, and procedural knowledge for emergency response. Adolescent education shifts toward risk recognition and decision-making in real-world contexts, addressing both accidental exposures and intentional misuse scenarios, with particular emphasis on peer pressure resistance skills and understanding of actual versus perceived substance risks.

Teachable moment utilization represents an evidence-based approach capitalizing on heightened receptivity to prevention information during specific circumstances creating personal relevance. Following a poisoning exposure (even if minor), caregivers demonstrate significantly enhanced motivation to implement prevention strategies, creating an ideal opportunity for targeted education addressing specific household risk patterns identified during the incident evaluation. Healthcare visits for related conditions similarly provide contextual relevance increasing information receptivity, such as well-child visits coinciding with developmental transitions to new mobility stages, or chronic condition management requiring home medication use creating exposure risk for all household members. Community events following high-profile poisoning incidents provide population-level teachable moments where public attention and concern create receptiveness to prevention messaging that might otherwise receive limited engagement. Implementation approaches at individual, healthcare system, and community levels involve identifying these high-receptivity periods and delivering appropriately tailored prevention messaging when it demonstrates highest likelihood of behavior change implementation.

Diverse outreach strategies address the recognized limitations of traditional educational approaches that often fail to reach highest-risk populations including those with limited healthcare access, language or literacy barriers, or socioeconomic constraints affecting implementation capacity. Community-based models deliver prevention education through trusted local organizations including religious institutions, community centers, and cultural organizations, with content and delivery methods adapted to specific community contexts and values. Technology-based outreach employs social media platforms, smartphone applications, and online resources reaching populations who may not engage with traditional prevention programming through healthcare or educational settings. Peer education approaches train community members to deliver information within their social networks, leveraging established trust relationships and cultural understanding beyond what external educators might achieve. These diverse strategies recognize that effective prevention education requires both appropriate content and delivery through channels accessible and acceptable to target populations, particularly those demonstrating highest poisoning risk who may have limited engagement with conventional healthcare systems providing traditional anticipatory guidance.

Community-Based Approaches

Poison center services provide both emergency response capabilities and prevention resources, with demonstrated cost-effectiveness and public health impact. Direct emergency consultation offers real-time exposure assessment, triage recommendations, and management guidance to both caregivers and healthcare providers, preventing unnecessary emergency department visits for non-toxic exposures while ensuring appropriate medical evaluation for potentially significant poisonings. Prevention resources include educational materials, community outreach programs, and data collection supporting surveillance activities identifying emerging hazards requiring targeted intervention. Pediatric-specific services include developmentally appropriate protocols recognizing distinctive management considerations across age groups, specialized educational materials addressing age-specific risk patterns, and data analysis identifying exposure trends requiring prevention focus. Implementation challenges include sustainable funding models as these services typically operate as public health resources rather than traditional healthcare reimbursement structures, awareness barriers limiting utilization particularly among vulnerable populations demonstrating highest poisoning risk, and integration with evolving healthcare delivery systems including electronic health records and telemedicine platforms.

Safe medication disposal programs address both pediatric poisoning risk from unused medications and broader public health concerns including environmental contamination and diversion potential. Take-back events provide periodic community collection opportunities for unused medications, while permanent collection sites at pharmacies, healthcare facilities, or law enforcement locations offer ongoing disposal options. Mail-back programs provide alternatives for individuals with mobility limitations or in rural areas with limited collection site access. In-home disposal methods including medication deactivation systems employ containment with activated charcoal or other binding agents rendering medications non-retrievable and non-active before standard waste disposal. These approaches demonstrate effectiveness in removing significant medication quantities from household accessibility, though challenges include awareness limitations, convenience barriers affecting utilization, and sustainable funding models for program maintenance. Pediatric poisoning prevention benefits occur through reduced medication availability for exploratory ingestion, while additional public health advantages include decreased environmental impact from improper disposal and reduced diversion potential for medications with misuse liability.

School-based prevention programs leverage educational settings reaching broad pediatric populations across socioeconomic categories. Curriculum integration embeds poisoning prevention within broader health education, science instruction, or safety programming rather than isolated presentations, creating multiple exposure opportunities reinforcing key concepts. Peer leadership models engage older students in developing and delivering age-appropriate prevention messaging to younger children, leveraging both the educational benefit for peer leaders who must master content for teaching and the enhanced receptivity of younger students to near-peer messaging compared to adult instruction. Parent engagement components extend program impact beyond the classroom through take-home materials, family homework assignments requiring caregiver-child interaction around safety concepts, and school-sponsored family education events addressing household safety practices. Effectiveness evaluation suggests greatest impact from comprehensive approaches combining classroom instruction, environmental modification within school settings, policy development supporting prevention practices, and explicit connection to household implementation rather than isolated knowledge-focused interventions.

Home visitation programs provide intensive individualized prevention support through direct observation and intervention in the child's actual environment. These programs employ trained visitors including nurses, social workers, or community health workers delivering structured prevention curricula while simultaneously conducting environmental assessment identifying specific household hazards. Intervention approaches include direct assistance with implementing recommended modifications such as installing cabinet locks, providing storage containers, or reorganizing household arrangements to reduce exposure risk. Follow-up visits ensure sustained implementation and address evolving hazards as the child develops new capabilities. These intensive approaches demonstrate particular benefit for high-risk populations including first-time parents, families with limited resources or support systems, and households with identified risk factors including substance use disorders or mental health conditions affecting supervision capacity. While resource requirements limit widespread implementation, targeted application addressing highest-risk scenarios shows favorable cost-benefit profiles considering the substantial economic and human costs associated with significant poisoning events.

Coalition-based approaches integrate diverse stakeholders including healthcare providers, educators, government agencies, community organizations, and industry representatives addressing poisoning prevention through coordinated multi-level interventions. These collaborative structures enable comprehensive strategies combining educational initiatives, environmental modifications, policy development, and social norm evolution rather than isolated single-method approaches demonstrating limited sustainable impact. Effective coalitions incorporate community member participation ensuring cultural appropriateness and implementation feasibility, rather than exclusively professional-driven program development. Implementation typically follows assessment-planning-intervention-evaluation cycles, with data-driven problem identification, evidence-based strategy selection, coordinated implementation leveraging complementary partner capabilities, and rigorous evaluation informing continuous improvement. This integrated approach addresses the recognized limitations of isolated interventions through coordinated strategies simultaneously addressing multiple risk and protective factors, creating systems-level change supporting sustained prevention impact beyond what individual organizations or sectors could achieve independently.

Summary

Pediatric toxicology addresses the unique physiological, developmental, and exposure characteristics that differentiate children from adults in toxic exposures. Age-specific concerns include altered toxicokinetics, with infants and young children having proportionally larger body surface area, higher total body water content, underdeveloped blood-brain barrier, immature hepatic enzyme systems, and variable renal clearance. These factors often increase vulnerability to toxins while producing different clinical manifestations than seen in adults. Developmental considerations affect exposure patterns and risk assessment: infants experience toxicity primarily through caregiver medication errors or passive environmental exposures; toddlers and preschoolers suffer exploratory ingestions of household products, medications, and plants due to oral exploration and increasing mobility; school-age children face risks from medication errors and increasing intentional experimentation; and adolescents demonstrate adult-pattern exposures including substance abuse and self-harm attempts. Common pediatric exposures include household cleaning products, analgesics (particularly acetaminophen), vitamins and supplements, antihistamines, cardiovascular medications, and topical preparations. Treatment modifications necessitate weight-based dosing calculations, careful fluid management to prevent hyponatremia, adjusted activated charcoal dosing, smaller equipment for procedures, and antidote adaptations. Supportive care must address children's smaller airways, decreased glycogen reserves affecting glucose homeostasis, and immature thermoregulation. Prevention strategies incorporate developmental stage-specific approaches including proper storage practices with child-resistant packaging, caregiver education regarding age-appropriate supervision, environmental assessment for potential toxins, and age-appropriate safety education for children and adolescents. Effective management requires recognizing red flags suggesting non-accidental poisoning including inconsistent history, inappropriate delay in seeking care, multiple previous episodes, and symptoms inconsistent with reported exposure

Self-Assessment Questions

1. Explain how developmental differences in hepatic enzyme systems affect acetaminophen metabolism in infants versus older children, and discuss the implications for toxicity risk and treatment.
2. Analyze the factors that make exploratory ingestions particularly common in toddlers, and describe evidence-based prevention strategies for this age group.
3. Describe the calculation methods for determining appropriate doses of activated charcoal, antidotes, and intravenous fluids for pediatric patients of different ages and weights.
4. Compare and contrast the management approach to iron poisoning in children versus adults, including risk assessment, diagnostic testing, and chelation therapy considerations.
5. Discuss the challenges in recognizing and managing adolescent intentional overdoses, including assessment of suicidality, confidentiality considerations, and follow-up requirements.
6. Analyze how the clinical manifestations of common toxins (such as anticholinergics, sympathomimetics, and opioids) may differ between pediatric and adult patients.
7. Describe the approach to management of button battery ingestions in children, including risk stratification based on battery size, location, and time since ingestion.
8. Explain how to recognize potential non-accidental poisoning in the pediatric population, including concerning history elements, physical findings, and appropriate intervention steps.
9. Discuss the special considerations in managing toxic exposures in neonates, including pharmacokinetic differences, manifestation of toxicity, and treatment modifications.
10. Evaluate the effectiveness of different prevention strategies including child-resistant packaging, caregiver education, poison prevention programs, and policy interventions in reducing pediatric poisonings

Bibliography

1. Koren G. Medications which can kill a toddler with one tablet or teaspoonful. J Toxicol Clin Toxicol. 1993;31(3):407-413.
2. Gouin S, Patel H. Unusual manifestations of acetaminophen toxicity in children: a case report. Pediatrics. 1996;97(6 Pt 1):918-920.
3. Mowry JB, Spyker DA, Cantilena LR Jr, McMillan N, Ford M. 2013 Annual Report of the American Association of Poison Control Centers' National Poison Data System (NPDS): 31st Annual Report. Clin Toxicol (Phila). 2014;52(10):1032-1283.
4. Ozanne-Smith J, Day L, Parsons B, Tibballs J, Dobbin M. Childhood poisoning: access and prevention. J Paediatr Child Health. 2001;37(3):262-265.
5. Bond GR. The role of activated charcoal and gastric emptying in gastrointestinal decontamination: a state-of-the-art review. Ann Emerg Med. 2002;39(3):273-286.
6. Bar-Oz B, Levichek Z, Koren G. Medications that can be fatal for a toddler with one tablet or teaspoonful: a 2004 update. Paediatr Drugs. 2004;6(2):123-126.
7. Liebelt EL, Shannon MW. Small doses, big problems: a selected review of highly toxic common medications. Pediatr Emerg Care. 1993;9(5):292-297.
8. Calello DP, Henretig FM. Pediatric toxicology: specialized approach to the poisoned child. Emerg Med Clin North Am. 2014;32(1):29-52.
9. Osterhoudt KC, Shannon M, Henretig FM. Toxicologic emergencies. In: Fleisher GR, Ludwig S, Henretig FM, editors. Textbook of pediatric emergency medicine. 7th ed. Philadelphia: Wolters Kluwer; 2016. p. 1154-1196.
10. Schueler HE, Beckett MW, Gettler G. Novel case of maternal, fetal, and neonatal cardiomyopathy due to ingestion of eucalyptus oil. Clin Toxicol (Phila). 2018;56(10):955-957.

CHAPTER 11

OCCUPATIONAL TOXICOLOGY

Author

Mr. Wilberforce Kasangaki, PG Scholar,
Department of Regulatory Affairs, Ramanbhai Patel College of Pharmacy, CHARUSAT, Changa, Gujarat, India

Abstract

Occupational toxicology addresses workplace chemical exposures that affect millions of workers across diverse industries, requiring specialized approaches to identification, management, and prevention. Workplace exposures occur through inhalation, dermal contact, and ingestion routes, with inhalation predominating in industrial settings where particulates, gases, vapors, and fumes present significant hazards. Industry-specific risks include silica and asbestos in construction, solvents and heavy metals in manufacturing, pesticides in agriculture, and chemotherapeutic agents in healthcare. Protection measures follow a hierarchical approach prioritizing elimination of the hazard, substitution with safer alternatives, engineering controls like ventilation systems, administrative controls including work rotation, and personal protective equipment as the final defense. Biological monitoring assesses internal dose through biomarkers in blood or urine, while environmental monitoring quantifies workplace contaminant levels using various sampling methods. Medical surveillance programs combine periodic examinations, function testing, and exposure records to detect adverse effects before clinically apparent disease develops. Regulatory frameworks establish permissible exposure limits, require hazard communication through standardized systems, mandate monitoring for certain substances, and establish medical removal provisions for workers showing early signs of toxicity. Occupational toxicologists must understand these complex interactions between workplace hazards, individual susceptibility factors, and regulatory requirements to effectively prevent, recognize, and manage work-related toxic exposures.

Keywords: *Occupational Exposure, Industrial Hygiene, Biomonitoring, Permissible Exposure Limits, Hazard Communication, Respiratory Protection*

Learning Objectives

After completion of the chapter, the learners should be able to:

- Identify common toxicants associated with specific industries and occupations, including their exposure routes, mechanisms of toxicity, and target organs.
- Apply the hierarchy of controls framework to develop comprehensive protection strategies for workplace chemical hazards.
- Design appropriate biological and environmental monitoring programs for specific occupational exposures, including selection of appropriate biomarkers and sampling strategies.
- Interpret occupational exposure limits including Permissible Exposure Limits (PELs), Threshold Limit Values (TLVs), and Short-Term Exposure Limits (STELs) in relation to workplace assessment and regulatory compliance.
- Develop medical surveillance programs tailored to specific workplace hazards, including appropriate screening tests, examination frequency, and action levels for intervention.
- Evaluate the effectiveness of personal protective equipment including respirators, chemical-resistant clothing, and gloves for specific workplace exposures, addressing selection, fit, maintenance, and limitations.

WORKPLACE EXPOSURES

Occupational environments present unique toxicological challenges through potential for prolonged, high-concentration exposure to diverse chemical, physical, and biological hazards.

Industrial Chemicals

Solvents represent among the most ubiquitous chemical exposures in industrial settings, with applications spanning degreasing, cleaning, extraction, paint and coating formulation, adhesives, and chemical synthesis across numerous industries. These compounds typically share properties including volatility creating inhalation exposure potential, lipid solubility enhancing dermal absorption and nervous system effects, and capacity to dissolve or extract other substances. Aliphatic hydrocarbons including hexane, heptane, and mineral spirits demonstrate primary toxicity through central nervous system depression, with n-hexane additionally causing peripheral neuropathy through its metabolite 2,5-hexanedione. Aromatic hydrocarbons including benzene, toluene, and xylene create more complex toxicity profiles: benzene demonstrates established hematopoietic toxicity including bone marrow depression and leukemogenicity through reactive metabolites; toluene produces both acute central nervous system effects and chronic manifestations including cognitive dysfunction and hearing loss; while xylene isomers create similar neurological effects with reduced hematological concerns. Chlorinated solvents including trichloroethylene, perchloroethylene, and methylene chloride produce hepatorenal toxicity alongside central nervous system depression, with additional specific concerns including cardiac sensitization to catecholamines, recognized carcinogenic potential for specific compounds, and carbon monoxide generation through metabolic pathways.

Work practices significantly influence exposure patterns, with particular high-risk scenarios including confined space operations where vapor accumulation creates both acute toxicity and oxygen displacement risks; spray applications generating respiratory-sized particles alongside vapor components; manual cleaning operations without local exhaust ventilation; and maintenance operations involving solvent-containing systems without adequate lockout/tagout and decontamination procedures. Exposure assessment employs industrial hygiene methodologies including air sampling with personal monitoring in the breathing zone, biological monitoring measuring either parent compounds or their metabolites in blood or urine, and dermal exposure assessment using specialized sampling techniques or fluorescent tracers with ultraviolet visualization. Multiple exposure routes necessitate comprehensive evaluation beyond air monitoring alone, as significant absorption may occur through dermal contact with both liquid and vapor forms of lipophilic solvents. Risk management approaches include substitution with less hazardous alternatives when feasible, engineering controls focusing on enclosure and ventilation, work practice modifications emphasizing closed transfer systems, and personal protective equipment including respiratory protection and chemical-resistant gloves selected based on specific solvent permeation characteristics.

Heavy metals continue creating significant occupational exposure concerns despite increasing regulation, with workers in mining, metallurgy, manufacturing, construction, electronics, and recycling industries demonstrating particular risk. Lead exposure occurs in battery manufacturing, radiator repair, metal recycling, construction involving older structures, and shooting range operations, with toxicity affecting hematopoietic, nervous, renal, reproductive, and cardiovascular systems. Contemporary understanding emphasizes health effects at blood lead levels previously considered acceptable, driving progressively lower occupational exposure limits.

Table 11.1: High-Risk Occupational Exposures by Industry

Industry	Common Toxicants	Primary Health Effects	Exposure Routes
Construction	Silica, asbestos, lead, solvents, wood dust	Pneumoconiosis, mesothelioma, neurotoxicity, cancer	Inhalation, dermal, ingestion
Healthcare	Anesthetic gases, chemotherapy drugs, disinfectants, latex	Reproductive effects, asthma, dermatitis, liver toxicity	Inhalation, dermal, needlestick
Agriculture	Pesticides, fertilizers, diesel exhaust, grain dust	Cholinergic toxicity, respiratory disease, dermatitis	Inhalation, dermal, ingestion
Manufacturing	Solvents, metals, plastics, engineered nanoparticles	Neurotoxicity, cancer, respiratory disease, dermatitis	Inhalation, dermal
Mining	Silica, coal dust, diesel exhaust, metals	Pneumoconiosis, COPD, cancer, heavy metal toxicity	Inhalation, dermal
Welding	Metal fumes, gases (ozone, nitrogen oxides)	Metal fume fever, pneumonitis, chronic lung disease	Inhalation, ocular

Cadmium exposures in nickel-cadmium battery production, metal plating, pigment manufacturing, and electronic waste processing create nephrotoxicity and carcinogenic risk through mechanisms including metallothionein binding and oxidative stress. Mercury exposure in chloralkali production, artisanal gold mining, dental amalgam handling, and certain manufacturing processes produces neurobehavioral effects through mechanisms targeting sulfhydryl-containing proteins and disrupting cellular redox status. Chromium compounds in metal plating, stainless steel welding, pigment production, and leather tanning create exposure risk primarily to hexavalent forms demonstrating respiratory irritation, sensitization potential, and carcinogenicity through DNA damage mechanisms.

> **Remember**
>
> **Industry-specific hazards include pneumoconioses from mineral dusts in mining and construction, neurotoxicity from solvents in manufacturing, cholinergic toxicity from pesticides in agriculture, and diverse chemical exposures in healthcare settings.**

Exposure routes vary by specific process and material state, with inhalation predominating for fume, dust, and vapor forms while ingestion typically occurs through hand-to-mouth transfer from contaminated surfaces or inadequate hygiene practices. Secondary exposure affecting family members through take-home contamination on work clothing and vehicles represents a recognized concern, particularly affecting children whose developing systems demonstrate enhanced vulnerability. Biological monitoring provides exposure assessment integrating all routes, with specific markers including blood lead levels, urinary cadmium, urinary mercury, and various chromium measurements in blood, urine, or exhaled breath condensate depending on the specific exposure scenario. Medical surveillance protocols incorporate both exposure biomarkers and early effect indicators potentially identifying subclinical toxicity before irreversible damage occurs, with specific programs tailored to particular metals and target organ concerns. Control strategies emphasize engineering approaches including enclosed systems, local exhaust ventilation, and wet methods reducing dust generation; work practices addressing hygiene, separate clean and dirty areas preventing cross-contamination, and proper cleaning procedures; and comprehensive personal protective equipment programs when other controls cannot achieve adequate exposure reduction.

Isocyanates, reactive chemicals containing the functional group N=C=O, create distinctive occupational health challenges through their widespread industrial use and significant sensitization potential. Major applications include polyurethane production for foams, elastomers, adhesives, and coatings, with common compounds including toluene diisocyanate (TDI), methylene diphenyl diisocyanate (MDI), and hexamethylene diisocyanate (HDI). Primary health effects involve respiratory sensitization potentially resulting in occupational asthma, with additional concerns including irritant effects on respiratory tract, skin, and mucous membranes; allergic contact dermatitis; and hypersensitivity pneumonitis with certain exposure patterns. The immunological mechanism involves isocyanate reactivity with biological proteins creating hapten-carrier complexes capable of triggering immune responses, with both IgE-mediated and non-IgE pathways implicated in respiratory sensitization. Particularly concerning work scenarios include spray application creating respirable aerosols with potential for both pulmonary deposition and skin exposure; heated processes volatilizing isocyanates from supposedly "safe" prepolymers; and grinding or cutting of cured polyurethane potentially liberating unreacted isocyanates.

Exposure assessment presents significant challenges due to isocyanates' high reactivity, tendency to polymerize, occurrence in multiple physical forms, and sensitizing potential at concentrations below many analytical method detection limits. Current approaches employ specialized sampling techniques including derivatization to stabilize the isocyanate group for analysis, with methodologies tailored to specific isocyanate species and exposure scenarios. Medical surveillance focuses on respiratory symptoms and function, with periodic questionnaires, spirometry, and occasionally specific inhalation challenge testing in specialized centers. Management strategies emphasize rigorous exposure control due to sensitization risk even at low concentrations, with approaches including closed systems where feasible, highly efficient local exhaust ventilation, respiratory protection programs with supplied air systems for higher-risk operations, comprehensive skin protection preventing dermal sensitization, and worker education regarding the irreversible nature of sensitization necessitating stringent exposure prevention.

Pesticides in occupational settings create complex toxicological challenges due to their intentional biocidal activity, diverse chemical classes with varying mechanisms, and multiple exposure routes. Agricultural workers experience exposure during mixing, loading, and application operations; reentry into treated areas; and harvesting activities. Additional occupational scenarios include pest control operations in structural, landscape, and public health applications; manufacturing and formulation facilities; and transportation and retail handling. Major chemical classes include organophosphates and carbamates inhibiting cholinesterase with resulting cholinergic effects; pyrethroids affecting sodium channels with predominantly neurological and dermal manifestations; neonicotinoids targeting nicotinic acetylcholine receptors; phenoxy herbicides with concerns regarding contaminants like dioxins in older formulations; and various fungicides with class-specific effects ranging from irritant properties to specific organ system toxicity.

Exposure assessment employs both environmental monitoring techniques including air sampling, surface wipe sampling, and patch or whole-body dosimetry for dermal exposure quantification; and biological monitoring measuring either parent compounds, specific metabolites, or effect biomarkers like cholinesterase activity for certain classes. Exposure determinants include application method, with backpack spraying typically creating higher exposure than mechanized systems; environmental conditions, particularly temperature and humidity affecting both dermal absorption and respiratory exposure patterns; use of personal protective equipment, with effectiveness highly dependent on proper selection, fit, condition, and decontamination practices; and work practices including hygiene behaviors, storage and handling procedures, and adherence to restricted entry intervals. Management approaches incorporate integrated pest management reducing overall pesticide use; engineering controls including closed mixing and loading systems; administrative controls focusing on training, supervision, and work scheduling to minimize exposure; and comprehensive personal protective equipment programs addressing the multiple exposure routes associated with pesticide handling.

Nanomaterials represent an emerging occupational exposure category with distinctive toxicological considerations resulting from their extremely small size (at least one dimension less than 100 nanometers) creating unique physical and chemical properties compared to their bulk material counterparts. Occupational exposures occur in research and development facilities, manufacturing operations producing raw nanomaterials, downstream incorporation into products, and increasingly in processing or disposal of nano-enabled products. Health concerns derive from nanomaterials' ability to deposit in the deep lung with limited clearance mechanisms, potential translocation across biological barriers including lung epithelium and blood-brain barrier, enhanced reactivity due to high surface area to mass ratio, and capacity to generate reactive oxygen species. Specific materials of concern include carbon nanotubes with asbestos-like morphology raising fibrogenic and carcinogenic potential; metal and metal oxide nanoparticles demonstrating various organ system effects; and quantum dots containing toxic metal components in highly bioavailable forms.

Exposure assessment employs specialized methodologies addressing the limitations of conventional industrial hygiene approaches when applied to nanoscale materials. Direct-reading instruments measure particle number concentrations and size distributions, though with limited capacity to distinguish engineered nanomaterials from background ultrafine particles. Electron microscopy provides definitive characterization but with significant analytical complexity and cost limitations for routine monitoring. Control banding approaches categorize processes and materials based on hazard and exposure potential when quantitative data remain unavailable. Risk management follows a precautionary framework emphasizing engineering controls including enclosed systems and specialized ventilation designs; administrative controls focusing on training, standard operating procedures, and housekeeping practices preventing particle resuspension; and personal protective equipment programs with attention to potential penetration of conventional protective materials by nanoscale particles. This evolving field continues developing both toxicological understanding and appropriate control methodologies as nanomaterial applications expand across industrial sectors.

Physical and Biological Hazards

Ionizing radiation creates occupational exposure concerns across diverse industries beyond obvious nuclear applications. Medical settings involve diagnostic radiology, nuclear medicine, and radiation oncology exposing healthcare workers through both primary and scatter radiation. Industrial applications include industrial radiography inspecting welds and structural components, gauge technologies incorporating radioactive sources for level and density measurement, and well logging in petroleum exploration. Research laboratories utilize various radioisotopes as tracers and analytical tools, while naturally occurring radioactive materials (NORM) create exposure potential in industries including oil and gas production, mining operations, and phosphate processing. Biological effects depend on radiation type (alpha, beta, gamma, neutron), energy level, dose rate, and tissue-specific sensitivity, with mechanisms predominantly involving direct DNA damage and indirect effects through free radical generation from water radiolysis.

Exposure assessment employs both personal dosimetry measuring accumulated dose and area monitoring identifying potential exposure zones. Dosimeter technologies include traditional film badges, thermoluminescent dosimeters (TLDs), optically stimulated luminescence (OSL) devices, and electronic personal dosimeters providing real-time readings. Biological dosimetry methods, primarily chromosomal aberration analysis, provide exposure assessment in situations without conventional monitoring data. Control measures follow the fundamental principles of time, distance, and shielding: minimizing exposure duration near sources; maximizing distance from radiation sources utilizing remote handling tools when practical; and implementing appropriate shielding materials matched to specific radiation types (lead for gamma, acrylic for beta, concrete or water for neutrons). These engineering approaches combine with administrative controls including restricted access systems, operational procedures minimizing exposure time, and comprehensive training programs ensuring worker understanding of both hazards and control strategies.

Non-ionizing radiation spans a broad electromagnetic spectrum portion including radiofrequency and microwave radiation, infrared radiation, visible light, and ultraviolet radiation, with distinct health effects depending on frequency, energy, and exposure pattern. Ultraviolet radiation in welding operations, sterilization processes, and outdoor work creates both acute effects including photokeratitis ("welder's flash") and photodermatitis, and chronic concerns including accelerated skin aging and increased skin cancer risk. Radiofrequency and microwave radiation from communication equipment, industrial heaters, and medical diathermy devices primarily creates thermal effects through tissue heating, with additional concerns regarding potential non-thermal biological effects though with less established evidence base. Infrared radiation from molten metal, glass operations, and certain industrial heating processes produces ocular concerns including corneal and retinal burns acutely and potential cataract formation with chronic exposure. Intense visible light, particularly blue-light wavelengths, from welding arcs, lasers, and high-intensity lighting systems creates retinal hazards through both photothermal and photochemical mechanisms.

Exposure assessment methodology varies across the non-ionizing radiation spectrum, with specialized instrumentation measuring specific parameters including power density, electric and magnetic field strength, and spectral characteristics matched to particular frequency bands. Biological monitoring remains limited for most non-ionizing radiation forms, though ultraviolet exposure assessment occasionally employs biological dosimeters including polysulphone films mimicking skin response. Control approaches emphasize engineering solutions including enclosure of radiation sources, specialized shielding materials matched to specific radiation types, and equipment design minimizing emission outside operational areas. Personal protective equipment includes specialized eyewear filtering specific wavelengths, skin coverings appropriate to the radiation type, and in some cases, radiofrequency-protective clothing for high-exposure scenarios. Administrative controls incorporate exposure time limitations, designated access restrictions to high-field areas, and worker education regarding both immediate and long-term effects associated with specific radiation types.

Noise represents among the most prevalent occupational hazards worldwide, affecting workers across manufacturing, construction, mining, transportation, agriculture, and numerous other sectors. Health effects extend beyond the obvious noise-induced hearing loss to include cardiovascular effects through stress pathway activation, sleep disturbance affecting recovery and general health, and safety concerns through communication interference and warning signal masking. Noise-induced hearing loss typically develops gradually through cochlear hair cell damage from metabolic and mechanical effects, with characteristics including initial loss in the 3000-6000 Hz range (particularly 4000 Hz notch), bilateral symmetrical pattern (unless exposure conditions create asymmetry), and irreversible progression with continued exposure. Additional auditory effects include tinnitus, hyperacusis, and accelerated age-related hearing loss (presbycusis) among noise-exposed populations.

Exposure assessment employs sound level measurements using either sound level meters for area monitoring or personal noise dosimeters capturing exposure throughout work shifts, with results compared against established damage-risk criteria typically specifying both exposure intensity and duration limits based on equal energy principles. These measurements require attention to factors including impulse components requiring specialized peak measurement capabilities, low-frequency components potentially underestimated by A-weighting scales, and exposure variability necessitating appropriate sampling strategies. Audiometric testing programs monitor hearing thresholds over time, ideally detecting temporary threshold shifts before they progress to permanent damage. Control approaches follow the hierarchy from engineering controls including equipment redesign, enclosure, barriers, and vibration dampening; administrative controls such as work scheduling limiting exposure duration and quiet areas for recovery periods; to personal hearing protection devices including earmuffs, earplugs, and semi-insert devices, with selection based on attenuation characteristics, comfort for consistent use, and compatibility with communication requirements and other personal protective equipment.

Biological hazards in occupational settings span diverse categories including infectious agents, allergenic proteins, toxic substances from biological sources, and bioaerosols containing multiple components. Healthcare workers experience exposure risk to bloodborne pathogens including hepatitis B virus, hepatitis C virus, and HIV through sharps injuries and body fluid exposures; airborne infectious agents including Mycobacterium tuberculosis and various respiratory viruses through close patient contact; and contact-transmitted pathogens causing healthcare-associated infections. Laboratory workers handling infectious materials or biological specimens face similar risks through potential exposures during specimen processing, culture manipulation, and waste handling. Agricultural workers encounter zoonotic disease transmission from animal handling; organic dust exposures from grain, hay, and silage potentially causing hypersensitivity pneumonitis; and potential exposure to endotoxins from gram-negative bacteria associated with respiratory inflammation.

Exposure assessment approaches vary with specific biological hazard categories, including air sampling with specialized bioaerosol collection devices, surface sampling identifying contamination and potential cross-transmission routes, and occasionally direct infection metrics through reported sharps injuries or confirmed occupational infections. Control strategies emphasize source elimination or substitution where feasible, as with vaccination programs preventing susceptible host populations; engineering controls including biosafety cabinets, negative pressure isolation rooms, and ventilation systems designed for bioaerosol control; work practice controls focusing on standard precautions in healthcare, aseptic techniques in laboratories, and proper animal handling procedures in agricultural settings; and personal protective equipment ranging from gloves and fluid-resistant clothing to respiratory protection matched to specific biological exposure risks. Comprehensive biological exposure management requires integration of these control approaches with administrative systems including exposure response protocols, post-exposure prophylaxis programs where applicable, and medical surveillance identifying exposure effects before significant health impact occurs.

Extreme thermal environments create physiological stress through both heat and cold exposure across numerous industries. Heat exposure in foundries, glass manufacturing, bakeries, laundries, outdoor work in hot climates, and various other settings produces a spectrum of health effects including heat rash from persistent moisture, heat cramps from electrolyte imbalances, heat exhaustion from cardiovascular strain during blood redistribution, and potentially fatal heat stroke when thermoregulatory mechanisms become overwhelmed. Individual susceptibility varies with acclimatization status, physical fitness, hydration, medical conditions, medication use, and personal factors including age and body composition. Cold exposure in outdoor winter work, refrigerated environments, food processing, and cryogenic operations similarly creates progressive effects from discomfort through frostnip and frostbite involving tissue freezing, to potentially fatal hypothermia with core temperature depression. Additional cold exposure concerns include non-freezing cold injuries from prolonged wet exposure and increased accident risk through reduced dexterity and cognitive effects.

Exposure assessment employs specialized thermal indices integrating temperature with relevant environmental and metabolic factors. Heat stress evaluation typically utilizes the Wet Bulb Globe Temperature (WBGT) index incorporating air temperature, humidity, radiant heat, and air movement, with results compared against work-rest regimens based on metabolic demands. Cold stress assessment employs the Wind Chill Temperature index for outdoor exposures or direct temperature measurements for indoor cold environments, with exposure limits considering both whole-body and extremity protection requirements. Physiological monitoring occasionally supplements environmental measurement, with core temperature, heart rate, and body weight changes (indicating fluid loss) providing individual strain assessment during heat exposure. Control approaches include engineering solutions such as radiant heat barriers, spot cooling systems, local exhaust ventilation, heated or cooled rest areas, and process modifications reducing heat generation or cold requirements; administrative controls including work-rest scheduling, acclimatization programs, altered work timing avoiding temperature extremes, buddy systems, and hydration protocols; and appropriate protective clothing selected based on specific thermal challenges, with particular attention to balancing heat protection against the potential for heat strain from impaired evaporative cooling with certain protective ensembles.

Exposure Assessment Methods

Industrial hygiene air sampling methodologies provide quantitative exposure assessment through systematic collection and analysis of airborne contaminants in workplace environments. Personal sampling, conducted in the breathing zone of workers, offers the most representative exposure measurement by capturing the air actually available for inhalation during task performance. Sampling media selection depends on the specific contaminant properties, with options including filters for particulate collection (further specified by pore size, material compatibility, and analytical requirements); solid sorbents like activated charcoal, silica gel, or specialized resins for vapor collection; impingers containing collection solutions for water-soluble contaminants; and direct-reading instruments for real-time measurement of specific substances or classes. Sampling strategies must address temporal variation through appropriate duration and timing decisions, with options including grab samples capturing momentary conditions; short-term samples (typically 15-30 minutes) assessing peak exposures during specific tasks; full-shift samples measuring time-weighted average exposure across entire work periods; and extended sampling over multiple days capturing variation between shifts or production cycles.

Sample analysis employs diverse methodological approaches matched to specific contaminants, including gravimetric analysis for total dust determination; size-selective analysis for respirable or inhalable fractions; microscopy techniques for asbestos and other fibers; atomic absorption or inductively coupled plasma methodologies for metals; gas or liquid chromatography for organic compounds; infrared spectroscopy for functional group identification; and mass spectrometry providing both identification and quantification capabilities. Quality assurance procedures incorporate field blanks identifying potential contamination sources; duplicate samples assessing precision; spiked samples evaluating recovery efficiency; and calibration verification ensuring measurement accuracy. Results interpretation requires comparison with established occupational exposure limits while considering sampling and analytical error, task representativeness, and potential interactions between multiple contaminants. This comprehensive approach provides objective documentation of exposure conditions, identifies highest risk operations for control prioritization, demonstrates regulatory compliance, and establishes baseline conditions for evaluating intervention effectiveness.

Biological monitoring measures toxicants or their metabolites in biological specimens, providing integrated exposure assessment across all routes and accounting for individual factors affecting absorption, distribution, metabolism, and elimination. Common sampling matrices include urine, with advantages including non-invasive collection and suitability for repeated sampling; blood, providing direct measurement of circulating toxicant levels though with greater collection barriers; exhaled breath, particularly valuable for volatile compounds eliminated through pulmonary routes; and occasionally hair, nails, or adipose tissue for compounds with appropriate pharmacokinetic properties for long-term deposition. Timing considerations significantly influence interpretation, with options including pre-shift samples assessing baseline conditions or prior shift carryover; post-shift samples capturing daily exposure accumulation; next-morning samples reflecting longer elimination phase components; and end-of-workweek samples for substances with multi-day accumulation patterns. Methodologies must address confounding factors including dietary sources, environmental exposures, medication use, and individual metabolic variation potentially affecting biomarker levels independent of occupational exposure.

Interpretation frameworks include Biological Exposure Indices (BEIs) established by the American Conference of Governmental Industrial Hygienists, Biological Guidance Values from various European agencies, and similar reference values from other organizations worldwide. These values typically represent biomarker levels expected in workers exposed at the corresponding airborne occupational exposure limit, though with recognition of the complex relationship between external exposure and internal dose. Some biomarkers directly measure the parent compound (blood benzene, urinary mercury), while others assess metabolites (urinary hippuric acid for toluene exposure, urinary methylhippuric acids for xylene). Effect biomarkers measure biochemical changes resulting from exposure, exemplified by cholinesterase depression monitoring for organophosphate exposure and various markers of oxidative stress, DNA damage, or protein adducts. This integrated exposure assessment approach complements environmental monitoring by addressing actual absorbed dose across all routes while accounting for individual factors affecting toxicokinetics, though with limitations including invasiveness, analytical complexity, and interpretation challenges for substances without established reference values.

Direct-reading instruments provide real-time exposure information enabling immediate hazard recognition and control implementation without the delay inherent in laboratory-based methodologies. Gas and vapor monitoring technologies include photoionization detectors measuring compounds with ionization potentials below the lamp energy; infrared analyzers detecting compounds absorbing specific wavelengths; electrochemical sensors generating signals proportional to target gas oxidation or reduction; and metal oxide semiconductors whose conductivity changes with adsorption of target gases. Aerosol monitoring instruments employ various principles including light scattering photometers measuring particle concentration through scattered light intensity; condensation particle counters growing submicron particles to optically detectable size through controlled condensation; optical particle counters providing size distribution information through scattered light analysis; and direct-reading respirable dust monitors employing cyclone pre-separators with real-time mass measurement. Specialized technologies address specific exposures, exemplified by real-time monitoring for noise (sound level meters, noise dosimeters), radiation (survey meters, electronic personal dosimeters), and various physical stressors (heat stress monitors, vibration analyzers).

These instruments offer significant advantages including immediate feedback identifying exposure sources and effectiveness of control measures; capability for continuous monitoring with alarm functions warning of dangerous concentrations; and data-logging functions capturing exposure patterns over time. Limitations include cross-sensitivity to interferent compounds; limited specificity compared to laboratory methods; calibration requirements affecting accuracy; and in some cases, higher detection limits than comparable laboratory techniques. Effective implementation requires understanding both technical specifications and operational considerations including appropriate calibration procedures, environmental factors affecting performance, maintenance requirements, and interpretation frameworks translating instrument readings to health-relevant exposure metrics. Integration of direct-reading instruments with traditional sampling approaches provides complementary information combining the temporal resolution of real-time monitoring with the specificity and sensitivity of laboratory analysis.

Exposure modeling employs mathematical approaches estimating exposure when direct measurement proves impractical due to resource limitations, process changes under consideration, or future scenario evaluation. Deterministic models incorporate physical and chemical principles governing contaminant generation, transport, and control, with complexity ranging from simple two-zone models representing near-field and far-field compartments to computational fluid dynamics simulations detailing airflow patterns and contaminant distribution throughout complex spaces. Empirical models derive exposure estimates from statistical relationships identified in existing measurement datasets, employing various regression techniques relating workplace characteristics and process parameters to expected exposure levels. Bayesian approaches integrate prior knowledge with limited measurement data, particularly valuable when complete sampling campaigns remain unfeasible but some data exists for model calibration. Pharmaco-Toxicokinetic modeling extends beyond exposure estimation to predict tissue doses and biological monitoring results based on exposure scenarios, workplace conditions, and human physiological parameters.

Model application requires appropriate validation establishing prediction accuracy within the intended operational domain, careful consideration of input parameter quality and associated uncertainty, and recognition of model limitations including boundary conditions beyond which predictions may become unreliable. Effective implementation often employs tiered approaches beginning with simple screening models identifying potential concerns, followed by progressively more sophisticated modeling for scenarios warranting detailed analysis. This exposure assessment methodology provides valuable perspective when direct measurement data remains unavailable, enables evaluation of control options before implementation, facilitates exposure reconstruction for epidemiological investigations or compensation determinations, and supports comprehensive understanding of exposure determinants beyond what measurement alone might reveal.

Exposure Limits and Guidelines

Occupational exposure limits (OELs) represent airborne contaminant concentrations considered acceptable for healthy worker populations with regular exposure throughout working lifetimes. These values serve multiple functions including regulatory compliance benchmarks, design targets for engineering controls, effectiveness metrics for exposure reduction programs, and decision frameworks for personal protective equipment implementation. Different jurisdictions establish legally enforceable standards through various regulatory mechanisms, exemplified by Permissible Exposure Limits (PELs) from the U.S. Occupational Safety and Health Administration, Workplace Exposure Limits (WELs) from the U.K. Health and Safety Executive, and similar standards from regulatory bodies worldwide. Complementing these regulatory values, scientific and professional organizations develop recommended limits without direct regulatory authority but often with more current scientific foundations, including Threshold Limit Values (TLVs) from the American Conference of Governmental Industrial Hygienists, Recommended Exposure Limits (RELs) from the National Institute for Occupational Safety and Health, and Derived No-Effect Levels (DNELs) under the European REACH framework.

Various exposure limit categories address different exposure patterns and health effect considerations. Time-weighted average limits apply to standard 8-hour workdays and 40-hour workweeks, representing concentrations not expected to create adverse effects with repeated daily exposure. Short-term exposure limits (typically 15-minute averages) address health effects developing from brief high-concentration exposures that might occur within otherwise acceptable daily averages. Ceiling limits specify concentrations that should never be exceeded even momentarily, typically applied to rapidly-acting substances with immediate serious effects. Peak limitations specify maximum allowable concentrations for defined durations and frequencies, addressing substances with significant short-term effects but where complete concentration measurement throughout all work periods proves impractical. Skin notations identify significant dermal absorption potential requiring control measures beyond respiratory protection, while sensitizer designations alert to potential immunological effects occurring below irritation thresholds.

Exposure limit development methodologies incorporate various scientific foundations with specific approaches determined by available evidence quality and mechanistic understanding. Health-based limits derive from epidemiological studies establishing exposure-response relationships in human populations, animal toxicology studies with appropriate uncertainty factors addressing interspecies extrapolation and human variability, or occasionally controlled human exposure studies with volunteer subjects. Analytical limits reflect detection capabilities of available sampling and analytical methodologies when health effect thresholds remain undetermined or appear below reliable quantification levels. Technologically-based limits consider feasibility of control measures in specific industries when health-based approaches suggest values difficult to achieve with current technology. Mixed approaches often represent the practical reality, with scientific foundation establishing initial values subsequently modified through feasibility considerations and stakeholder input during development processes.

Recognized limitations affect exposure limit application and interpretation in workplace settings. Many limits address only single substances despite common workplace scenarios involving multiple contaminant exposures potentially creating additive, synergistic, or antagonistic effects inadequately addressed through individual substance evaluation. Established limits typically assume standard exposure conditions including 8-hour workdays and 40-hour workweeks, with limited adjustment guidance for extended work schedules increasingly common in many industries. Individual susceptibility variations mean exposure within established limits may not protect all workers equally, with factors including genetic polymorphisms affecting metabolic capacity, pre-existing medical conditions, medication use, age, and gender creating potential vulnerability not fully addressed in population-based limit development. Historical development patterns mean many regulatory limits reflect outdated scientific understanding due to procedural barriers limiting update frequency, creating potential protection gaps between regulatory compliance and current health protection knowledge.

Implementation frameworks address these limitations through pragmatic approaches maintaining worker protection despite imperfect exposure limit systems. Additive effect models combine exposures to multiple substances affecting similar organ systems, particularly valuable for mixtures with comparable mechanisms like central nervous system depressants or upper respiratory irritants. Action level concepts implement control measures at exposure fractions (typically 50%) below regulatory limits, providing safety margins addressing measurement uncertainty and individual susceptibility. Work schedule adjustment calculations modify standard exposure limits for non-traditional schedules through various models including simple proportional adjustment based on weekly exposure duration, pharmacokinetic approaches considering biological half-lives, or recovery time models incorporating physiological recovery periods between exposures. These practical application frameworks enhance worker protection while acknowledging the inherent limitations of standardized exposure limits applied across diverse workplace conditions and worker populations.

PROTECTION MEASURES

Comprehensive occupational toxicant protection requires systematic implementation of control measures throughout workplace environments.

Engineering Controls

Substitution and process modification represent the highest hierarchy level of exposure control, eliminating or reducing hazards at their source rather than managing contaminants after generation. Material substitution replaces toxic substances with less hazardous alternatives while maintaining process functionality, exemplified by replacement of benzene with toluene or xylene in many solvent applications, substitution of water-based for solvent-based coating systems, and replacement of lead compounds with less toxic alternatives in various industrial applications. Process modification changes operational methodologies to reduce exposure potential while achieving equivalent production outcomes, including automation replacing manual handling of hazardous materials, wet methods reducing dust generation during cutting or grinding operations, and temperature reduction minimizing vapor generation from volatile compounds. Implementation effectiveness depends on comprehensive hazard evaluation for replacement options, as historical examples demonstrate potential for regrettable substitution when replacement materials later demonstrated unanticipated toxicity or environmental concerns. Successful implementation requires multidisciplinary collaboration between industrial hygienists, process engineers, production personnel, and management addressing both technical feasibility and productivity considerations alongside health protection goals.

Ventilation systems provide exposure reduction through contaminant capture, dilution, or removal from workplace environments. Local exhaust ventilation (LEV) captures contaminants at or near generation sources before they enter the broader workplace atmosphere, with components including hoods designed for specific process geometries and contaminant behavior characteristics; ducting sized for appropriate transport velocity preventing material settling; air cleaning devices matched to contaminant properties; and fans providing necessary air movement while overcoming system resistance. Capture efficiency depends on hood design optimization considering both contaminant release characteristics and work process requirements, with options including enclosing hoods completely surrounding emission sources; exterior hoods positioned outside processes capturing contaminants through induced air movement; receiving hoods utilizing natural contaminant movement properties; and low-volume high-velocity systems employing minimal airflow with precisely directed capture.

Table 11.2: Occupational Exposure Controls Hierarchy

Control Type	Examples	Advantages	Limitations
Elimination	Process redesign, material substitution	Completely removes hazard	May affect product quality, often high initial cost
Substitution	Less toxic alternatives, water-based instead of solvent-based products	Reduces hazard at source	May have performance trade-offs, requires toxicity evaluation of alternatives
Engineering	Ventilation systems, enclosed processes, automation	Consistent protection, minimal worker involvement	Initial cost, maintenance requirements, may limit production flexibility
Administrative	Training, job rotation, work scheduling, hygiene practices	Lower implementation cost, addresses work practices	Relies on worker compliance, less reliable than higher-level controls
Personal Protective Equipment	Respirators, gloves, protective clothing	Immediately implementable, adaptable to changing conditions	Last line of defense, requires proper selection, fit, and consistent use

General dilution ventilation provides secondary protection by introducing clean air diluting contaminant concentrations below harmful levels, particularly appropriate for lower toxicity materials released from numerous or mobile sources where local exhaust proves impractical. Effective implementation requires regular performance evaluation through visualization techniques, air velocity measurements, capture testing, and occasionally tracer gas studies verifying continued system effectiveness despite inevitable modifications, maintenance variations, and operational changes affecting initial design parameters.

Enclosure and isolation strategies physically separate hazardous processes from workers, creating barriers preventing contaminant release into occupied areas. Complete enclosures surround emission sources within sealed structures, with materials entering and exiting through controlled transfer mechanisms while maintaining negative pressure preventing outward leakage. Robotics and remote operation capabilities allow process operation and maintenance without direct worker presence in hazardous zones, particularly valuable for highly toxic materials or extreme environmental conditions. Glove box systems permit manual operations within enclosed environments through sealed glove ports maintaining separation between workers and hazardous materials, commonly employed in pharmaceutical, nuclear, and certain chemical manufacturing operations. Control room isolation locates operators in positively pressurized, separately ventilated spaces overseing processes through visual monitoring systems and instrumentation rather than direct presence. When complete isolation proves impractical, partial enclosures with optimized local exhaust capture particles and vapors that escape containment, while barrier systems including acrylic shields, vinyl strip curtains, or air curtains create partial separation reducing exposure without complete process isolation. Implementation requires attention to human factors considerations ensuring ergonomic access for necessary operations, maintenance requirements maintaining isolation integrity, and emergency response provisions addressing worker protection during abnormal conditions or system failures.

Process control automation reduces exposure through minimizing direct worker interaction with hazardous materials or processes. Automated material handling systems replace manual transfer operations for bulk chemicals, powders, and other hazardous substances, eliminating exposure during loading, unloading, and transport activities. Closed transfer systems prevent vapor release and direct contact during liquid movement between containers, vessels, and process equipment. Continuous monitoring technologies with automated response capabilities detect developing problems before significant contaminant release occurs, implementing corrective actions without worker presence in potentially hazardous areas. Remote maintenance technologies including condition monitoring sensors, robotic inspection capabilities, and design features supporting external service reduce exposure during repair and maintenance activities traditionally creating highest exposure potential. While typically requiring significant capital investment, these engineering approaches often demonstrate favorable long-term economics through combined benefits of exposure reduction, productivity improvement, quality enhancement, and reduced personal protective equipment requirements. Implementation success depends on comprehensive hazard analysis identifying appropriate automation targets, thorough worker training supporting effective system utilization, and ongoing evaluation ensuring continued performance as operational conditions evolve over time.

Dust control technologies address solid particle exposure through specialized engineering approaches targeting generation, transport, and removal mechanisms. Water spray systems suppress dust through several mechanisms: wetting particles increasing their mass and preventing reaerosolization; agglomeration creating larger particles with faster settling velocities; and direct particle capture through impaction with water droplets. Foam-based systems enhance dust control through extended moisture retention, reduced water consumption, and improved adhesion to hydrophobic materials. Vacuum collection systems capture particles at generation sources, particularly effective for fixed processing operations like grinding, cutting, or woodworking equipment. Electrostatic precipitation employs charged plates attracting and collecting oppositely charged particles, while cyclonic separation utilizes centrifugal force separating particles from air streams based on mass differences. Equipment design modifications reduce dust generation through features including enclosed transfer points minimizing material free-fall distances, reduced drop heights limiting impact fragmentation, appropriate belt cleaner systems preventing material carryback, and optimized material flow characteristics minimizing turbulence and associated particle entrainment. Road dust control in mining, construction, and similar operations employs specialized approaches including chemical stabilizers, polymer-based dust suppressants, and engineered surfacing materials reducing dust generation from vehicle traffic. These diverse engineering solutions require selection and implementation based on specific process characteristics, material properties, and operational constraints, often with multiple complementary technologies providing effective comprehensive control.

Administrative Controls

Exposure monitoring programs provide systematic assessment of workplace contaminant levels, supporting administrative control effectiveness through data-driven decision making. Comprehensive monitoring strategies establish baseline exposure profiles across operations and job classifications; identify highest risk activities guiding control prioritization; verify compliance with regulatory requirements; evaluate control measure effectiveness; and provide documentation supporting medical surveillance, training programs, and hazard communication. Implementation approaches include initial comprehensive surveys establishing exposure profiles across operations; routine monitoring maintaining current exposure characterization as processes evolve; targeted assessments addressing specific concerns or evaluating intervention effectiveness; and personal exposure monitoring documenting individual worker exposures for comparison with established limits. Effective programs incorporate clearly defined data quality objectives; appropriate sampling strategies addressing both routine operations and non-routine activities like maintenance or upset conditions; standardized documentation systems; trend analysis identifying developing concerns before they become serious hazards; and results communication ensuring workers, management, and health professionals receive information in formats supporting appropriate decision making within their respective roles.

Work practice modifications reduce exposure through changed behavior patterns while maintaining existing process equipment and materials. Standard operating procedures formalize optimal work techniques minimizing exposure, with elements including specific tool and equipment use instructions; proper chemical handling methodologies; defined cleaning and housekeeping protocols; and standardized approaches for routine operations. Job rotation distributes exposure across multiple workers rather than concentrating it on specific individuals, particularly valuable for stressors lacking effective engineering control options or during transitional periods while permanent controls undergo implementation. Modified work scheduling separates high-exposure operations from other activities either spatially or temporally, reducing secondary exposure to uninvolved workers. Break scheduling provides recovery periods during high-exposure tasks, particularly important for stressors like heat, noise, or ergonomic challenges where physiological recovery periods enhance tolerance. Housekeeping programs prevent contaminant accumulation on surfaces where it might become resuspended or transferred through hand-to-surface-to-mouth pathways, with elements including appropriate cleaning methodologies matched to specific contaminants; scheduled cleaning frequency preventing buildup; proper waste handling procedures; and designated clean and dirty areas preventing cross-contamination. While typically considered secondary to engineering controls, these administrative approaches often provide significant exposure reduction through relatively low-cost implementation when developed through collaborative processes incorporating worker knowledge alongside professional expertise.

Training and hazard communication programs ensure workers understand workplace hazards and appropriate protective measures. Regulatory frameworks including OSHA's Hazard Communication Standard and the Globally Harmonized System establish minimum requirements for information provision, while comprehensive programs extend beyond compliance to create genuine risk awareness and protective behavior adoption. Content elements include specific chemical hazard information; health effects associated with workplace exposures; warning sign and symptom recognition; appropriate control measure utilization; emergency response procedures; and resources for additional information or concern reporting. Delivery methodologies must address diverse educational backgrounds, language considerations, and learning style preferences, with approaches including traditional classroom instruction; hands-on demonstration and practice; computer-based interactive modules; and ongoing reinforcement through toolbox talks, safety meetings, and similar brief focused sessions. Effectiveness evaluation extends beyond simple attendance documentation to include knowledge verification through testing; behavior observation confirming application in actual work settings; and ongoing reinforcement addressing knowledge decay over time. This administrative control category creates essential foundation for other protection measures, as engineering controls and personal protective equipment demonstrate limited effectiveness without appropriate worker understanding and utilization.

Medical surveillance provides systematic health monitoring identifying potential exposure effects before significant or irreversible damage occurs. Program design elements include baseline examinations establishing pre-exposure health status; periodic assessments at intervals appropriate to specific hazard properties and toxicity mechanisms; targeted testing addressing organs systems affected by workplace exposures; and termination examinations documenting health status at employment conclusion. Examination components vary based on specific workplace hazards, with examples including spirometry evaluating lung function for workers exposed to respiratory toxicants; audiometric testing monitoring hearing among noise-exposed workers; biological monitoring measuring toxicants or their metabolites in blood or urine specimens; and specialized testing for specific concerns such as nerve conduction studies for neurotoxin-exposed populations. Implementation requires appropriate medical direction ensuring test selection matches specific hazard concerns; standardized testing protocols maintaining comparability across time; confidentiality protections encouraging honest symptom reporting; and effective communication systems ensuring relevant findings reach both individual workers and those responsible for workplace hazard control without compromising medical confidentiality. Integration with exposure monitoring data enables identification of potential problem areas before clinical disease manifests, creating opportunity for intervention through enhanced controls or reassignment before permanent health impacts develop.

Emergency response planning addresses potential high-exposure scenarios resulting from system failures, accidents, or unexpected events. Comprehensive plans incorporate hazard identification determining potential emergency scenarios based on materials present and process characteristics; response procedure development addressing containment, evacuation, medical intervention, and other necessary actions; equipment and supply procurement ensuring availability of necessary resources including personal protective equipment, first aid supplies, decontamination materials, and communication devices; personnel role assignment establishing clear responsibilities for alarm activation, evacuation coordination, headcount verification, and other critical functions; and coordination with external response agencies including fire departments, hazardous materials teams, and medical facilities that might become involved during actual emergencies. Regular drills and exercises verify plan functionality, identify improvement opportunities, and maintain response readiness among all personnel. Small-scale precursor events including minor spills, limited releases, or near-miss incidents provide valuable learning opportunities to strengthen systems before major events occur. This administrative control component addresses residual risk remaining after implementation of primary preventive approaches, recognizing that even well-designed systems occasionally experience failures requiring prepared response to minimize health impacts during abnormal conditions.

Personal Protective Equipment

Respiratory protection provides the final control level for airborne contaminants when engineering and administrative approaches cannot achieve adequate exposure reduction. Selection processes match respirator capabilities with specific hazard characteristics including contaminant type, concentration, and physical properties; warning properties indicating breakthrough; and oxygen availability. Air-purifying respirators remove contaminants through various mechanisms: particulate filters employing mechanical interception, impaction, diffusion, and electrostatic attraction for solid or liquid aerosols; chemical cartridges utilizing activated carbon or specialized sorbents for vapor and gas adsorption; and combination systems addressing multiple contaminant types simultaneously. Atmosphere-supplying respirators provide clean breathing air from external sources, with options including supplied-air respirators connected to compressed air sources through hoses; self-contained breathing apparatus carrying compressed air in portable cylinders; and powered air-purifying respirators using battery-powered blowers enhancing air movement through purifying elements. Selection factors include protection factor requirements based on contaminant concentration relative to exposure limits; physiological burden considerations including breathing resistance, weight, and heat stress potential; work requirement compatibility including communication needs, mobility requirements, and duration limitations; and practical implementation factors such as fit testing capability, maintenance provisions, and storage facilities.

Comprehensive respiratory protection programs extend beyond equipment provision to include additional elements ensuring effective implementation. Medical evaluation verifies individual capacity to safely wear respirators, considering both physical conditions like respiratory or cardiovascular disorders and psychological factors like claustrophobia potentially affecting safe usage. Fit testing employs either qualitative methods using detectable agents like saccharin or Bitrex with subjective response, or quantitative approaches measuring actual protection factors through instrumental methods, ensuring proper sealing between respirator and facial features. Proper use training covers donning and doffing procedures, user seal checks before each use, appropriate wear conditions including facial hair limitations, and recognition of warning signs indicating potential malfunction. Maintenance and storage programs ensure continued equipment functionality through appropriate cleaning procedures, component replacement schedules, inspection protocols, and proper storage conditions maintaining shape and cleanliness between uses. Program evaluation monitors overall effectiveness through elements including workplace monitoring verifying adequate protection, periodic review of hazard assessments ensuring appropriate selection decisions as conditions change, and compliance verification confirming consistent proper usage throughout covered operations. This comprehensive approach addresses the recognized limitations of respiratory protection as a primary control strategy, creating systems supporting effective implementation despite the inherent challenges of equipment requiring active user participation and consistent proper usage for effective protection.

Chemical protective clothing prevents dermal exposure through creating barriers between skin and workplace contaminants. Material selection matches protective properties with specific chemical hazards, considering factors including permeation resistance measuring chemical movement through intact materials at molecular level; penetration resistance addressing bulk flow through seams, closures, or imperfections; degradation resistance evaluating physical property maintenance upon chemical contact; and practical considerations including flexibility, durability, heat dissipation characteristics, and cost-effectiveness for the specific application. Clothing design incorporates appropriate coverage for exposure risk areas while maintaining wearer functionality, with options ranging from limited coverage items like gloves, sleeves, or aprons for splash protection to fully encapsulating suits for environments with severe exposure potential. Glove selection represents particularly critical decision points given the frequency of hand contact with contaminants, with material options including butyl rubber resistant to ketones and esters; nitrile offering petroleum derivative and chlorinated hydrocarbon protection; neoprene providing acid, base, and solvent resistance; polyvinyl alcohol demonstrating excellent organic solvent protection though with water sensitivity limitations; and various specialized laminates or composites addressing specific challenging chemical classes. Implementation programs incorporate selection guidance matching protection with specific workplace chemicals; inspection protocols identifying damage before protection becomes compromised; defined replacement schedules based on demonstrated chemical breakthrough times; appropriate decontamination procedures preventing cross-contamination; and proper disposal methods for contaminated items.

Limitations affecting chemical protective clothing effectiveness require recognition and management through comprehensive programs. Heat stress represents a significant concern as impermeable materials prevent normal evaporative cooling, potentially creating hazardous core temperature elevation particularly during strenuous work or in high temperature environments. Mitigation approaches include work-rest scheduling providing cooling periods; cooling systems ranging from ice vests to air-conditioned garments; and physiological monitoring identifying developing problems before serious health effects occur. Dexterity and mobility limitations affect task performance capabilities, productivity, and potentially safety when protective materials restrict normal movement patterns or tactile feedback. Ergonomic concerns include increased metabolic demands while wearing protective equipment; altered center of gravity affecting balance and fall risk; and potential for fatigue affecting both judgement and physical capabilities during extended wear periods. Psychological barriers including claustrophobia, communication difficulties, and isolation feelings may affect compliance and performance, particularly with higher protection level ensembles. Comprehensive implementation programs address these limitations through appropriate garment selection balancing protection requirements against human factors considerations; medical fitness evaluation ensuring individual capacity to safely wear required protection; training addressing both technical usage aspects and recognition of physiological warning signs; and supervision ensuring adherence to defined work-rest schedules and other protective measures against secondary risks created by the protective equipment itself.

Eye and face protection prevents exposure to chemical splashes, particulates, radiation, and other hazards potentially damaging these sensitive tissues. Selection criteria match protective properties with specific workplace hazards: safety glasses with side shields address moderate impact hazards and limited particle concerns; chemical goggles provide splash protection through indirect ventilation systems or unvented designs; face shields offer expanded face coverage while typically requiring underlying eye protection; laser safety eyewear incorporates specialized filtering matched to specific laser wavelengths; welding helmets combine radiation filtering with impact and spark protection; and specialized eyewear addresses specific concerns like ultraviolet protection during germicidal lamp operation or infrared filtering for furnace operations. Prescription safety eyewear accommodates vision correction requirements while maintaining protective properties, through either purpose-manufactured prescription safety glasses or cover goggles designed for wear over regular prescription eyewear. Implementation programs include hazard assessment identifying specific eye and face protection requirements for each operation; selection guidance matching protection type with identified hazards; fitting provisions ensuring proper positioning and coverage; maintenance procedures including cleaning, disinfection, and damage inspection; and training addressing both proper usage techniques and importance of consistent wear in designated areas. Integration with other personal protective equipment requires compatibility evaluation, particularly between eye protection and respiratory devices where proper fitting of both simultaneously often presents challenges requiring specific compatible models or unified systems incorporating multiple protection elements within integrated designs.

Hearing protection devices reduce noise exposure through creating barriers attenuating sound transmission to the inner ear. Earplugs insert into the ear canal, with varieties including premolded styles in various sizes; formable foam types expanding to fit individual ear canal geometry; custom-molded options created from individual ear impressions; and semi-insert or canal caps supported by lightweight bands. Earmuffs enclose the entire external ear with sound-attenuating cups containing acoustic insulation and soft cushions creating seals against the head, attached by adjustable headbands accommodating various head sizes and configurations. Selection factors include required attenuation based on workplace noise levels and exposure duration; comfort considerations affecting likelihood of consistent proper wear; compatibility with other required personal protective equipment; communication requirements during work tasks; and environmental factors including temperature, humidity, and hygiene conditions affecting appropriate device types. Noise Reduction Rating (NRR) values provide standardized attenuation metrics, though with recognition that laboratory-derived ratings typically overestimate real-world protection due to fitting variations, wear time inconsistency, and deterioration over usage periods.

Hearing conservation programs integrate protection devices within comprehensive approaches addressing noise exposure. Elements include exposure assessment identifying areas and operations requiring protection; engineering control evaluation determining feasibility of noise reduction at sources before relying on personal protection; appropriate device selection matching protection levels with exposure characteristics; training covering proper insertion or fitting techniques, care and maintenance procedures, and importance of consistent usage; fit testing verifying adequate attenuation for individual users with their specific devices; and audiometric testing monitoring hearing thresholds over time to verify program effectiveness. Field verification techniques including microphone in real ear measurements or field attenuation estimation systems provide actual attenuation assessment under workplace conditions, addressing the recognized limitations of laboratory-derived ratings in predicting real-world protection levels. Communication accommodations within high-noise environments include specialized systems ranging from simple earmuffs with communication capability to sophisticated devices allowing normal conversation while still providing protection against hazardous noise levels. This integrated approach addresses the inherent limitations of hearing protection devices as primary noise control strategies, recognizing that actual protection achieved typically falls substantially below rated values without comprehensive supporting programs ensuring proper selection, fitting, and consistent usage throughout all noise exposures.

SURVEILLANCE

Occupational health surveillance systems monitor worker populations for exposure patterns and health outcomes, supporting prevention through early identification of developing concerns.

Medical Surveillance

Hazard-based surveillance programs monitor specific worker populations with known or suspected exposure to particular toxic agents, implementing structured health assessment protocols matched to toxicant properties and potential health effects. Design elements include target population definition based on exposure assessment or job classification data; examination component selection addressing organ systems affected by workplace exposures; appropriate testing frequency considering both exposure patterns and expected latency for potential health effects; and action level criteria defining findings requiring intervention through either individual medical management or workplace control enhancement. Implementation typically follows tiered approaches with screening test administration to broader populations followed by more detailed evaluation for individuals with abnormal findings. Surveillance for specific hazards includes elements like spirometry monitoring pulmonary function in workers exposed to respiratory toxicants; audiometric testing tracking hearing thresholds among noise-exposed populations; and specialized testing for specific concerns such as blood lead monitoring, cholinesterase activity measurement for organophosphate-exposed workers, or bladder cancer screening for certain aromatic amine exposures. Effectiveness depends on several factors: appropriate test selection matching surveillance components to specific health endpoints associated with workplace exposures; standardized testing protocols ensuring results comparability across time and different providers; consistent participation among exposed populations avoiding selection bias from differential testing patterns; and integration with exposure data establishing connections between workplace conditions and observed health patterns.

Outcome-based surveillance monitors worker populations for health conditions potentially associated with occupational exposures, identifying patterns suggesting workplace contributions to disease burden. Approaches include symptom surveys systematically collecting self-reported health information across worker populations; focused physical examinations targeting specific organ systems based on potential work-related effects; analysis of administrative datasets including workers' compensation claims, absenteeism records, or health insurance utilization patterns; and occasionally establishment of specialized surveillance mechanisms for specific high-concern conditions such as cancer registries with occupational information collection.

> **Remember**
>
> **Surveillance combines environmental monitoring measuring workplace contaminant levels, biological monitoring assessing internal dose through biomarkers, and medical surveillance detecting early health effects before clinical disease develops.**

Statistical methods comparing disease rates within workplaces to appropriate reference populations help distinguish occupational contributions from background rates, though with recognition of challenges including healthy worker effects potentially masking workplace associations, latency periods complicating temporal connections, and multi-factorial disease etiology creating attribution difficulties. Implementation challenges include data access limitations, particularly for health information protected by confidentiality provisions; participation barriers affecting response rates for voluntary components; resource requirements for comprehensive program maintenance; and reluctance to identify potential work-relatedness for liability or regulatory compliance concerns. Despite these challenges, outcome-based surveillance provides essential complementary perspective to hazard-based approaches, potentially identifying unexpected exposure-disease relationships not captured through monitoring focused solely on known hazards.

Biological monitoring involves systematic measurement of chemical substances or their metabolites in biological specimens, providing integrated exposure assessment across all routes and accounting for individual factors affecting absorption, distribution, metabolism, and elimination. Program design requires decisions addressing several elements: appropriate biomarker selection among options including parent compound measurement, metabolite assessment, or effect biomarkers measuring biochemical alterations resulting from exposure; sampling matrix determination considering accessibility, stability, pharmacokinetic characteristics, and relationship to target organs; timing optimization based on toxicokinetic properties including absorption rates, distribution patterns, metabolism timeframes, and elimination characteristics; appropriate reference values for interpretation including biological exposure indices from professional organizations or regulatory guidelines; and decision criteria establishing action levels for individual intervention or workplace control enhancement. Implementation challenges include collection logistics for appropriate specimen timing; analytical laboratory capability for sometimes complex methodologies; interpretation complexity when results reflect combined occupational and environmental exposures; and worker acceptance concerns particularly for invasive sampling procedures.

Table 11.3: Occupational Exposure Monitoring Approaches

Monitoring Type	Methods	Applications	Interpretation Considerations
Personal air sampling	Breathing zone sampling pumps, passive badges	Evaluating individual worker exposure, regulatory compliance	Must consider task representativeness, sampling duration, analytical method limitations
Area monitoring	Fixed station monitors, grab samples	Identifying emission sources, evaluating engineering controls	May not reflect actual worker exposure
Biological monitoring	Blood, urine, exhaled breath analysis for toxicants or metabolites	Assessing actual absorbed dose across all routes	Results affected by individual metabolism, timing relative to exposure, non-occupational sources
Medical surveillance	Spirometry, blood tests, audiometry, specific toxin biomarkers	Early detection of health effects, evaluating control effectiveness	Requires baseline data, may detect effects only after significant exposure
Real-time monitoring	Direct-reading instruments for gases, vapors, particulates	Immediate feedback, identifying peak exposures, emergency response	Lower specificity, potential interferences, requires proper calibration

Effective programs address these challenges through approaches including field-appropriate collection protocols; quality assurance programs ensuring analytical accuracy; interpretation frameworks accounting for non-occupational contributions; and comprehensive communication addressing both confidentiality protections and result meaning. Integration with environmental monitoring creates complementary perspectives combining workplace concentration measurement with actual absorbed dose assessment, providing more comprehensive understanding than either approach alone could achieve.

Fitness for duty evaluation determines individual capability to safely perform job functions without unreasonable risk to themselves or others, particularly important for positions involving exposure to workplace toxicants where pre-existing conditions might create enhanced susceptibility or functional limitations affecting safe work performance. Components include preplacement examinations establishing baseline health status and identifying potential concerns before work commencement; periodic assessments monitoring for developing conditions potentially affecting safe performance; functional capacity evaluation determining physical capabilities relative to job demands; and occasionally specific testing assessing capabilities directly relevant to exposure scenarios, such as respirator clearance evaluations or assessment of biotransformation capacity for substances with metabolism-dependent toxicity. Ethical implementation requires careful balance between legitimate safety considerations and inappropriate discrimination, with principles including job-relatedness requiring direct connection between medical standards and actual job functions; individualized assessment evaluating specific capabilities rather than applying category-based exclusions; reasonable accommodation exploration before disqualification decisions; confidentiality maintenance separating medical information from general personnel records; and consistent application across similarly situated individuals avoiding selective enforcement patterns. Legal frameworks including the Americans with Disabilities Act in the United States and similar provisions internationally significantly influence implementation approaches, generally requiring focus on actual functional capabilities rather than diagnosis-based exclusions. When properly implemented, these programs support both individual worker protection through appropriate placement decisions and broader workforce safety through ensuring capability to safely implement necessary protection measures.

Quality assurance principles ensure medical surveillance generates reliable, comparable data supporting valid interpretation and appropriate intervention decisions. Elements include standardized testing protocols establishing consistent procedures across providers and time periods; instrument calibration and maintenance programs ensuring measurement accuracy; provider training and certification for specialized testing components like spirometry or audiometry; appropriate quality control procedures including duplicate testing, blinded sample submission, or other verification mechanisms; and comprehensive documentation systems maintaining result comparability across evaluation periods. Interpretation frameworks incorporate statistical process control concepts identifying variation exceeding expected random patterns, suggesting either quality problems or genuine health status changes requiring investigation. Common implementation challenges include provider variation when multiple clinicians perform examinations; instrument drift affecting measurement consistency; participant compliance issues creating missing data patterns potentially biasing results; and resource limitations affecting program maintenance across extended time periods necessary for chronic health effect monitoring. Addressing these challenges requires systematic approaches including detailed procedure manuals; regular provider training and competency verification; maintenance of consistent equipment when possible or detailed cross-calibration when changes become necessary; and dedicated program management ensuring continued prioritization despite changing organizational conditions or competing resource demands. This quality foundation creates essential credibility for medical surveillance findings, supporting appropriate workplace intervention when concerning patterns emerge while avoiding unnecessary actions based on artifactual findings or measurement inconsistencies rather than genuine health changes.

Exposure Surveillance

Workplace exposure monitoring systematically assesses airborne contaminant concentrations, providing objective documentation of exposure conditions, identifying highest risk operations, demonstrating regulatory compliance, and establishing baseline conditions for evaluating intervention effectiveness. Comprehensive programs incorporate several elements: representative sampling strategies addressing spatial variation across work areas and temporal patterns throughout production cycles; appropriate methodologies matched to specific contaminant physical and chemical properties; quality assurance procedures ensuring measurement reliability; and interpretation frameworks comparing results with established occupational exposure limits while considering potential additive or synergistic effects from multiple contaminant exposures. Implementation approaches include baseline comprehensive surveys establishing exposure profiles across operations; routine monitoring maintaining current exposure characterization as processes evolve; task-based assessment identifying specific high-exposure activities within broader job classifications; and worker notification systems ensuring appropriate result communication to affected employees. Integration with production data enables identification of exposure determinants—specific process parameters, equipment conditions, or operational variables significantly influencing exposure levels—creating opportunities for targeted control implementation rather than generalized approaches. Statistical analysis techniques including multiple regression modeling, bayesian methodology, and mixed effects models increasingly support sophisticated understanding of exposure patterns and their determinants, enhancing prevention through identification of modifiable factors most strongly associated with elevated exposure conditions.

Job-exposure matrices organize occupational exposure information through systematic frameworks linking job titles, tasks, or work areas with specific contaminant exposure assessments, facilitating epidemiological research and supporting exposure estimation for situations lacking direct measurement data. Development methodologies include expert assessment approaches utilizing industrial hygienist judgment based on process knowledge; direct measurement incorporation organizing available monitoring results by job or department classification; and hybrid approaches combining limited measurement data with expert judgment for comprehensive coverage. Matrix structures vary from simple job-exposure tables indicating presence/absence or qualitative exposure levels to sophisticated probabilistic frameworks incorporating exposure intensity distribution parameters, frequency estimates, and confidence ratings. These tools support numerous applications including retrospective exposure assessment for epidemiological studies linking past work conditions with current health outcomes; exposure estimation for similar exposure groups without complete monitoring data; identification of high-priority groups for targeted monitoring or intervention programs; and evaluation of control technology effectiveness through comparing exposure estimates before and after implementation. Limitations include potential misclassification when job titles inadequately represent actual task performance; temporal changes in exposure conditions as processes and controls evolve; and generalization challenges when matrices developed in one setting apply to different facilities or time periods. Despite these limitations, job-exposure matrices provide valuable tools supporting exposure assessment across broader populations than direct measurement alone could address, particularly valuable for understanding relationships between working conditions and health outcomes developing over extended time periods.

Sentinel event surveillance identifies individual cases or clustered occurrences suggesting significant exposure potential requiring further investigation and intervention. This approach employs various trigger indicators including unusual disease presentations potentially indicating workplace etiology; biological monitoring results exceeding action thresholds; reported symptoms clustered within specific work areas or job classifications; incidents involving chemical releases, spills, or control system failures; and occasionally community reports like unusual odors or visible emissions suggesting containment problems. Investigation protocols follow systematic approaches identifying exposure sources, affected populations, and appropriate control strategies, typically with escalating response intensity proportional to event severity or recurrence patterns. Implementation systems include reporting mechanisms ensuring appropriate information reaches responsible parties; triage protocols establishing investigation priorities based on severity indicators and potential population impact; standardized assessment methodologies ensuring comprehensive evaluation; and intervention tracking monitoring control implementation and effectiveness. Advantages compared to ongoing monitoring include resource efficiency through targeted investigation rather than continuous measurement; capacity for addressing emerging concerns not included in routine surveillance protocols; and often enhanced worker participation when investigations respond directly to reported concerns rather than following pre-established schedules. This targeted approach complements rather than replaces systematic exposure monitoring, providing responsive capacity for unexpected developments while ongoing programs maintain baseline condition assessment.

Exposure registries maintain systematic documentation of worker exposure to specific hazardous agents, supporting both individual worker protection through exposure history preservation and population-level analysis identifying potential health patterns associated with particular exposure circumstances. Registry components include worker identification information; exposure characterization detailing agents, concentrations, duration, and circumstances; employment information establishing temporal relationships; and occasionally follow-up health status tracking for registries with research components. Implementation approaches range from facility-specific systems maintained by individual employers to industry-wide programs covering multiple workplaces with similar exposures to government-maintained registries for specific high-concern substances like asbestos, benzene, or certain carcinogens. Operational considerations include data quality assurance ensuring accurate and complete information; confidentiality protections maintaining appropriate privacy while enabling necessary information access; and sustainable maintenance systems ensuring continued functionality across potentially extended timeframes matching latency periods for chronic health effects. Practical applications include documentation supporting workers' compensation claims or other exposure-related benefits; research resource creation enabling epidemiological investigation of exposure-disease relationships; exposure reconstruction supporting risk assessment for substances with emerging health concerns; and program evaluation examining effectiveness of control measures or regulatory standards through longitudinal exposure pattern assessment. While implementation challenges include resource requirements for system maintenance, potential participation barriers from privacy concerns, and sometimes complex governance considerations for multi-employer registries, these systems provide valuable infrastructure supporting both individual worker protection through exposure documentation and broader occupational health advancement through facilitating research into exposure-disease relationships.

Trend analysis methodologies examine exposure patterns across time, identifying directional changes, cyclical variations, and potential determinants supporting proactive intervention before adverse outcomes develop. Statistical approaches include simple linear regression establishing overall direction and magnitude of exposure changes; time series analysis identifying cyclical patterns, seasonal variations, or trend components within apparently random fluctuations; change-point analysis detecting significant shifts in exposure distributions potentially indicating process changes or control system modifications; and multivariate methods examining relationships between exposure metrics and potential explanatory variables including production volume, staffing patterns, maintenance schedules, or control system parameters. Visualization techniques including control charts adapted from quality management, cumulative summation (CUSUM) plots sensitive to subtle directional changes, and various graphical representations support both technical analysis and communication with diverse stakeholders including workers, management, and regulatory authorities. Implementation challenges include data quality requirements for meaningful trend identification; statistical power limitations when analyzing infrequent measurements or small worker populations; potential confounding from unrecognized process changes or measurement methodology modifications; and occasionally resistance to identifying adverse trends due to regulatory or liability concerns. Addressing these challenges requires approaches including standardized measurement protocols maintaining methodological consistency; appropriate statistical techniques accounting for data limitations; comprehensive process documentation capturing potential explanatory variables; and organizational cultures supporting transparency even when findings suggest problems requiring attention. When effectively implemented, trend analysis provides powerful preventive tool supporting intervention before overt health effects develop, aligning with fundamental industrial hygiene philosophy emphasizing anticipation and prevention rather than merely responding to established problems.

Epidemiological Methods

Occupational cohort studies follow defined worker populations over time, comparing disease occurrence rates with expected values or examining exposure-response relationships within the cohort. This methodology offers several advantages for occupational health surveillance: capacity for examining diseases with extended latency periods through retrospective cohort designs accessing historical records; ability to calculate absolute risk measures including incidence rates and cumulative incidence; opportunity to examine multiple health outcomes potentially associated with specific exposures; and reduced selection bias compared to voluntary participation studies when comprehensive workforce records provide the cohort definition frame. Implementation approaches include retrospective cohort studies assembling historical employment records and determining subsequent health outcomes through methods including mortality records, cancer registries, or medical insurance claims; prospective designs enrolling current workers with planned follow-up through either passive record linkage or active periodic contact; and sometimes hybrid approaches combining historical cohort assembly with prospective follow-up for recent periods. Analytical methods include standardized mortality or incidence ratio calculations comparing observed case numbers with expected values derived from general population rates adjusted for demographic characteristics; internal comparisons examining disease rates across exposure categories within the cohort; and exposure-response analyses evaluating relationships between quantitative or qualitative exposure metrics and disease risk, potentially identifying threshold effects or other non-linear patterns.

Occupational cohort studies present specific methodological challenges requiring careful consideration during design and interpretation. The healthy worker effect represents systematic bias when comparing worker populations with general reference populations, as employment typically requires baseline health status above population averages, potentially masking occupational disease risk through artificially lowered expected disease rates. Addressing approaches include internal comparison groups exposed to different levels of the agent under study but otherwise similar working conditions; adjustment techniques incorporating employment duration or time-since-hire variables; and occasionally alternative reference populations with comparable employment status but different exposure circumstances. Exposure assessment limitations affect many occupational studies, with historical operations often lacking systematic monitoring data, necessitating retrospective estimation through job-exposure matrices, expert assessment, or surrogate measures like employment duration in specific departments. Left truncation occurs when workers with early disease manifestation exit the workforce before study inclusion, potentially creating survival bias particularly problematic for rapidly progressive conditions. Despite these challenges, well-designed occupational cohort studies provide crucial evidence regarding exposure-disease relationships, supporting both evaluation of existing workplace standards and identification of emerging concerns requiring intervention.

Case-control studies compare exposure histories between individuals with specific health conditions (cases) and appropriately selected comparison groups without those conditions (controls), offering advantages including feasibility for rare diseases where cohort approaches would require impractically large populations; efficiency for conditions with long latency periods by focusing on existing cases rather than waiting for disease development; and opportunity for detailed exposure assessment through direct participant interview rather than relying solely on existing records. Occupational applications include investigation of potential work-related causes for specific diseases; evaluation of risk factors for conditions too rare for cohort study feasibility; and exploration of exposure-disease relationships when comprehensive employment records for cohort definition remain unavailable. Implementation approaches include nested case-control designs identifying cases and controls within defined cohorts, combining cohort study efficiency with more detailed exposure assessment for selected participants; hospital-based approaches recruiting cases from clinical settings with various control selection strategies; and population-based designs identifying cases through registries or surveillance systems with community-based control selection, typically offering greater generalizability though often with implementation challenges. Exposure assessment methods include structured occupational history interviews; job-exposure matrices converting employment information to exposure estimates; review of available industrial hygiene records; and occasionally novel approaches including molecular markers of specific exposures or direct workplace observation for current exposures.

Case-control studies face several methodological challenges requiring careful consideration during design and interpretation. Selection bias occurs when case or control recruitment produces groups with systematically different exposure opportunities unrelated to the studied disease relationship. Recall bias represents differential accuracy or completeness in exposure reporting between cases potentially motivated to identify explanations for their condition and controls without similar motivation. Confounding from non-occupational factors requires appropriate data collection and analytical adjustment approaches, particularly challenging when occupational exposures correlate with lifestyle factors or socioeconomic characteristics also associated with disease risk. Addressing these challenges requires approaches including standardized exposure assessment methods applied identically across case and control groups; validation substudies comparing reported information with objective data sources when available; appropriate matching or statistical adjustment for potential confounding variables; and careful interpretation acknowledging remaining limitations. Despite these challenges, case-control methodology provides valuable contributions to occupational health surveillance, particularly for outcomes too rare for practical cohort study approaches or situations requiring more detailed exposure assessment than typically available through existing records alone.

Cross-sectional studies simultaneously assess both exposure and health status at a single time point, offering advantages including relatively rapid implementation making them suitable for initial hypothesis exploration; feasibility for examining multiple exposure-outcome relationships within single study designs; and opportunity for incorporating both objective measurements and subjective symptom assessment providing complementary perspectives. Occupational applications include hazard surveillance evaluating prevalence of specific exposures across industries or job classifications; health surveillance assessing prevalence of work-related conditions within defined populations; exposure-response analysis examining relationships between current exposure levels and biological markers or functional assessments; and initial investigation of newly recognized potential hazards requiring rapid assessment. Implementation approaches include workplace-based studies examining current employees through various assessment methods including questionnaires, physical examinations, biological monitoring, or physiological testing; industry-wide surveys sampling workers across multiple facilities within specific sectors; and occasionally community-based studies incorporating occupational exposure assessment within broader health examination programs. Analytical approaches include simple prevalence comparisons across exposure categories; multiple regression techniques examining relationships between exposure metrics and continuous outcome variables like pulmonary function parameters or biological marker levels; and logistic regression evaluating associations between exposure circumstances and binary outcomes such as specific symptoms or clinical diagnoses.

Cross-sectional studies have significant limitations requiring consideration during design and interpretation. Temporal ambiguity represents their fundamental limitation, as simultaneous assessment of exposure and outcome creates uncertainty regarding causal direction—particularly problematic when health conditions might influence exposure patterns through job transfer, work modification, or employment termination. This healthy worker survivor effect creates potential for substantial underestimation of exposure-disease relationships when affected workers exit the workforce or transfer to lower-exposure positions before study participation. Prevalence-incidence bias occurs because cross-sectional designs capture existing (prevalent) rather than new (incident) cases, potentially obscuring relationships for conditions with either very short or very long duration. These limitations make cross-sectional studies generally inappropriate for definitive causal inference, particularly for chronic conditions with substantial latency or diseases affecting continued employment capability. Despite these limitations, cross-sectional studies provide valuable contributions to occupational health surveillance through their efficiency for initial hypothesis generation, capacity for examining current workplace conditions, and ability to incorporate detailed examination components sometimes impractical for larger longitudinal designs, serving as important components within comprehensive surveillance strategies incorporating complementary methodological approaches addressing different aspects of exposure-disease relationships.

Proportionate mortality and morbidity studies examine the distribution of causes of death or disease within occupational groups, comparing observed patterns with expected distributions based on general population statistics. This approach offers distinct advantages when denominator information establishing the at-risk population size remains unavailable, as is often the case for occupational groups without comprehensive employment records or dispersed workers without centralized tracking systems. Implementation involves calculating proportionate mortality or morbidity ratios (PMRs) comparing the percentage of deaths or cases from specific causes within the occupational group to corresponding percentages in appropriate reference populations, with values exceeding 100 indicating greater proportion than expected. Applications include surveillance for occupational groups without well-defined population bases such as union members, licensed professionals, or workers identified through certification registries; preliminary investigation of potentially hazardous industries suggesting more resource-intensive cohort studies when elevated proportions appear; and monitoring disease patterns among former workers lost to direct follow-up but identifiable through death certificates or disease registries. Analytical refinements include stratification by demographic characteristics accounting for population structure differences between occupational and reference groups; multiple cause analysis incorporating contributing conditions beyond the underlying cause of death; and case-control approaches within PMR frameworks comparing occupational histories between specific causes of death and selected control conditions presumed unrelated to occupational factors.

These proportionate methods have significant limitations requiring careful interpretation. Most fundamentally, they measure only relative distribution of causes rather than absolute risk, potentially producing elevated ratios for specific causes when other major causes are reduced within the occupational group—a particular concern when examining worker populations likely exhibiting healthy worker effects with reduced overall mortality from major causes like cardiovascular disease. This limitation means a condition might show elevated proportions without actually occurring at higher absolute rates than reference populations. Additional challenges include potential referent population inappropriateness when comparing specialized worker groups with general populations having substantially different demographic compositions or risk factor distributions; information quality concerns when relying on death certificates or similar administrative records with known classification inconsistencies; and limited exposure assessment capability when occupation information comes solely from final employment rather than comprehensive work histories. Despite these limitations, proportionate mortality and morbidity studies provide valuable surveillance tools when more rigorous designs remain infeasible due to denominator information unavailability, serving important roles in identifying potential occupational hazards warranting further investigation through more definitive methodologies when elevated proportions suggest possible workplace associations requiring additional evaluation.

REGULATIONS

Regulatory guidelines establish legal requirements for occupational exposure management, creating enforceable standards protecting worker health.

Regulatory Agencies

The Occupational Safety and Health Administration (OSHA) serves as the primary federal agency responsible for workplace health regulation in the United States, established through the Occupational Safety and Health Act of 1970 with the mandate to ensure "safe and healthful working conditions for working men and women." Regulatory authority encompasses standard-setting establishing legally enforceable exposure limits and workplace practice requirements; enforcement through inspections, citation issuance, and penalty assessment; record-keeping requirements for workplace injuries, illnesses, and exposure monitoring; and consultation services providing compliance assistance particularly for smaller employers. Standard-setting processes involve several mechanisms: notice-and-comment rulemaking publishing proposed standards with opportunities for stakeholder input before finalization; emergency temporary standards addressing grave dangers requiring immediate intervention; national consensus standard adoption incorporating externally developed guidelines into regulatory framework; and occasionally negotiated rulemaking bringing diverse stakeholders together for collaborative standard development. Enforcement approaches include programmed inspections targeting high-hazard industries or specific emphasis areas; unprogrammed inspections responding to complaints, referrals, or reported incidents; and follow-up visits verifying abatement of previously identified violations. Penalties vary with violation classification including de minimis conditions with minimal safety impact; non-serious violations presenting workplace hazards with unlikely death or serious injury potential; serious violations creating substantial probability of death or serious harm; willful violations involving intentional disregard or plain indifference to requirements; and repeat violations for substantially similar conditions previously cited within five years, with penalty structures incorporating both statutory maximums and adjustment factors including employer size, good faith efforts, and compliance history.

The National Institute for Occupational Safety and Health (NIOSH) functions as the research agency for occupational safety and health within the U.S. federal government, established alongside OSHA through the same 1970 legislation but with fundamentally different roles reflecting research and recommendation focus rather than regulatory authority. Core functions include conducting research identifying occupational hazards and developing prevention strategies; providing recommendations to OSHA and the Mine Safety and Health Administration regarding appropriate exposure limits and control technologies; investigating potentially hazardous working conditions through Health Hazard Evaluation program responding to requests from employers, employees, or their representatives; developing and disseminating educational materials promoting workplace health protection; and maintaining various surveillance systems monitoring occupational illness and injury patterns. The Recommended Exposure Limits (RELs) developed through NIOSH research provide science-based guidance, though without direct regulatory enforcement capability unless adopted by regulatory agencies through their standard-setting processes. Additional programs include the National Occupational Research Agenda establishing research priorities through stakeholder collaboration; various certification programs for personal protective equipment including respirators and hearing protection devices; and training initiatives including Education and Research Centers supporting graduate education in occupational health disciplines. This complementary relationship between NIOSH research functions and OSHA regulatory authority creates institutional framework separating scientific assessment from regulatory enforcement, though with ongoing interaction through various consultation and advisory mechanisms ensuring research relevance to practical workplace protection needs.

The Environmental Protection Agency (EPA) influences occupational health through several regulatory programs addressing chemical manufacturing, distribution, and environmental releases with workplace implication. The Toxic Substances Control Act (TSCA) provides authority for evaluating new and existing chemicals, requiring pre-manufacture notification with toxicity and exposure information, enabling restrictions when substances present unreasonable risks, and mandating various reporting requirements including substantial risk information when manufacturers discover significant hazards. Recent TSCA amendments strengthen EPA's ability to require testing, evaluate existing chemicals, and implement risk management measures potentially affecting workplace exposures alongside consumer and environmental applications. The Federal Insecticide, Fungicide, and Rodenticide Act (FIFRA) establishes registration requirements for pesticide products, including occupational exposure assessment, appropriate labeling specifying protective measures for workers, and sometimes specific restrictions on application methods or protective equipment requirements based on toxicity concerns. Worker Protection Standards developed under FIFRA specifically address agricultural worker protection through requirements including safety training, notification of pesticide applications, restricted entry intervals after treatment, and provision of decontamination supplies and emergency assistance. While focused primarily on environmental protection rather than occupational health as primary mission, these EPA regulatory frameworks significantly affect workplace chemical exposures through restricting market availability of highly toxic substances, requiring hazard information generation and dissemination, and establishing specific protection requirements for certain chemical classes, complementing OSHA's workplace-focused regulatory approach with broader chemical management systems influencing which substances enter commercial channels and under what conditions.

State-level occupational safety and health agencies operate under federal OSHA approval in approximately half of U.S. states, implementing programs required to be "at least as effective as" federal standards while permitted to establish more stringent requirements addressing state-specific concerns. These "State Plan" programs must cover both private and public sector employees (with limited exceptions for states covering only public employees), maintain qualified personnel, provide consultation services, and incorporate whistleblower protections equivalent to federal provisions. Regulatory approaches vary considerably across State Plan jurisdictions, with some closely mirroring federal standards while others implement significant additional protections including more stringent exposure limits, industry-specific standards addressing regional concerns, or enhanced reporting and documentation requirements beyond federal baselines. California's program exemplifies expanded protection through its Permissible Exposure Limits covering approximately 200 substances not addressed by federal standards, many with more protective values than federal counterparts, alongside specific standards addressing hospital ergonomics, wildfire smoke exposure, heat illness prevention, and other hazards without dedicated federal regulations. State programs often demonstrate greater agility implementing new protections compared to federal processes, sometimes establishing standards later adopted nationally after demonstrating effectiveness at state level. This federal-state regulatory partnership creates system balancing national consistency through baseline requirements while enabling regional adaptation addressing specific industry patterns, workforce characteristics, and hazard prevalence variations across different states, though with resulting complexity for employers operating across multiple jurisdictions potentially subject to differing regulatory requirements.

International regulatory frameworks demonstrate considerable variation in structure, coverage, and enforcement approaches across different countries and regions, reflecting diverse legal systems, economic development levels, and cultural approaches to occupational risk management. The European Union employs framework legislation establishing general principles, supplemented by specific directives addressing particular hazards or sectors, with implementation through member state legislation creating generally consistent approaches across European countries while maintaining national administrative systems. This structure incorporates precautionary principles requiring demonstration of safety rather than proven harm before intervention, mandatory risk assessment requirements regardless of specific exposure limits, and strong worker consultation rights throughout hazard management processes. Canadian regulations operate through federal legislation covering approximately 10% of workers in federally regulated industries alongside provincial systems covering remaining workplaces, with the Canadian Centre for Occupational Health and Safety providing research and information similar to NIOSH functions though without direct regulatory authority. Australian model Work Health and Safety laws create template legislation implemented with some variation across individual states and territories, incorporating risk management principles, consultation requirements, and "reasonably practicable" standards for hazard control. Developing nations demonstrate widely varying regulatory frameworks, from comprehensive systems with limited enforcement capacity to minimal structures addressing only basic safety concerns, often with significant informal economy sectors operating outside regulatory oversight. These diverse international approaches create complex compliance environments for multinational employers while offering comparative perspective on alternative regulatory strategies potentially informing domestic policy development through identifying effective practices from other systems addressing similar workplace protection challenges through different regulatory mechanisms.

Standard-Setting Process

The evidence base for occupational exposure limits integrates diverse information sources including epidemiological studies, toxicological research, case reports, and occasionally controlled human exposure investigations under ethical oversight. Epidemiological evidence provides direct human relevance through examining actual workplace populations, with strengths including real-world exposure patterns, integration of multiple exposure routes, and demonstration of effects relevant to working populations rather than requiring cross-species extrapolation. Limitations include exposure characterization challenges, particularly for retrospective studies; healthy worker effects potentially masking adverse outcomes; confounding from non-occupational factors; and often insufficient sample sizes for detecting rare outcomes or small effect magnitudes. Toxicological studies offer complementary perspective through controlled exposure conditions, precise dose characterization, ability to evaluate mechanisms of action, and capacity for identifying effects with long latency periods within reasonable study timeframes. However, interspecies extrapolation introduces uncertainty regarding human relevance, laboratory exposure conditions may poorly represent workplace patterns, and most animal studies cannot incorporate lifetime exposure durations commensurate with working careers. Case reports provide sentinel information about potential hazards, particularly valuable for rare or unusual effects unlikely detected through systematic studies, though with limitations including uncertain exposure characterization, potential reporting biases, and inability to establish background rates for comparison. Integration approaches increasingly employ systematic review methodologies with explicit criteria for study quality assessment, evidence synthesis procedures addressing conflicting findings, weight of evidence determinations identifying most reliable information sources, and transparent documentation of decision processes translating scientific evidence into numerical exposure limits or other regulatory requirements.

Risk assessment frameworks provide structured approaches translating scientific evidence into practical exposure limits through sequential analysis of available information. Hazard identification evaluates whether substances demonstrate capacity for causing adverse effects regardless of exposure circumstances, considering evidence strength across human, animal, and mechanistic studies while classifying agents into categories like "known human carcinogen," "probable carcinogen," or "reproductive toxicant" based on established criteria. Dose-response assessment examines relationships between exposure levels and effect probabilities or severities, identifying critical effects occurring at lowest exposure levels, determining points of departure from available studies (typically NOAELs, LOAELs, or benchmark doses), and applying appropriate uncertainty factors addressing data limitations. These factors typically include 10-fold adjustments for interspecies extrapolation from animal studies to humans; intraspecies variation accounting for human susceptibility differences; LOAEL to NOAEL extrapolation when no-effect levels remain unidentified; subchronic to chronic extrapolation for studies with exposure durations shorter than working lifetimes; and database insufficiency when significant information gaps create additional uncertainty. Exposure assessment evaluates typical workplace conditions, including exposure frequency, duration, and intensity across different industries, job classifications, and control technology implementation levels. Risk characterization integrates these elements, determining whether current or anticipated exposures exceed levels associated with acceptable risk based on regulatory frameworks, with carcinogen assessment often employing 1/1,000 to 1/10,000 lifetime excess risk as benchmark ranges, while non-cancer effects typically utilize hazard quotients comparing exposure estimates with health-based reference values.

Feasibility considerations introduce economic and technical factors into standard-setting processes, recognizing practical implementation constraints alongside health protection objectives. Technological feasibility assessment evaluates whether exposure control to proposed limit levels can be achieved with available engineering approaches, considering evidence from facilities already achieving such levels, control technology effectiveness in similar applications, and reasonable timeframes for implementation when current capabilities require enhancement. Economic feasibility examines financial impact on affected industries, including capital investment requirements for control equipment installation; ongoing operational costs for maintenance, energy consumption, and consumable supplies; productivity effects from control implementation; and overall industry economic characteristics assessing capacity to absorb compliance costs without significant business viability impacts. Approaches balancing health protection with feasibility concerns include phased implementation providing extended timelines for industries facing significant challenges; alternative compliance options offering flexibility in implementation approaches; exemptions for specific applications where substitution proves impossible and exposure remains minimal; and occasionally differential standards across industry sectors reflecting varying control capabilities or economic circumstances. While criticized by some stakeholders as potentially compromising health protection, feasibility analysis remains legally required component of many regulatory frameworks, with court decisions consistently upholding its relevance while establishing boundaries ensuring health considerations maintain primary importance within appropriate balance reflecting statutory mandates.

Stakeholder participation significantly influences regulatory development through various mechanisms incorporating diverse perspectives throughout standard-setting processes. Formal notice-and-comment rulemaking solicits written input on proposed standards, with agencies legally required to consider substantive comments and provide reasoned responses addressing significant issues raised. Public hearings provide forums for oral testimony from affected parties, creating opportunities for direct exchange between regulators and stakeholders while establishing public record documenting diverse viewpoints.

Advisory committees bring together representatives from science, industry, labor, and public interest organizations for structured discussion of technical issues, regulatory approaches, and implementation considerations, providing consensus recommendations when possible or at minimum clarifying areas of agreement and remaining disagreement. Negotiated rulemaking represents more intensive collaboration, convening balanced stakeholder groups to collectively develop regulatory language addressing identified hazards while incorporating practical implementation considerations from those directly affected. Pre-proposal stakeholder meetings conducted before official rulemaking begins allow early input shaping initial regulatory concepts, potentially identifying innovative approaches or implementation challenges before significant resource investment in specific regulatory language. These participatory mechanisms serve multiple functions: enhancing technical quality through diverse expertise incorporation; building implementation support by addressing practical concerns during development rather than after finalization; fulfilling democratic principles regarding public input on governmental actions; and occasionally developing creative solutions beyond what regulators might independently devise through collaborative problem-solving among parties with different perspectives but shared interest in establishing workable protection systems.

Regulatory impact analysis systematically evaluates anticipated effects of proposed regulations, typically including both quantitative and qualitative assessment of costs, benefits, and distributional impacts across affected populations. Cost assessment addresses compliance expenditures including capital investment for engineering controls; ongoing operational expenses for maintenance, monitoring, and administrative requirements; productivity effects from work practice modifications or equipment changes; and potential innovation impacts when resources direct toward compliance rather than other business objectives. Benefits evaluation quantifies positive outcomes including reduced occupational illness and injury; decreased medical treatment costs; lowered workers' compensation expenses; enhanced productivity through reduced absenteeism and turnover; and occasionally secondary benefits like improved product quality from better controlled processes or environmental improvements from reduced emissions. Monetization approaches assign financial values to health outcomes through various methodologies including willingness-to-pay studies measuring individuals' valuation of risk reduction; cost-of-illness calculations incorporating medical expenses and productivity losses; and occasionally value-of-statistical-life figures derived from wage-risk studies or stated preference research. Uncertainty analysis acknowledges limitations in both cost and benefit projections, typically presenting ranges rather than point estimates while identifying key variables most significantly affecting outcomes. Distributional assessment examines how costs and benefits distribute across different stakeholders, including various industry sectors, business sizes, geographical regions, and worker populations, with particular attention to potential disparate impacts on economically vulnerable groups or communities with pre-existing environmental justice concerns. While sometimes criticized as overly emphasizing quantifiable factors at the expense of more difficult-to-measure health and social benefits, these analyses provide structured framework for considering regulatory consequences, supporting informed decision-making that considers both protection effectiveness and implementation impacts across diverse affected populations.

Summary

Occupational toxicology addresses workplace chemical exposures that affect millions of workers across diverse industries, requiring specialized approaches to recognition, evaluation, management, and prevention. Workplace exposures occur through inhalation, dermal contact, and ingestion routes, with inhalation predominating in industrial settings where particulates, gases, vapors, and fumes present significant hazards. Toxicological effects range from acute poisoning to chronic diseases with long latency periods, complicating recognition of causality. Industry-specific risks include silica and asbestos in construction and mining leading to pneumoconiosis and malignancies; solvents and heavy metals in manufacturing causing neurotoxicity, hepatotoxicity, and nephrotoxicity; pesticides in agriculture producing acute cholinergic crisis and potential chronic neurological effects; and unique healthcare exposures to chemotherapeutic agents, anesthetic gases, and disinfectants. Protection measures follow a hierarchical approach prioritizing elimination or substitution of hazardous substances when feasible, followed by engineering controls such as ventilation systems and process enclosure, administrative controls including work rotation and exposure monitoring, and personal protective equipment as the final defense line. Respiratory protection ranges from simple filtering facepieces to powered air-purifying respirators and supplied-air systems based on contaminant properties and concentration. Surveillance encompasses both environmental monitoring measuring workplace contaminant levels and biological monitoring assessing internal dose through biomarkers in blood, urine, or exhaled air. Medical surveillance programs combine periodic examinations, function testing, and exposure records to detect adverse effects before clinically apparent disease develops. Regulatory frameworks establish permissible exposure limits, require hazard communication through standardized systems like the Globally Harmonized System, mandate monitoring for certain substances, and establish medical removal provisions for workers showing early signs of toxicity. Occupational toxicologists must understand these complex interactions between workplace hazards, individual susceptibility factors, and regulatory requirements to effectively prevent, recognize, and manage work-related toxic exposures.

Self-Assessment Questions

1. Describe the hierarchy of controls approach to occupational exposures and provide specific examples of each control level for a workplace solvent exposure.
2. Compare and contrast the mechanisms, clinical manifestations, and management approaches for acute versus chronic occupational lead exposure.
3. Analyze the principles and implementation of a comprehensive biological monitoring program for workers exposed to organic solvents, including selection of appropriate biomarkers and interpretation guidelines.
4. Explain the pathophysiology, recognition, and management of occupational asthma, including both sensitizer-induced and irritant-induced mechanisms.
5. Discuss the special concerns and protection measures needed for hazardous drug handling in healthcare settings, including antineoplastic agents, hormonal medications, and other high-risk pharmaceuticals.
6. Describe the approach to evaluating workers with suspected occupational toxicity, including essential history elements, appropriate diagnostic testing, and determination of work-relatedness.
7. Analyze how regulatory exposure limits including Permissible Exposure Limits (PELs), Threshold Limit Values (TLVs), and Short-Term Exposure Limits (STELs) are established, utilized, and enforced.
8. Explain the principles of respiratory protection selection, including considerations for different contaminant types, concentration levels, and work conditions.
9. Discuss the challenges in recognizing and managing chronic low-level exposures to neurotoxicants in the workplace, including early detection strategies and prevention approaches.
10. Describe how occupational toxicologists contribute to disaster response scenarios involving chemical releases, including exposure assessment, decontamination decisions, and medical monitoring of responders

Bibliography

1. Blanc PD, Toren K. Occupation in chronic obstructive pulmonary disease and chronic bronchitis: an update. Int J Tuberc Lung Dis. 2007;11(3):251-257.
2. Bener A, Dogan M, Lestringant GG, Pasha MA, Al-Humaidi TR, Al-Ketbi J. Occupational and non-occupational risk factors for asthma and respiratory symptoms in adults. Eur J Intern Med. 2000;11(3):164-169.
3. Balmes J, Becklake M, Blanc P, Henneberger P, Kreiss K, Mapp C, et al. American Thoracic Society Statement: occupational contribution to the burden of airway disease. Am J Respir Crit Care Med. 2003;167(5):787-797.
4. Cullen MR, Redlich CA, Beckett WS, Weltmann B, Sparer J, Jackson G, et al. Feasibility study of respiratory questionnaire and peak flow recordings in autobody shop workers exposed to isocyanate-containing spray paint: observations and limitations. Occup Med (Lond). 1996;46(3):197-204.
5. Rosenstock L, Cullen MR, Brodkin CA, Redlich CA. Textbook of clinical occupational and environmental medicine. 2nd ed. Philadelphia: Elsevier Saunders; 2005.
6. Leung CC, Yu IT, Chen W. Silicosis. Lancet. 2012;379(9830):2008-2018.
7. Szeinuk J, Beckett WS, Clark N, Hailoo WL. Medical evaluation for respirator use. Am J Ind Med. 2000;37(1):142-157.
8. Cullen MR, Kominsky JR, Rossman MD, Cherniack MG, Rankin JA, Balmes JR, et al. Chronic beryllium disease in a precious metal refinery. Clinical epidemiologic and immunologic evidence for continuing risk from exposure to low level beryllium fume. Am Rev Respir Dis. 1987;135(1):201-208.
9. Cowie HA, Creely KS, Miller BG, Fowler K, Hurley F, Groat S, et al. A review of the literature on global dermal occupational exposure, with a focus on hand-arm-only exposures, to determine the suitability of undertaking a biological monitoring approach to exposure assessment. Edinburgh: Institute of Occupational Medicine; 2007.
10. National Toxicology Program. 14th Report on Carcinogens. Research Triangle Park, NC: U.S. Department of Health and Human Services, Public Health Service; 2016..

CHAPTER 12

ADDICTION AND SUBSTANCE ABUSE

Author

Miss Mishthi Prajapati, PharmD Scholar, Department of Pharmacy Practice, Parul Institute of Pharmacy & Research, Faculty of Pharmacy, Parul University, Vadodara, Gujarat, India

Abstract

E Addiction and substance abuse represent significant public health concerns with complex biological, psychological, and social dimensions requiring comprehensive understanding and management. Common drugs of abuse span multiple categories with distinct characteristics: stimulants like cocaine and amphetamines produce euphoria, increased energy, and sympathomimetic effects; opioids generate analgesia and euphoria while risking respiratory depression; sedative-hypnotics including benzodiazepines and alcohol cause anxiolysis and sedation; hallucinogens alter perception and cognition; and novel psychoactive substances continuously emerge to evade legal restrictions. Clinical manifestations of substance use disorders follow recognized patterns including compulsive use despite consequences, tolerance requiring escalating doses, withdrawal symptoms upon cessation, and neurobiological adaptations reflecting altered reward circuitry functioning. Acute intoxication and overdose present with substance-specific syndromes requiring targeted interventions, while chronic use leads to characteristic medical, psychological, and social complications. Treatment approaches incorporate pharmacological interventions including medication-assisted treatment for opioid and alcohol use disorders, psychosocial therapies spanning cognitive-behavioral approaches and motivational enhancement, and recovery support services delivered across a continuum from outpatient to residential settings. Prevention programs target different population levels, with universal strategies addressing entire communities, selective approaches focusing on high-risk groups, and indicated interventions targeting individuals showing early substance use patterns, all within a framework that addresses risk factors while enhancing protective factors.

Keywords: *Substance Use Disorder, Addiction, Medication-Assisted Treatment, Withdrawal, Intoxication, Harm Reduction*

Learning Objectives

After completion of the chapter, the learners should be able to:

- Differentiate between major categories of commonly abused substances based on their pharmacological properties, clinical effects, and patterns of use.
- Recognize the clinical manifestations of substance intoxication, withdrawal, and use disorders across different drug classes.
- Implement appropriate acute interventions for substance overdose including naloxone for opioids, benzodiazepines for stimulant toxicity, and supportive care tailored to specific substances.
- Develop comprehensive treatment plans incorporating pharmacological approaches, psychosocial interventions, and recovery support services appropriate to patient needs and substance use patterns.
- Compare the efficacy, indications, and limitations of medication-assisted treatments including methadone, buprenorphine, naltrexone, acamprosate, and disulfiram.
- Design evidence-based prevention strategies addressing substance use across the spectrum from primary prevention to harm reduction, with attention to developmental stages and population needs.

COMMON DRUGS OF ABUSE

Substance use disorders represent complex biopsychosocial conditions with diverse clinical presentations, neurobiology, and treatment implications across different substance categories.

Opioids

Opioids encompass both naturally occurring compounds derived from the opium poppy (Papaver somniferum), including morphine and codeine; semi-synthetic derivatives such as heroin, oxycodone, and hydrocodone; and fully synthetic agents including fentanyl, methadone, and tramadol. These substances produce their effects primarily through interaction with the μ-opioid receptor, with secondary activity at δ and κ receptors contributing to their complex pharmacological profile. Activation of these G-protein coupled receptors inhibits adenylyl cyclase, decreases neuronal excitability through potassium channel modulation, and reduces neurotransmitter release, collectively producing analgesia, euphoria, respiratory depression, and other characteristic effects. Acute intoxication typically manifests with pupillary constriction (miosis), reduced consciousness ranging from sedation to coma, respiratory depression, and constipation, though tolerance to many effects develops rapidly with repeated exposure. Individual substances demonstrate significant pharmacokinetic variation, with heroin (diacetylmorphine) showing rapid brain penetration through enhanced lipophilicity before metabolic conversion to active morphine; fentanyl and analogs demonstrating extreme potency (50-10,000 times morphine) through efficient receptor binding; and methadone exhibiting prolonged half-life (24-36 hours) creating both extended therapeutic duration and withdrawal challenges.

> **Remember**
>
> **Substance use disorders involve neurobiological changes in reward circuitry, executive function, and stress response systems, making addiction a chronic brain disorder requiring comprehensive medical and psychosocial treatment rather than simply a behavioral problem**

The evolving opioid epidemic demonstrates distinct phases reflecting changing availability and use patterns. Initial prescription opioid misuse expanded substantially in the late 1990s and early 2000s, driven by increased pharmaceutical marketing, shifting pain treatment paradigms emphasizing opioid therapy, and prescription practices often exceeding appropriate indications or durations. As regulatory restrictions and prescribing practice changes reduced prescription opioid availability, many individuals transitioned to heroin, which offered greater accessibility and lower cost despite increased use risks including uncertain purity, adulterant exposure, and injection-related complications. The current phase involves synthetic opioids, particularly illicitly manufactured fentanyl and its analogs, which have infiltrated both the heroin supply and counterfeit prescription tablet market. These highly potent compounds create extreme overdose risk due to their narrow therapeutic window, variability in illicit products, and rapid onset potentially outpacing naloxone rescue capability. This dynamic landscape necessitates evolving prevention, harm reduction, and treatment approaches addressing these shifting patterns while recognizing the persistent risk for cross-substance transition when availability changes occur.

Opioid tolerance, dependence, and addiction represent distinct but interrelated phenomena with important clinical implications. Tolerance develops through multiple mechanisms including receptor desensitization, internalization, and various intracellular adaptations, manifesting as diminishing effect with repeated dosing and requiring increased amounts to achieve comparable outcomes. Physical dependence represents neuroadaptation to continuous opioid presence, with homeostatic adjustments creating a new equilibrium state requiring continued substance exposure for normal functioning. Withdrawal emerges when this dependence faces abrupt discontinuation, producing a syndrome typically including autonomic hyperactivity (diaphoresis, piloerection, mydriasis), gastrointestinal distress (nausea, vomiting, diarrhea), generalized pain, and intense craving. While both tolerance and dependence represent expected physiological adaptations to repeated opioid exposure, addiction involves additional behavioral, cognitive, and psychological dimensions including compulsive use despite harmful consequences, impaired control over consumption, and preoccupation with obtaining and using the substance. This distinction explains why patients receiving appropriate long-term opioid therapy may develop tolerance and dependence without necessarily demonstrating addiction, though these phenomena certainly increase vulnerability when additional genetic, psychological, and environmental risk factors exist.

Overdose represents the most immediate life-threatening consequence of opioid misuse, with fatality primarily resulting from respiratory depression through μ-receptor mediated effects on brainstem respiratory centers. Risk factors include high-potency formulations, particularly illicitly manufactured fentanyl analogs; combined depressant use, especially with benzodiazepines or alcohol creating synergistic respiratory effects; decreased tolerance following periods of abstinence such as incarceration or treatment; solitary use without others present to intervene; and comorbid conditions affecting respiratory function including chronic obstructive pulmonary disease or sleep apnea. Clinical presentation typically involves the classic triad of respiratory depression, central nervous system depression, and miosis, though mixed presentations may occur with co-ingestants or in cases of severe hypoxia where pupillary response becomes less reliable. Management centers on respiratory support and opioid antagonism through naloxone, which competitively displaces opioids from receptors restoring respiratory drive. While historically administered primarily by medical personnel, expanding community-based naloxone distribution has demonstrated effectiveness in reducing overdose fatalities through enabling bystander response before professional assistance arrives. Implementation considerations include appropriate dosing for high-potency synthetic opioids potentially requiring multiple administrations; recognition of naloxone's shorter duration compared to many opioids necessitating extended monitoring; and withdrawal precipitation potentially causing distress and rarely, acute pulmonary edema or catecholamine surge with associated cardiovascular complications.

Table 12.1: Commonly Abused Substances and Their Effects

Substance Class	**Examples**	**Acute Effects**	**Chronic Effects**
Opioids	Heroin, fentanyl, oxycodone	Euphoria, sedation, respiratory depression, miosis	Physical dependence, constipation, immunosuppression
Stimulants	Cocaine, methamphetamine, MDMA	Euphoria, hyperalertness, tachycardia, hypertension, hyperthermia	Psychosis, cardiovascular disease, weight loss, dental problems
Sedative-hypnotics	Benzodiazepines, barbiturates, alcohol	Anxiolysis, sedation, disinhibition, respiratory depression	Cognitive impairment, physical dependence, tolerance
Cannabis	Marijuana, hashish, concentrates	Euphoria, relaxation, altered perception, increased appetite	Amotivational syndrome, potential cognitive effects, cannabinoid hyperemesis
Hallucinogens	LSD, psilocybin, DMT	Perceptual alterations, synesthesia, emotional lability	Hallucinogen persisting perception disorder (rare)

Stimulants

Cocaine, derived from Erythroxylum coca leaves, produces stimulant effects primarily through blocking reuptake of monoamine neurotransmitters (dopamine, norepinephrine, and serotonin) at synaptic sites, resulting in increased neurotransmitter availability and prolonged receptor activation. This mechanism differs from amphetamine-type stimulants, which both block reuptake and actively promote neurotransmitter release from presynaptic terminals, creating somewhat different clinical profiles though with substantial overlap. Available forms include cocaine hydrochloride powder typically used intranasally or dissolved for intravenous administration, and alkaloidal "crack" cocaine created through basic extraction enabling vaporization and inhalation. These different preparations create distinct pharmacokinetic profiles, with crack cocaine demonstrating particularly rapid onset (seconds) and brief duration (5-10 minutes) contributing to its highly reinforcing nature and characteristic binge use patterns. Acute effects include euphoria, increased energy, alertness, intense pleasure, and psychomotor agitation alongside physiological manifestations of sympathetic nervous system activation including tachycardia, hypertension, hyperthermia, mydriasis, and diaphoresis. Cocaine-associated medical emergencies primarily involve cardiovascular complications including arrhythmias, myocardial infarction, and hemorrhagic stroke resulting from combined vasoconstrictive effects, platelet activation, enhanced clotting cascade, and direct myocardial toxicity. Additional concerns include seizures through lowered seizure threshold, hyperthermia with potential progression to rhabdomyolysis and renal failure, and psychiatric manifestations including stimulant-induced psychosis characterized by paranoia, agitation, and occasionally hallucinations. Chronic use creates risk for nasal septum perforation with intranasal administration, pulmonary damage with inhalational use, and endocarditis or bloodborne infections with injection. Treatment approaches emphasize supportive care during acute intoxication, with benzodiazepines addressing agitation, seizures, and autonomic hyperactivity, while long-term management remains predominantly psychosocial with no FDA-approved pharmacotherapy specifically for cocaine use disorder.

Amphetamine-type stimulants include both pharmaceutical preparations (dextroamphetamine, lisdexamfetamine, methamphetamine) primarily prescribed for attention-deficit/hyperactivity disorder and narcolepsy, and illicitly manufactured forms, particularly crystal methamphetamine. These compounds increase synaptic concentrations of monoamine neurotransmitters through multiple mechanisms: inhibiting reuptake through transporter proteins, displacing stored neurotransmitters from vesicles, and directly reversing transporter direction causing neurotransmitter efflux into synapses.

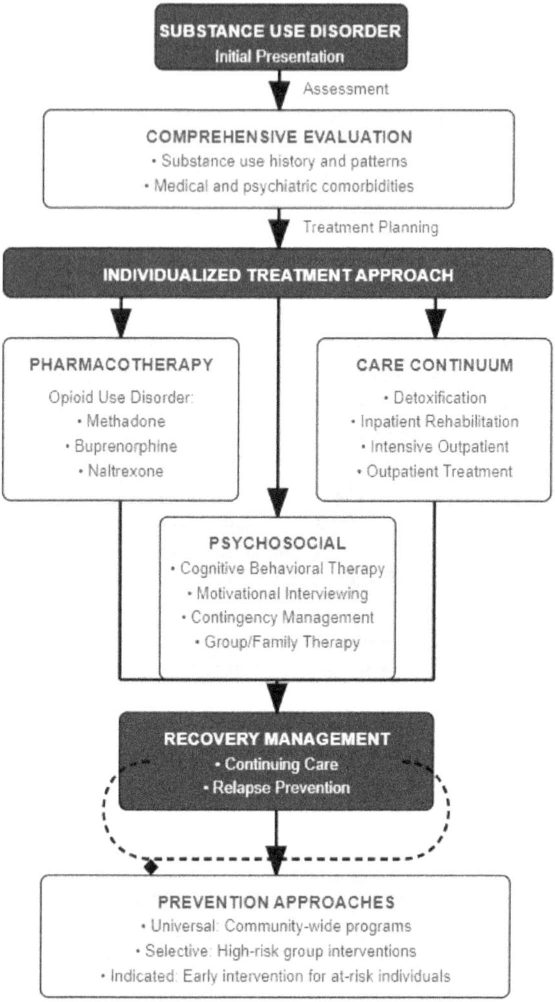

Figure 12.1: Substance Use Disorder Management

Methamphetamine demonstrates high lipophilicity creating rapid brain penetration and prolonged effects, with elimination half-life exceeding 12 hours compared to approximately 2 hours for dextroamphetamine. Route of administration significantly affects pharmacokinetics and associated risks, with oral consumption producing gradual onset over 30-60 minutes; intranasal use creating more rapid effects within 5-10 minutes; smoking enabling almost immediate central nervous system effects similar to intravenous administration while avoiding injection-related complications; and intravenous use creating most rapid and intense effects with associated infectious and vascular risks. Acute intoxication presents with sympathomimetic symptoms including tachycardia, hypertension, hyperthermia, mydriasis, and diaphoresis alongside behavioral manifestations ranging from increased energy, confidence, and sociability to agitation, paranoia, and occasionally frank psychosis with hallucinations and delusions. Medical complications mirror those of cocaine though with typically longer duration reflecting extended half-life, including cardiovascular emergencies, seizures, hyperthermia, and rhabdomyolysis. Distinctive to methamphetamine, chronic use frequently manifests with severe dental deterioration ("meth mouth") resulting from combined xerostomia, bruxism, poor oral hygiene, and sugar cravings; formication with resulting excoriation from sensation of insects crawling under the skin; and distinctive physical appearance changes through combined weight loss, skin picking, and premature aging. Treatment approaches primarily involve behavioral interventions, with limited evidence supporting certain pharmacotherapies including bupropion and naltrexone for reducing use and craving, though none have achieved FDA approval specifically for methamphetamine use disorder.

Novel psychoactive stimulants represent an evolving category including synthetic cathinones (colloquially termed "bath salts") and various phenethylamine derivatives designed to mimic traditional stimulant effects while temporarily circumventing drug control laws through structural modifications. Cathinone, the prototype compound naturally occurring in khat plant (*Catha edulis*) leaves, undergoes various synthetic alterations creating compounds including mephedrone, methylone, and 3,4-methylenedioxypyrovalerone (MDPV). These substances primarily increase synaptic monoamine concentrations through mechanisms similar to cocaine and amphetamines, though with varying selectivity for specific neurotransmitter systems creating diverse effect profiles. Typically marketed under misleading labels as "bath salts," "plant food," or "research chemicals" with deceptive "not for human consumption" disclaimers, these products gained popularity for their initial legal status, easy internet purchasing, and absence from standard drug screens. Clinical presentations generally resemble traditional stimulant intoxication but often with more pronounced psychiatric manifestations including severe agitation, paranoia, hallucinations, and occasionally violent behavior requiring physical restraint and chemical sedation. Medical complications mirror those of other stimulants but sometimes with greater severity, including hyperthermia, rhabdomyolysis, seizures, and cardiovascular emergencies potentially culminating in multi-organ failure. Management focuses on supportive care with benzodiazepines providing first-line treatment for agitation and autonomic hyperactivity, occasionally requiring addition of antipsychotics for severe psychiatric symptoms, while addressing specific complications including active cooling for hyperthermia, fluid resuscitation for rhabdomyolysis, and appropriate seizure management. Long-term treatment follows principles for other stimulant use disorders, though complicated by limited research specifically addressing these newer compounds and frequent polysubstance use patterns among affected individuals.

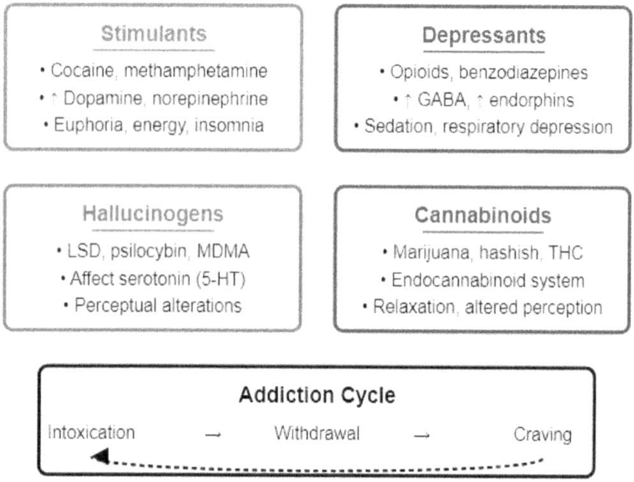

Figure 12.2: Common Drugs of Abuse and Their Effects

Prescription stimulants, primarily methylphenidate and amphetamine derivatives used in attention-deficit/hyperactivity disorder and narcolepsy treatment, create distinct patterns of misuse particularly among adolescents and young adults. Common motivations include performance enhancement through improved concentration during academic work; weight control through appetite suppression; recreational use seeking euphoria, particularly when administered through non-prescribed routes; and occasionally to counteract effects of other substances like alcohol, enabling greater consumption without sedation. While sharing basic pharmacological mechanisms with illicit stimulants, these pharmaceutical products contain known quantities of pure substances with predictable effects, creating somewhat lower risk profiles than illicitly manufactured counterparts, though still with significant concern for cardiovascular complications, psychiatric effects, and dependence with heavy use. Routes of non-medical administration include oral consumption of higher-than-prescribed doses; intranasal use through crushing tablets; and occasionally injection after dissolving tablets, with each non-oral route creating more rapid onset, greater intensity, and additional route-specific risks including nasal septum damage or injection-related complications. Prevention approaches focus on appropriate prescribing practices including thorough evaluation before initiation, regular monitoring during treatment, prescription drug monitoring program utilization, and education regarding diversion risks; educational initiatives targeting common misperceptions regarding safety of prescription versus illicit stimulants; and collegiate programs addressing academic pressure and providing alternative stress management approaches beyond substance use. Treatment primarily involves behavioral interventions similar to other stimulant use disorders, with particular attention to addressing underlying motivations including possible undiagnosed attention-deficit/hyperactivity disorder warranting appropriate evaluation and potentially legitimate pharmacotherapy rather than unmonitored self-medication.

Sedative-Hypnotics

Benzodiazepines represent a widely prescribed medication class with significant misuse potential, acting primarily through potentiation of gamma-aminobutyric acid (GABA) at GABAA receptors, enhancing chloride ion influx and resulting neuronal inhibition. Individual agents demonstrate substantial pharmacokinetic variation, with ultra-short-acting compounds (midazolam, triazolam) showing rapid onset and brief effect duration; intermediate-acting agents (alprazolam, lorazepam) with moderate duration; and long-acting compounds (diazepam, clonazepam) demonstrating prolonged effects often enhanced by active metabolites with extended half-lives. This pharmacokinetic diversity creates different clinical applications but also affects dependence development, withdrawal characteristics, and overall misuse patterns. Legitimate therapeutic indications include anxiety disorders, insomnia, seizure disorders, muscle spasms, alcohol withdrawal, and procedural sedation, though prescribing often extends beyond evidence-based applications into various off-label uses. Misuse patterns include medication overuse beyond prescribed parameters; recreational use for euphoric or calming effects; self-medication of untreated psychiatric conditions; and frequently, co-use with other substances either enhancing desired effects (typically with opioids or alcohol) or mitigating undesired effects of stimulants. Physical dependence develops relatively rapidly with regular use through adaptations in GABA receptor composition and function, creating risk for withdrawal syndromes ranging from rebound anxiety and insomnia with short-term use to potentially life-threatening complications including seizures and delirium with abrupt discontinuation after extended high-dose consumption. This withdrawal potential necessitates gradual tapering rather than abrupt cessation, with typical schedules reducing dosage by 5-10% weekly, though sometimes requiring much slower reductions for long-term, high-dose users. Management of benzodiazepine use disorder involves careful, supervised tapering, occasionally substituting longer-acting agents for short-acting compounds to reduce withdrawal fluctuations; addressing underlying conditions potentially driving use including untreated anxiety or insomnia; and implementing alternative evidence-based treatments for these conditions including cognitive-behavioral therapy and appropriate non-benzodiazepine pharmacotherapy.

Non-benzodiazepine sedative-hypnotics, including "Z-drugs" (zolpidem, zaleplon, eszopiclone) and older agents such as barbiturates and methaqualone, act primarily through GABA system modulation though with varying receptor subtype selectivity and binding sites creating somewhat different clinical profiles. Z-drugs were initially marketed as improvements over benzodiazepines with claims of reduced dependence potential and fewer next-day cognitive effects, though subsequent research demonstrated substantial similarity in both therapeutic and adverse effect profiles when equivalent doses were compared. These agents show particular popularity for insomnia treatment, with misuse patterns including dose escalation beyond prescribing parameters; intentional resistance to sleep onset to experience euphoriant effects; and use primarily for anxiolytic properties despite predominant marketing for insomnia. Barbiturates, while currently prescribed much less frequently than in previous decades, maintain limited legitimate indications including certain seizure disorders, procedural sedation, and occasionally severe insomnia unresponsive to safer alternatives. Their narrow therapeutic index creates significant overdose risk, particularly when combined with other central nervous system depressants, explaining their substantially reduced prescribing compared to historical patterns. Barbiturates maintain relevance in contemporary substance use treatment primarily through their inclusion in certain multi-ingredient products and occasionally being sought specifically for their more profound sedation compared to benzodiazepines. Methaqualone, though no longer legally manufactured in most countries, occasionally appears in illicit markets under various names including "Quaaludes," with continued demand reflecting its historical reputation for creating distinctive relaxation and sexual disinhibition. Management approaches for these diverse sedative-hypnotics follow principles similar to benzodiazepines, with gradual tapering for dependence, supportive care with possible flumazenil consideration for acute overdose (though with caution regarding seizure risk), and addressing underlying conditions driving use through evidence-based alternatives including cognitive-behavioral therapy for insomnia and appropriate non-sedative pharmacotherapy for anxiety disorders when indicated.

Gamma-hydroxybutyrate (GHB) and its precursors gamma-butyrolactone (GBL) and 1,4-butanediol (BD) represent substances with both limited legitimate medical applications and significant misuse patterns. GHB functions as an endogenous neurotransmitter at specific GHB receptors while also affecting GABA systems, creating a complex pharmacological profile. At lower doses, effects include euphoria, sociability, and mild disinhibition somewhat resembling alcohol intoxication; at higher doses, profound sedation and anesthesia can occur, with extremely narrow margin between desired effects and dangerous sedation explaining frequent overdose presentations. Legitimate medical uses include treatment of narcolepsy with cataplexy (sodium oxybate) and historically, surgical anesthesia in some European countries, while illicit use occurs primarily in nightlife settings and among bodybuilders for supposed growth hormone effects. Particularly concerning applications include use as a "date rape drug" due to rapid sedative properties, amnesia induction, and quick elimination limiting detection capability. Distinct from many sedative-hypnotics, GHB demonstrates extremely short half-life (30-60 minutes) creating characteristic brief but intense intoxication and, with regular use, a unique withdrawal syndrome necessitating frequent dosing to prevent symptoms. This withdrawal pattern creates considerable management challenges, potentially involving hourly dosing during initial stages, with symptoms including autonomic instability, tremor, anxiety, insomnia, and occasionally psychosis or delirium potentially persisting 1-2 weeks. Treatment approaches include benzodiazepines at high doses typically exceeding those for alcohol withdrawal; occasionally baclofen which affects GABA-B receptors similarly to GHB; and inpatient management for significant cases given the potential severity and rapid onset of withdrawal symptoms. Prevention efforts include both substance-focused education regarding narrow therapeutic window and detecting potential drink tampering, alongside environmental approaches in nightlife settings including improved monitoring, staff training regarding overdose recognition, and ensuring appropriate medical response capability for this uniquely challenging substance.

Alcohol, despite its legal status and cultural integration, functions pharmacologically as a sedative-hypnotic substance acting primarily through GABA enhancement and NMDA receptor inhibition, with complex additional effects on various neurotransmitter systems including dopamine, serotonin, and endogenous opioids explaining its diverse behavioral effects. Acute intoxication progresses from initial disinhibition, mild euphoria, and sociability at lower blood concentrations to significantly impaired coordination, judgment, and emotional regulation at moderate levels, potentially culminating in respiratory depression, unconsciousness, and rarely death at extremely high concentrations. Chronic heavy use creates adaptive changes throughout the central nervous system, including GABA receptor downregulation and NMDA receptor upregulation, establishing a new homeostatic state requiring alcohol presence for normal functioning. When alcohol is suddenly removed from this adapted system, withdrawal emerges with manifestations ranging from relatively mild symptoms (tremor, anxiety, insomnia, nausea) to severe presentations including seizures, hallucinations, and delirium tremens characterized by profound autonomic instability, confusion, and occasionally cardiovascular collapse. This withdrawal potential necessitates careful medical management, typically through benzodiazepine administration following symptom-triggered or fixed-schedule protocols, with dosing requirements occasionally reaching extremely high levels for individuals with significant tolerance. Beyond acute management, alcohol use disorder treatment typically involves psychosocial interventions including motivational enhancement, cognitive-behavioral approaches, and mutual help group participation, potentially supplemented by pharmacotherapy options including naltrexone reducing rewarding effects through opioid receptor antagonism; acamprosate normalizing glutamate neurotransmission; and disulfiram creating aversive reactions when alcohol is consumed through acetaldehyde accumulation. Long-term complications include hepatic disease ranging from fatty infiltration to cirrhosis; neurological damage manifesting as peripheral neuropathy, cerebellar degeneration, or cognitive impairment; cardiomyopathy; and significantly increased cancer risk at multiple sites including oropharyngeal, esophageal, hepatic, and colorectal tissues. This extensive complication profile combined with widespread availability and social acceptance creates unique challenges for both prevention and treatment, requiring integrated approaches addressing individual vulnerability, cultural factors, policy considerations, and healthcare system responses.

Cannabis and Hallucinogens

Cannabis contains numerous pharmacologically active compounds, with delta-9-tetrahydrocannabinol (THC) and cannabidiol (CBD) representing the most extensively studied constituents, though over 100 additional cannabinoids and various terpenes contribute to the complex effects profile. THC primarily acts as a partial agonist at cannabinoid

CB1 receptors concentrated in the central nervous system, while CBD demonstrates minimal direct CB1 activity but affects numerous other systems including serotonin receptors, GPR55, and various ion channels. Acute effects typically include euphoria, relaxation, altered sensory perception, impaired short-term memory, attention difficulties, increased appetite, dry mouth, conjunctival injection, and tachycardia. Individual responses vary considerably based on several factors: specific cannabis strain and resulting cannabinoid/terpene profile; THC:CBD ratio, with CBD potentially mitigating certain THC-induced effects including anxiety and psychosis; administration route affecting absorption rate and first-pass metabolism; individual tolerance status; and set and setting including expectations, environment, and psychological state. Available forms have diversified substantially with legalization in various jurisdictions, expanding beyond traditional plant material to include high-potency extracts like butane hash oil containing 60-90% THC compared to 15-25% in typical flower; manufactured edibles with delayed onset creating risk for overconsumption before initial effects manifest; and various vaporization methodologies reducing some respiratory risks associated with combustion while potentially introducing others through additives and heating element interactions. Medical applications continue expanding with varying evidence quality across conditions, including relatively strong support for chemotherapy-induced nausea, certain pain syndromes, and multiple sclerosis spasticity, alongside numerous conditions with more preliminary evidence. Potential complications include cannabis use disorder affecting approximately 10% of users with regular consumption patterns; cannabis hyperemesis syndrome characterized by cyclic vomiting paradoxically improved with hot showers and typically resolving with abstinence; exacerbation of certain psychiatric conditions, particularly psychotic disorders and possibly anxiety in vulnerable individuals; bronchitis and respiratory symptoms with smoked routes; potential developmental impacts with adolescent use; and driving impairment lasting several hours after consumption. Treatment approaches for cannabis use disorder remain predominantly psychosocial, including motivational enhancement, cognitive-behavioral therapy, and contingency management, with no currently approved pharmacotherapy despite investigation of various agents including N-acetylcysteine, gabapentin, and cannabinoid replacement approaches.

Classic hallucinogens, including lysergic acid diethylamide (LSD), psilocybin, mescaline, and dimethyltryptamine (DMT), produce their characteristic effects primarily through serotonin 5-HT2A receptor agonism, though with additional activity at various other serotonin receptor subtypes and sometimes dopaminergic or adrenergic systems.

These substances induce profound alterations in perception, cognition, and emotion without causing true hallucinations (perceptions without stimuli) in the strict sense, instead typically producing illusions, synesthesia (sensory cross-activation), and intensified perception of actually present stimuli. Physical effects remain relatively minimal compared to psychological manifestations, typically limited to pupillary dilation, modest increases in heart rate and blood pressure, occasionally tremor, and sometimes nausea particularly with plant-derived compounds like psilocybin mushrooms or peyote cactus containing mescaline. Psychologically, effects progress from initial sensory intensification and emotional lability to deeper alterations in thought processes, self-perception, and occasionally mystical-type experiences characterized by unity, transcendence, and ineffability at higher doses. Individual substances demonstrate different duration profiles: LSD typically lasting 8-12 hours; psilocybin 4-6 hours; DMT producing very brief but intense effects when smoked (15-30 minutes) or extended experiences lasting 3-5 hours when consumed as ayahuasca with monoamine oxidase inhibitors preventing gastrointestinal degradation. Adverse reactions primarily involve psychological distress including anxiety, paranoia, or frightening experiences during intoxication, with long-term complications generally uncommon except in vulnerable individuals with pre-existing or family history of psychotic disorders. Hallucinogen persisting perception disorder represents a rare but documented phenomenon involving continued visual disturbances sometimes persisting months or years after hallucinogen use, typically as visual snow, halos, or geometric patterns. Management of acute adverse reactions ("bad trips") emphasizes supportive care in calm environments with reassurance that effects will resolve, occasionally supplemented by benzodiazepines for severe anxiety or agitation when non-pharmacological approaches prove insufficient. Unlike many substances of abuse, classic hallucinogens demonstrate minimal addiction potential due to their non-dopaminergic mechanism, rapid tolerance development, and often psychologically challenging nature discouraging frequent use, though contemporary research investigating their therapeutic potential for conditions including depression, anxiety, and substance use disorders under controlled conditions represents a significant paradigm shift from previous research restrictions.

Dissociative anesthetics, including phencyclidine (PCP), ketamine, and dextromethorphan (DXM), produce altered consciousness characterized by detachment from environment and self through primarily uncompetitive NMDA receptor antagonism, though with additional effects on opioid, dopamine, and other neurotransmitter systems creating substance-specific effect profiles. Ketamine, originally developed as an anesthetic and maintaining legitimate medical applications including procedural sedation, treatment-resistant depression, and pain management, produces dose-dependent effects ranging from mild dissociation and mood elevation at lower doses to profound dissociation with immobility and perceived out-of-body experiences (the "k-hole") at higher amounts. PCP, though now rarely encountered compared to its 1970s-1980s prevalence, creates more pronounced sympathomimetic effects, longer duration (12-24 hours versus 1-2 hours for ketamine), and greater propensity for agitation and occasionally violent behavior during intoxication. Dextromethorphan, widely available in over-the-counter cough preparations, produces dissociative effects only at doses substantially exceeding therapeutic recommendations, typically staged by users from mild euphoria and perceptual changes at lower recreational doses to profound dissociation comparable to ketamine or PCP at high amounts. Complications include hypertensive emergencies, hyperthermia, rhabdomyolysis, and urinary tract pathology (particularly with chronic ketamine use), alongside behavioral risks during dissociated states potentially leading to accidents or victimization due to impaired judgment and motor control. Management of acute intoxication emphasizes supportive care addressing physiological disturbances, with benzodiazepines for agitation or sympathomimetic excess, while recognizing that excessive restraint of agitated individuals may worsen metabolic complications including hyperthermia and rhabdomyolysis. Treatment for chronic use focuses primarily on psychosocial interventions, though ketamine use disorder presents unique challenges through complex motivation patterns including self-medication for depression, recreational use for dissociative experiences, and sometimes legitimate prescribed use for treatment-resistant psychiatric conditions requiring careful differentiation between therapeutic application and problematic patterns.

Novel hallucinogens and designer psychedelics represent an evolving category including compounds developed to mimic classic hallucinogens while temporarily circumventing regulatory control through structural modifications. NBOMe compounds (25I-NBOMe, 25C-NBOMe) represent potent phenethylamine derivatives active at microgram doses similar to LSD but with significantly greater physiological complications including vasoconstriction, tachycardia, hypertension, hyperthermia, and seizures creating substantial morbidity and occasional mortality compared to traditional hallucinogens' relatively benign physiological profile. Synthetic cannabinoids, sometimes marketed as "Spice" or "K2," bind cannabinoid receptors with full agonist activity unlike THC's partial agonism, potentially creating more profound and unpredictable effects including psychosis, seizures, myocardial infarction, stroke, and kidney injury depending on the specific compound, which frequently changes as regulatory agencies identify and schedule particular formulations. These novel substances create substantial clinical challenges including unpredictable effects due to varying potency and composition even within products sharing identical branding; limited detection through standard toxicology screening necessitating specialized testing often unavailable in emergency settings; and evolving clinical presentations as new compounds continuously emerge replacing scheduled predecessors. Management emphasizes symptom-directed supportive care rather than specific antidotes, with benzodiazepines addressing agitation, seizures, and excessive sympathetic activation; active cooling for hyperthermia; and occasionally antipsychotics for severe psychiatric manifestations unresponsive to benzodiazepines alone. Prevention efforts include regulatory approaches rapidly scheduling identified compounds, though often struggling to keep pace with novel analog development; education regarding unpredictability and potentially severe complications compared to traditional counterparts; and addressing underlying factors driving use including curiosity, mislabeled products, or intended evasion of drug testing programs detecting more established substances.

CLINICAL MANIFESTATIONS

Substance use disorders manifest through characteristic patterns affecting biological, psychological, and social functioning across different stages of development and progression.

Acute Intoxication

The neurobiological basis of acute intoxication reflects diverse pharmacological mechanisms across substance classes, with manifestations reflecting specific receptor interactions and resulting neurotransmitter system alterations. Central nervous system depressants, including alcohol, benzodiazepines, and opioids, primarily enhance inhibitory neurotransmission through various mechanisms: alcohol potentiates gamma-aminobutyric acid (GABA) activity while inhibiting excitatory glutamate function; benzodiazepines specifically modulate GABAA receptors increasing chloride ion influx and resulting neuronal inhibition; and opioids activate mu-opioid receptors reducing neurotransmitter release throughout affected circuits. These inhibitory effects manifest as progressive central nervous system depression with dose-dependent impairment in psychomotor functioning, coordination, judgment, and eventually respiratory drive with sufficient doses. Stimulants including cocaine, amphetamines, and methylphenidate produce their characteristic effects through increasing synaptic concentrations of monoamine neurotransmitters (primarily dopamine, norepinephrine, and to varying degrees, serotonin) either by blocking reuptake transporters or stimulating release from neuronal storage vesicles. The resulting hyperactivation of these neurotransmitter systems creates both central manifestations including euphoria, increased alertness, and occasionally psychosis with higher doses, alongside peripheral sympathomimetic effects through noradrenergic stimulation. Hallucinogens and cannabis demonstrate more complex mechanisms: classic hallucinogens primarily affect serotonergic systems through 5-HT2A receptor agonism creating perceptual alterations and cognitive changes without significant vital sign abnormalities; while cannabis acts through cannabinoid receptor activation with additional effects across multiple neurotransmitter systems. This neurobiological diversity explains the distinctive intoxication syndromes across substance classes, though with considerable individual variation based on specific agent properties, dose, administration route, metabolism, and various host factors including genetic polymorphisms affecting drug-metabolizing enzymes.

Clinical assessment of acute intoxication integrates history, physical examination, and laboratory findings with recognition of characteristic toxidrome patterns. History collection, often challenging due to patient impairment or unreliable reporting, ideally addresses substance type, quantity, route, timing, and co-ingestion of other substances, supplemented by collateral information from companions, first responders, or available prescription databases.

Physical examination focuses on vital signs, mental status, pupillary response, and specific system findings suggesting particular substance involvement: miosis, respiratory depression, and decreased bowel sounds with opioids; mydriasis, hyperreflexia, hyperthermia, and diaphoresis with stimulants; horizontal nystagmus, ataxia, and dysarthria with sedative-hypnotics; and conjunctival injection with cannabis. Laboratory assessment may include toxicology screening though with important limitations including false positives, false negatives, varying detection windows across substances, and inability to establish causality between detected substances and clinical presentation. Additional testing focuses on potential complications including electrolyte disturbances, acid-base abnormalities, rhabdomyolysis, and end-organ damage based on specific substance properties. Intoxication assessment requires integration of these findings with knowledge of typical substance presentations, careful consideration of differential diagnoses including medical conditions mimicking intoxication (hypoglycemia, neurological emergencies, infectious processes), and recognition that polysubstance use frequently creates mixed clinical pictures not matching typical single-substance toxidromes.

Table 12.2: Diagnostic Criteria and Clinical Manifestations of Substance Use Disorders

Domain	Criteria	Clinical Indicators
Impaired control	Taking larger amounts than intended, unsuccessful attempts to cut down, excessive time spent obtaining/using/recovering, craving	Failed promises to limit use, increasing time dedicated to substance, intrusive thoughts about use
Social impairment	Failure to fulfill major role obligations, continued use despite social problems, reduced important activities	Work/school problems, relationship conflicts, abandoning hobbies
Risky use	Use in physically hazardous situations, continued use despite physical/psychological problems	DUI, using while operating machinery, continued use despite medical advice
Pharmacological indicators	Tolerance, withdrawal	Needing increased amounts for effect, characteristic withdrawal syndromes
Severity classification	Mild: 2-3 criteria Moderate: 4-5 criteria Severe: ≥6 criteria	Progressive impairment across multiple life domains

Management priorities in acute intoxication address immediate safety concerns while providing appropriate level of care based on presentation severity. Initial assessment follows standard emergency medicine principles emphasizing airway, breathing, and circulation with specific attention to respiratory depression with opioids and sedative-hypnotics; cardiovascular complications with stimulants; and aspiration risk with any substantial consciousness impairment. Specific antidotes or reversal agents apply in limited circumstances: naloxone for opioid-induced respiratory depression; flumazenil for isolated benzodiazepine overdose in appropriate clinical scenarios; and occasionally sodium bicarbonate for membrane-stabilizing agent toxicity. More commonly, management emphasizes supportive care addressing specific physiological disturbances: benzodiazepines for stimulant-induced agitation, hypertension, and hyperthermia; active cooling measures for severe hyperthermia; intravenous fluids for dehydration or hypotension; and occasionally chemical sedation or physical restraint when absolutely necessary for patient and staff safety with severely agitated presentations. Disposition decisions consider intoxication severity, presence of complications requiring specific interventions, co-occurring medical or psychiatric conditions, and social circumstances affecting safe discharge planning. This might range from brief emergency department observation with discharge once clinically stable for uncomplicated presentations, to intensive care admission for severe toxicity or complications, to psychiatric hospitalization when intoxication resolves but reveals underlying mental health concerns requiring immediate intervention.

Complications of acute intoxication vary significantly across substance classes, with recognition and prevention representing critical management components. Respiratory complications predominate with central nervous system depressants, ranging from hypoxemia through hypoventilation to complete respiratory arrest, particularly with combined depressant use creating synergistic effects beyond what individual substances might produce alone. Cardiovascular emergencies occur more commonly with stimulants, including arrhythmias, acute coronary syndromes, aortic dissection, and stroke through mechanisms including coronary vasospasm, enhanced platelet aggregation, increased myocardial oxygen demand, and blood pressure surges. Hyperthermia represents a particularly dangerous complication associated with stimulants, serotonergic agents, and certain novel psychoactive substances, potentially progressing to life-threatening levels through combined direct hypothalamic effects, increased muscle activity, and impaired heat dissipation mechanisms. Secondary trauma frequently complicates intoxication through impaired coordination, judgment, and risk perception, creating vulnerability for falls, motor vehicle accidents, and various injuries whose management may take precedence over the underlying intoxication. Mental status changes spanning from mild confusion to profound agitation or coma create risk for various complications including aspiration, rhabdomyolysis from prolonged immobility, self-injury during delirious states, and occasionally violent behavior threatening both patient and provider safety. Management approaches addressing these diverse complications must balance competing priorities including patient dignity, autonomy, and therapeutic relationship establishment with safety considerations, recognizing that overly restrictive or confrontational approaches may escalate rather than ameliorate behavioral disturbances while potentially creating additional iatrogenic complications.

Medical emergencies requiring specific recognition and management approaches occur with particular substance classes and use patterns. Stimulant-associated excited delirium represents a potentially life-threatening hyperadrenergic state characterized by hyperthermia, agitation, unusual strength, pain insensitivity, and acidosis, requiring aggressive intervention with benzodiazepines, active cooling, and careful attention to positional asphyxia risk during restraint. Opioid overdose with respiratory depression necessitates naloxone administration, with dosing considerations including the specific opioid involved (higher doses often required for fentanyl and analogs), previous opioid tolerance affecting withdrawal precipitation risk, and naloxone's shorter duration compared to many opioids potentially requiring repeated dosing or continuous infusion. Serotonin syndrome, occasionally occurring with various substances including certain antidepressants, MDMA, and some novel psychoactive compounds, presents with the triad of mental status changes, neuromuscular abnormalities (particularly clonus and hyperreflexia), and autonomic instability, requiring discontinuation of serotonergic agents and occasionally specific treatment with cyproheptadine for moderate to severe cases. Withdrawal syndromes emerging during intoxication assessment, particularly with alcohol or sedative-hypnotics, may necessitate appropriate prophylaxis or treatment alongside management of the presenting intoxication. Wernicke encephalopathy, an acute neurological emergency associated with alcohol use disorder, requires immediate thiamine administration before glucose to prevent precipitation or worsening of symptoms including encephalopathy, oculomotor dysfunction, and ataxia. Recognition and appropriate management of these specific emergencies requires both substance-specific knowledge and systematic assessment approaches identifying potentially life-threatening complications requiring immediate intervention beyond general supportive care.

Withdrawal Syndromes

Depressant withdrawal syndromes, including those associated with alcohol, benzodiazepines, and other sedative-hypnotics, represent potentially life-threatening conditions requiring careful assessment and often medical management. The underlying pathophysiology involves adaptive changes during chronic exposure, primarily GABAA receptor downregulation and NMDA receptor upregulation, creating a new homeostatic state dependent on continued substance presence. When the substance is removed, the resulting inhibitory/excitatory imbalance produces characteristic manifestations progressing from initial autonomic hyperactivity (tachycardia, hypertension, diaphoresis, tremor) and anxiety to more serious complications including seizures and delirium in severe cases. Alcohol withdrawal typically develops within 6-24 hours after last consumption, peaking around 24-72 hours and generally resolving within 5-7 days, though protracted symptoms may persist weeks longer. Benzodiazepine withdrawal follows similar patterns but with timeline dependent on specific agent half-life—short-acting compounds like alprazolam producing more rapid and intense withdrawal, while long-acting agents like diazepam creating more gradual but extended syndromes. Assessment employs both clinical evaluation and standardized tools like the Clinical Institute Withdrawal Assessment for Alcohol (CIWA-Ar) quantifying severity through measures of various symptoms including tremor, anxiety, agitation, headache, nausea, visual and auditory disturbances, and disorientation. Management typically involves benzodiazepine administration following either symptom-triggered protocols based on assessment scores or fixed-schedule approaches with gradual dose reduction, with specific considerations including cross-tolerance between different GABA-modulating substances; higher dosing requirements for individuals with significant tolerance; and adjunctive medications addressing specific symptoms including beta-blockers for autonomic hyperactivity, anticonvulsants for seizure prophylaxis, and antipsychotics for severe agitation or hallucinations when benzodiazepines alone prove insufficient. Nutritional support represents another critical component, particularly for alcohol withdrawal, with thiamine, folate, multivitamins, and electrolyte repletion addressing common deficiencies and reducing complication risk.

Opioid withdrawal, while not typically life-threatening unlike sedative-hypnotic withdrawal, creates significant morbidity and represents a major barrier to recovery through its severe discomfort driving continued use despite adverse consequences. Physiologically, chronic opioid exposure produces compensatory adaptations including upregulation of adenylyl cyclase activity, which becomes unmasked during withdrawal when opioid inhibition suddenly ceases. The resulting noradrenergic hyperactivity primarily drives withdrawal manifestations including rhinorrhea, lacrimation, piloerection, diaphoresis, mydriasis, gastrointestinal distress (nausea, vomiting, diarrhea), abdominal cramping, muscle and joint pain, anxiety, and intense craving. Onset timing depends on specific opioid properties—short-acting agents like heroin typically producing symptoms within 8-12 hours after last use, while longer-acting substances like methadone may not produce significant withdrawal until 24-48 hours after discontinuation. Duration similarly varies by specific agent, generally 5-7 days for short-acting opioids but potentially several weeks with methadone. Assessment employs both clinical evaluation and standardized tools including the Clinical Opiate Withdrawal Scale (COWS) quantifying severity through measures of various signs and symptoms including pulse rate, pupillary dilation, gastrointestinal distress, tremor, yawning, anxiety, and pain. Management approaches include both symptomatic treatment and opioid replacement strategies. Symptomatic approaches employ medications addressing specific manifestations: clonidine or lofexidine for autonomic symptoms; antiemetics for nausea; loperamide for diarrhea; NSAIDs or acetaminophen for pain; and occasionally trazodone or hydroxyzine for insomnia. Alternatively, opioid agonist therapy with methadone or buprenorphine effectively prevents withdrawal while providing opportunity for stabilization, developing treatment engagement, and potentially long-term maintenance preventing return to illicit use. These approaches are not mutually exclusive, with many programs employing adjunctive medications alongside agonist therapy, particularly for breakthrough symptoms during induction or dose adjustment periods.

Stimulant withdrawal, often termed "crash" or "comedown," primarily manifests through neurovegetative symptoms including fatigue, hypersomnia, increased appetite, anhedonia, dysphoria, and intense craving, reflecting neuroadaptation to chronic dopaminergic stimulation with subsequent depletion after substance discontinuation. While lacking the potentially dangerous physiological manifestations of depressant withdrawal, stimulant abstinence creates significant psychological distress and functional impairment through profound mood disturbance occasionally reaching severity warranting suicidality assessment. Methamphetamine withdrawal typically lasts longer than cocaine (potentially 2-3 weeks versus 7-10 days) reflecting different half-lives and neurochemical effects, though with substantial individual variation based on use patterns, amount, and duration. Assessment focuses primarily on clinical evaluation without widely validated standardized scales comparable to those used for opioid or alcohol withdrawal, though some specialized tools like the Amphetamine Withdrawal Questionnaire provide structured evaluation frameworks. Management approaches remain largely supportive without FDA-approved medications specifically for stimulant withdrawal, typically including structured daily activities minimizing isolation and rumination; supportive counseling addressing intense craving; sleep hygiene measures addressing initial insomnia often followed by hypersomnia; and nutritional support addressing both appetite changes and often significant self-neglect during active use periods. Various medications have undergone investigation without clear consensus regarding efficacy, including modafinil for fatigue and cognitive impairment; mirtazapine or trazodone for sleep disturbance; antipsychotics for agitation or psychotic symptoms sometimes persisting during early abstinence; and various dopaminergic agents hypothetically addressing reward system dysregulation. Regardless of specific pharmacological approach, recognition of post-acute withdrawal extending beyond acute physical symptoms represents a critical factor in treatment planning, with persistent anhedonia, executive function impairment, and episodic craving potentially continuing months into recovery and requiring ongoing support and monitoring during this vulnerable period.

Cannabis withdrawal has gained increasing recognition alongside changing usage patterns, with higher-potency products, increased daily consumption, and concentrated extracts creating greater physiological dependence potential than historically observed. The syndrome typically emerges within 24-72 hours after cessation in heavy users, peaking around days 4-6 and gradually resolving over 1-2 weeks, though sleep disturbance and other subtle symptoms occasionally persist longer. Common manifestations include irritability, anxiety, depressed mood, restlessness, insomnia or disturbing dreams, decreased appetite, headache, and various somatic symptoms including sweating, chills, and gastrointestinal discomfort. While rarely requiring medical management, cannabis withdrawal creates significant discomfort potentially undermining abstinence attempts, particularly when individuals misattribute symptoms to underlying conditions that cannabis was supposedly treating rather than recognizing them as temporary withdrawal manifestations. Assessment primarily involves clinical evaluation, though standardized instruments including the Cannabis Withdrawal Scale provide structured documentation and severity quantification useful for both clinical management and research contexts. Management approaches include psychological support and education regarding expected symptoms and timeline; temporary symptomatic medications addressing specific manifestations like sleep disturbance or anxiety when severe; and occasionally gradual tapering rather than abrupt cessation for highly dependent individuals. Various pharmacological interventions have undergone investigation without definitive evidence supporting any single approach, including dronabinol (synthetic THC) for suppressing withdrawal through replacement similarly to nicotine replacement in tobacco cessation; gabapentin for addressing irritability and sleep disturbance; and various mood stabilizers or antidepressants targeting emotional symptoms. The most important clinical considerations involve accurately diagnosing withdrawal rather than misattributing symptoms to other conditions; providing realistic expectations regarding duration and intensity; and distinguishing withdrawal management from longer-term cannabis use disorder treatment, which typically requires more extensive psychosocial intervention addressing underlying use motivations and developing alternative coping strategies beyond temporary withdrawal symptom management.

Atypical and polysubstance withdrawal presents particular clinical challenges through complex symptom patterns, unpredictable timelines, and potential medical complications beyond those typically associated with single-substance withdrawal. Hallucinogen and dissociative withdrawal remains somewhat controversial, with classic hallucinogens like LSD and psilocybin demonstrating minimal evidence for physiological dependence or withdrawal syndromes despite their profound acute effects. However, MDMA and related entactogens may produce post-use syndromes including depressed mood, fatigue, and cognitive impairment reflecting serotonin depletion, though these typically resolve spontaneously with abstinence and supportive care. Dissociative substances like ketamine and phencyclidine demonstrate more clearly established withdrawal phenomena with regular use, including anxiety, tremor, autonomic instability, and intense craving potentially complicated by perceptual disturbances during early abstinence. Novel psychoactive substances create particularly unpredictable withdrawal presentations due to limited clinical experience, unknown specific pharmacological properties, and frequent adulteration or misrepresentation of products. Polysubstance dependence, extremely common in clinical practice, creates compound withdrawal syndromes requiring careful assessment to identify all contributing substances and prioritize management based on relative danger and symptom severity. Particular challenges include distinguishing between manifestations of different substance withdrawals occurring simultaneously; identifying appropriate medication approaches when cross-tolerance exists between substances; and managing potentially dangerous interactions between withdrawal states, such as the epileptogenic potential of stimulant withdrawal potentially exacerbating seizure risk during concurrent sedative-hypnotic withdrawal. Management approaches necessarily involve comprehensive assessment identifying all substances used regularly; prioritization addressing most medically dangerous withdrawals first (typically alcohol and sedative-hypnotics); careful monitoring for emerging symptoms of secondary withdrawals as primary symptoms resolve; and flexible treatment planning capable of addressing unexpected manifestations as they develop. These complex presentations typically benefit from inpatient or residential management settings providing continuous monitoring and immediate intervention capability rather than outpatient approaches more suitable for predictable single-substance withdrawal with lower complication risk.

Long-Term Effects

Neurobiological adaptations to chronic substance use create persistent changes affecting cognitive function, emotional regulation, and behavioral control beyond acute intoxication or withdrawal. Structurally, various substances produce distinctive patterns of brain volume alterations visible through neuroimaging: alcohol typically demonstrates ventricular enlargement, cortical thinning particularly in frontal regions, and cerebellar volume reduction; stimulants including cocaine and methamphetamine show reduced gray matter volume in prefrontal cortex, striatum, and limbic structures; and opioids associate with white matter abnormalities and altered connectivity between reward regions and prefrontal control areas. Functionally, these structural changes manifest through disrupted neural circuits involved in reward processing, executive function, stress response, and interoceptive awareness. The mesocorticolimbic dopamine system, central to reward processing and motivation, undergoes significant adaptation with chronicity including receptor downregulation, altered dopamine release patterns, and compensatory changes in downstream signaling cascades. These adaptations help explain various clinical phenomena including diminished response to natural rewards (anhedonia), enhanced salience of substance-related cues (craving), and impaired inhibitory control over consumption. Importantly, these neurobiological changes demonstrate significant but incomplete reversibility with sustained abstinence, with recovery trajectories varying substantially based on specific substance, use duration and intensity, individual genetic factors, and various protective elements including cognitive reserve and neuroplasticity capacity. Understanding these neuroadaptive changes provides biological context for behavioral manifestations observed clinically while supporting conceptualization of substance use disorders as chronic brain conditions requiring long-term management approaches rather than expecting immediate normalization upon achieving initial abstinence.

Cognitive impairment associated with substance use disorders spans multiple domains with both substance-specific patterns and common features across different agents. Executive function deficits represent particularly consistent findings, manifesting as difficulties with planning, working memory, cognitive flexibility, response inhibition, and decision-making—functions predominantly supported by prefrontal cortical regions particularly vulnerable to substance-related neurotoxicity. Memory impairment varies across substances, with alcohol demonstrating both encoding and retrieval deficits potentially progressing to Korsakoff syndrome with thiamine deficiency; cannabis showing immediate recall impairment with relative preservation of delayed recall; and MDMA associated with verbal memory deficits correlating with use frequency and lifetime consumption. Processing speed reductions commonly occur with multiple substances including alcohol, methamphetamine, and heroin, while attention deficits demonstrate particular prominence with stimulant withdrawal despite these substances' acute attention-enhancing effects. Importantly, cognitive deficits significantly impact treatment outcomes through multiple mechanisms: impairing comprehension of therapeutic material; reducing benefit from cognitive-behavioral interventions requiring abstract reasoning and cause-effect analysis; limiting medication adherence through prospective memory difficulties; and creating functional impairments potentially triggering relapse when frustration tolerance diminishes. Clinical approaches addressing these cognitive manifestations include cognitive rehabilitation techniques; cognitive remediation therapy targeting specific deficit areas; psychoeducation helping patients understand cognitive symptoms as substance effects rather than personal failings; structured approaches compensating for executive dysfunction through external organizational systems; and occasionally pharmacological interventions although with limited evidence for most agents beyond treating comorbid conditions like ADHD or depression potentially contributing to cognitive symptoms. Longitudinal studies demonstrate significant but typically incomplete cognitive recovery with sustained abstinence, with improvement trajectories varying across domains—attention and processing speed often showing earlier improvement than more complex executive functions requiring extended neural network reorganization.

Medical complications of chronic substance use create significant morbidity and mortality while frequently complicating addiction treatment through bidirectional interactions where substance use worsens medical conditions while medical symptoms potentially trigger continued use for self-medication or pain relief. Cardiovascular complications include cardiomyopathy and arrhythmias with alcohol and stimulants; bacterial endocarditis with injection drug use; coronary artery disease accelerated by cocaine and methamphetamine; and hypertension exacerbated by various substances including alcohol and stimulants. Pulmonary manifestations range from chronic bronchitis and emphysema with smoked substances including tobacco, cannabis, and crack cocaine, to pulmonary arterial hypertension with stimulants, to various infectious complications including tuberculosis and pneumonia occurring at higher rates among individuals with substance use disorders. Hepatic disease predominantly associates with alcohol (fatty liver, alcoholic hepatitis, cirrhosis) and injection drug use (viral hepatitis), while renal complications occur with various substances including heroin-associated focal segmental glomerulosclerosis and cocaine-induced accelerated hypertensive nephropathy. Infectious disease burden among individuals with substance use disorders substantially exceeds general population rates, reflecting combined immunological effects of certain substances, injection-related exposures, and various social determinants including homelessness, incarceration, and healthcare access barriers. Neurological complications include peripheral neuropathy (alcohol, certain opioids), seizure disorders (alcohol withdrawal, stimulant use), and cerebrovascular events (stimulants, particularly cocaine). Endocrine disruption manifests variously including alcohol-related hypogonadism, opioid-induced hypogonadism and adrenal insufficiency, and cannabis effects on reproductive hormones. Integrating addiction and medical care becomes essential given these complex interactions, with approaches including coordinated care models addressing both conditions simultaneously; medication-assisted treatment options compatible with medical comorbidities; pain management strategies appropriate for individuals with opioid use disorders; and comprehensive harm reduction addressing infectious disease risks alongside substance use intervention.

Psychiatric comorbidity represents the norm rather than exception among individuals with substance use disorders, with bidirectional relationships where mental health conditions increase addiction vulnerability while substance use exacerbates psychiatric symptoms. Epidemiological data consistently demonstrate elevated rates of major depressive disorder, bipolar disorder, anxiety disorders, post-traumatic stress disorder, attention-deficit/hyperactivity disorder, and personality disorders among individuals with substance use disorders compared to general population rates. These associations reflect multiple potential mechanisms including shared genetic vulnerability factors; self-medication of psychiatric symptoms; substance-induced neurobiological changes affecting emotional regulation circuits; and common environmental risk factors including trauma exposure, early life adversity, and chronic stress. Diagnostic challenges include distinguishing between independent psychiatric conditions versus substance-induced disorders that may remit with sustained abstinence;

recognizing the potential for substances to mimic psychiatric symptoms during intoxication or withdrawal; and evaluating psychiatric symptoms during periods of active substance use when manifestations frequently appear mixed or atypical. Treatment approaches for co-occurring disorders have evolved substantially from sequential models (treating one condition before addressing the other) to parallel models (separate treatment systems simultaneously addressing each condition) to contemporary integrated approaches addressing both conditions within unified treatment frameworks. Evidence supports several principles for effective management including comprehensive assessment before definitive psychiatric diagnosis; stabilization of acute substance use before finalizing psychiatric treatment plans when feasible; consideration of medication options less likely to be misused or with lower interaction risk; psychotherapeutic approaches addressing both conditions such as integrated cognitive-behavioral therapy; and longitudinal monitoring recognizing that symptom presentations may shift substantially during early recovery requiring treatment plan adjustments. Despite significant advances in understanding these complex relationships, implementation gaps remain with many treatment systems still inadequately equipped to address the full spectrum of co-occurring psychiatric and substance use conditions.

Social and functional consequences of substance use disorders extend beyond direct physiological and psychological effects, often persisting long after achieving abstinence and creating significant barriers to recovery. Occupational impacts include reduced productivity, increased absenteeism, workplace accidents, and employment instability, potentially progressing to long-term unemployment with associated financial distress, skill erosion, and diminished self-efficacy. Relationship disruption spans family, romantic, and social connections, with substance-centered behavior patterns, emotional unavailability, trust violations, and sometimes financial exploitation or interpersonal violence creating profound relationship damage requiring extended healing even after establishing stable recovery. Legal consequences ranging from criminal charges directly related to substance possession or distribution to secondary legal issues including driving under the influence, public intoxication, or various offenses committed while obtaining or using substances create barriers including incarceration, criminal records limiting housing and employment opportunities, financial penalties depleting recovery resources, and ongoing legal system involvement through probation or parole requirements. Housing instability and homelessness disproportionately affect individuals with substance use disorders through combined factors including income reduction, relationship dissolution eliminating shared housing options, discrimination from potential landlords, and eviction histories. Stigma compounds these functional impacts through both public stigma creating systematic discrimination and self-stigma internalizing negative societal views, potentially leading to diminished help-seeking, identity narrowing to substance-using roles, and reduced hope for meaningful recovery. Comprehensive treatment approaches must address these multidimensional consequences through interventions including vocational rehabilitation, family therapy, legal assistance, supportive housing programs, stigma reduction initiatives, and community integration support helping individuals rebuild functional lives beyond abstinence alone. Recovery capital—the internal and external resources supporting sustained recovery—provides a useful framework for assessing and enhancing these social and functional domains, recognizing that building stable recovery typically requires addressing these broader life dimensions rather than focusing exclusively on substance use itself.

TREATMENT METHODS

Effective addiction treatment integrates multiple modalities addressing the complex biological, psychological, and social dimensions of substance use disorders.

Detoxification and Stabilization

Medically supervised withdrawal management provides safe transition from active substance use to abstinence through systematic monitoring and appropriate pharmacotherapy addressing withdrawal syndromes. Alcohol withdrawal management typically employs benzodiazepines following either symptom-triggered protocols based on standardized assessment tools like the Clinical Institute Withdrawal Assessment for Alcohol (CIWA-Ar), or fixed-schedule approaches with predetermined dosing and gradual tapering. Benzodiazepine selection considerations include long-acting agents like diazepam or chlordiazepoxide providing smoother withdrawal through self-tapering metabolites versus shorter-acting agents like lorazepam or oxazepam offering advantages for patients with hepatic impairment. Adjunctive medications addressing specific symptoms include anticonvulsants providing seizure prophylaxis while potentially reducing benzodiazepine requirements; beta-blockers or clonidine for autonomic hyperactivity; and occasionally antipsychotics for severe agitation or hallucinations unresponsive to adequate benzodiazepine dosing. Opioid withdrawal management employs either abstinence-based approaches using adjunctive medications addressing specific symptoms (clonidine or lofexidine for autonomic symptoms, NSAIDs for pain, antiemetics for nausea), or opioid agonist approaches using methadone or buprenorphine to prevent withdrawal while enabling stabilization. Sedative-hypnotic withdrawal requires careful assessment identifying specific agents involved, typical consumption patterns, and previous withdrawal history, with management typically involving substituting longer-acting benzodiazepines for shorter-acting agents or other GABAergic substances, followed by gradual dose reduction at rates of approximately 10-25% weekly depending on individual factors. Setting determination weighs multiple factors including withdrawal severity, medical comorbidities, psychiatric stability, previous withdrawal complications, social support, and outpatient monitoring feasibility, with options ranging from outpatient management for less severe presentations to inpatient or residential care for complex cases or those with significant risk factors for complicated withdrawal.

> **Remember**
>
> **Medication-assisted treatment combines pharmacotherapy with psychosocial interventions, with established efficacy for opioid use disorder (methadone, buprenorphine, naltrexone) and alcohol use disorder (naltrexone, acamprosate, disulfiram).**

Pharmacological approaches for maintaining abstinence and reducing relapse risk vary substantially across different substance use disorders. For alcohol use disorder, FDA-approved medications include naltrexone (oral or extended-release injectable) blocking opioid receptors and reducing alcohol's rewarding effects; acamprosate normalizing glutamate neurotransmission disrupted by chronic alcohol exposure; and disulfiram creating aversive reactions when alcohol is consumed through acetaldehyde accumulation, though with limited evidence for effectiveness outside highly structured settings ensuring medication adherence. For opioid use disorder, medication treatment options include methadone, a full μ-opioid receptor agonist administered through specialized opioid treatment programs; buprenorphine, a partial agonist available through office-based prescribing by qualified providers; and extended-release naltrexone, an opioid antagonist requiring complete abstinence before initiation. These medications demonstrate substantial evidence for reducing illicit opioid use, overdose risk, infectious disease transmission, and overall mortality, with effect sizes exceeding many other medical interventions. For tobacco use disorder, nicotine replacement therapies in various formulations (patch, gum, lozenge, inhaler, nasal spray) reduce withdrawal symptoms while eliminating combustion-related toxins; bupropion affects dopaminergic and noradrenergic systems reducing craving and withdrawal; and varenicline acts as a partial agonist at nicotinic acetylcholine receptors, both reducing withdrawal symptoms and blocking reward from smoking if relapse occurs. Despite extensive research, no FDA-approved pharmacotherapies currently exist specifically for stimulant, cannabis, or hallucinogen use disorders, though various medications including modafinil, bupropion, naltrexone, and topiramate have shown limited or mixed evidence requiring further investigation. Off-label prescribing addressing specific symptoms, cravings, or comorbid conditions frequently occurs in clinical practice despite limited disorder-specific evidence, highlighting the need for continued medication development research addressing these treatment gaps.

Psychosocial interventions during early recovery focus on establishing initial abstinence, developing immediate coping strategies, addressing ambivalence, and building therapeutic alliance supporting continued treatment engagement. Motivational interviewing employs a directive yet client-centered approach exploring and resolving ambivalence about change through reflective listening, developing discrepancy between current behavior and broader goals, rolling with resistance rather than direct confrontation, and supporting self-efficacy. This approach shows particular value during initial engagement when ambivalence remains high, with evidence supporting both standalone effectiveness for milder substance use disorders and enhanced outcomes when integrated with other treatment modalities for more severe presentations. Contingency management provides tangible reinforcement for specific target behaviors, typically documented abstinence through biological testing, with reinforcers including vouchers exchangeable for retail goods, prize drawings, or clinic privileges. This approach demonstrates among the largest effect sizes of any behavioral intervention across multiple substances, though implementation challenges include funding limitations for reinforcers, sustainability concerns after contingencies end, and occasional philosophical objections to providing external rewards for recovery behaviors. Cognitive-behavioral approaches address substance-related thoughts and behaviors through structured interventions identifying high-risk situations, developing coping skills, challenging dysfunctional beliefs, and practicing alternative responses. These interventions demonstrate effectiveness across various substances and delivery formats, with particular value for developing specific skills addressing individual relapse vulnerabilities. Acceptance and commitment therapy, a third-wave cognitive-behavioral approach, emphasizes psychological flexibility through mindfulness, acceptance of urges without acting on them, clarification of personal values, and committed action aligned with these values rather than controlled by momentary urges. This approach offers particular advantages for individuals struggling with traditional thought-challenging approaches or experiencing intense cravings that prove difficult to directly suppress or control.

Withdrawal complications requiring specialized management approaches occur across different substance classes, necessitating careful monitoring and appropriate intervention protocols. Alcohol withdrawal delirium (delirium tremens) represents a medical emergency characterized by profound confusion, hallucinations, severe autonomic instability, and potential progression to cardiovascular collapse if inadequately treated. Management requires aggressive benzodiazepine administration, often at doses substantially exceeding typical therapeutic ranges, with potential need for intensive care monitoring addressing complications including fluid and electrolyte disturbances, hyperthermia, and occasionally respiratory support. Benzodiazepine withdrawal seizures typically occur early in the withdrawal course, requiring both immediate seizure management and evaluation for underlying seizure threshold-lowering factors potentially complicating standard withdrawal protocols. Protracted withdrawal syndromes extending beyond acute physiological stabilization create significant relapse risk, with manifestations varying across substances: post-acute alcohol withdrawal potentially including anxiety, insomnia, and cognitive difficulties persisting weeks to months; protracted opioid abstinence syndrome featuring dysphoria, sleep disturbance, and temperature dysregulation; and extended cannabis withdrawal occasionally including mood disturbance and sleep architecture disruption beyond expected acute withdrawal resolution. Management approaches include patient education normalizing these experiences as expected recovery phases rather than permanent conditions or signs of underlying pathology; targeted symptomatic medication for specific manifestations significantly impacting functioning or recovery engagement; and occasionally consideration of maintenance pharmacotherapy when protracted symptoms create substantial relapse risk despite adequate psychosocial support. Polysubstance withdrawal creates particular complexity through overlapping or sequential syndromes requiring careful assessment distinguishing between manifestations of different substance withdrawals versus complications or emerging psychiatric symptoms, with management typically prioritizing most medically dangerous withdrawals first while maintaining vigilance for emerging symptoms of secondary withdrawals as initial symptoms resolve.

Transitional services bridging the gap between detoxification and longer-term treatment represent critical components addressing the vulnerability period following physiological stabilization. Patient placement criteria guide appropriate level of care determination based on multiple dimensions including acute intoxication/withdrawal potential, biomedical conditions, emotional/behavioral conditions, readiness for change, relapse potential, and recovery environment.

Table 12.3: Evidence-Based Treatment Approaches for Substance Use Disorders

Treatment Type	Specific Interventions	Applications
Pharmacotherapy	Opioid use disorder: Methadone, buprenorphine, naltrexone Alcohol use disorder: Naltrexone, acamprosate, disulfiram Tobacco use disorder: NRT, bupropion, varenicline	Moderate to severe physical dependence, relapse prevention
Behavioral therapies	Cognitive-behavioral therapy Contingency management Motivational enhancement therapy 12-step facilitation Community reinforcement	Addressing psychological aspects, developing coping skills, enhancing motivation
Psychosocial supports	Recovery housing Peer support services Vocational services Case management	Social stabilization, ongoing recovery support
Treatment settings	Outpatient Intensive outpatient Partial hospitalization Residential/inpatient Medically managed inpatient	Setting should match severity, withdrawal risk, comorbidities, and recovery environment

These criteria support matching treatment intensity to individual needs rather than applying uniform approaches across heterogeneous patient populations. Integrated assessment during withdrawal management evaluates factors beyond immediate physiological stabilization, including psychiatric comorbidity, cognitive functioning, social support systems, housing stability, and readiness for different treatment approaches. Case management services coordinate transition between levels of care, addressing practical barriers potentially interrupting treatment continuity including transportation needs, insurance authorization, childcare arrangements, and employment considerations. Motivational enhancement during this transition period addresses the common phenomenon of waning motivation once acute withdrawal resolves, with specific focus on developing personalized understanding of substance-related consequences, exploring ambivalence, and establishing concrete next steps maintaining treatment momentum. Overdose prevention education provides crucial harm reduction intervention before discharge, including naloxone distribution and training for individuals with opioid use disorders, recognition of tolerance reduction following abstinence periods, and specific guidance regarding particular risk factors including polysuppressant use and using when alone. These transitional components collectively address the substantial drop-off commonly occurring between detoxification completion and longer-term treatment engagement, recognizing that physiological stabilization alone rarely provides sufficient intervention for sustainable recovery without appropriate continuing care addressing the complex psychological, social, and behavioral dimensions of substance use disorders.

Behavioral Therapies

Cognitive-behavioral approaches represent extensively studied interventions addressing the thoughts, emotions, and behaviors maintaining substance use disorders. Core elements include functional analysis identifying specific triggers for substance use, thoughts and beliefs surrounding substances, and reinforcement patterns maintaining behavior; skills training developing alternative coping strategies for high-risk situations previously handled through substance use; cognitive restructuring challenging distorted thinking patterns supporting continued use despite consequences; and relapse prevention planning identifying potential high-risk situations and developing specific response strategies before these situations arise. Evidence supports effectiveness across various substances, with particular strength for alcohol, stimulants, cannabis, and tobacco use disorders. Implementation formats range from individual therapy allowing personalized focus on specific triggers and patterns, to group delivery offering peer feedback, shared problem-solving, and modeling opportunities. Specific cognitive-behavioral variants include Relapse Prevention focusing on identifying and managing high-risk situations; Coping Skills Training developing specific behavioral alternatives for situations previously managed through substance use; and integrated approaches addressing co-occurring psychiatric conditions alongside substance use. Critical therapeutic elements include collaborative goal-setting respecting patient priorities rather than imposing clinician-determined objectives; skills practice through role-play, behavioral rehearsal, and homework assignments between sessions; and gradual exposure to triggers in controlled contexts developing mastery over previously overwhelming cues. These cognitive-behavioral approaches demonstrate both standalone effectiveness and enhanced outcomes when combined with appropriate pharmacotherapy, particularly for alcohol and opioid use disorders where combined treatment consistently outperforms either modality alone.

Contingency management interventions systematically reinforce target behaviors, typically abstinence demonstrated through biological verification, although increasingly employed for other recovery-oriented behaviors including treatment attendance, medication adherence, or skill practice completion. Implementation approaches include voucher-based reinforcement providing monetary-equivalent vouchers exchangeable for retail goods or services; prize-based contingency management where negative biological tests earn draws from a prize bowl containing reinforcers of varying values; and clinic privileges models where program benefits like reduced clinic attendance frequency or take-home medication doses are contingent on documented abstinence. Effectiveness research demonstrates robust outcomes across various substances with particularly strong evidence for stimulants, opioids, and cannabis, often showing superior short-term abstinence rates compared to other psychosocial interventions, though with ongoing research addressing post-contingency maintenance of behavioral changes. Key implementation elements include clear behavioral targets objectively verified through appropriate biological testing; immediate reinforcement delivery following target behavior demonstration; and escalating reinforcement schedules where consecutive positive behaviors receive increasing reinforcement value while reset contingencies following non-compliance provide immediate consequences without entirely sacrificing future reinforcement opportunity. Implementation barriers include funding limitations for reinforcement costs; philosophical objections regarding external reward provision; and occasionally practical challenges establishing appropriate monitoring protocols, particularly for substances with short detection windows requiring frequent testing. Recent innovations addressing these barriers include lower-cost prize-based approaches maintaining effectiveness with reduced financial burden; technology-enabled monitoring through smartphone applications and remote testing capabilities; and integration of contingency management principles into existing program structures like medication take-home schedules without requiring additional dedicated funding streams.

Motivational approaches recognize ambivalence as normal within behavior change processes while employing structured techniques helping individuals resolve this ambivalence in favor of healthier choices. Motivational Interviewing represents the most extensively studied approach, employing specific principles including expressing empathy through reflective listening; developing discrepancy between current behavior and broader goals or values; rolling with resistance rather than direct confrontation; and supporting self-efficacy through recognizing strengths and previous successful changes. These principles manifest through specific techniques including open-ended questioning, affirmations, reflective listening, and summarizing (collectively forming the acronym OARS), alongside strategic focus on change talk—client statements supporting motivation for change. Evidence supports motivational interviewing effectiveness across substances, with particular strength as engagement strategy for individuals with limited initial change readiness, as a precursor to more action-oriented treatments, and as an integration element within other therapeutic approaches. Motivational Enhancement Therapy represents a more structured application incorporating standardized assessment feedback within a typically brief (2-4 session) intervention format, showing effectiveness particularly for alcohol use disorders. Implementation considerations include maintaining appropriate balance between client autonomy and direction toward health-promoting choices; addressing sustaining talk (arguments against change) without creating defensiveness or opposition; appropriately addressing the common phenomenon of verbal commitment without corresponding behavioral follow-through; and recognizing when to transition from motivational approaches to more action-oriented interventions once commitment to change solidifies. Recent developments include adaptations for group delivery formats; cultural modifications enhancing relevance across diverse populations; and integration with digital health technologies providing motivational support between formal clinical encounters.

Mindfulness-based interventions address substance use disorders through developing non-judgmental awareness of present-moment experiences including cravings, negative emotional states, and habitual reactive patterns that typically trigger substance use. Core components include formal meditation practices developing attention control and present-moment awareness; informal mindfulness applications during daily activities; specific techniques addressing substance-related experiences like urge surfing, where individuals observe and describe cravings without automatically responding; and values clarification helping align behavior with deeper priorities beyond immediate discomfort relief. Mindfulness-Based Relapse Prevention integrates traditional cognitive-behavioral relapse prevention elements with mindfulness practices, particularly addressing automatic pilot responses and creating space between triggers and reactions. Acceptance and Commitment Therapy applies mindfulness principles alongside psychological flexibility development, helping individuals accept difficult internal experiences without necessarily acting on them while committing to behaviors aligned with personally meaningful values. Evidence supports these approaches across substances including alcohol, stimulants, opioids, and tobacco, with particular effectiveness for reducing intensity and frequency of cravings, developing alternative responses to negative emotional states previously managed through substances, and addressing shame and self-criticism potentially perpetuating relapse cycles. Implementation considerations include appropriate practice duration and frequency balancing ideal development with realistic patient capabilities; addressing common misconceptions regarding mindfulness as relaxation technique rather than awareness practice; culturally sensitive adaptations recognizing diverse spiritual and contemplative traditions; and integration with other treatment components including pharmacotherapy and environmental modifications. Recent developments include abbreviated protocols making mindfulness more accessible within standard treatment timeframes; applications specifically addressing chronic pain alongside substance use, particularly relevant for opioid use disorders; and digital adaptations providing guided practice opportunities between formal treatment sessions.

Family and social network interventions recognize the profound influence of interpersonal relationships on both substance use patterns and recovery processes. Community Reinforcement Approach and Family Training (CRAFT) targets concerned significant others of treatment-resistant individuals, teaching strategies for encouraging treatment entry, reducing inadvertent substance use reinforcement, enhancing reinforcement for non-using behavior, and improving relationship quality independent of substance use changes. Evidence demonstrates CRAFT's superior effectiveness for engaging previously treatment-resistant individuals compared to traditional approaches like Al-Anon or confrontational interventions. Behavioral Couples Therapy addresses substance use alongside relationship functioning through interventions including daily sobriety contracts, communication skills training, and shared positive activities rebuilding relationship quality damaged through substance use. This approach consistently demonstrates improved outcomes for both substance use and relationship functioning compared to individual treatment alone. Multidimensional Family Therapy, primarily developed for adolescent substance use disorders, addresses individual adolescent factors, parent functioning, family interaction patterns, and extra-familial systems including schools and juvenile justice, showing effectiveness for both substance use reduction and improved family functioning. Network Therapy engages selected family and friends as a support network actively participating in treatment through regular network sessions alongside individual therapy, leveraging natural support systems while providing education and skills helping network members effectively support recovery. Contemporary implementations increasingly recognize family diversity beyond traditional structures, with adaptations for various family configurations including single-parent households, blended families, same-sex partnerships, and extended kinship networks relevant for many cultural contexts. These approaches collectively demonstrate the value of addressing substance use disorders within social context rather than as purely individual phenomena, particularly given the substantial research demonstrating both familial influence on substance use development and the critical role supportive relationships play in maintaining recovery.

Pharmacotherapy

Medications for opioid use disorder (MOUD) represent among the most effective interventions in addiction treatment, with substantial evidence demonstrating reduced mortality, illicit opioid use, infectious disease transmission, and criminal activity. Methadone, a full μ-opioid receptor agonist, provides 24-36 hour prevention of withdrawal and craving through daily oral dosing, typically administered through specialized opioid treatment programs under federal and state regulations. Evidence supports flexible individualized dosing generally ranging from 60-120 mg daily, with higher doses within this range typically demonstrating superior outcomes compared to lower doses inadequately addressing craving throughout the dosing interval. Buprenorphine, a partial μ-opioid receptor agonist, demonstrates similar effectiveness while offering different pharmacological properties including ceiling effect on respiratory depression creating enhanced safety profile, office-based prescribing capability through qualified providers, and formulation options including sublingual tablets/films and extended-release monthly injections. Naltrexone, a μ-opioid receptor antagonist available in both oral and extended-release injectable formulations, blocks opioid effects through competitive receptor binding without producing physical dependence or withdrawal upon discontinuation, though requiring complete abstinence before initiation to avoid precipitated withdrawal. Comparative effectiveness research indicates superior retention with agonist treatments (methadone, buprenorphine) compared to antagonist treatment (naltrexone), though with similar effectiveness regarding illicit opioid use reduction among patients who remain engaged.

Implementation considerations include addressing stigma and misconceptions regarding these evidence-based treatments, including persistent myths about "replacing one addiction with another" despite substantial evidence demonstrating normalization of physiology and function with appropriate MOUD; regulatory barriers affecting methadone access through limited treatment program availability in many regions; prescriber limitations for buprenorphine requiring specific training and patient limits; and insurance barriers including prior authorization requirements, dosing restrictions, and time limitations unsupported by medical evidence. Duration of treatment remains individualized rather than predetermined, with research demonstrating significantly higher relapse rates following arbitrary time-based discontinuation compared to maintenance approaches based on stability and patient readiness, supporting conceptualization of opioid use disorder as a chronic condition potentially requiring long-term management similar to other chronic medical disorders.

Pharmacotherapy for alcohol use disorder encompasses several FDA-approved medications with different mechanisms and clinical applications. Naltrexone, available in both oral and extended-release injectable formulations, blocks opioid receptors reducing alcohol's rewarding effects and subsequent craving, with particular effectiveness for individuals reporting significant euphoria or "high" from drinking and those with a family history of alcohol use disorder suggesting genetic susceptibility to endogenous opioid system involvement. The oral formulation requires daily administration at 50 mg, while the extended-release injection provides monthly coverage at 380 mg, addressing adherence challenges common with daily oral medications. Acamprosate normalizes glutamate neurotransmission disrupted by chronic alcohol exposure, reducing post-acute withdrawal symptoms like anxiety, insomnia, and dysphoria that frequently trigger relapse, with standard dosing of 666 mg three times daily and renal dose adjustment requirements for impaired kidney function. Disulfiram inhibits aldehyde dehydrogenase creating acetaldehyde accumulation when alcohol is consumed, resulting in unpleasant reactions including flushing, nausea, vomiting, and headache, serving as aversive deterrent rather than craving reduction or withdrawal management. Its effectiveness depends heavily on supervised administration ensuring consistent dosing, with typical regimens of 250-500 mg daily. Off-label medications with varying evidence include topiramate, which affects both glutamate and GABA systems showing promise particularly for reducing heavy drinking days; gabapentin, primarily addressing alcohol withdrawal symptoms but with some evidence for maintained drinking reduction; and baclofen, a GABA-B agonist with mixed evidence across studies but potential applications particularly for patients with comorbid liver disease contraindicated for other options. Implementation considerations include systematic screening identifying appropriate candidates; addressing provider knowledge gaps regarding medication effectiveness and appropriate prescribing practices; integrating pharmacotherapy with psychosocial interventions which enhances outcomes compared to either approach alone; and clarifying that abstinence represents only one possible treatment goal, with significant harm reduction benefits possible through substantial drinking reduction even without complete abstinence. Despite substantial evidence supporting these medications, utilization remains remarkably low with fewer than 10% of eligible patients receiving appropriate pharmacotherapy, highlighting significant implementation gaps between evidence and practice.

Pharmacotherapy for stimulant use disorders represents an area of active research with promising approaches but currently no FDA-approved medications specifically for cocaine, methamphetamine, or prescription stimulant use disorders. Replacement or agonist-like approaches have investigated various dopaminergic agents including methylphenidate, modafinil, and extended-release amphetamine formulations, with mixed results showing some benefit in subpopulations but insufficient evidence for general clinical recommendations. Antagonist approaches have examined agents blocking stimulant reward mechanisms, including dopamine receptor antagonists and various anticonvulsants affecting glutamate systems, again with limited consistent evidence across studies. Provocative recent research demonstrates potential for combination pharmacotherapy approaches where concurrent administration of extended-release mixed amphetamine salts with the opioid antagonist naltrexone produced significant methamphetamine use reduction compared to placebo, potentially creating synergistic effects addressing both dopamine depletion and opioid system involvement in stimulant use disorders. This combination approach requires further research but represents an important paradigm shift from single-mechanism medications toward combination therapy addressing multiple neurotransmitter systems involved in stimulant addiction. Current clinical practice frequently employs off-label prescribing addressing specific symptoms associated with stimulant use disorders, including antidepressants for post-withdrawal depression; antipsychotics for stimulant-induced psychosis or severe agitation; and various agents targeting craving including bupropion, naltrexone, and topiramate, though with recognition that evidence remains preliminary for most approaches. Management of comorbid attention-deficit/hyperactivity disorder in patients with stimulant use disorders presents particular challenges balancing appropriate ADHD treatment against misuse potential, typically employing non-stimulant options including atomoxetine, bupropion, or guanfacine when possible, or extended-release stimulant formulations with lower diversion potential when non-stimulant options prove inadequate. Future pharmacotherapy development will likely require innovative approaches considering the complex neurobiology of stimulant use disorders, including medications addressing neuroplasticity and recovery of reward system function beyond simple replacement or antagonism strategies.

Pharmacotherapy for tobacco use disorder employs various medication classes addressing nicotine withdrawal, craving reduction, and relapse prevention. Nicotine replacement therapy (NRT) provides controlled nicotine doses without the numerous toxins in tobacco smoke, available in multiple formulations including transdermal patches providing steady nicotine levels over 16-24 hours; gum, lozenges, and inhalers delivering more immediate but shorter-duration relief particularly valuable for breakthrough cravings; and nasal spray offering the most rapid delivery approximating cigarette inhalation pharmacokinetics. These formulations can be used alone or in combination, with evidence supporting superior outcomes using long-acting patches concurrently with short-acting forms addressing breakthrough cravings compared to single-product approaches. Bupropion, an atypical antidepressant affecting dopaminergic and noradrenergic systems, reduces withdrawal intensity and nicotine craving while potentially addressing post-cessation depressive symptoms, typically administered at 150 mg sustained-release formulation twice daily starting 1-2 weeks before the quit date. Varenicline acts as a partial agonist at nicotinic acetylcholine receptors, both reducing withdrawal symptoms through modest receptor activation and blocking rewarding effects if smoking occurs through competitive binding, administered in titrated dosing reaching 1 mg twice daily with meals, ideally starting 1 week before the target quit date. Combination pharmacotherapy approaches, particularly varenicline with nicotine replacement, demonstrate enhanced effectiveness compared to monotherapy in more heavily dependent smokers. Implementation considerations include appropriate patient education regarding medication usage, as improper administration (particularly with nicotine replacement) significantly reduces effectiveness; addressing misconceptions regarding safety, including unfounded concerns about cardiovascular risk with properly used nicotine replacement; and duration of treatment, with extended therapy beyond traditional 8-12 week courses showing enhanced long-term abstinence rates, particularly for more dependent smokers. While e-cigarettes contain nicotine and are used by some for cessation purposes, insufficient evidence exists regarding their effectiveness as cessation aids compared to established pharmacotherapy, with ongoing concerns regarding long-term health effects and potential for sustained nicotine dependence rather than complete cessation. Pharmacotherapy selection should consider individual factors including previous quit experiences, comorbid conditions, contraindications, medication interactions, and patient preferences, within comprehensive treatment approaches integrating behavioral support with medication management.

Psychiatric medication management in patients with co-occurring substance use disorders requires specialized approaches addressing the complex interactions between substances and psychiatric symptoms. Diagnosis timing represents an initial consideration, ideally allowing sufficient abstinence period (typically 2-4 weeks when feasible) before establishing psychiatric diagnoses, distinguishing between substance-induced conditions potentially resolving with continued abstinence versus independent disorders requiring specific psychiatric treatment. When immediate psychiatric medication appears necessary despite ongoing substance use, selection factors include abuse potential (avoiding benzodiazepines, stimulants, and certain sedating medications when possible); interaction risk with actively used substances (particularly considering respiratory depression risk with combined central nervous system depressants); and medication characteristics affecting adherence probability, including dosing frequency, adverse effect profile, and cost. Specific diagnostic considerations include depression treatment preferentially employing medications with lower sedation potentially exacerbating substance-induced cognitive impairment; anxiety disorders often managed with serotonergic antidepressants rather than benzodiazepines despite their slower onset; bipolar disorder typically requiring mood stabilizers with attention to specific substance interactions including valproate effects on alcohol metabolism and carbamazepine induction potentially affecting methadone levels; and psychotic disorders requiring antipsychotic selection considering both acute presentation and substance-specific risks, including QT prolongation with methadone combinations or seizure threshold lowering with stimulant withdrawal. Medication monitoring requires enhanced vigilance addressing both typical considerations and substance-specific concerns, including liver function with alcohol use disorder; QT prolongation with methadone and certain antipsychotics; and medication adherence challenges common in early recovery when cognitive function, daily structure, and health prioritization may remain compromised. Integrated treatment approaches addressing both psychiatric symptoms and substance use simultaneously demonstrate superior outcomes compared to sequential or parallel treatment models, with particular effectiveness when prescribers maintain expertise in both domains or work within collaborative care models ensuring effective communication between psychiatric and addiction treatment providers.

PREVENTION PROGRAMS

Substance use disorder prevention encompasses comprehensive strategies addressing risk and protective factors across multiple levels from individuals to broader social environments.

Primary Prevention

School-based prevention programs represent the most extensively implemented and evaluated approaches, with evolution from ineffective information-only and fear-based models toward evidence-based curricula addressing specific risk and protective factors. Effective programs share several characteristics including interactive teaching methods promoting active student engagement rather than passive lecture formats; developmentally appropriate content matched to cognitive capabilities and relevant social contexts across different age groups; sufficient program intensity and duration, with research suggesting minimum thresholds of 10-15 sessions with reinforcement in subsequent years; social influence approaches addressing peer pressure resistance skills through modeling and guided practice; normative education correcting misperceptions regarding peer substance use prevalence typically overestimated by adolescents; comprehensive content addressing substance-specific information alongside broader life skills development; and fidelity-enhancing elements ensuring consistent implementation as designed rather than selective component delivery. Specific evidence-based curricula include Life Skills Training, employing cognitive-behavioral techniques developing self-management, social skills, and substance resistance across multiple sessions spanning several school years; Strengthening Families Program, addressing both youth skills and parenting practices through parallel and joint parent-child sessions; and Good Behavior Game, a classroom management approach implemented in early elementary grades that demonstrably reduces subsequent substance use despite not directly addressing substances, highlighting the impact of early self-regulation development on later substance use vulnerability. Implementation challenges include competing demands within educational settings, sustainable funding limitations, maintaining program fidelity across diverse school contexts, and addressing cultural relevance across different communities. Recent innovations include integration with digital technologies providing interactive components and personalized feedback; cultural adaptations maintaining core components while enhancing relevance for specific populations; and implementation science approaches identifying optimal dissemination strategies translating research programs into sustainable real-world applications.

> **Remember**
>
> **Effective prevention approaches address risk and protective factors across individual, family, peer, school, and community domains, with strategies matched to developmental stage and targeted to appropriate universal, selective, or indicated populations.**

Family-based prevention approaches address critical risk and protective factors within family systems, recognizing the substantial influence of family functioning on substance use initiation and progression. Effective programs employ various mechanisms including enhancing parent-child communication quality and frequency, particularly regarding substances and related behaviors; developing consistent and appropriate monitoring and supervision practices; establishing clear expectations and consequences regarding substance use; strengthening family bonding and attachment; and modeling healthy attitudes and behaviors regarding substances. Implementation formats range from universal programs offered to general populations regardless of risk status, to selective programs targeting families with specific risk factors such as parental substance use disorders or children demonstrating early behavioral problems, to indicated programs for families already showing preliminary signs of concern including early substance experimentation or conduct issues. Specific evidence-based interventions include Strengthening Families Program providing parallel parent and child skill development sessions followed by joint family practice; Family Check-Up offering motivational assessment-based feedback identifying specific family strengths and challenges followed by tailored parenting support; and Functional Family Therapy addressing both family communication patterns and broader contextual factors maintaining problematic behaviors. Effectiveness evidence demonstrates both direct substance use reduction and improvements in mediating factors including enhanced parental monitoring, reduced family conflict, improved communication, and strengthened attachments. Implementation challenges include recruitment and retention of families, particularly those facing multiple stressors potentially limiting participation capacity; cultural acceptability of parenting interventions that may conflict with traditional practices in some communities; and sustainable delivery systems extending beyond time-limited research initiatives. Contemporary adaptations increasingly incorporate flexible delivery methods including online formats, home visiting options, and abbreviated versions addressing practical barriers to traditional multi-session, in-person programs while maintaining core effective components.

Environmental prevention strategies address substance availability, policies, social norms, and community factors beyond individual or family-level interventions. Regulatory approaches include age restrictions limiting legal purchase age for alcohol and tobacco, typically 21 and 18-21 years respectively in most jurisdictions; outlet density policies limiting the concentration of alcohol retailers in specific geographic areas; zoning regulations regarding locations of cannabis dispensaries, liquor stores, or nightlife venues; taxation policies increasing prices and subsequently reducing consumption, particularly among price-sensitive youth; and specific substance controls including prescription drug monitoring programs tracking controlled substance prescriptions to identify inappropriate prescribing patterns or potential diversion. Enforcement measures include compliance checks verifying age verification practices among retailers; sobriety checkpoints reducing impaired driving; and consequence systems for violations that meaningfully impact business operations rather than representing minimal operational costs. Media campaigns and counter-marketing efforts address social norms and attitudes, with effectiveness evidence suggesting targeted approaches addressing specific behaviors and audiences outperform general awareness campaigns; inclusion of specific action recommendations rather than simply highlighting problems; and sufficient exposure intensity and duration to influence established attitudes. Community mobilization approaches engage diverse stakeholders including schools, law enforcement, healthcare, businesses, faith communities, and citizen groups in coordinated prevention efforts addressing local priorities through comprehensive strategies rather than isolated interventions. Implementation considerations include policy development processes engaging key stakeholders while addressing potential opposition from commercial interests; enforcement resources ensuring policies extend beyond symbolic measures to actual practice change; cultural and contextual factors affecting appropriateness of specific approaches across different communities; and sustainability mechanisms maintaining efforts beyond initial implementation periods. Evidence supports environmental approaches as essential components within comprehensive prevention systems, often demonstrating population-level impacts exceeding individually-focused interventions alone, particularly when multiple complementary strategies address different aspects of the environment simultaneously.

Selective and indicated prevention targets higher-risk populations rather than universal approaches addressing entire communities regardless of risk status. Selective prevention focuses on subgroups with elevated risk based on biological, psychological, or social factors including children of parents with substance use disorders; youth experiencing early life adversity or trauma; individuals with certain psychiatric conditions increasing vulnerability including ADHD, conduct disorder, or early-onset depression; and communities experiencing concentrated disadvantage, high availability of substances, or limited protective resources. Implementation approaches include mentoring programs pairing at-risk youth with stable adult role models; skills-focused curricula specifically addressing vulnerability factors common in targeted populations; case management connecting families with needed resources addressing underlying stressors; and community-based programs creating alternative activities and support systems in high-risk neighborhoods. Indicated prevention addresses individuals already demonstrating early warning signs including initial substance experimentation, problem behaviors, or early symptoms not yet meeting diagnostic criteria for substance use disorders. Approaches include screening and brief interventions identifying concerning patterns before they progress to disorders; individualized counseling addressing specific emerging issues; family-focused interventions targeting both youth behavior and family dynamics; and specialized school-based programs for students demonstrating academic or behavioral problems associated with increased substance use vulnerability. Implementation considerations include stigma concerns potentially affecting participation willingness; appropriate balance between targeting based on risk while avoiding labeling or self-fulfilling prophecies; ethical issues regarding intervention without diagnosed conditions; and resource allocation questions balancing higher costs per participant of selective and indicated approaches against potentially greater per-person impact compared to universal programs. Evidence suggests optimal prevention systems integrate universal, selective, and indicated approaches creating comprehensive coverage addressing different population segments according to risk level and specific needs, rather than relying exclusively on any single prevention tier.

Digital and technology-based prevention represents an evolving approach leveraging electronic platforms to deliver prevention content, enhance engagement, and extend reach beyond traditional programs. Computer-based and internet prevention programs adapt evidence-based curricula for digital delivery, enabling standardized implementation, personalized feedback based on individual responses, and flexible access outside structured settings like schools or community centers. Mobile applications provide various prevention functions including substance education through interactive formats; skill-building exercises developing refusal techniques, stress management, and decision-making capabilities; personalized feedback comparing individual substance use to peer norms; and goal-setting with progress tracking reinforcing positive choices. Social media approaches leverage these platforms' influence on youth culture through both counter-marketing challenging pro-substance messages and positive content promoting healthy alternatives, protective behaviors, and accurate information correcting misperceptions. Virtual reality applications create immersive environments for practicing resistance skills in simulated high-pressure situations or experiencing consequences of different choices without real-world risks. Evidence regarding effectiveness shows promising results for technology-based approaches, particularly when incorporating elements of effective traditional programs including interactive components rather than passive information delivery; personalized feedback addressing individual risk and protective factors; sufficient program "dosage" through multiple sessions or extended engagement; and some form of human connection or guidance rather than entirely automated delivery. Implementation considerations include accessibility across socioeconomic status addressing digital divide concerns; privacy and data security particularly for programs collecting sensitive information; integration with broader prevention systems rather than standalone technology solutions; and rapid technological evolution potentially requiring frequent updates maintaining both technical functionality and cultural relevance. These approaches offer particular advantages including appeal to digital natives comfortable with technology-mediated communication; cost-effective delivery after initial development investments; implementation fidelity through standardized delivery; and potential for broad reach including populations facing barriers to traditional program participation.

Screening and Early Intervention

Screening tools for substance use and substance use disorders have evolved from simple yes/no questions to validated instruments balancing brevity with sufficient sensitivity and specificity for clinical utility. Brief screening instruments widely implemented in various settings include the Alcohol Use Disorders Identification Test (AUDIT), a 10-item questionnaire assessing consumption patterns, dependence symptoms, and harmful consequences with demonstrated validity across diverse populations and clinical contexts; the Drug Abuse Screening Test (DAST), available in versions ranging from 10 to 28 items evaluating drug-related problems and consequences; and the CAGE questionnaire providing an ultra-brief 4-item screen primarily for alcohol use disorders focusing on key dependence indicators. Newer instruments addressing limitations of earlier screens include the Alcohol, Smoking and Substance Involvement Screening Test (ASSIST) developed by the World Health Organization providing comprehensive coverage across substance categories while distinguishing between use, risky use, and likely dependence; the Tobacco, Alcohol, Prescription medication, and other Substance use (TAPS) tool designed specifically for primary care settings with validated self-administration capability; and the CRAFFT (Car, Relax, Alone, Forget, Friends, Trouble) developed specifically for adolescents with age-appropriate language and content. Implementation approaches include universal screening where all patients in particular settings undergo screening regardless of presentation; targeted screening focusing on higher-risk populations including pregnant women, patients with specific medical conditions frequently complicated by substance use, or those presenting with suspicious symptoms; and opportunistic screening incorporated into routine healthcare encounters like annual examinations or new patient assessments. Electronic screening through tablet computers or kiosks in waiting areas demonstrates particular promise addressing both efficiency concerns and patient comfort disclosing sensitive information. Critical implementation elements include non-judgmental framing explaining screening as routine healthcare similar to blood pressure measurement rather than targeted questioning; privacy considerations ensuring confidential response collection and appropriate information sharing; workflow integration minimizing disruption to clinical operations; and established protocols connecting positive screens to appropriate assessment and intervention resources rather than simply documenting results without action.

Brief interventions represent time-limited counseling approaches designed for non-treatment-seeking individuals identified through screening, typically delivered in healthcare or other non-specialty settings. The core model follows the FRAMES structure: Feedback regarding personal risk based on screening results; emphasis on personal Responsibility for change; clear Advice regarding behavior change; a Menu of options for reducing use or associated harms; Empathic counseling style avoiding confrontation or judgment; and Self-efficacy enhancement supporting confidence in change capability. Implementation typically involves 1-5 sessions ranging from 5-60 minutes, with evidence suggesting even single-session interventions produce measurable effects, particularly for unhealthy alcohol use. Motivational interviewing provides the predominant theoretical framework, employing techniques including reflective listening, developing discrepancy between current behavior and broader goals, and supporting change talk—patient statements favoring behavior change. Evidence most strongly supports brief interventions for unhealthy alcohol use in primary care settings, with meta-analyses demonstrating consistent reductions in weekly drinking and binge episodes, though with more modest evidence for illicit drug use and limited evidence for tobacco compared to more intensive tobacco cessation interventions. Implementation considerations include provider training requirements ensuring appropriate motivational style rather than confrontational or purely educational approaches; role definition regarding which staff members (physicians, nurses, behavioral health specialists, or others) deliver interventions within specific settings; documentation and reimbursement procedures supporting sustainability within healthcare systems; and appropriate expectations recognizing brief interventions as harm reduction and early intervention tools rather than treatment for established severe substance use disorders. Recent adaptations include computer-assisted brief interventions combining standardized electronic assessment with provider-delivered counseling; stepped care models providing initial brief intervention with escalation to more intensive approaches for non-responders; and culturally adapted versions addressing specific beliefs, values, and contexts across diverse populations.

Screening, Brief Intervention, and Referral to Treatment (SBIRT) represents an integrated public health approach systematically identifying and addressing substance use across a spectrum from risky use to severe disorders. This comprehensive model incorporates universal screening using validated tools; brief intervention for individuals screening positive for risky use but not meeting criteria for substance use disorders; brief treatment for moderate risk cases requiring more extended intervention than typical brief interventions provide; and referral to specialty treatment for high-risk individuals meeting criteria for substance use disorders requiring more intensive care. Implementation settings include primary care practices, emergency departments, trauma centers, college health services, employee assistance programs, and various community settings encountering individuals not actively seeking substance use treatment. Evidence demonstrates effectiveness for reducing alcohol consumption and alcohol-related consequences across diverse settings, with more limited but growing evidence for other substances. Cost-effectiveness analyses indicate positive returns on investment through reduced healthcare utilization, decreased hospitalizations, and prevention of progression to more severe conditions requiring intensive treatment. Implementation support systems developed to enhance adoption include standardized protocols and clinical decision support tools embedded in electronic health records; reimbursement mechanisms through both public and private insurance; training programs preparing diverse providers for appropriate implementation; and quality improvement approaches addressing common implementation barriers. Critical success factors include leadership commitment creating organizational culture supporting SBIRT implementation; workflow redesign integrating screening and intervention within existing clinical processes rather than adding disconnected components; community partnerships ensuring appropriate referral resources for identified high-risk cases; and monitoring systems tracking both implementation fidelity and clinical outcomes. Recent innovations include telehealth-delivered SBIRT extending reach to underserved areas; peer-delivered models incorporating individuals with lived experience alongside clinical staff; and automated systems using artificial intelligence to guide personalized intervention approaches based on specific risk factors and responses.

Secondary prevention addresses early-stage substance use problems before they progress to severe disorders, employing various approaches beyond SBIRT models. Indicated prevention programs target adolescents and young adults demonstrating early substance use or related risk behaviors, including interventions like Project ALERT combining resistance skills training with normative education and motivational enhancement; Life Skills Training developing general and substance-specific competencies reducing vulnerability to progression; and Adolescent Community Reinforcement Approach addressing both substance use and associated life problems through behavioral skill development and positive reinforcement for non-using activities. Educational interventions for specific violation contexts include mandated programs for college students receiving alcohol violations and specialized curricula for youth facing initial legal consequences for substance-related offenses, designed as early intervention opportunities rather than simply punitive responses. Workplace programs implement regular screening alongside employee assistance programs providing confidential assessment and brief counseling, with evidence supporting both health improvements and economic benefits through reduced absenteeism and improved productivity. Digital early intervention approaches include online assessment with automated personalized feedback comparing individual use to normative data; mobile applications tracking consumption patterns while providing motivational support for moderation goals; and social media campaigns targeting individuals displaying interest in substance-related content with resources for evaluation and assistance. Specialized early intervention models address unique population needs, including pregnant women with Screening, Brief Intervention, and Referral to Treatment for Maternal Substance Use programs incorporating prenatal care coordination; military personnel through mandatory post-deployment assessments addressing substance use alongside other reintegration challenges; and adolescents through school-based student assistance programs providing counseling, support groups, and family interventions before problems require formal treatment. These diverse secondary prevention approaches collectively aim to interrupt progression toward severe substance use disorders through early identification and intervention when behavior remains more modifiable and before substantial consequences accumulate creating additional barriers to change.

Community-Based Programs

Community coalitions bring together diverse stakeholders creating coordinated prevention efforts addressing substance use issues through systematic change processes rather than isolated interventions. Effective coalitions typically include representation from various sectors including schools, healthcare, law enforcement, businesses, faith communities, youth organizations, government agencies, media, parents, and youth themselves. Implementation follows structured processes beginning with comprehensive community assessment identifying local substance use patterns, risk and protective factors, existing resources, and gaps in services. Strategic planning translates assessment findings into clear goals, measurable objectives, and specific strategies systematically addressing identified priorities, with selection guided by both local relevance and evidence regarding effectiveness. Action plans detail implementation steps, responsible parties, timelines, required resources, and anticipated barriers. Evaluation mechanisms monitor both implementation fidelity and outcome achievement, with results informing continuous improvement through regular plan adjustments. Evidence from initiatives like Communities That Care, Drug-Free Communities Support Program, and PROSPER (PROmoting School-community-university Partnerships to Enhance Resilience) demonstrates effectiveness in reducing youth substance use, delinquency, and associated risk behaviors when coalitions maintain fidelity to structured processes and implement comprehensive strategies rather than isolated programs. Implementation challenges include maintaining diverse engagement beyond initial enthusiasm; navigating power dynamics between professional and community members; securing sustainable funding beyond initial grant periods; balancing fidelity to evidence-based approaches with local adaptation addressing specific community contexts; and maintaining focus on environmental and policy changes rather than defaulting exclusively to individual education programs with more limited population impact.

Media campaigns and social marketing approaches attempt to influence knowledge, attitudes, and behaviors regarding substances through strategic communication across various platforms. Evidence-supported principles include clear behavioral focus on specific actions rather than general awareness or attitude change; targeted message development addressing particular audience segments based on demographics, current behavior, and psychosocial characteristics; sufficient exposure intensity and duration to achieve meaningful impact; complementary components addressing both individual knowledge and environmental contexts; and integration with broader prevention initiatives rather than standalone media efforts. Effective campaigns typically progress through systematic development processes including formative research understanding target audience perspectives; message development and pretesting ensuring relevance, credibility, and impact; strategic dissemination through channels reaching intended audiences; and outcome evaluation measuring actual behavior change rather than simply message recall or attitude shifts. Contemporary approaches increasingly leverage digital and social media complementing traditional channels, with capabilities including precise audience targeting based on interests and demographics; interactive engagement rather than passive message reception; peer-to-peer message amplification through sharing functions; and real-time analytics enabling message refinement based on audience response. Counter-marketing efforts specifically addressing industry promotion of harmful products like tobacco, alcohol, or cannabis employ strategies including exposing deceptive marketing tactics; highlighting industry targeting of vulnerable populations including youth and marginalized communities; and reframing substance use as a public health issue rather than simply individual choice. The effectiveness evidence for media campaigns demonstrates modest but meaningful effects when properly designed and implemented, with particularly strong evidence for tobacco counter-marketing campaigns and emerging support for targeted campaigns addressing prescription drug misuse, though with more limited evidence for general substance use prevention messaging.

Regulatory and policy approaches address substance accessibility, normative environments, and consequences associated with harmful use through various mechanisms operating at community levels. Alcohol policies with demonstrated effectiveness include maintaining minimum legal drinking age at 21; limiting outlet density through licensing restrictions; enforcing responsible beverage service through server training and liability laws; implementing and enforcing blood alcohol concentration limits for driving; and restricting promotional activities particularly targeting young people. Tobacco control policies with strong evidence include comprehensive smoke-free air laws prohibiting smoking in workplaces and public spaces; significant taxation increasing prices beyond youth purchasing power; counter-marketing campaigns highlighting industry tactics and health consequences; and retail access restrictions including minimum age enforcement, licensing requirements, and product placement limitations. Prescription drug policies addressing diversion and misuse include prescription drug monitoring programs tracking controlled substance prescribing and dispensing; safe storage and disposal initiatives preventing household medication access; prescriber education programs promoting appropriate prescribing practices; and "pill mill" laws addressing inappropriate high-volume prescribing. Cannabis policy represents an evolving area as jurisdictions implement various regulatory frameworks, with emerging evidence suggesting importance of potency limitations, packaging requirements preventing youth appeal, advertising restrictions, outlet density controls, and preventing industry dominance over regulatory processes. Implementation considerations include enforcement resources ensuring policies extend beyond symbolic measures to actual practice change; addressing potential displacement effects where restrictions in one community may increase problems in neighboring areas; equity impacts ensuring policies do not disproportionately burden disadvantaged communities; and evaluation systems monitoring both intended outcomes and potential unintended consequences.

Community-driven culturally specific approaches recognize that substance use patterns, risk and protective factors, and effective prevention strategies may vary substantially across cultural contexts. Indigenous or Native American communities have developed various culture-centered prevention approaches including revitalization of traditional practices and ceremonial activities that strengthen cultural identity and connection; healing circles addressing historical trauma and its relationship to substance use; community-based participatory research ensuring programs address locally identified priorities rather than externally imposed frameworks; and adaptation of evidence-based programs incorporating cultural elements enhancing relevance and effectiveness. Latino/Hispanic communities have implemented family-centered prevention approaches emphasizing familismo (family interconnectedness) and respeto (respect across generations); faith community partnerships leveraging religious institutions' influence and reach; and promotora models utilizing community health workers from within the community to deliver culturally congruent prevention messages and services. African American communities have developed approaches emphasizing strengths-based frameworks rather than deficit perspectives; incorporating historical context and resilience messaging; utilizing respected community institutions including churches, barber shops, and beauty salons as prevention settings; and addressing environmental justice concerns affecting community health and substance use vulnerability. Asian American and Pacific Islander programs address the heterogeneity across numerous cultural subgroups through tailored approaches respecting specific beliefs and practices regarding substances; incorporating appropriate language and communication styles; addressing intergenerational acculturation gaps potentially creating family conflict and youth vulnerability; and working within appropriate community authority structures. Evidence increasingly demonstrates that culturally grounded prevention approaches developed with meaningful community participation demonstrate enhanced engagement, retention, and effectiveness compared to simply translating mainstream programs for diverse populations, highlighting the importance of cultural humility, community voice, and recognition of unique protective factors within different cultural contexts

Summary

Addiction and substance use disorders represent complex biopsychosocial conditions characterized by compulsive substance use despite negative consequences, with neurobiological underpinnings involving reward pathway dysregulation. Common drugs of abuse span multiple categories with distinct pharmacological properties: stimulants like cocaine and amphetamines increase synaptic concentrations of monoamines producing euphoria, increased energy, and sympathomimetic effects; opioids including heroin, prescription analgesics, and synthetic compounds activate mu receptors generating analgesia and euphoria while risking respiratory depression; sedative-hypnotics such as benzodiazepines and alcohol enhance GABA activity causing anxiolysis and sedation; hallucinogens alter perception through serotonergic and other mechanisms; and cannabinoids produce relaxation and perceptual changes through cannabinoid receptor activation. Clinical manifestations of substance use disorders follow recognizable patterns including compulsive use despite consequences, tolerance requiring escalating doses, withdrawal syndromes upon cessation, and neurobiological adaptations reflecting altered reward circuitry functioning. Acute intoxication presents with substance-specific syndromes requiring targeted interventions, while chronic use leads to characteristic medical, psychological, and social complications. Treatment approaches incorporate pharmacological interventions including medication-assisted treatment (methadone, buprenorphine, and naltrexone for opioid use disorder; acamprosate, naltrexone, and disulfiram for alcohol use disorder), psychosocial therapies spanning cognitive-behavioral approaches, motivational enhancement, contingency management, and twelve-step facilitation, and recovery support services delivered across a continuum from outpatient to residential settings based on individual needs and severity. Prevention programs target different population levels, with universal strategies addressing entire communities, selective approaches focusing on high-risk groups, and indicated interventions targeting individuals showing early substance use patterns, all within a framework addressing risk factors while enhancing protective factors through evidence-based approaches including family-based programs, school-based prevention, community coalitions, and policy interventions affecting availability, price, and normative environment.

Self-Assessment Questions

1. Describe the neurobiological changes that occur in the brain's reward system with chronic substance use, and explain how these changes contribute to the clinical features of addiction.
2. Compare and contrast the pharmacology, clinical effects, and overdose management for stimulants, opioids, sedative-hypnotics, and hallucinogens.
3. Analyze the clinical manifestations, assessment tools, and treatment approaches for alcohol use disorder, including both pharmacological and psychosocial interventions.
4. Explain the principles of medication-assisted treatment for opioid use disorder, including the pharmacology, indications, contraindications, and implementation considerations for methadone, buprenorphine, and naltrexone.
5. Describe the clinical presentation and management approach for withdrawal syndromes from different substance classes, with particular attention to potentially life-threatening withdrawals.
6. Discuss the evidence base for different psychosocial interventions in substance use disorders, including cognitive-behavioral therapy, motivational interviewing, and contingency management.
7. Analyze the relationship between substance use disorders and co-occurring mental health conditions, including assessment approaches and integrated treatment strategies.
8. Explain the principles of harm reduction in substance use disorder management, including specific interventions and their evidence base.
9. Describe the components of effective prevention programs for different developmental stages from childhood through young adulthood.
10. Discuss the unique challenges in identifying and managing substance use disorders in special populations including pregnant women, adolescents, older adults, and healthcare professionals.

Bibliography

1. Koob GF, Volkow ND. Neurobiology of addiction: a neurocircuitry analysis. Lancet Psychiatry. 2016;3(8):760-773.
2. Kampman K, Jarvis M. American Society of Addiction Medicine (ASAM) national practice guideline for the use of medications in the treatment of addiction involving opioid use. J Addict Med. 2015;9(5):358-367.
3. Volkow ND, Koob GF, McLellan AT. Neurobiologic advances from the brain disease model of addiction. N Engl J Med. 2016;374(4):363-371.
4. D'Onofrio G, O'Connor PG, Pantalon MV, Chawarski MC, Busch SH, Owens PH, et al. Emergency department-initiated buprenorphine/naloxone treatment for opioid dependence: a randomized clinical trial. JAMA. 2015;313(16):1636-1644.
5. Jonas DE, Amick HR, Feltner C, Bobashev G, Thomas K, Wines R, et al. Pharmacotherapy for adults with alcohol use disorders in outpatient settings: a systematic review and meta-analysis. JAMA. 2014;311(18):1889-1900.
6. Carvalho AF, Heilig M, Perez A, Probst C, Rehm J. Alcohol use disorders. Lancet. 2019;394(10200):781-792.
7. Bahorik AL, Satre DD, Kline-Simon AH, Weisner CM, Campbell CI. Alcohol, cannabis, and opioid use disorders, and disease burden in an integrated health care system. J Addict Med. 2017;11(1):3-9.
8. Hasin DS, O'Brien CP, Auriacombe M, Borges G, Bucholz K, Budney A, et al. DSM-5 criteria for substance use disorders: recommendations and rationale. Am J Psychiatry. 2013;170(8):834-851.
9. Miller WR, Rollnick S. Motivational interviewing: helping people change. 3rd ed. New York: Guilford Press; 2013.
10. McLellan AT, Lewis DC, O'Brien CP, Kleber HD. Drug dependence, a chronic medical illness: implications for treatment, insurance, and outcomes evaluation. JAMA. 2000;284(13):1689-1695.

CHAPTER 13

POISON CONTROL CENTERS

Author

Miss Reetu Singh, Assistant Professor,
Department of Pharmacy, Shri Rama Krishna College of Pharmacy, Satna, Madhya Pradesh, India

Abstract

Poison Control Centers provide essential toxicological expertise through 24/7 telephone consultation services that significantly reduce healthcare costs while improving patient outcomes. Organizationally, these centers maintain specialized staffing with certified Specialists in Poison Information (typically pharmacists or nurses with advanced training) supervised by medical toxicologists who provide clinical leadership and protocol development. Support personnel manage data systems, educational initiatives, and quality improvement programs. Operational protocols guide call management from initial triage through substance identification, risk assessment, management recommendations, and follow-up calls. Centers employ sophisticated electronic documentation systems and toxicological databases to support accurate, evidence-based advice across diverse exposure scenarios. Documentation captures essential elements including substance characteristics, exposure circumstances, clinical effects, interventions, recommendations, and outcomes, serving both immediate clinical needs and long-term surveillance functions. Centers contribute critical public health services through real-time toxicosurveillance detecting emerging threats like novel recreational drugs, medication tampering, or chemical incidents. Educational outreach targets healthcare providers, public safety personnel, and community members with poison prevention messaging and clinical toxicology updates. Research activities analyze exposure patterns, intervention efficacy, and economic impacts. Through these integrated functions, Poison Control Centers serve as sentinel systems for toxic exposures while providing cost-effective consultation that reduces unnecessary emergency department visits and improves poisoning outcomes across diverse populations.

Keywords: *Poison Control Centers, toxicosurveillance, Specialists in Poison Information, telephone consultation, poison prevention, National Poison Data System*

Learning Objectives

After completion of the chapter, the learners should be able to:

- Describe the organizational structure of Poison Control Centers, including staffing requirements, certification standards, and functional roles of key personnel.
- Analyze the operational workflow for poison exposure calls from initial contact through triage, assessment, recommendations, and follow-up processes.
- Implement comprehensive documentation practices capturing essential toxicological, clinical, and epidemiological elements required for both patient care and surveillance purposes.
- Explain how Poison Control Centers contribute to public health through toxicosurveillance, outbreak detection, and disaster response coordination.
- Evaluate the economic and clinical impact of Poison Control Centers on healthcare resource utilization and poisoning-related outcomes.
- Utilize Poison Control Center resources effectively as a healthcare provider, including appropriate consultation timing, essential information sharing, and implementation of recommendations

ORGANIZATION

Poison control centers serve as specialized healthcare resources providing expert toxicology information and management recommendations to healthcare facilities, first responders, and the general public.

Historical Development

The evolution of poison control centers reflects changing patterns of poisoning exposures, advances in toxicology knowledge, and developments in healthcare delivery systems. The first formal poison information service was established in Chicago in 1953 by Louis Gdalman, a hospital pharmacist responding to increasing pediatric poisoning cases during the post-World War II proliferation of household chemicals and medications. This initial service consisted primarily of a card file containing treatment information for common toxins, accessible through a dedicated telephone line. Similar local initiatives rapidly developed across the United States, with early centers typically operating independently within individual hospitals, staffed by pharmacists, physicians, or nurses with variable training and resources.

These early centers functioned without standardization regarding staff qualifications, reference materials, documentation practices, or quality assurance processes, creating inconsistent service delivery and recommendations. The American Association of Poison Control Centers (AAPCC) formed in 1958 to address these inconsistencies, initially focusing on information sharing and gradually developing into a certification and standard-setting organization.

Table 13.1: Poison Control Center Organizational Structure

Component	Personnel	Primary Functions
Clinical Operations	Specialists in Poison Information (SPIs), Medical Directors	24/7 telephone consultation, exposure management
Medical Direction	Board-certified medical toxicologists	Case consultation, protocol development, quality assurance
Administration	Managing Director, Administrative Staff	Financial management, staffing, strategic planning
Education	Education Coordinators	Professional education, public outreach, prevention programs
Data/Surveillance	Data Managers, IT Personnel	Data collection, analysis, surveillance, NPDS participation
Quality Assurance	QA Coordinators	Case review, performance improvement, certification maintenance

Significant evolution occurred during the 1970s and 1980s, with several developments shaping modern poison center operations. The establishment of medical toxicology as a recognized specialty created a formal knowledge base and training pathway for poison center medical direction. Federal initiatives including the Poison Prevention Packaging Act of 1970 and increased funding for poison prevention activities recognized the public health significance of poisoning. Technological advances enabled more systematic information management, initially through microfilm and microfiche systems replacing card files, later through computerized databases, and eventually through specialized poison center management software.

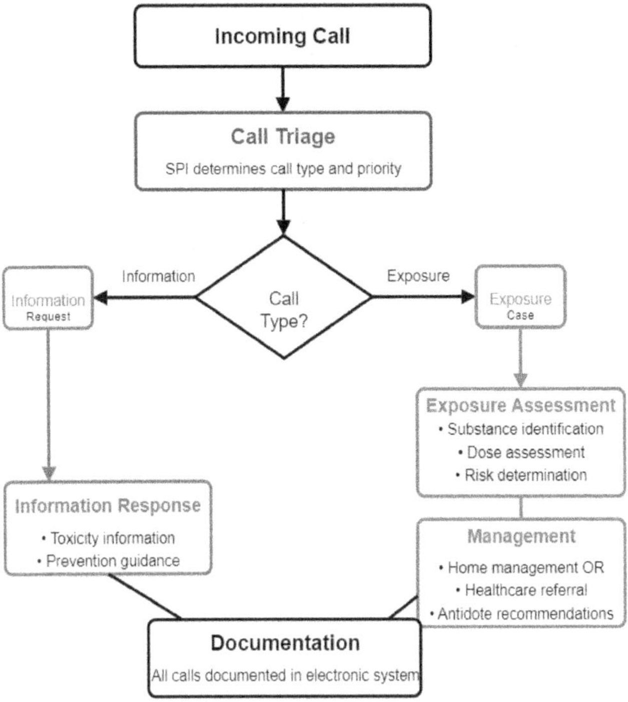

Figure 13.1: Poison Center Call Flow and Operations

Economic pressures and recognition of service duplication led to regional consolidation, with the number of centers decreasing from over 600 in the 1970s to approximately 55 certified centers currently serving the United States. This consolidation created economies of scale supporting more comprehensive services, 24/7 operations with specialized staff, enhanced quality assurance processes, and participation in national data collection. Contemporary poison centers now function as regional resources within integrated healthcare systems rather than isolated hospital departments, with mandates extending beyond direct clinical consultation to encompass public health surveillance, disaster response, research, and education. This evolution represents a transformation from informal, localized information services to sophisticated regional toxicology resources addressing both individual patient care and broader public health objectives.

International poison center development demonstrates both similarities and important variations compared to the United States model. European centers typically evolved from academic toxicology departments or emergency hospital services, often with closer integration to regulatory authorities addressing chemical safety. The European Association of Poisons Centres and Clinical Toxicologists (EAPCCT) serves as a coordinating body analogous to the AAPCC, though with less direct regulatory or certification authority. Developing nations face particular challenges establishing poison centers, including limited toxicology expertise, funding constraints, telecommunications infrastructure limitations, and sometimes insufficient political recognition of poisoning as a public health priority. The World Health Organization supports international poison center development through technical guidelines, training programs, and advocacy emphasizing the cost-effectiveness of centralized toxicology expertise compared to distributed management of poisoning cases without specialized guidance. Contemporary international collaboration occurs through several mechanisms including harmonized data collection enabling cross-national poisoning surveillance; shared access to specialized toxicology databases; international consultation networks addressing rare or emerging toxins; and collaborative research examining cross-cultural variations in poisoning epidemiology. Despite substantial variation in organizational structures, funding mechanisms, and scope of activities, international consensus increasingly recognizes essential poison center functions including 24/7 emergency consultation, toxicovigilance, healthcare professional education, and public outreach regardless of specific organizational models.

The economic foundation of poison centers has evolved through several models reflecting both service value recognition and funding challenges. Initially, centers operated primarily as hospital departments supported through institutional budgets, essentially subsidized by the hosting facility's general operations. As service regionalization extended reach beyond individual hospitals, funding mechanisms necessarily evolved to reflect broader service populations. Contemporary poison centers typically operate with diverse funding streams including state government appropriations recognizing public health service; federal grants supporting specific activities like surveillance or disaster preparedness; telecommunications surcharges or fees on specific services providing stable dedicated funding; contracts with healthcare systems, managed care organizations, or military facilities receiving services; and occasionally foundation or corporate support for specific educational or research initiatives. Despite demonstrated cost-effectiveness through prevention of unnecessary emergency department visits and healthcare resource optimization, poison centers face recurring funding challenges with multiple factors contributing to this paradox: services primarily prevent rather than create healthcare utilization, making value demonstration more complex than revenue-generating departments; benefits often accrue to different entities than funding providers; public perception occasionally views centers as primarily addressing pediatric accidents rather than complex adult exposures or healthcare facility consultations; and fragmented responsibility across healthcare, public health, and emergency preparedness sectors creates coordination challenges for sustainable support. These economic realities necessitate ongoing value demonstration, creative funding approaches, and effective articulation of the comprehensive service role beyond public perception of a simple telephone hotline.

> **Remember**
>
> **Poison Control Centers are staffed by certified Specialists in Poison Information (primarily pharmacists and nurses with specialized training) and medical toxicologists who provide 24/7 telephone consultation for both public and healthcare provider calls.**

Certification and accreditation processes establish minimum standards ensuring service quality and consistency across centers. The American Association of Poison Control Centers administers the certification program requiring centers to meet specific structural standards including: 24/7 operation with immediate accessibility by telephone; staffing by specialists in poison information with appropriate credentials; board-certified medical toxicologist direction; comprehensive toxicology information resources; quality improvement processes; documented algorithms and protocols; standardized documentation systems; educational program participation; and contribution to the National Poison Data System. Certification requires initial application demonstrating compliance with all standards, followed by periodic re-certification reviewing continued adherence and service quality. Beyond organizational certification, individual staff certification as Specialists in Poison Information (SPI) occurs through the American Association of Poison Control Centers, requiring appropriate professional background (typically pharmacy, nursing, or physician assistant training), minimum experience handling poison exposures, and successful completion of a comprehensive certification examination testing toxicology knowledge and poison center practice. Medical directors typically require board certification in medical toxicology through either the American Board of Emergency Medicine or the American Board of Pediatrics, following completion of accredited medical toxicology fellowships. These layered certification processes—

encompassing organizational structure, staff credentials, and medical leadership—collectively ensure standardized capability across the national poison center network, creating a system where callers receive evidence-based, consistent recommendations regardless of geographical location, while still allowing for regional variations addressing local needs, toxicological concerns, and healthcare delivery systems.

Staffing and Structure

Specialists in Poison Information (SPIs) serve as the primary service providers in poison centers, managing approximately 90% of exposure calls without requiring direct physician consultation. These professionals typically come from pharmacy, nursing, or physician assistant backgrounds, bringing valuable clinical knowledge regarding medication mechanisms, patient assessment, and healthcare operations. SPI responsibilities include comprehensive exposure assessment through systematic questioning; toxin identification often requiring detective work with incomplete information; risk assessment based on substance properties, exposure circumstances, and patient characteristics; development of appropriate management recommendations considering both toxicological principles and practical implementation constraints; effective communication of recommendations to various audiences from laypersons to healthcare specialists; thorough documentation of all interactions; and appropriate follow-up ensuring outcome determination. The specialized knowledge required extends far beyond general healthcare training, necessitating extensive orientation typically lasting 3-6 months, ongoing continuing education, and formal certification through the American Association of Poison Control Centers. This certification process requires minimum experience handling at least 2,000 human exposure cases, successful completion of a comprehensive examination covering clinical toxicology, poison management principles, and poison center operations, and ongoing recertification through continuing education and practice requirements. The specialized training creates professionals with unique capabilities addressing the distinctive challenges of toxicology consultation, including management of exposures rarely encountered in general healthcare practice, development of assessment skills suited to telephone consultation without direct patient examination, familiarity with thousands of commercial and pharmaceutical products, and ability to provide recommendations across the entire healthcare spectrum from home management through critical care.

Medical directors and clinical toxicologists provide advanced clinical expertise, consultation for complex cases, and overall medical leadership within poison centers. These physicians typically possess board certification in medical toxicology following specialized fellowship training beyond their primary specialty, most commonly emergency medicine or pediatrics.

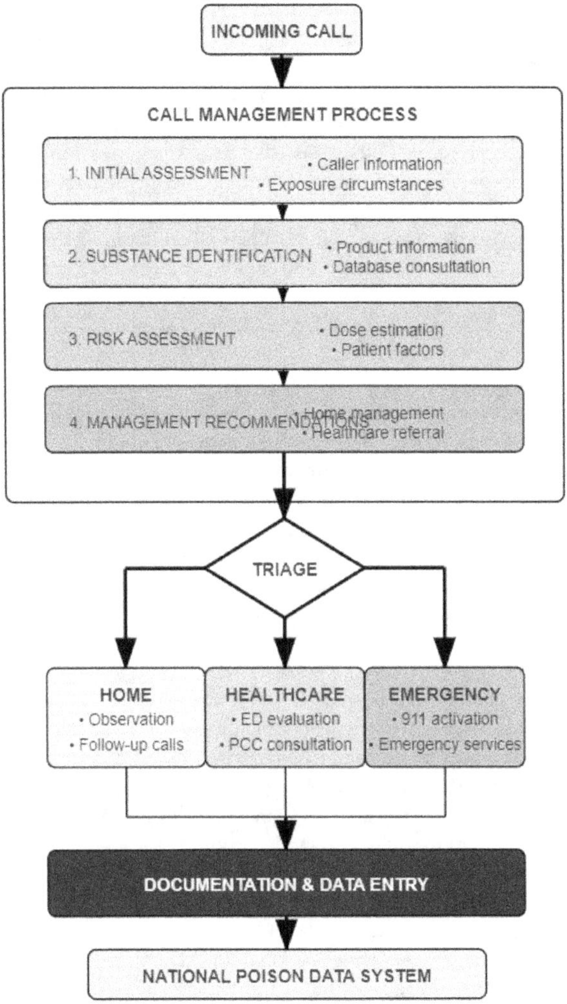

Figure 13.2: Poison Control Center Operations

Responsibilities include availability for consultation regarding high-risk, unusual, or complex exposures; development and approval of management protocols and algorithms guiding SPI practice; quality assurance review ensuring appropriate management recommendations; liaison with regional healthcare facilities establishing toxicology consultation relationships; education for both poison center staff and external healthcare providers; participation in research regarding emerging toxicological concerns; and administrative leadership regarding clinical operations. The relationship between SPIs and medical toxicologists represents a collaborative practice model where routine exposures receive management from SPIs working within established protocols, while specific case categories automatically trigger toxicologist consultation, including life-threatening exposures, unusual toxins without established management protocols, pregnancy-related exposures, complex pediatric cases, situations involving multiple conflicting clinical priorities, and cases where initial management recommendations have not produced expected improvement. This tiered approach optimizes resource utilization, allowing SPIs to manage straightforward cases while ensuring appropriate physician involvement for situations requiring advanced expertise. Beyond direct poison center responsibilities, medical toxicologists often fulfill broader roles within regional healthcare systems, potentially including emergency department consultation, inpatient toxicology services, occupational medicine practice, forensic toxicology consultation, and public health advisory functions. This integration within broader healthcare and public health systems strengthens poison center capabilities through enhanced institutional relationships, continuous clinical experience with diverse toxicological presentations, and maintenance of advanced management expertise applicable to poison center consultation.

Administrative leadership within poison centers addresses the complex operational requirements extending beyond clinical toxicology expertise. Management positions typically include a managing director or executive director overseeing overall center operations; education coordinator developing and implementing professional and public education programs; quality assurance coordinator monitoring service quality and compliance with established standards; data manager ensuring appropriate information collection, analysis, and reporting; and various administrative support roles addressing telecommunications systems, information technology infrastructure, financial management, and human resources. These administrative functions support core clinical services while enabling broader poison center roles in public health, education, and research. Managing directors specifically navigate complex responsibilities including: securing and maintaining diverse funding streams essential for operational sustainability; developing strategic partnerships with healthcare systems, public health agencies, emergency management organizations, and educational institutions; ensuring regulatory compliance across telecommunications, healthcare information, and public health domains; managing staff recruitment, retention, and development within a specialized field with limited candidate pools; and articulating poison center value to various stakeholders including funders, healthcare partners, and policy makers. The most effective administrative leadership combines understanding of clinical toxicology practice with healthcare administration expertise, enabling appropriate balancing of clinical quality, fiscal responsibility, and strategic positioning within evolving healthcare and public health systems. This comprehensive administrative capability becomes increasingly important as poison centers expand beyond traditional clinical consultation roles to encompass broader responsibilities in healthcare system optimization, public health surveillance, and emergency preparedness, requiring sophisticated organizational management beyond toxicological expertise alone.

Organizational structures for poison centers vary based on host institution type, historical development, funding mechanisms, and regional healthcare system characteristics. The most common institutional affiliations include academic medical centers, providing advantages through connection with toxicology training programs, research infrastructure, and specialty consultation availability; freestanding non-profit organizations, allowing focused mission and independent operations though sometimes with resource limitations; public health departments, facilitating integration with broader public health services while sometimes creating bureaucratic constraints; and hospital systems, providing stable institutional support though potentially with competing priorities affecting resource allocation. Regardless of specific institutional affiliation, effective organizational structures typically include several key elements: clearly defined reporting relationships establishing appropriate authority and accountability; medical direction with sufficient authority ensuring clinical quality while respecting specialized SPI expertise; formal relationships with regional healthcare facilities supporting smooth consultation processes; integration with emergency management systems enabling effective disaster response; advisory boards including diverse stakeholders guiding strategic development; and quality assurance systems with authority to implement practice improvements when indicated. Governance models range from direct hospital department structures with traditional hierarchical oversight, to independent non-profit organizations with boards of directors, to government agency divisions within public health or emergency management frameworks. Each model presents different advantages and challenges regarding operational flexibility, funding stability, and integration with related services. The optimal organizational structure balances sufficient independence allowing specialized toxicology service focus against appropriate integration with complementary healthcare and public health systems, while ensuring sustainable funding, appropriate oversight, and capability for rapidly responding to emerging toxicological threats or changing service needs.

Quality assurance systems ensure consistent, evidence-based service delivery while facilitating continuous improvement through systematic evaluation, feedback, and practice modification. Comprehensive quality assurance programs typically include several components: case review processes examining representative samples of exposure cases for appropriate assessment, management recommendations, documentation, and follow-up; focused reviews targeting high-risk exposure categories, unusual circumstances, or cases with unexpected outcomes; continuous monitoring of key performance indicators including telephone accessibility metrics, documentation completeness, follow-up completion rates, and clinical outcome concordance with expectations; periodic knowledge assessment ensuring staff maintain current toxicology expertise; and systematic processes translating quality findings into practice improvements through protocol revisions, educational interventions, or system modifications. Implementation approaches include real-time quality assurance during case management, with medical directors or senior SPIs available for immediate consultation regarding complex or high-risk exposures; retrospective review examining randomly selected cases and specifically flagged exposures; regular case conferences discussing challenging cases, unusual toxins, or evolving management approaches; and formal morbidity and mortality reviews for cases with adverse outcomes. The most effective systems maintain appropriate balance between ensuring adherence to evidence-based protocols while respecting professional judgment in complex cases without clear algorithm-driven solutions. Beyond individual case quality, broader programmatic evaluation examines accessibility for diverse populations including language minorities, the elderly, and disadvantaged communities; appropriateness of healthcare resource utilization recommendations balancing patient safety against unnecessary emergency department referrals; and effectiveness of broader poison center initiatives including surveillance activities, disaster response capabilities, and educational programs. These comprehensive quality assurance processes ensure that poison centers maintain the highest standards of toxicology practice while continuously adapting to evolving knowledge, changing exposure patterns, and emerging management approaches.

OPERATIONS

Poison control centers employ systematic processes for exposure assessment, management recommendation development, and follow-up ensuring appropriate care while generating valuable public health data.

Call Management

Telephone triage represents the initial process determining appropriate service pathway based on exposure circumstances, affected individual characteristics, and presenting symptoms. This structured assessment begins with fundamental determinations: whether the contact involves actual exposure versus information-only request; human versus animal exposure; exposure acuity and timing; intentional versus unintentional nature; and preliminary severity assessment based on substance, quantity, and initial symptoms. These basic parameters guide subsequent triage decisions, including call prioritization when multiple simultaneous contacts occur; appropriate staff assignment based on case complexity and expertise requirements; physician notification necessity; and preliminary disposition recommendation between home management, healthcare evaluation, or emergency services activation. Implementation typically follows structured protocols ensuring consistent decision-making while supporting professional judgment application for atypical scenarios. Critical triage considerations include recognition of immediate life threats requiring emergency service activation before detailed assessment; identification of exposures with delayed symptom onset potentially creating false reassurance during initial evaluation; recognition of exposure characteristics suggesting higher severity risk despite current clinical stability; and appropriate balancing between unnecessarily alarming callers versus ensuring adequate concern for potentially serious exposures.

Special population considerations significantly influence triage decisions, with pediatric patients, pregnant women, elderly individuals, and those with significant comorbidities or medication regimens typically receiving more conservative recommendations than otherwise healthy adults with similar exposures. Effective telephone triage represents a specialized skill balancing protocol adherence ensuring standardization with clinical judgment applying principles to unique situations, requiring both comprehensive toxicology knowledge and refined communication capabilities gathering essential information efficiently while establishing rapport supporting subsequent recommendation adherence.

Exposure assessment methodology employs structured questioning gathering essential information supporting accurate risk determination and appropriate management recommendations. Critical information elements include substance identification with as much specificity as possible, including product names, active ingredients, concentrations, and formulation characteristics; exposure circumstances including route (ingestion, inhalation, dermal, ocular, parenteral), duration, and context providing insights into potential quantity and intent; patient characteristics including age, weight, pregnancy status, medical conditions, and current medications potentially affecting toxin susceptibility or management approaches; symptom evaluation addressing presence, severity, progression, and organ systems involved; interventions already attempted before poison center contact; and available resources including transportation capability, home care capacity, and proximity to healthcare facilities.

Remember

The systematic approach to poison exposure calls includes substance identification, dose assessment, risk determination based on toxicokinetics and patient factors, triage decisions, management recommendations, and follow-up calls to assess outcomes.

Information gathering approaches employ specific techniques enhancing accuracy despite the challenging telephone assessment environment, including open-ended questioning encouraging detailed description rather than interpretation; directed questioning for specific high-value details when spontaneous provision proves insufficient; clarification of ambiguous terminology ensuring mutual understanding; reflective listening confirming accurate information capture; and timeline establishment determining relationship between exposure, symptom onset, and progression pattern. Particular attention focuses on substance identification challenges, with strategies including careful spelling confirmation preventing sound-alike errors; location determination helping narrow possibilities when exact identification remains uncertain; visual description of packaging, pills, or materials when product names are unknown; exploration of context potentially suggesting likely exposures when direct identification proves impossible; and occasionally guidance for digital image transmission enabling visual assessment by poison center staff. This systematic exposure assessment creates the essential foundation for subsequent risk assessment and management recommendation development, representing a fundamental poison center function requiring both specialized knowledge and refined interviewing skills.

Risk assessment processes translate exposure information into determination of potential toxicity, expected clinical course, and appropriate intervention level.

Table 13.2: Call Management and Response Protocols

Call Type	Initial Assessment	Information Resources
Exposure	Substance, quantity, route, time, symptoms, patient demographics	POISINDEX, TOMES, product databases
Information Request	Type of information needed, urgency, context	Databases, reference texts, manufacturer information
Healthcare Provider Consultation	Patient status, treatment already initiated, specific questions	Primary literature, specialized databases, toxicologist consultation
Environmental/Public Health	Exposure scenario, population at risk, setting	CHEMM, WISER, hazardous materials databases
Follow-Up	Previous case number, interim developments, current status	Original case record, additional resources as needed

This analysis integrates multiple factors including specific toxin properties and toxic dose considerations; individual patient characteristics affecting susceptibility; exposure circumstances influencing actual absorbed dose; time relationship between exposure and evaluation; current clinical status; and trajectory suggesting stability, improvement, or deterioration. Toxin-specific considerations include known toxic mechanisms; dose-response relationships established through literature, databases, and experience; specific organ system vulnerabilities associated with particular agents; expected onset and progression timing for toxic effects; potential delayed manifestations requiring monitoring despite current asymptomaticity; available antidotes or specific therapeutic interventions; and anticipated clinical course with and without interventions. Patient factors significantly influencing assessment include age-related vulnerabilities, particularly in very young and elderly populations; pregnancy considerations including both maternal and fetal risk; medical comorbidities affecting toxin metabolism, elimination, or target organ reserve; medication regimens creating potential interactions; and genetic factors when known to influence toxin susceptibility. Exposure analysis examines circumstances affecting actual dose absorption, including formulation characteristics influencing dissolution and absorption rates; exposure route determining bioavailability and absorption kinetics; timing relative to food consumption for ingestions; duration and concentration for inhalational or dermal exposures; and decontamination or interventions already performed potentially reducing effective dose. These multidimensional considerations support development of risk determinations typically categorized as minimal or nontoxic exposure requiring observation only; minor effects expected with symptomatic management; moderate toxicity requiring specific interventions; major or life-threatening exposure necessitating aggressive management; or confirmed non-exposure based on circumstantial analysis. This risk stratification directly informs subsequent management recommendation development, creating the critical link between exposure assessment and appropriate intervention guidance.

Management recommendation development translates risk assessment into practical guidance addressing both optimal toxicological management and implementation feasibility within specific circumstances. Home management recommendations apply to approximately 70% of exposures, appropriate for minimal toxicity situations, minor symptoms amenable to symptomatic care, or certain moderate exposures where home observation with poison center follow-up provides safe, cost-effective alternatives to healthcare facility evaluation. These recommendations typically include observation parameters with specific concerning symptoms warranting reevaluation; appropriate home interventions which may include limited decontamination measures, symptomatic care, or monitoring practices; explicit instruction regarding interventions to avoid, particularly addressing common misconceptions like induced vomiting; follow-up scheduling establishing continued poison center monitoring; and circumstances that should trigger emergency services activation if clinical changes occur. Healthcare facility referrals, representing approximately 30% of exposures, include specific guidance regarding appropriate transportation method based on current stability and anticipated progression; triage level recommendation balancing appropriate urgency against unnecessarily alarming language; preview of likely interventions helping facilities prepare for patient arrival; relevant laboratory studies or diagnostic evaluations warranting consideration; specific management recommendations including decontamination approaches, antidotes, enhanced elimination techniques, or particular monitoring parameters; and notation of poison center availability for ongoing consultation during treatment. Special situations requiring customized recommendations include exposures in remote locations with limited healthcare access; patients refusing recommended evaluation despite concerning exposure characteristics; vulnerable populations including children, pregnant women, and elderly individuals potentially requiring more conservative management; suspected self-harm attempts needing both toxicological and psychiatric considerations; mistrust situations where caller skepticism threatens recommendation adherence; and cases where social service or law enforcement notification obligations arise from exposure circumstances. Effective recommendation development considers not only ideal toxicological management but also practical implementation factors including caller capabilities, resource availability, geographic constraints, and likelihood of recommendation adherence, creating realistic, contextually appropriate guidance rather than rigid protocol application regardless of individual circumstances.

Follow-up processes represent essential components of poison center practice, serving multiple functions including outcome determination, management plan adjustment based on clinical progression, continued guidance as cases evolve, and data completeness for surveillance and research purposes. Implementation typically involves systematic scheduling based on risk assessment, with higher toxicity potential warranting more frequent and extended monitoring compared to minimal risk exposures. Home-managed cases typically receive follow-up calls timed to coincide with expected symptom onset or progression periods, enabling reevaluation when toxicity might develop rather than arbitrary timing. Healthcare facility cases receive follow-up contacts coordinated with expected clinical progression points, balancing information needs against excessive contact potentially burdening busy clinical staff. Follow-up assessment includes systematic reevaluation of clinical status focusing on symptom presence, severity, and trajectory; intervention implementation and apparent effectiveness; new concerns or questions arising since initial contact; and appropriate closure determination based on clinical resolution or stability. Documentation practices ensure comprehensive outcome recording including observed clinical effects organized by organ system; interventions performed with apparent results; laboratory or diagnostic findings when available; clinical course description including duration, severity, and complications; final medical outcome categorized using standardized classifications from no effect through major effect or death; and case closure determination when either clinical resolution occurs or further follow-up would not affect management or outcome determination. Special considerations apply to various scenarios including cases lost to follow-up despite attempts; situations where initial recommendations were not followed requiring alternative management development; unexpected outcomes prompting reevaluation of initial assessment; prolonged toxicity requiring extended monitoring beyond typical patterns; and cases involving substances with limited toxicity information where detailed outcome documentation provides valuable reference data for future exposures. This systematic follow-up process transforms poison centers from simple consultation services into comprehensive case management systems supporting patients throughout toxicological emergencies while generating valuable data regarding exposure outcomes across diverse substances and circumstances.

Information Delivery

Telephone communication effectiveness significantly influences both information gathering accuracy and recommendation implementation likelihood, requiring specialized techniques addressing the challenges of critical health communication without visual cues or direct patient assessment. Initial rapport establishment creates foundation for effective interaction through appropriate introduction establishing professional identity and service purpose; expression of concern demonstrating empathy regardless of exposure circumstances; and non-judgmental approach even with scenarios involving preventable accidents, substance misuse, or self-harm attempts. Information gathering employs techniques balancing efficiency with comprehensiveness, including open-ended questions encouraging detailed description followed by specific inquiries addressing critical details; reflective listening confirming accurate understanding; and appropriate pacing allowing sufficient response time while maintaining conversation direction. Language adaptation ensures comprehension across diverse educational levels, cultural backgrounds, and native languages, with strategies including avoidance of medical jargon when speaking with laypersons; confirmation of understanding through technique like "teach-back" where callers rephrase recommendations in their own words; appropriate technical terminology with healthcare professionals enabling precise communication; and integration of translation services for non-English speakers ensuring accurate information exchange despite language barriers. Emotional management represents another essential communication element, with approaches addressing caller anxiety through calm, confident tone; recognition and validation of legitimate concerns; factual reassurance when appropriate without minimizing valid worries; and structured information delivery preventing overwhelming cognitive processing capacity during stressful situations. Recommendation delivery employs specific techniques enhancing adherence likelihood, including clear prioritization distinguishing critical actions from supplementary measures; explicit rationale explanation connecting recommendations to health concerns; anticipatory guidance preparing callers for expected developments; and concrete action steps rather than general principles. Documentation of communication includes verbatim quotation of critical information provided by callers ensuring accuracy without interpretation bias; notation of specific recommendations delivered including any alternatives discussed; recording of apparent comprehension level and agreement with recommendations; and documentation of any barriers identified potentially affecting implementation capability. These specialized communication techniques collectively address the challenges inherent in telephone consultation, supporting both accurate assessment and effective intervention despite the absence of direct patient examination or visual clinical assessment typically available in traditional healthcare settings.

Healthcare professional interactions require specialized approaches different from general public communication, reflecting professional knowledge base, clinical responsibilities, and collaborative consultation relationships rather than directive guidance typical with laypersons. Effective consultation with healthcare providers begins with appropriate role establishment as collaborative toxicology resource rather than authoritative director, recognizing the treating provider's ultimate responsibility for patient care while offering specialized expertise supporting clinical decision-making. Information exchange employs medical terminology enabling precise communication; recognition of clinical data already collected avoiding redundant questioning; efficient communication focusing on assessment and management rather than educational digressions; and appropriate acknowledgment of referring provider's expertise and initial management steps. Recommendation delivery employs evidence-based approach with literature or database references when appropriate; clear distinctions between standard recommendations based on established toxicology principles versus suggestions for unusual scenarios with limited evidence; explicit risk-benefit discussions for interventions with potential complications; and appropriate framing recognizing healthcare resource constraints, competing clinical priorities, and practical implementation considerations within specific practice environments. Specialized documentation for healthcare professional interactions includes credentials of both consulting and consulted parties; specific clinical questions prompting consultation; detailed management recommendations provided; apparent plan implementation intention from consulting provider; arrangements for continued case collaboration including follow-up timing and communication mechanisms; and explicit notation of any recommendation disagreements or alternative approaches selected by treating providers. These professional-to-professional interactions represent an important poison center function distinct from public access services, requiring different communication approaches, modified recommendation framing, specialized documentation, and recognition of collaborative rather than directive relationships supporting optimal patient care through effective toxicology expertise integration within broader healthcare delivery systems.

Documentation standards ensure comprehensive, accurate recording of all poison center interactions supporting both individual case management and broader surveillance, research, and quality improvement functions. Core documentation elements include contact information facilitating follow-up and case continuity; demographic data supporting epidemiological analysis; exposure details including substance, route, circumstances, and timing; assessment findings covering symptoms, interventions before contact, and risk determination; recommendations provided including specific guidance, warnings, and follow-up arrangements; management course throughout the case including interventions, clinical progression, and outcome determination; and administrative elements including staff identification, case classification, and record linkage information for related contacts. Implementation typically employs structured electronic systems with standardized fields ensuring consistent data collection alongside free text capabilities allowing narrative documentation of unique case aspects not captured in categorical elements. Quality standards address several dimensions including factual accuracy ensuring reliable information recording; completeness capturing all essential elements supporting both clinical management and data utilization; timeliness with real-time documentation during active case management; appropriate detail balancing comprehensive recording against excessive documentation consuming time needed for direct service provision; confidentiality protection through appropriate access controls and information sharing limitations; and standardized terminology facilitating accurate coding for surveillance and research purposes. Special considerations apply to various scenarios including particularly complex or high-risk cases warranting enhanced documentation detail; cases with potential medical-legal implications requiring meticulous recording of all communications and recommendations; cases involving suspected abuse, self-harm, or criminal activity triggering mandatory reporting obligations; and unusual exposures or emerging substances where detailed documentation provides valuable reference information for future similar situations. Beyond supporting individual case management, this comprehensive documentation creates the essential data foundation for broader poison center functions including toxicosurveillance identifying emerging hazards, quality improvement activities enhancing service delivery, research expanding toxicological knowledge, and value demonstration supporting operational sustainability.

Information confidentiality represents an essential consideration balancing appropriate information utilization for patient care, public health, and operational purposes against privacy protection obligations. Legal frameworks governing poison center operations include Health Insurance Portability and Accountability Act (HIPAA) requirements regarding protected health information; state-specific privacy regulations which may extend beyond federal standards; specific poison center confidentiality statutes in many jurisdictions providing enhanced protection for toxicology consultation records; and federal confidentiality regulations for substance use disorder information when applicable to specific cases. Implementation approaches address several dimensions including appropriate information sharing with healthcare providers directly involved in patient care; limited data set creation for surveillance and research activities with removal of direct identifiers; mandatory reporting compliance for situations including suspected child abuse, elder abuse, or certain infectious diseases; appropriate response to legal demands including subpoenas, court orders, or law enforcement requests; and internal access controls ensuring staff members access only records necessary for their specific responsibilities. Special considerations apply to various scenarios including adolescent confidentiality with complex parent/guardian access considerations; cases involving illicit substance use where additional stigma and potential legal concerns exist; situations where public health and safety concerns potentially justify broader information sharing than typical clinical scenarios; and cases involving public figures or high-profile incidents creating enhanced media interest and confidentiality challenges. Balancing these considerations requires carefully developed policies, staff training regarding confidentiality obligations, appropriate technical safeguards within information systems, and regular privacy practice review ensuring continued compliance with evolving legal requirements. This structured approach supports both individual privacy protection and appropriate information utilization for legitimate patient care, public health, and operational purposes, maintaining public trust essential for poison center utilization while enabling valuable data utilization beyond direct service provision.

Public Access Services

Public education programs represent essential poison center functions addressing prevention, appropriate emergency response, and service awareness through diverse initiatives targeted to specific populations and risk factors. Childhood poisoning prevention represents a traditional focus, with programming addressing several dimensions: developmental risk recognition helping parents anticipate and address changing exposure risks as children develop new capabilities; safe storage practices for medications, household chemicals, and other potential toxins; appropriate use of safety packaging while recognizing its limitations; supervision strategies balancing vigilance against impractical constant monitoring expectations; and specific high-risk substance education addressing particularly dangerous common household toxins. General public initiatives extend beyond childhood focus to address broader population needs including medication safety for adults addressing polypharmacy risks, look-alike product confusion, and dosing error prevention; household chemical safety covering proper storage, use according to label instructions, and ventilation requirements; food safety focusing on proper preparation, storage, and recognition of potential contamination; plant safety addressing identification of toxic species and appropriate placement relative to children and pets; seasonal hazard education targeting risks associated with specific annual patterns like carbon monoxide during heating seasons or plant exposures during spring foraging; and emerging risk communication addressing newly recognized hazards requiring rapid public awareness. Healthcare provider education includes both formal programs like continuing education courses and informal knowledge transfer through routine consultations, covering topics like current management recommendations for common toxins; recognition of toxidromes supporting accurate diagnosis; appropriate use of diagnostic testing including toxicology screens; antidote availability, indications, and administration guidance; and emerging substance awareness for new drugs of abuse or pharmaceutical agents. Implementation approaches span diverse methodologies including traditional printed materials like brochures, magnets, and posters; digital content through websites, social media, and mobile applications; mass media campaigns utilizing radio, television, and print outlets; community presentations at schools, senior centers, health fairs, and community events; and targeted outreach to specific high-risk populations identified through surveillance data analysis. Effectiveness evaluation increasingly employs outcome measures beyond simple distribution counts, examining actual knowledge acquisition, behavior change, and ultimately exposure rate modification within targeted categories, supporting continuous program refinement based on demonstrated impact rather than simply activity volume.

Table 13.3: Poison Center Public Health Contributions

Function	**Activities**	**Partner Organizations**
Toxicosurveillance	Real-time data analysis, pattern recognition, aberration detection	CDC, FDA, state health departments
Disaster Response	Surge capacity, specialized information, triage support	Emergency management agencies, FEMA, HazMat teams
Cost Avoidance	Home management when appropriate, healthcare utilization optimization	Healthcare systems, insurers, Medicaid/Medicare
Outbreak Investigation	Case finding, exposure characterization, intervention recommendations	CDC, state/local health departments, FDA
Public Health Education	Risk communication, prevention messaging, healthcare provider training	Schools, community organizations, healthcare facilities

Awareness campaigns ensure that potential service users know about poison center availability, access methods, and appropriate utilization circumstances. These initiatives address several awareness dimensions: universal access information communicating the national poison help line (1-800-222-1222) automatically routing callers to their regional center; service scope clarification addressing common misconceptions by explaining both emergency response for actual exposures and information availability for prevention questions; confidentiality assurance addressing privacy concerns potentially limiting utilization, particularly for sensitive exposure circumstances; cost clarification emphasizing free availability regardless of insurance status or immigration status; and appropriate utilization guidance helping the public distinguish between situations warranting poison center contact versus those requiring immediate emergency services activation. Implementation approaches include permanent environmental placement through refrigerator magnets, phone stickers, and programmed smartphone contacts ensuring access information availability during emergencies; digital presence optimization ensuring high search result visibility when potential users seek poisoning information online; integration within healthcare settings through materials in emergency departments, primary care offices, and pharmacies; targeted outreach to underutilized populations identified through demographic analysis of service utilization patterns; language-appropriate materials addressing diverse linguistic communities within service regions; and strategic partnerships with complementary organizations including childcare providers, schools, senior services, and community health workers extending reach beyond direct poison center capabilities. Evaluation metrics examine both general population awareness through surveys assessing knowledge of services and access methods, and more specific utilization patterns analyzing service penetration across geographic regions, demographic categories, and exposure types, identifying potential awareness gaps requiring targeted intervention. These comprehensive awareness initiatives represent essential complements to actual service provision, as poison centers can only deliver value to individuals who know about availability and access methods during poisoning emergencies or when seeking preventive information.

Telephone information services address non-emergency inquiries regarding potential toxicity, proper use of potentially hazardous substances, and prevention strategies. These services differ from emergency exposure management through their informational rather than interventional nature, though employing similar toxicology expertise. Common inquiry categories include medication information requests addressing proper dosing, potential side effects, interaction concerns, and appropriate administration methods; household product questions regarding proper use, potential hazards, safe storage, and disposal recommendations; plant and mushroom identification assisting with determining potential toxicity of species found in yards, homes, or wild settings; environmental exposure concerns addressing contaminants in water, air, or soil; occupational chemical information regarding workplace substance hazards and appropriate protective measures; animal toxicity questions addressing potential pet exposures or comparative toxicology issues; pregnancy and lactation inquiries regarding medication safety, environmental exposures, or household chemical concerns during these vulnerable periods; and general prevention information supporting proactive risk reduction through environmental modification and appropriate safety practices. Response approaches emphasize clear information provision balancing comprehensive hazard communication against unnecessarily alarmist messaging; appropriate knowledge limitations acknowledgment when questions exceed available toxicological information; educational communication style developing caller risk assessment capabilities rather than simply providing singular answers; referral to appropriate specialized resources for questions beyond poison center scope; and documentation supporting both quality assurance and identification of common information needs potentially warranting broader educational initiatives. These information services provide valuable public health benefits through accurate toxicology information accessibility, misconception correction, unnecessary emergency department referral prevention for perceived but non-actual hazards, and relationship building with community members before emergency situations occur. While less dramatic than emergency exposure management, these informational services represent important poison center functions supporting rational risk assessment and appropriate precautionary behavior through expert toxicology information access outside emergency contexts.

Special services address unique needs beyond standard exposure management and information provision, extending poison center capabilities to meet specific community requirements. Language accessibility services ensure meaningful access for diverse linguistic populations through several approaches: direct multilingual staffing with specialists fluent in commonly encountered languages; telephone interpretation services providing real-time translation for less frequently encountered languages; translated educational materials addressing common prevention topics and basic service information; culturally adapted messaging recognizing that effective communication involves not only language translation but also cultural context understanding; and community partnerships with organizations serving specific linguistic populations extending trusted information channels. Hearing impaired accessibility includes telecommunications relay services, text-based communication options, and video remote interpreting for sign language users, ensuring equitable service access regardless of hearing status. Industry and occupational services provide specialized support for workplace exposures through enhanced information regarding industrial chemicals, appropriate occupational exposure response protocols, and coordination with occupational health providers, particularly valuable for facilities working with unusual or high-hazard materials. Disaster response capabilities include surge capacity for mass exposure events; specialized information regarding chemical, biological, radiological, nuclear, and explosive agents; integration with emergency management systems through established communication channels and response protocols; decontamination guidance for first responders and healthcare facilities; and participation in community preparedness planning before events occur. School health program support includes specialized resources for school nurses managing common childhood exposures in educational settings; curriculum materials supporting poison prevention education appropriate for various grade levels; and consultation availability addressing school-specific scenarios like science laboratory incidents or medication administration errors. These specialized services demonstrate poison center adaptability addressing diverse community needs beyond core exposure management functions, reflecting evolution from simple telephone advice services to comprehensive toxicology resources responsive to varied stakeholder requirements across healthcare, public health, occupational, educational, and emergency management domains.

PUBLIC HEALTH ROLE

Poison control centers serve essential public health functions extending beyond individual exposure management to broader population health protection, surveillance, and education.

Toxicovigilance

Active surveillance systematically analyzes poison center data identifying concerning patterns requiring public health intervention before widespread harm occurs. Methodological approaches include: aberration detection algorithms continuously analyzing incoming data for statistically unusual patterns comparing current activity against historical baselines; spatial analysis identifying geographical clustering potentially indicating localized exposure sources; temporal trend monitoring detecting gradual changes in specific exposure types, severity, or demographic patterns; syndromic surveillance grouping cases by symptom constellations rather than reported substances, potentially identifying unknown toxins through characteristic effect patterns; sentinel event monitoring flagging individual cases with unusual characteristics warranting investigation despite lacking statistical clustering; and integrated surveillance combining poison center data with complementary sources including emergency department visits, hospital admissions, medical examiner reports, and laboratory test results. Implementation typically involves automated analytical systems performing continuous data review with alert generation when predefined thresholds are exceeded; toxicologist or epidemiologist review determining actual versus statistical anomalies; coordinated investigation with public health authorities when concerning patterns are confirmed; and continuous refinement improving detection sensitivity while minimizing false positives consuming limited investigative resources. Applications include early identification of contaminated consumer products before widespread distribution; detection of emerging drugs of abuse before recognition through traditional monitoring systems; identification of medication packaging or labeling problems creating systemic error risks; recognition of occupational exposure clusters suggesting workplace hazards; and detection of potential bioterrorism or chemical terrorism events through unusual exposure patterns. This proactive surveillance transforms routine poison center documentation into valuable public health intelligence, supporting early intervention preventing additional exposures rather than simply managing consequences after widespread impact has occurred. This population health protection function represents a critical poison center contribution beyond individual patient care, creating public health value far exceeding direct service provision alone through systematic pattern recognition identifying emerging threats before they become major public health emergencies.

Outbreak investigation capabilities enable poison centers to rapidly characterize and respond to unusual exposure clusters, complementing traditional public health infrastructure with specialized toxicological expertise. When surveillance activities identify potential clusters, structured investigation processes typically include case definition development specifying clinical, laboratory, and epidemiological criteria distinguishing related cases from background occurrences; case finding extending beyond initially identified cases through healthcare provider alerts, media announcements, or database searching; detailed exposure assessment through enhanced information collection regarding potential sources, circumstances, and timelines; laboratory coordination facilitating appropriate testing identifying responsible agents; clinical guidance development supporting consistent management across affected healthcare facilities; and collaboration with regulatory agencies addressing product removal, facility closure, or other interventions preventing additional exposures. Implementation strengths include poison centers' 24/7 availability supporting rapid response regardless of timing; established relationships with healthcare facilities enabling efficient information exchange; toxicological expertise guiding appropriate testing and management approaches; standardized documentation systems supporting systematic data collection; and experience managing unusual or unknown toxins when initial agent identification remains uncertain. Case examples demonstrating this capability include identification of contaminated medications through unusual adverse effect patterns; characterization of foodborne illness outbreaks from toxin-producing organisms; investigation of illness clusters from contaminated dietary supplements; identification of occupational exposure incidents affecting multiple workers; and assessment of environmental contamination events affecting community residents. These outbreak investigation capabilities transform poison centers from passive recipients of individual exposure reports into active public health response agencies capable of rapidly characterizing and addressing population exposure threats. This function represents valuable public health infrastructure extending traditional health department capabilities through specialized toxicological expertise, 24/7 availability, and established healthcare system relationships supporting rapid response to emerging threats before widespread harm occurs.

> **Remember**
>
> **Beyond direct consultation, Poison Control Centers fulfill critical public health roles including toxicosurveillance for emerging threats, disaster response coordination, healthcare provider education, and public poison prevention outreach.**

Hazard identification and risk communication processes translate surveillance findings and investigation results into actionable information preventing additional exposures. When concerning patterns are identified, systematic assessment determines appropriate response level based on factors including exposure severity, population vulnerability, spread potential, intervention availability, and evidence certainty. For situations warranting active response, structured communication processes typically include targeted notification alerting specific groups at heightened risk through established channels such as health alert networks reaching healthcare providers, direct communication with affected industries or facilities, or specialized notifications to vulnerable populations; broader public communication when appropriate through media releases, social media alerts, or website announcements balancing adequate warning against unnecessary alarm; specific guidance development addressing recommended actions, exposure recognition, and appropriate response if exposure occurs; and coordination with regulatory agencies ensuring consistent messaging across public health, healthcare, and regulatory communications. Implementation considerations include message development balancing technical accuracy with public comprehensibility; appropriate urgency level conveying seriousness without creating panic; specific actionable recommendations rather than vague warnings; sensitivity to potential economic or psychological impacts of warnings; and follow-up communications updating information as investigations proceed or situations resolve. These risk communication capabilities transform surveillance data and investigation findings from passive information into active exposure prevention through appropriate translation of technical findings into practical guidance for affected populations, healthcare providers, and responsible authorities. This communication function represents an essential component of comprehensive toxicovigilance, as even the most sophisticated detection systems create little public health value without effective mechanisms translating findings into appropriate preventive action through timely, accurate, and actionable risk communication reaching those in position to implement protective measures before additional exposures occur.

Environmental health partnerships connect poison center toxicological expertise with agencies addressing chemical safety, occupational exposures, and environmental contamination, creating synergistic capability exceeding either individual system alone. These collaborative relationships typically include formal arrangements with environmental protection agencies supporting joint investigation of chemical releases, spills, or contamination incidents; occupational safety and health authorities addressing workplace exposure patterns identified through surveillance; consumer product safety agencies investigating potentially hazardous products identified through unusual exposure reports; and public health environmental divisions addressing community-wide exposure concerns. Operational models include data sharing agreements enabling systematic information exchange while maintaining appropriate confidentiality protections; joint response protocols establishing coordinated investigation and intervention processes for chemical incidents; mutual consultation arrangements providing toxicological expertise to environmental agencies while gaining environmental assessment capabilities for poison centers; and sometimes co-located personnel facilitating seamless collaboration through physical proximity. Implementation examples include poison center identification of unusual pesticide exposure patterns triggering environmental investigation of application practices or regulatory compliance; coordinated response to chemical spills or releases with poison centers providing healthcare guidance while environmental agencies address containment and remediation; collaborative assessment of clusters suggesting indoor air quality concerns in specific buildings or facilities; joint investigation of possible water contamination incidents identified through unusual symptom reports; and combined response to natural disasters creating complex chemical exposure scenarios through infrastructure damage, displaced hazardous materials, or interrupted utility services. These environmental health partnerships transform isolated regulatory, environmental, and medical systems into integrated chemical safety networks addressing the full spectrum from exposure prevention through consequence management. This collaborative approach recognizes that effective chemical safety requires both the toxicological expertise and healthcare system connections of poison centers and the regulatory authority, environmental monitoring capability, and remediation resources of environmental agencies, creating comprehensive protection exceeding what either system could provide independently.

Disaster Response

Chemical incident response capabilities enable poison centers to provide critical toxicological expertise during hazardous materials emergencies, industrial accidents, transportation spills, and other acute chemical release scenarios. Core functions typically include: agent identification support through database access, chemical property information, and recognition of characteristic toxidromes when unknown substances present; exposure risk assessment evaluating potential health impacts based on substance properties, release characteristics, environmental conditions, and population proximity; decontamination guidance addressing appropriate methods, priorities, and resource requirements for exposed individuals; triage recommendations supporting efficient resource allocation distinguishing between patients requiring immediate intervention versus observation only; treatment consultation providing specific management recommendations for confirmed or suspected exposures; healthcare facility preparation alerting potentially receiving hospitals regarding agent information, expected clinical effects, and management approaches; and public information support developing accurate, actionable guidance for affected communities. Implementation strengths include 24/7 availability ensuring immediate response regardless of timing; established relationships with emergency medical services, hazardous materials teams, and emergency departments facilitating effective communication during high-stress situations; comprehensive toxicology information resources supporting rapid guidance development even for unusual chemicals; and surge capacity managing multiple simultaneous consultations during large-scale incidents. Operational arrangements typically include formal integration within emergency management systems through designated roles in emergency operations plans; predetermined communication channels ensuring information flow during incidents when routine systems may be overwhelmed; regular participation in disaster exercises testing response capabilities before actual events; and sometimes dedicated disaster response protocols streamlining operations during declared emergencies. These chemical incident capabilities transform poison centers from routine healthcare consultants into essential emergency response assets providing specialized expertise critical for effective management of hazardous materials incidents, industrial accidents, and other acute chemical emergencies potentially affecting population health.

Radiological and nuclear incident support leverages poison center operational infrastructure and healthcare system connections to assist response efforts during these specialized emergency scenarios. While specific radiological expertise typically resides with specialized agencies like the Radiation Emergency Assistance Center/Training Site (REACTS) or state radiation control programs, poison centers provide complementary capabilities including: communication hub functionality connecting healthcare facilities with radiological experts through established consultation processes; triage support distinguishing between potentially exposed individuals requiring assessment versus those seeking evaluation due to concern alone; decontamination guidance regarding appropriate methods based on specific radionuclide properties and exposure circumstances; countermeasure information addressing appropriate use of potassium iodide, Prussian blue, DTPA, or other specific medical countermeasures; treatment recommendations for combined injuries involving both radiological contamination and conventional trauma; and public information support developing appropriate guidance balancing necessary precautions against excessive anxiety. Implementation arrangements typically include predefined relationships with specialized radiological resources ensuring rapid connection during emergencies; basic radiological education for poison center staff supporting appropriate initial response before specialist consultation; predetermined roles within radiological emergency response plans clarifying responsibilities and communication channels; and sometimes specialized protocols addressing unique aspects of radiological emergencies compared to more common chemical exposures. These capabilities transform poison centers from chemical-focused resources into valuable assets during radiological incidents, particularly through their established healthcare system connections, 24/7 availability, and experience managing public concern during perceived exposure situations—functions complementing the specialized technical expertise of radiation safety authorities and creating more effective integrated response than either system could provide independently.

Biological incident consultation provides support during natural disease outbreaks, bioterrorism events, or other situations involving unusual infectious or biological toxin exposures. While primary expertise for infectious disease emergencies typically resides with public health departments and specialized centers like CDC, poison centers offer complementary capabilities including: initial pattern recognition through syndromic surveillance potentially identifying unusual symptom clusters before specific pathogen identification; differential diagnosis support distinguishing between chemical, biological, and radiological causes of presenting symptoms; exposure and prophylaxis information regarding concerns like anthrax, ricin, botulinum toxin, and other biological agents with toxicological dimensions; medication information addressing appropriate use of antibiotics, antivirals, or other countermeasures during public health emergencies; adverse effect management for countermeasures distributed during mass prophylaxis campaigns; and public information support handling individual concerns during community-wide biological incidents. Implementation arrangements typically include integration within broader bioterrorism response systems; predetermined roles within public health emergency plans; established communication channels with public health authorities and specialized biological expertise resources; and staff education regarding biological agents with toxicological dimensions enabling appropriate initial response before specialist consultation. During actual incidents, poison centers frequently manage substantial call volume from concerned individuals seeking guidance regarding symptoms, potential exposure, and appropriate actions, providing valuable public information services complementing official communications and reducing burden on emergency medical services and healthcare facilities. These biological incident capabilities transform poison centers from strictly chemical exposure resources into valuable assets during complex public health emergencies through their healthcare system connectivity, public accessibility, and experience managing situations involving both actual exposure concerns and public anxiety requiring appropriate contextualization and guidance.

Surge capacity management enables poison centers to maintain essential services during major incidents creating extreme call volume beyond normal operational parameters. Preparedness measures typically include scalable staffing models identifying additional qualified personnel available during emergencies, including off-duty staff, recently retired specialists, affiliated toxicologists, and sometimes poison center staff from unaffected regions through mutual aid arrangements; telecommunications systems designed for expansion handling multiple simultaneous incoming calls beyond normal volumes; predetermined triage protocols prioritizing calls during overwhelming situations ensuring most urgent cases receive immediate attention; standardized information sets addressing common questions for specific incident types enabling consistent, efficient response without requiring individualized specialist formulation for each contact; technology support including interactive voice response systems providing basic information for common questions, website resources offering standardized guidance, and sometimes social media monitoring identifying common concerns requiring proactive messaging; and coordination mechanisms with emergency management systems enabling appropriate resource request when center capabilities become overwhelmed despite internal surge measures. Implementation experience demonstrates that different incident types create distinct surge patterns, with sudden-onset events like chemical releases typically generating immediate, intense surge primarily from potentially exposed individuals seeking guidance, while evolving situations like food contamination incidents often produce extended moderate surge with substantial media-driven concern from individuals without actual exposure risk. Effective surge management transforms potentially overwhelming situations from operational failures into successful public service delivery through systematic preparation, appropriate resource scaling, and predetermined operational modifications matching response capacity to incident-driven demand patterns. This capability represents an essential element of comprehensive emergency preparedness, as even the most sophisticated response plans provide limited value if key communication nodes like poison centers become overwhelmed during implementation, creating public perception of system failure exactly when confident competence is most critical for public trust.

Educational Outreach

Professional education initiatives develop specialized toxicology knowledge among healthcare providers, first responders, and allied professionals, enhancing both direct patient care capability and appropriate poison center utilization. Target audiences include emergency medicine physicians and nurses as frontline poisoning management providers; primary care practitioners encountering various toxicological issues from medication interactions to environmental exposures; pediatric providers managing common childhood ingestions; emergency medical technicians and paramedics making field triage and intervention decisions; pharmacists addressing medication safety and adverse effect recognition; school nurses managing common exposure scenarios in educational settings; and various specialists encountering toxicological dimensions within their practice areas. Content typically includes toxidrome recognition supporting accurate diagnosis; initial management priorities before toxicology consultation; appropriate diagnostic testing selection avoiding unnecessary resource utilization; specific antidote utilization guidance; enhanced elimination technique indications and limitations; recognition of unusual or emerging toxic presentations; and effective consultation processes maximizing poison center value. Implementation approaches include formal continuing education programs through seminars, conferences, and online modules; rotations for medical, pharmacy, and nursing students developing both toxicology knowledge and appropriate consultation habits early in professional development; toxicology rounds at affiliated healthcare facilities addressing real cases with educational value; regular case conferences reviewing interesting or instructive exposures; distribution of toxicology bulletins highlighting emerging concerns or management updates; and "teachable moments" during actual case consultations extending beyond immediate management to broader educational principles. Evaluation increasingly employs outcome measures beyond simple participation counts, examining actual knowledge acquisition, practice pattern changes, and ultimately patient care improvement through appropriate toxicology management and consultation. These professional education initiatives transform poison centers from passive consultation resources into active participants in healthcare workforce development, creating systemic capacity for appropriate toxicological management extending beyond direct poison center service interactions to broader healthcare system enhancement through widespread toxicology knowledge dissemination.

Public education programs address prevention, appropriate emergency response, and poison center awareness through diverse initiatives targeting specific populations and risk factors. Prevention content typically includes developmental risk education helping parents anticipate and address changing exposure risks as children develop new capabilities; safe storage practices for medications, household chemicals, and other potential toxins; appropriate use of safety packaging while recognizing its limitations; supervision strategies balancing vigilance against impractical constant monitoring expectations; medication safety addressing dosing errors, look-alike product confusion, and polypharmacy risks; household chemical safety covering proper use, ventilation requirements, and hazardous mixture avoidance; seasonal hazard awareness targeting risks associated with specific annual patterns like carbon monoxide during heating seasons; food safety focusing on proper preparation, storage, and wild food precautions; and plant safety addressing identification of toxic species and appropriate placement relative to children and pets. Emergency response education covers immediate actions when exposures occur; appropriate poison center utilization guidance; common intervention misconceptions like induced vomiting; and recognition of symptoms warranting immediate medical evaluation. Implementation employs diverse approaches including traditional materials like brochures, refrigerator magnets, and posters; digital content through websites, social media, and mobile applications; media campaigns utilizing radio, television, and print outlets; community presentations at schools, senior centers, health fairs, and community events; and targeted outreach to specific high-risk populations identified through surveillance data. Linguistic and cultural considerations receive increasing attention, with materials developed in multiple languages and culturally adapted messaging addressing diverse communities' specific needs, beliefs, and practices. Evaluation increasingly examines actual knowledge acquisition, behavior change, and ultimately exposure rate modification within targeted categories rather than simply distribution metrics. These comprehensive public education initiatives transform poison centers from reactive emergency services into proactive prevention resources, creating value beyond direct exposure management through systematic risk reduction across diverse populations and exposure categories.

Policy and regulatory guidance leverages poison center toxicosurveillance data and clinical experience supporting evidence-based approaches to chemical safety, pharmaceutical regulation, and consumer protection. This advisory function typically includes data provision documenting actual exposure patterns, circumstances, and outcomes informing regulatory decisions with real-world experience rather than theoretical concerns alone; technical consultation during regulatory development providing practical toxicological perspective regarding proposed requirements; impact assessment evaluating implemented policies through longitudinal exposure pattern analysis; unintended consequence identification when regulatory changes create unexpected exposure scenarios or behavior modifications; emerging hazard notification alerting regulators to newly identified risks before widespread impact occurs; and sometimes expert testimony providing toxicological perspective during legislative or regulatory proceedings. Specific applications include pharmaceutical packaging and labeling requirements informed by documented confusion patterns or dosing errors; consumer product safety standards addressing identified hazard patterns in household items; chemical labeling systems balancing appropriate hazard communication against unnecessarily alarming language; protective equipment requirements for occupational settings based on documented exposure incidents; environmental standards regarding chemicals demonstrating actual human exposure consequences; storage and disposal regulations addressing identified diversion or environmental contamination patterns; and professional practice standards regarding appropriate prescribing, dispensing, or administration of high-risk medications. The most effective implementation establishes formal relationships with regulatory authorities creating systematic information flow rather than ad hoc consultation, with arrangements including data use agreements enabling appropriate surveillance information sharing; regular communication mechanisms ensuring awareness of emerging concerns;

advisory committee participation providing ongoing toxicological perspective within regulatory processes; and sometimes joint investigations addressing complex or high-impact situations requiring both toxicological expertise and regulatory authority. This policy advisory function transforms poison center surveillance data and clinical experience from isolated information into valuable regulatory intelligence supporting evidence-based approaches to chemical, pharmaceutical, and consumer product safety across multiple domains.

Media and risk communication initiatives translate toxicological knowledge into accessible public information, addressing both ongoing education needs and emerging hazard communication. Proactive media engagement includes regular features providing seasonal safety information, addressing common misconceptions, and highlighting prevention strategies; relationships with health reporters facilitating accurate toxicology coverage within news organizations; expert commentary availability for toxicology-related stories ensuring evidence-based perspective within public discourse; educational content development for various media platforms including print, broadcast, digital, and social channels; and media training for poison center representatives ensuring effective communication during both routine and emergency situations. Reactive media response addresses emerging situations requiring rapid, accurate information dissemination, with approaches including standardized press release templates for common scenarios enabling quick customization; predetermined messaging addressing frequently recurring issues like local mushroom poisonings or seasonal hazards; spokesperson designation ensuring consistent, authoritative communication; and coordination mechanisms with partner agencies supporting unified messaging during multi-agency response scenarios. Implementation considerations include message development balancing technical accuracy with public comprehensibility; appropriate uncertainty acknowledgment when complete information remains unavailable; actionable recommendations providing specific guidance rather than vague warnings; sensitivity to potential economic impacts of warnings on affected industries; and linguistic and cultural appropriateness ensuring effective communication across diverse communities. Media relationship management balances accessibility supporting accurate coverage against appropriate boundaries preventing sensationalism, particularly for unusual or dramatic poisoning cases potentially creating copycat behavior or unwarranted public alarm. These media and risk communication capabilities transform poison centers from simply technical resources into effective public communicators, translating complex toxicological information into accessible, actionable guidance reaching diverse populations through trusted information channels and supporting both routine safety education and emergency risk communication during acute toxicological threats.

Summary

Poison Control Centers provide 24/7 specialized toxicological expertise through telephone consultation services that significantly reduce healthcare costs while improving patient outcomes across diverse exposures. Organizationally, these centers maintain sophisticated infrastructures with certified Specialists in Poison Information (SPIs)—typically pharmacists or nurses with advanced toxicology training—supervised by board-certified medical toxicologists who provide clinical leadership and protocol development. Administrative directors manage operations, while support personnel maintain information systems, coordinate educational initiatives, and conduct quality improvement programs. Operational protocols guide systematic call management from initial triage through substance identification, risk assessment, management recommendations, and follow-up calls. Centers utilize sophisticated electronic documentation systems and extensive toxicological databases to support accurate, evidence-based recommendations across exposure scenarios ranging from pediatric ingestions to industrial chemical incidents. Documentation captures essential elements including substance characteristics, exposure circumstances, clinical effects, interventions, recommendations, and outcomes, serving both immediate clinical needs and long-term surveillance functions. This detailed information feeds into the National Poison Data System, enabling real-time toxicosurveillance to detect emerging threats like novel recreational drugs, medication tampering, chemical incidents, or foodborne outbreaks. Centers fulfill critical public health functions through proactive roles in disaster preparedness, participation in emergency response networks, professional education for healthcare providers, and public education campaigns on poison prevention. They serve as toxicology resources for healthcare facilities, public health agencies, industry, and regulatory bodies, while conducting research on exposure patterns, treatment efficacy, and prevention strategies. Through these integrated functions, Poison Control Centers serve as sentinel systems for toxic exposures while providing cost-effective consultation that reduces unnecessary emergency department visits and improves poisoning outcomes.

Self-Assessment Questions

1. Describe the organizational structure of Poison Control Centers, including the qualifications, certification requirements, and roles of key personnel such as Specialists in Poison Information and medical toxicologists.
2. Analyze the systematic approach used by Poison Control Centers when managing calls about potential toxic exposures, from initial contact through follow-up processes.
3. Explain how Poison Control Centers determine risk and appropriate triage for potentially toxic exposures, including factors considered in these assessments.
4. Discuss the essential elements captured in Poison Control Center documentation systems and how this information serves both clinical and public health functions.
5. Describe the National Poison Data System (NPDS) and how it facilitates real-time toxicosurveillance to identify emerging public health threats.
6. Analyze the evidence demonstrating the clinical and economic impact of Poison Control Centers on healthcare resource utilization and patient outcomes.
7. Explain how Poison Control Centers contribute to disaster preparedness and response for incidents involving chemical, biological, or radiological exposures.
8. Describe the educational initiatives conducted by Poison Control Centers for healthcare providers, including topics, formats, and objectives of these programs.
9. Discuss the public education strategies employed by Poison Control Centers to promote poison prevention and appropriate response to exposures across different age groups and settings.
10. Analyze how Poison Control Centers adapt their operations and recommendations to address emerging threats such as novel psychoactive substances, pharmaceutical adulterants, or new household products

Bibliography

1. Vassilev ZP, Marcus SM. The impact of a poison control center on the length of hospital stay for patients with poisoning. J Toxicol Environ Health A. 2007;70(2):107-110.
2. Gummin DD, Mowry JB, Beuhler MC, Spyker DA, Bronstein AC, Rivers LJ, et al. 2020 Annual Report of the American Association of Poison Control Centers' National Poison Data System (NPDS): 38th Annual Report. Clin Toxicol (Phila). 2021;59(12):1282-1501.
3. Blizzard JC, Michels JE, Richardson WH, Reeder CE, Schulz RM, Holstege CP. Cost-benefit analysis of a regional poison center. Clin Toxicol (Phila). 2008;46(5):450-456.
4. Wolkin AF, Martin CA, Law RK, Schier JG, Bronstein AC. Using poison center data for national public health surveillance for chemical and poison exposure and associated illness. Ann Emerg Med. 2012;59(1):56-61.
5. Litovitz T, Benson BE, Ford M, Krenzelok EP, Palmer R, Griffith JRK, et al. Evolution of the toxicall database: the American Association of Poison Control Centers database. Clin Toxicol (Phila). 2008;46(10):929-931.
6. Hoffman RS. Understanding the limitations of retrospective analyses of poison center data. Clin Toxicol (Phila). 2007;45(8):943-945.
7. Dart RC, Bronstein AC, Spyker DA, Cantilena LR, Seifert SA, Heard SE, et al. Poisoning in the United States: 2012 emergency medicine report of the National Poison Data System. Ann Emerg Med. 2015;65(4):416-422.
8. Miller TR, Lestina DC. Costs of poisoning in the United States and savings from poison control centers: a benefit-cost analysis. Ann Emerg Med. 1997;29(2):239-245.
9. Nelson LS, Perrone J, DeRoos F, Stork C, Hoffman RS. Poison control centers and emergency departments: partners in toxicosurveillance and public health. J Med Toxicol. 2019;15(2):126-130.
10. Hoppe-Roberts JM, Lloyd LM, Chyka PA. Poisoning mortality in the United States: comparison of national mortality statistics and poison control center reports. Ann Emerg Med. 2000;35(5):440-448.

CHAPTER 14

PREVENTIVE MEASURES

Author

Dr. Shaik Asha Begum, HOD and Associate Professor,
Department of Pharmaceutical Regulatory Affairs,
KVSR Siddartha College of Pharmaceutical Sciences, Vijayawada,
Andhra Pradesh, India

Abstract

Preventing toxic exposures requires integrated approaches spanning communication, engineering, education, and policy domains to address diverse hazards across populations. Risk communication strategies employ principles of clarity, transparency, and cultural sensitivity to effectively convey toxicological information through multiple channels while addressing audience-specific needs, perceptions, and literacy levels. Particular attention must focus on communicating uncertainty, balancing technical accuracy with understandability, and maintaining trust through consistent messaging during toxic emergencies. Safety measures follow a hierarchical framework prioritizing inherently safer chemical alternatives and designs, followed by engineering controls like child-resistant packaging and flow restrictors, warning systems including standardized labeling and hazard symbols, and administrative measures such as storage regulations. These technical interventions work synergistically with educational programs targeting developmental stage-appropriate content for children, specific hazard training for workers, professional education for healthcare providers, and general public awareness campaigns through diverse media. Policy development completes the preventive framework through regulatory approaches including chemical testing requirements, exposure limits, reporting mandates, product restrictions, and infrastructure supporting poison prevention. Implementation science principles guide the adaptation of evidence-based interventions to specific communities and settings, with evaluation mechanisms measuring process indicators, behavioral changes, and ultimate outcomes in terms of reduced poisoning incidence and severity. This comprehensive approach recognizes that effective prevention requires coordinated efforts across multiple sectors, addressing both individual behaviors and systemic factors contributing to toxic exposures.

Keywords: *Poison Prevention, Risk Communication, Child-Resistant Packaging, Safety Regulations, Hazard Labeling, Toxic Exposure Education*

Learning Objectives

After completion of the chapter, the learners should be able to:

- Design effective risk communication strategies for toxicological hazards that address audience characteristics, risk perception factors, and appropriate message framing.
- Apply the hierarchy of safety measures to develop comprehensive prevention strategies for specific toxic exposures in home, workplace, and community settings.
- Develop age-appropriate educational interventions addressing common toxic exposures across developmental stages from early childhood through adulthood.
- Analyze the role of regulatory approaches in poison prevention, including product safety standards, labeling requirements, and restricted access provisions.
- Implement evaluation methodologies to assess the effectiveness of prevention programs using appropriate process, behavioral, and outcome metrics.
- Create integrated prevention strategies that combine communication, engineering, education, and policy approaches to address specific toxicological hazards

RISK COMMUNICATION

Effective risk communication represents a critical component of toxicology prevention, enabling informed decision-making through appropriate hazard information transfer to diverse stakeholders.

Principles and Models

Risk communication fundamentally involves the exchange of information regarding potential harms, with theoretical frameworks evolving substantially over recent decades. Early models employed simple information deficit approaches assuming that providing technical information alone would produce appropriate risk-reduction behaviors. This transmission-focused model presumed that experts possessed objective risk knowledge while public audiences lacked information, creating a unidirectional flow of technical data without significant consideration of reception, interpretation, or contextual factors affecting implementation. Recognition of this model's limitations led to more sophisticated mental models approaches examining how target audiences conceptualize specific risks, often revealing fundamental differences between expert and public understanding that simple information provision failed to address. This recognition shifted practice toward identifying and addressing existing mental frameworks rather than assuming blank-slate recipients. Further evolution produced cultural cognition models acknowledging that risk perception operates within social and cultural contexts where worldviews, group identities, and cultural values fundamentally shape how risk information is received, interpreted, and applied. These models recognize that even identical information may produce dramatically different responses based on cultural factors, trust relationships, and alignment with existing values or identity frameworks. Contemporary approaches increasingly employ social amplification frameworks examining how risk information flows through social systems with various amplification or attenuation factors including media coverage, institutional responses, and community networks that collectively shape risk perception beyond the technical characteristics of the hazard itself. These evolving theoretical frameworks have transformed risk communication practice from simple information dissemination toward more nuanced approaches acknowledging the complex interplay between technical information, psychological processing, social context, and cultural frameworks determining how risk information translates into preventive behavior.

> **Remember**
>
> **Risk communication about toxic hazards must balance technical accuracy with comprehensibility, address perception factors influencing how people interpret risk information, and provide specific actionable recommendations tailored to the audience's needs and capabilities.**

Trust and credibility fundamentally determine risk communication effectiveness, with research consistently demonstrating their primacy in message reception and implementation. Source credibility derives from multiple dimensions including perceived expertise regarding the specific risk domain; demonstrated competence through previous accurate assessments and effective recommendations; objectivity reflected through balanced presentation acknowledging both risks and benefits; empathy demonstrating genuine concern for audience welfare beyond technical considerations; transparency regarding information limitations, uncertainties, or evolving understanding; and consistency across messages, communicators, and time periods avoiding contradictions that undermine confidence. Trust development requires sustained relationship building rather than crisis-limited interaction, with ongoing communication establishing reliability before emergency situations demand immediate action based on recommendations. When addressing distrustful audiences, effective approaches acknowledge past failures creating skepticism; demonstrate concrete changes addressing previous shortcomings; employ trusted intermediaries with established credibility in affected communities; provide verifiable information enabling independent confirmation; and recognize that trust restoration requires substantially more evidence and time than initial trust development.

These principles apply across various toxicological contexts including industrial facility communications with surrounding communities, regulatory agencies addressing consumer product risks, healthcare providers discussing medication hazards, and public health authorities managing chemical emergencies—all situations where technical information effectiveness depends fundamentally on the trust relationship between communicator and audience. This trust centrality represents a paradigm shift from earlier approaches assuming information quality alone determined effectiveness, recognizing instead that identical information from trusted versus distrusted sources produces dramatically different behavioral outcomes regardless of technical accuracy or presentation quality.

Message development for toxicological risk communication requires systematic attention to content, structure, and delivery characteristics supporting both comprehension and appropriate action. Effective content balances completeness against overwhelming complexity, providing sufficient detail for informed decision-making without creating information overload that paradoxically reduces understanding. Core content elements typically include hazard identification explaining the specific toxic agent and its characteristics; exposure pathway clarification addressing how the toxicant might contact individuals through various routes; dose-response information relating exposure magnitude to potential health effects; contextual comparison helping audiences understand relative risk magnitude compared to familiar reference points; practical prevention guidance translating technical information into actionable protective measures; and appropriate uncertainty acknowledgment distinguishing between well-established facts and more preliminary conclusions. Structural considerations include primacy placement with most critical information appearing first given attention limitations; appropriate hierarchical organization supporting both quick scanning for essential points and detailed review for those seeking comprehensive understanding; explicit connection between hazard information and recommended actions ensuring protective behavior motivation; and consistent formatting across similar communications enabling familiar navigation. Delivery characteristics include readability matched to audience education levels without unnecessary technical terminology; cultural appropriateness addressing language preferences, communication norms, and relevant analogies or examples; visual support through appropriate graphics enhancing comprehension beyond text alone; and emotional calibration matching tone to situation seriousness while avoiding both alarmism and inappropriate reassurance.

Table 14.1: Risk Communication Approaches by Audience and Context

Audience	Message Components	Effective Channels	Evaluation Metrics
General Public	Simple instructions, action-oriented guidance, context for risk level	Mass media, social media, websites	Message recall, behavior adoption, exposure reduction
Healthcare Providers	Technical information, management protocols, resource access	Professional journals, continuing education, clinical decision supports	Practice change, management protocol adherence
High-Risk Populations	Targeted prevention strategies, specific exposure scenarios, accessible language	Community outreach, trusted intermediaries, culturally appropriate materials	Exposure reduction in target population, knowledge improvement
Emergency Communication	Clear action directives, protective measures, information sources	Alert systems, broadcast media, social media	Protective action implementation, information-seeking behavior

Message testing before widespread dissemination allows refinement addressing comprehension barriers, unintended implications, or practical implementation challenges identified through representative audience feedback. This comprehensive approach transforms technical toxicological information into effective risk communication supporting informed decision-making and appropriate protective behavior across diverse audiences with varying education levels, cultural backgrounds, and prior risk experiences.

Audience analysis represents an essential foundation for effective risk communication, recognizing that different populations require tailored approaches based on their characteristics, concerns, and communication preferences. Demographic considerations include education levels affecting appropriate terminology, explanation depth, and assumed background knowledge; language proficiency determining translation needs, idiomatic adjustment, or simplified presentation; age-related factors influencing both risk perception and preferred information channels; cultural frameworks shaping hazard interpretation and valued information sources; and socioeconomic factors affecting both access to communication channels and practical prevention capability. Beyond these general characteristics, effective audience analysis examines specific knowledge and attitude dimensions including existing awareness about the particular hazard; mental models revealing how the audience conceptualizes the risk potentially revealing misconceptions requiring correction; emotional responses including fear, outrage, or apathy affecting message reception; competing concerns that might override risk information regardless of comprehension; and self-efficacy beliefs regarding ability to implement protective measures which significantly influence behavioral response regardless of risk perception. Implementation capacity represents another critical dimension including financial resources affecting affordability of recommended actions; time availability for information processing and protective measure implementation; technical capability for understanding and applying complex information; and environmental constraints limiting protective option feasibility regardless of individual motivation. Communication channel preferences also vary substantially across audiences, with considerations including traditional versus digital media usage patterns; trusted information sources within specific communities; formal versus informal information dissemination networks; and accessibility requirements for audiences with sensory, cognitive, or physical limitations. This multidimensional audience analysis transforms generic risk communication into targeted approaches addressing specific population characteristics, concerns, and capabilities, substantially enhancing the likelihood that toxicological information will translate into appropriate protective behavior rather than being ignored, misunderstood, or impractical within the audience's actual life circumstances.

Hazard Communication Systems

Globally Harmonized System of Classification and Labelling of Chemicals (GHS) represents an internationally standardized approach for communicating chemical hazards through consistent classification criteria, labeling elements, and safety data sheet formats. Developed under United Nations auspices to harmonize diverse national systems, GHS establishes uniform hazard classification based on physical properties (flammability, reactivity, explosivity), health effects (acute toxicity, carcinogenicity, reproductive toxicity), and environmental impacts. This classification determines standardized communication elements including pictograms with immediately recognizable symbols; signal words ("Danger" or "Warning") indicating relative severity; hazard statements describing specific risks in standardized language; and precautionary statements providing consistent handling, storage, and emergency response guidance. Implementation requires manufacturer or importer hazard determination through testing or available scientific literature; label development with appropriate GHS elements based on classification; and safety data sheet preparation following standardized 16-section format covering comprehensive information from chemical identification through disposal considerations. Workplace implementation includes maintaining current safety data sheets for all hazardous chemicals; ensuring proper labeling on all containers including secondary vessels; training employees regarding label interpretation and protective measure implementation; and appropriate program documentation demonstrating compliance. International adoption varies with some jurisdictions implementing comprehensive requirements across all sectors while others apply modified approaches based on existing regulatory frameworks, though with progressive movement toward global consistency. Benefits include enhanced worker protection through improved hazard recognition regardless of language barriers; reduced trade barriers through internationally consistent requirements; improved emergency response through standardized information availability; and comprehensive hazard profile availability supporting informed risk management decisions. While implementation challenges include transition costs updating existing documentation; training requirements ensuring effective system utilization; and sometimes limited literacy or comprehension despite standardized formats, the system represents significant improvement over previous fragmented approaches through establishing consistent global language for chemical hazard communication transcending national boundaries and language differences.

Consumer product labeling for toxicological hazards balances comprehensive risk communication against practical space limitations, literacy considerations, and regulatory requirements across diverse product categories. Approaches vary substantially by product type, with pharmaceuticals typically employing standardized formats including patient package inserts providing comprehensive information beyond label space constraints; household chemicals utilizing required warning statements, precautionary guidance, first aid instructions, and increasingly, prescribed pictograms communicating hazards visually; pesticides carrying detailed application instructions, safety precautions, environmental hazard information, and registration numbers enabling additional information access; and consumer goods containing potentially toxic components including appropriate hazard statements based on specific risk profiles. Effectiveness considerations include readability with appropriate font size, contrast, and reading level matching general population capabilities; formatting with strategic information organization prioritizing critical safety information; comprehensibility ensuring consumers actually understand rather than merely see provided information; and cultural considerations addressing linguistic diversity, varying risk perception frameworks, and different safety behavior norms across populations. Implementation challenges include limited space on small product containers; competing information including marketing elements potentially overshadowing safety information; varying literacy and language capabilities among consumers; balancing comprehensive hazard communication against creating information overload reducing overall comprehension; and appropriate representation of uncertain risks neither overstating nor understating potential concerns based on evolving scientific understanding. Evaluation research consistently demonstrates gaps between intended communication and actual consumer comprehension or behavior, with findings indicating that many consumers do not read labels before product use; struggle understanding technical terminology when they do read; fail connecting general warnings to specific behavioral changes; and face practical implementation barriers even when comprehension occurs. These findings have driven evolution toward more visual communication through standardized pictograms, simplified language focusing on concrete actions rather than technical hazard descriptions, and recognition that labeling represents only one component within broader product safety systems requiring complementary approaches including inherently safer design, packaging modifications reducing exposure potential, and public education beyond point-of-use information.

Workplace notification systems communicate toxicological hazards through multiple complementary mechanisms supporting worker protection through informed decision-making and appropriate protective measures. Beyond fundamental GHS requirements for container labeling and safety data sheet availability, comprehensive systems typically include hazard training programs ensuring workers understand specific risks, protective equipment requirements, exposure minimization procedures, and appropriate emergency response for materials in their work areas; warning signage identifying hazardous areas, required protective equipment, emergency equipment locations, and evacuation routes; exposure monitoring notifications informing workers about environmental measurements, personal sampling results, and their interpretation relative to established exposure limits; medical surveillance communications providing individuals with health monitoring results, their significance, and any indicated follow-up actions; and incident notification systems alerting workers about accidental releases, exposure events, or near-miss situations with preventive implications. Implementation considerations include language appropriateness addressing workforce diversity through multilingual materials or universal pictograms when literacy or language barriers exist; comprehension verification ensuring actual understanding rather than mere information provision; integration with existing workflow rather than creating separate "safety" functions disconnected from regular operations; refresher communication maintaining hazard awareness despite familiarity-induced complacency; and verification systems ensuring critical safety information actually reaches affected workers rather than remaining in binders or databases without practical utilization. Special considerations apply to contract workers, visitors, maintenance personnel, and others who may encounter workplace hazards without regular presence in affected areas, requiring modified approaches ensuring these populations receive appropriate hazard information despite their non-routine presence. Effectiveness evaluation examines both process metrics like information distribution and outcome measures including actual knowledge, appropriate protective behavior, and ultimately, reduced exposure incidents. These comprehensive workplace notification systems transform technical toxicological information into practical protection through systematic communication processes ensuring that those potentially exposed to workplace hazards receive, understand, and can implement appropriate protective information regardless of position, background, or specific job function.

Environmental risk notification addresses community hazards from industrial operations, contaminated sites, environmental releases, or ambient pollution through systems balancing public right-to-know principles against avoiding unwarranted alarm. Regulatory frameworks including the Emergency Planning and Community Right-to-Know Act (EPCRA) and corresponding international regulations establish requirements for hazard disclosure, release reporting, and emergency notification based on specific substance characteristics and quantity thresholds. Implementation typically involves multiple components including facility chemical inventories accessible to emergency planners and sometimes the general public; toxic release reporting documenting emissions into air, water, or land with public database availability; emergency notification systems alerting authorities and affected populations about accidental releases through sirens, reverse 911 systems, emergency broadcast networks, or mobile alerts; environmental monitoring disclosures providing ambient measurement data for air, water, or soil contaminants; and remediation communications addressing contaminated site cleanup activities, progress, and residual risks. Effectiveness considerations include appropriate detail balancing technical accuracy against public comprehensibility; trustworthy sources as information from distrusted entities often faces rejection regardless of content quality; meaningful context helping recipients interpret technical information through relevant comparisons, clear health implication explanations, and practical response guidance; and bidirectional communication enabling community questions, concerns, and perspectives to influence both information provision and response activities. Special challenges include communicating uncertain risks when complete health effect information remains unavailable; addressing outrage factors like involuntary exposure, unequal distribution, or dreaded outcomes that elevate perceived risk beyond statistical probability alone; managing stigma concerns where hazard information may affect property values or community identity; and balancing transparency against security considerations for potentially dangerous materials. Effective systems recognize these complexities through approaches including community advisory panels enabling ongoing dialogue rather than crisis-limited interaction; layered information providing both simplified overviews and detailed technical data matching different audience needs; trusted intermediaries when direct communication faces credibility barriers; and proactive engagement rather than legally-minimal disclosure that often generates suspicion rather than reassurance. These evolving approaches transform environmental hazard communication from adversarial information extraction toward collaborative risk governance where affected communities participate meaningfully in both information development and risk management decision-making.

Emergency Communication

Crisis communication during acute toxicological emergencies requires specialized approaches addressing the unique challenges of high-consequence, evolving situations where information may remain incomplete but action necessity remains immediate. Effective systems balance information accuracy against timeliness through phased communication acknowledging initial uncertainty while providing actionable guidance; develop message components including concise hazard description, specific protective actions, expected duration, and information update scheduling; establish pre-determined dissemination channels including emergency alert systems, media relationships, official websites, social media platforms, and community networks ensuring broad reach across diverse populations; identify appropriate spokespersons combining technical credibility with communication capability; and implement message coordination protocols preventing contradictory guidance from different authorities. Content considerations include message simplicity focusing on essential actions during high-stress situations where cognitive processing becomes impaired; specific behavioral guidance rather than general hazard information alone; explanation sufficiency providing enough rationale for recommended actions without overwhelming detail; appropriate uncertainty acknowledgment distinguishing between confirmed facts and evolving assessment; and cultural sensitivity addressing diverse risk perception frameworks, language requirements, and trusted information sources across affected populations. Common implementation challenges include rapidly evolving situations where initial information proves incomplete or inaccurate necessitating corrections that may undermine credibility; competing voices including unofficial sources, social media speculation, and sometimes deliberate misinformation complicating official message reception; technical complexity of many chemical hazards creating translation challenges for general audience comprehension; differential impacts across communities creating perception of inequitable protection or response; and sometimes conflict between public demand for absolute certainty and technical reality of incomplete information during early emergency phases. Evaluation research highlights several critical success factors including message consistency across different authorities and time periods; spokesperson credibility established before crisis situations develop; regular updates even when significant new information remains unavailable; appropriate empathy balancing technical information with recognition of emotional impact; and sufficient communication capacity avoiding overwhelming delays during peak information demand periods. These specialized approaches transform crisis communication from simple information broadcast toward strategic engagement supporting effective protective action across diverse populations despite the inherent challenges of uncertain, evolving, high-consequence toxicological emergencies.

Warning systems for imminent toxicological hazards alert potentially affected populations about immediate threats requiring protective action, with effectiveness determined by multiple factors beyond mere message transmission. Comprehensive systems address four essential dimensions: detection utilizing instrumentation, monitoring networks, and reporting systems identifying hazardous conditions requiring warning issuance; decision processes establishing authority, criteria, and protocols determining when warnings are justified based on detection information; dissemination through multiple channels including sirens, emergency alert systems, broadcast media, mobile technologies, and community networks ensuring message receipt regardless of location, time, or individual characteristics; and response capability supporting appropriate protective actions through both advance planning and real-time guidance. Technical considerations include detection sensitivity balancing false negative avoidance against false positive minimization; message specificity providing location-relevant information rather than generalized alerts covering unnecessarily broad areas; timing optimization maximizing protective action opportunity while ensuring sufficient verification preventing unwarranted alerts; channel redundancy ensuring critical warnings reach intended recipients despite individual channel failures; and appropriate termination notification when threats resolve preventing unnecessary protective measure continuation. Human factors significantly influence effectiveness, with key dimensions including comprehensibility ensuring messages convey clear meaning across diverse linguistic, educational, and cultural backgrounds; trust determining whether recipients accept warning legitimacy and implementation recommendations; confirmation tendencies where individuals typically seek additional information before acting regardless of message urgency; and practical response capability where theoretical protective actions may prove impossible for certain populations without appropriate assistance. Implementation challenges include cross-jurisdictional coordination when hazards cross administrative boundaries requiring multi-agency collaboration; special population considerations including those with mobility limitations, sensory impairments, institutional settings, or language barriers requiring targeted approaches; technology limitations where no single communication channel reaches entire populations necessitating layered systems; and maintaining system readiness through regular testing, updating, and exercising without creating alert fatigue diminishing future response. These multidimensional considerations transform warning systems from simple technologies toward comprehensive sociotechnical systems integrating detection capabilities, decision processes, communication channels, and community response planning into coordinated approaches supporting effective protective action during imminent toxicological threats.

Public health messaging addresses ongoing toxicological concerns through sustained communication campaigns rather than emergency-focused alerts, with approaches balancing hazard awareness against unneccesary anxiety creation. Effective campaigns develop comprehensive strategies identifying specific audiences, key messages, appropriate channels, and evaluation metrics before implementation; create message frameworks addressing hazard characteristics, exposure pathways, health implications, risk factors, and specific protective actions; select appropriate channels including traditional media, digital platforms, healthcare provider networks, community organizations, and educational institutions matching target audience communication preferences; establish timelines balancing sufficient exposure for message penetration against potential fatigue from excessive repetition; and implement evaluation processes measuring both reach metrics like exposure frequency and outcome indicators including knowledge acquisition, attitude change, and ultimately, behavior modification. Content considerations include appropriate hazard framing neither minimizing legitimate concerns nor creating excessive fear disproportionate to actual risk; personal relevance establishment connecting abstract hazards to specific audience concerns, values, or experiences; self-efficacy support emphasizing actions within individual capability rather than overwhelming problems without practical solutions; narrative approaches using stories and examples enhancing engagement beyond statistical information alone; and positive framing emphasizing health protection benefits rather than focusing exclusively on negative consequences. Implementation challenges include competing priorities in information-saturated environments where toxicological messages compete against numerous other concerns for limited attention; scientific uncertainty communication where complete information about risks or protective action effectiveness remains unavailable; addressing misinformation which may spread more rapidly or compellingly than more nuanced evidence-based guidance; sustainability maintaining appropriate attention for chronic hazards lacking the inherent urgency of emergency situations; and evaluation complexities where establishing direct causal connections between communication campaigns and behavior changes often proves methodologically challenging. Successful programs increasingly employ audience segmentation developing tailored approaches for different populations based on their specific characteristics, concerns, and communication preferences rather than one-size-fits-all messaging; pre-testing with representative audience members identifying potential comprehension barriers or unintended implications before widespread dissemination; storytelling approaches making abstract risks concrete through individual experiences or scenarios; and trusted messenger utilization where information from community-embedded sources may receive greater acceptance than external authorities regardless of identical content. These comprehensive approaches transform public health risk communication from simple information provision toward strategic engagement supporting sustained protective behavior adoption addressing toxicological hazards requiring ongoing attention rather than one-time emergency response.

Information coordination during complex toxicological incidents addresses the challenges of multiple organizations communicating about the same situation, where inconsistent or contradictory messaging can significantly undermine response effectiveness regardless of individual message quality. Effective coordination establishes clear roles delineating which entities have communication authority regarding different aspects of the situation; develops joint information systems where representatives from various organizations share information, align messages, and coordinate release timing; creates escalation protocols determining when information requires approval beyond operational levels before public release; establishes common terminology preventing confusion from different technical language or jargon across organizations; implements rumor control mechanisms identifying and addressing misinformation through coordinated correction; and develops pre-scripted message components for anticipated scenarios enabling rapid deployment without compromising quality or consistency. Organizational arrangements include joint information centers physically or virtually co-locating public information officers from different agencies during major incidents; crisis communication networks maintaining relationships and protocols during non-emergency periods; unified command structures establishing clear authority hierarchies including communication aspects; and sometimes formal mutual aid agreements specifying inter-organizational support including communication assistance during large-scale events. Implementation challenges include differing organizational cultures where various entities may have substantially different approaches to transparency, uncertainty acknowledgment, or public engagement; jurisdictional complexities where unclear authority boundaries create potential coordination gaps or overlaps; operational security concerns where some information may require restriction despite transparency preferences; political considerations potentially influencing communication strategies beyond technical response requirements; and resource disparities where organizations with limited communication capacity may struggle maintaining coordination with better-equipped partners despite willingness. Technological support increasingly includes shared digital platforms enabling real-time information exchange, collaborative message development, and coordinated dissemination tracking; social media monitoring tools providing situational awareness regarding public information environment and emerging concerns; and sometimes virtual operations support teams providing specialized communication expertise to resource-limited organizations during major incidents. These coordination mechanisms transform potentially fragmented, contradictory information from multiple sources into coherent guidance supporting effective public response during complex toxicological incidents where numerous organizations share communication responsibilities across different operational aspects, jurisdictional boundaries, and specialized knowledge domains.

Psychological Dimensions

Risk perception factors fundamentally influence how individuals interpret and respond to toxicological hazard information, with research identifying key dimensions extending far beyond statistical probability or objective harm potential. Dread characteristics significantly amplify perceived risk, with particularly strong effects from exposures perceived as catastrophic rather than chronic; potentially fatal rather than merely illness-causing; threatening future generations through reproductive or developmental effects; inequitably distributed affecting vulnerable populations disproportionately; and especially dreaded outcomes like cancer compared to other health effects of similar objective severity. Control factors similarly influence perception, with substantially amplified concern for involuntary exposures compared to voluntary risks; uncontrollable hazards where personal protective actions appear limited; unfamiliar substances lacking historical experience providing contextual understanding; and human-created rather than naturally occurring toxicants regardless of identical health effects. Knowledge characteristics also shape perception, with heightened concern for exposures with delayed or invisible effects making personal detection impossible; inadequately understood mechanisms creating scientific uncertainty; novel or exotic substances lacking extensive safety research; and risks perceived as unknown to science or hidden by authorities rather than openly acknowledged and investigated. These psychological dimensions explain why public risk rankings often diverge dramatically from expert assessments based primarily on statistical likelihood and harm magnitude, with substances like industrial chemicals, pesticides, and radiation typically generating concern exceeding their statistical mortality burden compared to more familiar, voluntary risks with higher objective harm rates. Effective risk communication acknowledges these psychological dimensions rather than dismissing them as irrational, addressing control concerns through actionable guidance, knowledge factors through transparent information sharing, and dread characteristics through appropriate context and comparison rather than exclusively statistical information. This psychological understanding transforms risk communication from frustrated attempts to align public perception with expert statistical assessment toward more effective approaches acknowledging and addressing the legitimate psychological dimensions influencing risk perception beyond pure probability or consequence magnitude.

Outrage management addresses the emotional dimensions of toxicological risk situations, recognizing that public responses often reflect perceived process injustice, institutional distrust, or violation of cultural values beyond technical hazard characteristics alone. This approach distinguishes between hazard (the technical risk potential) and outrage (the emotional response to surrounding circumstances), acknowledging that effective risk communication must address both dimensions rather than focusing exclusively on technical information which may prove ineffective when significant outrage exists. Common outrage factors include involuntary exposure where affected individuals had no choice regarding risk acceptance; inequitable distribution where certain communities bear disproportionate burden while others receive benefits; institutional arrogance through dismissive treatment of community concerns; process exclusion where affected populations lack meaningful participation in decisions affecting their exposure; and evidence of prior institutional failures undermining current credibility regardless of technical accuracy. Effective outrage management employs various strategies including explicit acknowledgment validating emotional responses as legitimate rather than irrational; genuine dialogue establishing two-way communication rather than one-directional information provision; process transparency demonstrating openness rather than suggesting information concealment; appropriate accountability accepting responsibility for past failures rather than defensive denial; power sharing through meaningful community involvement in decision processes; and concrete demonstration of responsiveness showing that public input actually influences actions rather than merely being collected without impact. Implementation challenges include institutional resistance to acknowledging emotional dimensions as legitimate communication considerations; difficulty balancing validation of emotions against avoiding reinforcement of technical misconceptions; organizational concerns about legal liability from acknowledgments; and sometimes fundamental value conflicts where complete resolution proves impossible rather than merely requiring better explanation. Research demonstrates that failure addressing outrage dimensions often proves counterproductive, as technical information from distrusted sources facing significant community outrage typically encounters rejection regardless of scientific validity, while addressing outrage factors creates receptivity to technical information that might otherwise face dismissal despite objective accuracy. This approach transforms risk communication from frustrated technical explanation toward more effective engagement acknowledging the legitimate emotional and process dimensions that significantly influence information reception, interpretation, and ultimately, protective behavior adoption regarding toxicological hazards.

Cultural factors significantly influence risk communication effectiveness, with research demonstrating that identical information produces dramatically different responses based on recipients' cultural frameworks, values, and identities. Cultural cognition theory explains these variations through two fundamental dimensions: hierarchical versus egalitarian worldviews affecting perceptions of appropriate authority and expertise sources; and individualist versus communitarian orientations influencing views on personal versus collective responsibility for both risk creation and mitigation. These cultural frameworks create distinctive risk-filtering patterns where individuals more readily accept information aligning with their existing worldview while scrutinizing or rejecting contrary information regardless of objective evidence quality. Beyond these broad dimensions, specific cultural characteristics significantly influence risk communication reception including language patterns affecting appropriate terminology, explanation structure, and communication formality; family structures influencing who makes health-related decisions and appropriate information targeting; religious frameworks potentially affecting interpretations of causality, responsibility, and appropriate response; historical experiences with institutions shaping trust relationships regardless of current communication quality; and community knowledge systems potentially offering valuable complementary understanding alongside technical scientific information. Effective cross-cultural communication employs various strategies including cultural knowledge development understanding specific audience frameworks before message creation; appropriate messenger selection utilizing trusted voices within particular communities; message tailoring addressing specific cultural values, concerns, and priorities; bidirectional engagement incorporating community perspectives rather than imposing external frameworks; and sometimes cultural bridging explicitly connecting technical information with existing belief systems rather than presenting them as competing knowledge frameworks. Implementation challenges include avoiding stereotyping while acknowledging meaningful cultural variations; balancing cultural appropriateness against core technical accuracy requirements; addressing historical distrust resulting from previous negative experiences; and developing sufficient communicator diversity reflecting the populations being served. These cultural considerations transform risk communication from standardized information dissemination toward culturally responsive engagement recognizing that effective information transfer requires addressing not merely what is said but the cultural context determining how that information is received, interpreted, and ultimately translated into protective behavior across diverse populations.

Media influence significantly shapes toxicological risk perception through various mechanisms extending beyond simple information provision to framing, amplification, and social context creation. News media affects risk perception through story selection determining which toxicological concerns receive public attention regardless of objective risk magnitude; issue framing establishing interpretive frameworks emphasizing particular aspects like uncertainty, conflict, or human impact; source selection determining whose voices receive amplification potentially privileging certain perspectives over others; narrative structure often favoring individual stories over statistical patterns despite their limited representativeness; and sometimes sensationalism prioritizing dramatic, frightening, or novel aspects potentially distorting risk magnitude perception. Social media creates additional influence dimensions including algorithm-driven exposure potentially creating filter bubbles reinforcing existing beliefs rather than providing balanced information; rapid information spread without traditional verification processes; powerful visual content potentially creating stronger emotional responses than text-based information alone; and peer endorsement where information from personal connections may receive greater credibility than official sources regardless of accuracy. Entertainment media similarly influences risk perception through fictional portrayals of chemical hazards often emphasizing worst-case scenarios; character depiction potentially creating stereotypes about affected populations or responsible parties; narrative resolution typically favoring dramatic, definitive outcomes rather than the scientific uncertainty characterizing many actual toxicological situations; and visual representation making abstract risks concrete though sometimes with limited technical accuracy. Effective risk communication within this complex media environment requires strategic approaches including proactive relationship development with journalists covering environmental health topics; rapid response capability addressing misinformation before widespread dissemination; development of compelling, accurate narratives competing effectively against misleading simplifications; visual communication creating appropriate impact without misrepresenting risk characteristics; social media monitoring providing early warning for emerging concerns or misinformation; and media literacy promotion helping audiences critically evaluate toxicological information across platforms. These approaches acknowledge media's powerful influence on risk perception while developing strategic engagement rather than merely lamenting sensationalism or inaccuracy, recognizing that effective risk communication must operate within the actual media environment where people receive information rather than idealized scenarios of direct, unmediated expert-to-public communication about toxicological hazards.

SAFETY MEASURES

Preventive interventions create defense layers addressing toxicological risks through engineering controls, administrative measures, and individual protection strategies.

Engineering Controls

Substitution and elimination represent the highest tier in the hierarchy of controls, fundamentally preventing exposure by removing or replacing hazardous substances rather than managing risks through exposure reduction strategies. This approach includes complete elimination removing particular toxic agents from processes entirely when their function proves non-essential; direct substitution replacing hazardous substances with less toxic alternatives performing identical functions; process modification achieving desired outcomes through fundamentally different methods avoiding particular toxicant use; and product reformulation maintaining desired characteristics while removing or reducing hazardous components. Implementation typically follows systematic methodology including comprehensive hazard identification establishing clear understanding of current toxic materials and their specific roles; alternative identification generating potential substitutes through literature review, supplier consultation, research database searching, and sometimes original research; comparative assessment evaluating alternatives across multiple dimensions including technical performance, toxicological profile, physical hazards, environmental impacts, and economic feasibility; pilot testing confirming practical implementation viability before full-scale conversion; and post-implementation monitoring verifying both technical success and actual exposure reduction. Technical challenges include finding alternatives matching all critical performance parameters, as substitutes may address toxicity concerns while introducing different limitations regarding effectiveness, durability, processing requirements, or physical properties; addressing multiple hazards simultaneously rather than creating risk trade-offs where reduced toxicity comes at the expense of increased flammability, reactivity, or environmental persistence; and sometimes limited alternatives for highly specialized applications with unique performance requirements.

Table 14.2: Engineering Controls and Safety Measures

Control Type	Applications	Implementation Considerations	Effectiveness Measures
Child-resistant packaging	Medications, household chemicals, cannabis products	Testing standards (PPPA), senior-friendly design, product-specific requirements	Exposure reduction rates, proper reclosure rates
Product reformulation	Concentrated laundry packets, antifreeze, medications	Maintaining product efficacy, cost implications, consumer acceptance	Toxic exposures per unit sold, severity reduction
Flow restrictors	Liquid medications, household chemicals	Universal design principles, tamper resistance, cost	Volume limitations during exposure events
Safety closures	Cleaning products, automotive fluids, pesticides	Ease of proper use, consumer education, manufacturing standards	Exposure reduction, proper usage rates
Locked storage	Medications, cannabis products, pesticides	Affordability, convenience, consumer compliance	Adoption rates, exposure reduction in homes with devices

Organizational challenges include economic concerns regarding conversion costs, potential productivity impacts during transition periods, or ongoing cost differentials; institutional inertia favoring familiar processes and materials despite hazards; technical knowledge limitations within organizations regarding potential alternatives; and sometimes competitive considerations where specific formulations represent proprietary advantages. Despite these challenges, successful implementation examples span diverse applications including solvents (replacing chlorinated compounds with aqueous or citrus-based alternatives), heavy metals (substituting non-toxic brighteners for cyanide in electroplating), pesticides (developing integrated pest management reducing chemical dependence), and consumer products (reformulating with non-toxic ingredients while maintaining performance). These substitution and elimination approaches transform toxicological risk management from exposure limitation toward fundamental prevention, addressing hazards at their source rather than managing consequences after introducing toxic materials into processes, products, or environments.

Process isolation creates physical separation between hazardous substances and potential receptors, preventing exposure while maintaining necessary material utilization when elimination or substitution proves impractical. Implementation approaches include complete enclosure surrounding processes within sealed systems preventing material escape into the broader environment; remote operation utilizing automation, robotics, or mechanical linkages allowing process control without direct worker presence in hazardous areas; barrier systems establishing physical separation through walls, shields, or enclosures permitting visual monitoring while preventing exposure; glove box technology enabling manual manipulation within sealed environments through integrated glove ports maintaining containment integrity; and controlled environment systems maintaining negative pressure ensuring airflow direction contains potential releases within designated areas. Technical considerations include material compatibility ensuring containment systems resist degradation from enclosed substances; maintenance accessibility allowing necessary service without compromising isolation integrity; emergency systems addressing potential containment failures through secondary controls; instrumentation providing process monitoring without breaching containment; and sometimes transfer systems enabling material movement into and out of isolated environments without direct exposure during transitions. Implementation challenges include capital cost requirements for sophisticated containment technologies; production rate impacts when isolated processes operate less efficiently than open systems; ergonomic limitations when physical barriers restrict movement, visibility, or tactile feedback; maintenance complexity often requiring specialized procedures for accessing equipment within containment; and sometimes quality control challenges when direct observation or intervention becomes limited by isolation systems. These isolation approaches demonstrate particular value for substances with significant health hazards at low concentrations, materials where engineering controls alone cannot reliably maintain safe atmospheric levels, processes where intermittent high-exposure activities create risk despite average concentration control, and highly toxic materials where redundant protection layers provide essential safety margins despite primary control effectiveness. Effective implementations transform exceptionally hazardous operations that would create unacceptable risk in open environments into manageable processes through systematic exposure prevention, maintaining necessary material utilization while ensuring worker protection through fundamental separation between hazards and potential receptors rather than attempting to control exposure after contamination occurs in shared spaces.

Ventilation systems represent critical engineering controls addressing airborne toxicants through contaminant removal, dilution, or directional airflow management. Local exhaust ventilation (LEV) captures contaminants at or near generation sources before dispersion into the broader environment, with components including capture hoods designed based on contaminant release characteristics and process geometry; ducting sized appropriately for transport velocity preventing material settling; air cleaning devices matched to specific contaminant properties; and fans providing necessary air movement overcoming system resistance. Design considerations include capture efficiency optimization through hood placement immediately adjacent to emission sources; appropriate face velocity ensuring effective contaminant capture without creating turbulence potentially reducing performance; transport velocity maintenance preventing material settling within ductwork; and appropriate air cleaning technology selection based on contaminant characteristics including filters for particulates, adsorption systems for gases and vapors, and sometimes specialized technologies for specific contaminants. General ventilation systems provide broader airborne contaminant management through dilution with clean air reducing concentrations below harmful levels; directional airflow ensuring contaminant movement away from breathing zones toward controlled exhaust points; and sometimes air cleaning when recirculation rather than single-pass systems prove necessary. These systems require careful design considerations including appropriate air exchange rates based on space volume and contaminant generation rate; supply and exhaust point positioning creating desired airflow patterns without short-circuiting or dead zones;

and sometimes pressure relationships maintaining predetermined airflow direction between connected spaces preventing cross-contamination. Implementation challenges include energy consumption concerns particularly in climate-controlled environments where conditioned air exhaustion creates significant costs; balancing ventilation requirements against other building systems including heating, cooling, and fire protection; performance degradation through modifications, maintenance lapses, or operational changes affecting original design parameters; and sometimes competing requirements when processes require specific environmental conditions conflicting with optimal ventilation arrangements. Performance verification represents another critical dimension, with methods including airflow visualization using smoke or similar tracers; velometer measurements confirming appropriate capture velocities; tracer gas testing quantifying capture efficiency under actual operating conditions; and sometimes computational fluid dynamics modeling predicting performance before installation or evaluating modification impacts without physical testing. These comprehensive ventilation approaches transform spaces containing airborne contaminant sources into controlled environments where exposure remains below harmful levels through systematic contaminant management, representing fundamental engineering controls applicable across diverse settings from industrial processes to laboratory operations to healthcare environments.

Process modification addresses toxicological hazards through fundamental changes to production methods, operational procedures, or manufacturing approaches rather than managing exposures within existing systems. These modifications include operational parameter adjustments altering temperature, pressure, or concentration reducing hazardous intermediate formation or volatile emissions; physical state changes using granular materials instead of powders reducing dust generation or employing paste forms rather than volatile liquids limiting evaporation; manufacturing sequence alterations performing hazardous steps earlier in production when materials remain contained within closed systems; reaction pathway modifications achieving identical end products through alternative chemical routes avoiding toxic intermediates; automation integration removing workers from direct interaction with hazardous process stages; and sometimes complete technology shifts achieving desired outcomes through fundamentally different approaches eliminating particular hazards entirely. Implementation methodology typically involves process hazard analysis identifying specific steps creating highest exposure potential; engineering assessment examining modification feasibility without compromising product quality or production efficiency; alternative development through scientific literature review, industrial benchmarking, or research collaboration; pilot implementation demonstrating practical viability before full-scale conversion; and performance verification confirming both reduced exposure and maintained production objectives. Successful examples span diverse applications including solvent reduction through advanced mixing technologies achieving dissolution with minimal quantities; dust control through pelletization or microencapsulation maintaining material functionality while eliminating respirable particles; toxic intermediate elimination through alternative synthesis pathways achieving identical end products without hazardous precursors; and automation implementation performing high-exposure tasks through robotics or enclosed systems without direct worker involvement. Implementation challenges include technical expertise requirements for fundamental process redesign often exceeding typical industrial hygiene resources; capital investment needs for equipment modifications or replacements; production interruption concerns during transition periods; product qualification requirements ensuring modified processes maintain critical quality parameters; and sometimes intellectual property limitations when optimal solutions involve proprietary technologies or methods. Despite these challenges, process modification often provides superior long-term solutions compared to exposure controls within inherently hazardous processes, addressing fundamental risk sources rather than attempting to manage consequences after hazard generation. This approach represents the practical application of prevention through design principles, integrating safety considerations into core process development rather than adding control measures to inherently dangerous systems after implementation.

Material handling systems provide specialized engineering controls addressing exposure during transport, transfer, and processing operations where containment breaches commonly occur. Closed transfer systems enable material movement between containers, vessels, or process equipment without open handling, utilizing various technologies including mechanical connectors creating sealed interfaces between vessels; vacuum transfer systems moving materials through negative pressure rather than pouring or scooping; peristaltic or diaphragm pumps maintaining material containment during liquid transfers; and gravity-fed systems with sealed connections preventing exposure during solid material movement. Automated dispensing technologies precisely deliver predetermined material quantities without manual handling, reducing both routine exposure during normal operations and spill potential from handling errors. Dust suppression systems address particulate exposures through methods including controlled vacuum systems capturing particles during handling operations; ventilated bagging or weighing stations containing dust within limited zones; moisture addition reducing dustiness while maintaining material functionality; and specialized dumping stations with integrated ventilation capturing particulates during highest exposure operations like bag emptying or container charging. Waste handling represents another critical exposure point addressed through engineered systems including closed drainage systems preventing volatile emission during liquid waste transfer; ventilated waste accumulation areas controlling emissions from collected materials; sealed containers preventing leakage or emission during temporary storage; and sometimes specialized solidification or stabilization technologies converting liquid wastes to less mobile forms before disposal. Implementation considerations include material compatibility ensuring system components resist degradation from handled substances; maintenance accessibility allowing necessary service without creating additional exposure; ergonomic design supporting efficient operation without awkward movements potentially compromising proper usage; cleaning provisions preventing cross-contamination between different materials; and appropriate fail-safe features ensuring containment during power failures or other abnormal conditions. These specialized material handling systems transform high-exposure operations like weighing, mixing, charging, transferring, and waste management into controlled processes with minimal worker contact, addressing critical exposure pathways often overlooked when focus remains exclusively on primary production processes despite their often greater contribution to actual worker exposure through frequent breaches of otherwise well-controlled systems during necessary material movement operations.

Administrative Controls

Exposure monitoring programs systematically assess toxicant levels in workplace environments, providing essential data supporting hazard identification, control effectiveness evaluation, and compliance verification. Comprehensive programs integrate multiple monitoring approaches including initial surveys establishing baseline exposure profiles across operations and job classifications; routine monitoring maintaining current exposure characterization as processes evolve; targeted assessments addressing specific concerns or evaluating intervention effectiveness; and personal exposure monitoring documenting individual worker exposures for comparison with established limits. Methodological considerations include sampling strategy development determining monitoring frequency, duration, and location based on exposure variability, process characteristics, and specific contaminant properties; appropriate sampling method selection considering analytical sensitivity, specificity, and practical implementation factors; quality assurance procedures ensuring reliable results through proper calibration, field blanks, and analytical method validation; data interpretation frameworks comparing results against applicable standards while considering sampling and analytical error; and comprehensive documentation maintaining results for regulatory compliance, trend analysis, and medical surveillance correlation. Implementation approaches typically follow tiered frameworks with initial screening using direct-reading instruments or simplified methods identifying potential concerns, followed by more comprehensive assessment where indicated using reference methods providing defensible quantification for comparison with established exposure limits. Beyond regulatory compliance, sophisticated programs utilize exposure data for multiple advanced applications including similar exposure group identification enabling efficient monitoring resource allocation; exposure determinant identification revealing specific process characteristics, work practices, or environmental factors most strongly influencing exposure levels; control effectiveness evaluation quantifying intervention impact rather than assuming reduction based on implementation alone; predictive model development forecasting exposure under varied conditions without comprehensive measurement; and sometimes epidemiological analysis relating exposure metrics to health outcomes within the specific workforce. These comprehensive monitoring approaches transform workplace health protection from assumption-based management toward evidence-driven decision-making supported by systematic exposure characterization, ensuring resources address actual rather than perceived risks while quantitatively demonstrating protection adequacy or identifying improvement needs through objective measurement rather than subjective assessment alone.

Standard operating procedures (SOPs) establish consistent work practices reducing exposure variability, preventing high-risk operations, and ensuring appropriate control utilization across different workers, shifts, and production scenarios. Effective SOPs address multiple exposure reduction dimensions including proper control system utilization with specific steps ensuring appropriate ventilation operation, containment system integrity, or other engineering controls before beginning operations; material handling protocols minimizing exposure during high-risk operations like container opening, weighing, mixing, or transfer between vessels; housekeeping requirements preventing contaminant accumulation on surfaces where it might become resuspended or transferred through secondary contact; emergency response actions addressing spills, leaks, or other unexpected releases with appropriate containment and decontamination methods; and proper maintenance procedures ensuring control systems receive necessary service without creating additional exposure during the maintenance process itself. Development methodology typically involves multidisciplinary collaboration including experienced operators providing practical knowledge, industrial hygienists addressing exposure control principles, process engineers contributing technical understanding, and sometimes medical personnel incorporating health protection considerations. Implementation success requires addressing multiple dimensions beyond mere document creation, including appropriate format using clear, concise language with logical organization and visual elements enhancing comprehension; training ensuring both procedural knowledge and understanding of underlying protection principles; accessibility making procedures readily available at point of operation rather than isolated in administrative offices; regular review maintaining relevance as processes, materials, or control technologies evolve; and compliance verification ensuring actual work practices match documented procedures rather than creating "paper programs" without operational implementation. Common challenges include balancing comprehensiveness against usability as excessively detailed procedures may face practical rejection; addressing procedural conflicts between production efficiency and optimal exposure control when tensions exist; ensuring continued adherence despite familiarity potentially breeding complacency over time; and adaptation for workforce diversity considering language limitations, educational differences, and varied learning styles affecting comprehension and implementation. Despite these challenges, well-designed and effectively implemented SOPs represent valuable administrative controls complementing engineering systems, particularly for operations where exposure potential significantly depends on specific work practices rather than being fully controlled through engineering systems alone regardless of operator behavior.

Training programs develop knowledge, skills, and motivation supporting appropriate exposure prevention behavior across the workforce. Comprehensive programs address multiple dimensions including hazard communication ensuring understanding of specific toxic substances, their health effects, and exposure routes; engineering control operation teaching proper use, limitations, and performance verification for installed systems; work practice training developing specific skills for exposure-minimizing techniques; personal protective equipment covering selection, fitting, inspection, maintenance, and limitations; emergency response preparation addressing appropriate actions during spills, releases, or other abnormal situations; regulatory compliance ensuring understanding of legal requirements and their practical implementation; and sometimes risk communication developing appropriate perspective balancing legitimate concern against unnecessary fear potentially interfering with effective operations. Instructional design considers adult learning principles through approaches including practical demonstration beyond theoretical explanation; hands-on practice developing actual skills rather than mere knowledge; problem-solving scenarios building critical thinking beyond rote procedure following; and connection to existing knowledge creating meaningful learning integrated with prior understanding rather than isolated information. Implementation effectively addresses diverse workforce characteristics through language-appropriate materials addressing non-native speakers; literacy-adjusted approaches ensuring comprehension regardless of reading ability; cultural considerations affecting risk perception, authority relationships, and communication styles; and sometimes computer literacy variations when technology-based training components are employed. Delivery methods balance various approaches including classroom instruction allowing interactive discussion and immediate question resolution; on-the-job training developing skills in actual work environments; computer-based modules allowing self-paced completion and standardized content; and sometimes simulation exercises creating realistic practice opportunities for emergency scenarios or high-hazard operations without actual exposure risk. Effectiveness evaluation extends beyond simple attendance documentation to include knowledge verification through testing; skill demonstration through performance observation; behavior change assessment through workplace practice monitoring; and ultimately outcome evaluation through exposure reduction or incident prevention. Refresher training maintains knowledge and skills addressing natural decay over time, process or material changes requiring updated information, and complacency development through extended hazard familiarity without negative consequences. These comprehensive training approaches transform worker behavior from uninformed risk-taking toward knowledge-based protective actions, creating essential human performance complement to engineering controls and establishing foundation for effective administrative control implementation through developed understanding, skill, and motivation rather than mere compliance with directives regardless of comprehension.

Medical surveillance programs systematically monitor worker health identifying potential exposure effects before significant or irreversible damage occurs. Comprehensive programs include multiple components: baseline examinations establishing pre-exposure health status before potential toxicant contact; periodic assessments at intervals appropriate to specific hazard properties and toxicity mechanisms;

targeted testing addressing organs systems affected by workplace exposures; and termination examinations documenting health status at employment conclusion. Specific examination elements vary based on potential exposures, with examples including pulmonary function testing for respiratory toxicant exposure; blood count and chemistry panels for substances affecting hematopoietic or hepatic systems; neurological assessment for neurotoxic agent exposure; specialized testing for specific concerns such as cholinesterase monitoring for organophosphate-exposed workers or biological monitoring measuring toxicants or their metabolites in blood or urine specimens; and sometimes advanced diagnostic procedures when standard screening suggests potential abnormalities requiring further evaluation. Implementation requires careful program design considering both individual and group surveillance dimensions: individual monitoring identifies potential health effects requiring medical intervention or exposure reduction for specific workers, while group analysis examines patterns across the workforce potentially revealing unrecognized exposure problems or control inadequacies despite compliance with established limits. Operational considerations include appropriate provider selection ensuring occupational health expertise beyond general clinical knowledge; standardized testing protocols maintaining result comparability across time; confidentiality protections encouraging honest symptom reporting while meeting regulatory requirements; effective communication systems ensuring relevant findings reach both individual workers and those responsible for workplace hazard control; integration with exposure monitoring data enabling identification of potential problem areas before clinical disease manifests; and appropriate action protocols when surveillance identifies potential work-related health effects. Particular challenges include distinguishing between occupational and non-occupational causes when health findings have multiple potential etiologies; addressing health effects with long latency periods potentially manifesting after employment termination; maintaining appropriate medical records supporting both current management and potential future claims; and balancing screening sensitivity against specificity preventing both missed cases and excessive false positives creating unnecessary concern. These comprehensive medical surveillance approaches transform occupational disease prevention from reactive response after manifest illness toward proactive identification during reversible stages, supporting early intervention through exposure reduction, medical treatment, or job modification before permanent health damage occurs while simultaneously providing feedback regarding control program effectiveness through systematic health outcome monitoring.

Hazard communication programs ensure workers receive,

understand, and can use information regarding toxic substances in their work environment. Beyond basic regulatory compliance with standards like OSHA's Hazard Communication Standard or GHS requirements, comprehensive programs address multiple information transfer dimensions including chemical inventory development identifying all hazardous substances present in the workplace; safety data sheet management ensuring current information availability for all hazardous materials; labeling systems maintaining identification throughout internal use including secondary containers; formal training programs developing general hazard communication understanding and specific knowledge regarding particular workplace toxicants; and supplemental communication methods addressing specialized needs beyond minimum requirements. Implementation effectiveness depends on several critical factors including information accessibility ensuring hazard data remains readily available when needed rather than isolated in administrative offices; comprehensibility addressing educational, language, and technical knowledge variations across the workforce; practical application guidance connecting general hazard information to specific protective measures within actual work operations; and psychological appropriateness balancing sufficient concern generating protective behavior against excessive fear potentially interfering with effective performance. Specific implementation approaches include electronic systems providing immediate safety data sheet access through barcodes, QR codes, or searchable databases; multilingual materials addressing workforce diversity; job-specific information summarizing critical hazard details and protective measures for particular operations rather than relying solely on comprehensive but complex safety data sheets; visual communication using standardized pictograms, color coding, or other non-text methods supporting understanding despite literacy limitations; and sometimes specialized communication for unique populations like maintenance workers who may encounter numerous materials across various operations without regular exposure to any single substance. Evaluation examines both process metrics like information distribution and outcome measures including actual knowledge, appropriate protective behavior, and ultimately, exposure reduction. These comprehensive hazard communication programs transform technical toxicological information into practical workplace protection through systematic information management and effective communication processes ensuring that workers not only have access to required information but actually understand and apply appropriate protective measures based on specific chemical hazards present in their work environment.

Personal Protective Equipment

Respiratory protection programs provide systematic approaches addressing airborne toxicant exposure when engineering controls cannot achieve sufficient exposure reduction alone. Comprehensive programs include multiple components: hazard assessment determining specific respiratory hazards, their concentrations, and physical properties guiding appropriate respirator selection; medical evaluation verifying individual capacity to safely wear respirators considering both physical conditions like respiratory or cardiovascular disorders and psychological factors like claustrophobia; appropriate selection matching respirator capabilities with specific hazard characteristics including contaminant type, concentration, and warning properties; fit testing ensuring proper sealing between respirator and facial features through either qualitative methods using detectable agents with subjective response or quantitative approaches measuring actual protection factors; proper use training covering donning and doffing procedures, user seal checks, appropriate wear conditions, and recognition of warning signs indicating potential malfunction; maintenance and storage establishing appropriate cleaning procedures, component replacement schedules, inspection protocols, and proper storage conditions; and program evaluation monitoring overall effectiveness through workplace monitoring, health surveillance, and compliance verification. Respirator types include air-purifying respirators removing contaminants through filters, cartridges, or canisters appropriate to specific hazard properties; supplied-air respirators providing clean air from external sources through airlines; self-contained breathing apparatus carrying breathing air supply with the user; and powered air-purifying respirators using battery-powered blowers enhancing air movement through purifying elements while reducing breathing resistance. Selection factors include protection factor requirements based on contaminant concentration relative to exposure limits; physiological burden considerations including breathing resistance, weight, and heat stress potential; work requirement compatibility including communication needs, mobility requirements, and duration limitations; and practical implementation factors such as fit testing capability, maintenance provisions, and storage facilities. Implementation challenges include ensuring consistent proper usage throughout exposure periods; addressing comfort concerns affecting compliance; managing beard restrictions necessary for proper face sealing; coordinating with other required personal protective equipment potentially affecting fit or function; and sometimes production pressure potentially compromising proper usage despite knowledge of requirements. Program administration requires significant resources including respiratory protection program administrator designation, detailed written programs documenting all program elements, regular evaluation ensuring continued effectiveness, and appropriate record-keeping maintaining required documentation. Despite these complexities, effective respiratory protection programs provide essential exposure reduction for scenarios where engineering controls remain impractical or insufficient, creating significant protection through properly selected, fitted, maintained, and consistently used respiratory protection equipment within comprehensive program frameworks ensuring these devices achieve their potential protection capability rather than creating false security through improper implementation.

Chemical protective clothing prevents dermal exposure to toxic substances through creating barriers between skin and workplace contaminants. Effective programs include multiple components: hazard assessment identifying specific chemical agents, their physical states, concentration, and potential contact scenarios; material selection matching protective properties with identified hazards considering permeation resistance measuring chemical movement through intact materials at molecular level, penetration resistance addressing bulk flow through seams or closures, and degradation resistance evaluating physical property maintenance upon chemical contact; garment selection determining appropriate coverage and design based on exposure patterns and work requirements; proper use training covering correct donning and doffing procedures, inspection before use, recognition of breakthrough or degradation indicators, and appropriate wear duration limitations; decontamination procedures preventing cross-contamination or secondary exposure during removal; storage and maintenance establishing appropriate cleaning, inspection, and storage requirements maintaining protective integrity between uses; and program evaluation verifying continued effectiveness through performance monitoring, exposure assessment, and compliance verification. Protective clothing types span various categories including gloves protecting against hand contact with selection factors including dexterity requirements, tactile sensitivity needs, and physical protection beyond chemical resistance; aprons providing frontal torso protection suitable for splash hazards with limited exposure potential; coveralls offering full body protection against more extensive exposure scenarios; and specialized ensembles including boots, hoods, and fully encapsulating suits for high-hazard environments requiring comprehensive protection. Material options include various polymers with specific chemical resistance profiles: nitrile offering petroleum derivative and solvent resistance; neoprene providing acid, base and solvent protection; butyl rubber resisting ketones and esters; polyvinyl chloride protecting against acids and caustics; natural rubber for biological hazards and water-based solutions; and various specialized laminates addressing specific challenging chemical classes. Selection methodology typically employs chemical compatibility charts matching materials with specific agents based on laboratory testing, permeation data comparing breakthrough times across material options, and sometimes field testing under actual use conditions evaluating practical performance beyond laboratory measurements. Implementation challenges include heat stress from impermeable materials preventing normal evaporative cooling; dexterity and mobility limitations affecting task performance; proper sizing across diverse workforce anthropometry; ensuring consistent proper usage throughout exposure periods; and sometimes conflicting requirements between optimal chemical protection and other considerations like fire resistance, physical hazard protection, or static electricity concerns. These comprehensive chemical protective clothing programs transform dermal exposure risks through systematic barrier implementation, providing essential protection against toxic substances capable of causing local skin effects or contributing to total body burden through dermal absorption when selected, maintained, and utilized within proper program frameworks ensuring theoretical protection translates into actual exposure reduction during workplace operations.

Eye and face protection prevents exposure to chemical splashes, vapors, and other hazards potentially damaging these sensitive tissues. Comprehensive programs include systematic hazard assessment identifying specific risks including splash potential, vapor concentrations, concurrent physical hazards like impacts or radiation, and environmental factors affecting selection; appropriate protection selection matching equipment characteristics to identified hazards with options including safety glasses with side shields for limited particle protection, chemical goggles providing splash protection through indirect ventilation or unvented designs, face shields offering expanded face coverage while typically requiring underlying eye protection, and specialized equipment addressing unique hazards like ultraviolet sources or laser operation; proper use training covering correct positioning, adjustment for individual fit, concurrent use with other protective equipment, and appropriate maintenance; cleaning and maintenance procedures ensuring continued visual clarity, structural integrity, and hygienic conditions; storage requirements preventing damage between uses; and program evaluation verifying continued effectiveness through performance assessment, incident analysis, and compliance monitoring. Selection considerations include optical quality maintaining visual acuity without distortion; compatibility with prescription eyewear for workers requiring vision correction; anti-fog properties preventing vision impairment from condensation; impact resistance when physical hazards exist alongside chemical concerns; comfort and fit affecting likelihood of consistent proper usage; and compatibility with other required protective equipment including respiratory protection or hearing protection potentially creating fit interference. Implementation challenges include ensuring consistent proper usage throughout exposure periods; addressing fogging issues in humid environments or during strenuous activity; maintaining appropriate replacement programs when scratches, cracks, or other damage compromise protection; and sometimes production pressure or convenience factors potentially compromising proper usage despite knowledge of requirements. Specific chemical considerations include compatibility between protective equipment materials and workplace chemicals preventing degradation compromising protection; appropriate coverage for specific exposure scenarios with different splash or vapor hazard patterns; and sometimes specialized requirements for particularly hazardous materials requiring heightened protection levels beyond standard equipment. These eye and face protection programs transform potential vision-threatening or permanently damaging exposures into controlled risks through systematic protection implementation, particularly critical given both the eye's exceptional vulnerability to chemical damage and the catastrophic functional impact of vision impairment, creating essential protection for sensitive tissues at particular risk during chemical handling, processing, or emergency situations.

Specialized protective equipment addresses unique toxicological exposures beyond standard respiratory, dermal, and eye protection programs. Hearing protection programs, while primarily addressing noise exposure, include components relevant to ototoxic chemical exposure which may potentiate noise-induced hearing loss or cause auditory damage through direct toxicity mechanisms. These programs include hazard assessment identifying combined noise and chemical exposure scenarios requiring enhanced protection; appropriate device selection considering attenuation requirements, comfort factors affecting compliance, and compatibility with other required protective equipment; training addressing proper insertion or fitting techniques and recognition of warning signs indicating potential auditory effects; and audiometric testing monitoring hearing thresholds over time verifying protection adequacy. Fall protection systems intersect with toxicological concerns in scenarios involving work at heights in chemical environments, confined space entry involving toxic atmospheres, or emergency response to chemical incidents at elevation. These programs require specialized consideration for chemical compatibility of harnesses, lanyards, and anchorage systems ensuring materials maintain structural integrity despite chemical exposure;

decontamination procedures preventing secondary exposure during equipment handling or storage; and sometimes specialized rescue planning for chemical exposure victims requiring simultaneous fall protection during extraction. Confined space protection specifically addresses toxic atmosphere concerns through atmospheric testing before entry; continuous monitoring during occupancy; appropriate respiratory protection selection for identified hazards; ventilation systems ensuring breathable atmosphere maintenance; and rescue capability addressing potential toxic exposure emergencies within space limitations. Heat stress management becomes particularly relevant with chemical protective clothing as impermeable materials preventing normal evaporative cooling significantly increase heat stress potential. These programs include acclimatization protocols developing physiological adaptation before full-shift impermeable garment usage; appropriate work-rest scheduling based on environmental conditions, work intensity, and specific ensemble characteristics; hydration protocols preventing fluid and electrolyte imbalances; physiological monitoring identifying developing heat stress before serious health effects occur; and sometimes cooling technologies ranging from ice vests to air-conditioned garments reducing heat stress during necessary impermeable ensemble usage. These specialized programs address the complex interactions between different workplace hazards, recognizing that toxic substance exposure often occurs within multifaceted environments requiring integrated protection strategies addressing chemical hazards alongside other workplace risks through coordinated approaches rather than isolated programs addressing individual hazard categories without consideration of their interactions and cumulative effects on worker protection needs.

Safety Management Systems

Hazard identification methodologies systematically recognize toxicological risks before exposure occurs, enabling proactive intervention rather than reactive response after harm manifestation. Comprehensive approaches employ multiple complementary techniques including process hazard analysis examining entire production systems identifying points where toxic materials could contact workers through normal operations, maintenance activities, or foreseeable abnormal conditions; job hazard analysis breaking work into discrete tasks evaluating each step for potential exposure through inhalation, skin contact, ingestion, or injection routes; walkthrough surveys directly observing workplace conditions identifying visible hazards, control deficiencies, or concerning work practices; industrial hygiene sampling quantifying actual exposure levels for comparison with established limits; safety data sheet review identifying hazardous properties of workplace materials; medical surveillance trend analysis revealing potential exposure patterns through health outcome evaluation; and incident investigation examining actual exposure events for systemic prevention opportunities. Implementation effectiveness depends on several critical factors including multidisciplinary participation engaging diverse perspectives from operations, maintenance, engineering, health and safety, and management rather than isolated assessment by specialists alone; worker involvement incorporating frontline experience with actual conditions beyond theoretical process understanding; systematic documentation ensuring comprehensive coverage without overlooking potential exposure scenarios; appropriate hazard ranking prioritizing intervention resources toward greatest risks; and regular reassessment maintaining current hazard understanding as processes, materials, and operations evolve. Advanced approaches increasingly incorporate emerging methodologies including predictive exposure modeling estimating potential exposures before process implementation; control banding providing structured risk assessment frameworks when detailed exposure data remains unavailable; biological monitoring assessing actual body burden complementing environmental sampling; and sometimes real-time monitoring technologies providing continuous exposure assessment rather than periodic sampling snapshots. These comprehensive hazard identification systems transform toxicological risk management from reactive response addressing manifest problems toward proactive prevention identifying and addressing potential exposures before harm occurs, creating foundation for effective risk management through systematic recognition of where, when, and how toxic substances might contact workers throughout complex operational systems rather than focusing exclusively on obvious high-visibility hazards while potentially overlooking significant exposure sources during routine operations, maintenance activities, abnormal conditions, or seemingly minor tasks cumulatively creating substantial exposure potential.

Risk assessment frameworks provide structured approaches evaluating identified hazards, determining their significance, and prioritizing intervention resources. Comprehensive methodologies address multiple dimensions including hazard characterization examining inherent toxicological properties through safety data sheet review, toxicological database consultation, and regulatory classification examination; exposure assessment determining potential magnitude, frequency, and duration of worker contact through industrial hygiene sampling, similar exposure group analysis, or modeling when direct measurement proves impractical; dose-response evaluation relating exposure levels to potential health outcomes based on established occupational exposure limits, toxicological literature, or epidemiological evidence; and risk characterization integrating these elements into holistic evaluation determining overall significance considering both exposure likelihood and potential consequence severity. Implementation typically employs matrix approaches plotting probability against severity creating risk categories guiding appropriate intervention levels, with variations including standard risk matrices using qualitative descriptors like "unlikely" or "severe"; semi-quantitative systems assigning numerical values to risk factors creating calculated risk scores; and occasionally fully quantitative approaches using statistical modeling estimating numerical risk probabilities. Critical success factors include appropriate uncertainty acknowledgment when complete information remains unavailable; consistent application preventing subjective bias affecting different hazard evaluations; regular updating as new information becomes available or workplace conditions change; and clear connection between assessment results and subsequent intervention prioritization ensuring resource allocation matches identified risk patterns. Advanced approaches increasingly incorporate sophisticated methodologies including benchmark dose modeling establishing exposure thresholds with defined confidence limits; physiologically based pharmacokinetic modeling estimating target tissue doses from external exposure measurements; probabilistic techniques addressing variability and uncertainty through distribution functions rather than point estimates; and occasionally molecular approaches examining specific toxicological mechanisms within affected worker populations. These structured risk assessment frameworks transform hazard information into actionable intelligence guiding intervention prioritization, ensuring limited resources address most significant risks rather than being allocated based on visibility, familiarity, ease of control, or other factors potentially disconnected from actual health risk magnitude. This systematic prioritization creates maximum health protection from available resources through objective, evidence-based decision frameworks determining where attention should focus within complex workplaces containing numerous potential hazards with varying significance levels.

Control verification and validation systems ensure that implemented protective measures actually deliver intended exposure reduction rather than merely existing as theoretical protections without practical effectiveness. Comprehensive approaches include multiple complementary techniques: initial verification confirming proper installation matching design specifications; performance testing measuring control effectiveness under actual operating conditions; exposure monitoring comparing worker exposure levels before and after implementation; visual examination identifying physical condition including damage, modification, or deterioration potentially compromising function; operational parameter checking verifying critical indicators like air flow, pressure differentials, or other measurements within specified ranges; worker feedback collecting user experience regarding practical effectiveness, usability issues, or operational challenges; and periodic reevaluation ensuring continued performance despite aging, process changes, or maintenance activities. Implementation methodologies vary by control type, with examples including ventilation system evaluation through smoke visualization revealing air flow patterns, air velocity measurement confirming appropriate capture or transport, tracer gas studies quantifying actual contaminant capture efficiency, and pressure differential monitoring ensuring proper directional flow maintenance; containment system validation through pressure testing verifying boundary integrity, leak detection identifying potential escape points, and sometimes tracer studies measuring actual containment effectiveness under operating conditions; personal protective equipment verification through fit testing measuring actual protection factors, inspection confirming material integrity, and occasionally workplace protection factor studies measuring performance under actual use conditions rather than laboratory testing alone; and administrative control validation through work practice observation, procedure compliance auditing, and effectiveness verification measuring whether theoretical protection translates into actual exposure reduction. Critical success factors include appropriate testing frequency balancing resource limitations against performance verification needs; test condition representativeness ensuring evaluation occurs under normal operating parameters rather than idealized scenarios; comprehensive coverage examining all critical system components rather than isolated elements alone; appropriate documentation maintaining performance records supporting both compliance demonstration and trend analysis; and effective corrective action systems addressing identified deficiencies through root cause analysis and systematic response beyond superficial repair. These verification and validation systems transform controls from paper compliance or theoretical protection toward demonstrated effectiveness, ensuring that implemented measures actually deliver intended exposure reduction rather than creating false security through apparent protection lacking practical effectiveness when subjected to objective performance evaluation under actual operating conditions.

Training effectiveness evaluation measures whether educational programs actually develop knowledge, skills, and behaviors necessary for appropriate exposure prevention rather than merely documenting attendance or completion. Comprehensive approaches employ multiple assessment dimensions reflecting progressive training impact levels: reaction evaluation measuring participant satisfaction, perceived relevance, and engagement; knowledge assessment verifying information acquisition through testing, demonstration, or skill performance; behavior change evaluation examining whether workplace practices actually reflect training content through observation, work product review, or performance monitoring; results measurement determining whether training ultimately affects exposure reduction, incident prevention, or health outcome improvement; and program improvement processes using evaluation findings to enhance future training effectiveness. Implementation methodologies include pre/post testing measuring knowledge change attributable to training intervention; skill demonstration through structured scenarios or simulations assessing capability beyond mere information recall; workplace observation determining whether learned practices transfer to actual job performance; exposure monitoring measuring whether behavior changes produce actual exposure reduction; and occasionally controlled comparison examining differences between trained and untrained groups when experimental designs prove practical. Critical success factors include appropriate evaluation design matching assessment methods to specific training objectives; reliable measurement tools producing consistent results across different evaluators or time periods; practical implementation balancing comprehensive assessment against resource limitations; clear success criteria establishing quantifiable targets rather than subjective judgments; and effective feedback mechanisms ensuring evaluation findings actually influence program improvement rather than merely documenting current effectiveness without driving enhancement. Advanced approaches increasingly incorporate innovative methodologies including performance-based evaluation focusing on demonstrated capability rather than knowledge testing alone; technology-enabled observation using video analysis, wearable sensors, or other tools capturing actual workplace behavior beyond limited direct observation periods; longitudinal assessment examining knowledge retention and behavior maintenance over extended timeframes rather than immediate post-training evaluation only; and sometimes return-on-investment analysis quantifying training value through comparing program costs against financial benefits from reduced exposure, prevented illness, or improved productivity. These comprehensive evaluation systems transform training from compliance activity documenting minimum regulatory requirements toward performance improvement tool verifying that educational interventions actually develop exposure prevention capability, providing both accountability demonstrating resource justification and continuous improvement guidance identifying enhancement opportunities for future programming based on systematic effectiveness assessment rather than anecdotal impression or participant satisfaction alone.

Management systems integration embeds toxicological risk management within broader organizational processes rather than maintaining isolated programs disconnected from core business operations. Comprehensive approaches establish systematic connections between toxic exposure prevention and various organizational dimensions including strategic planning incorporating health protection goals alongside production, quality, and financial objectives; resource allocation processes ensuring appropriate funding, staffing, and technology support for exposure control initiatives; performance management systems establishing accountability for health protection alongside other operational responsibilities; information systems capturing exposure data alongside production metrics enabling integrated analysis; continuous improvement mechanisms addressing toxicological hazards within broader operational enhancement processes; contractor management ensuring consistent protection across all workplace activities regardless of employment relationship; management of change processes evaluating potential exposure impacts before implementing process, material, or organizational modifications; and emergency management systems addressing toxicological release scenarios alongside other potential emergencies. Implementation methodologies include policy integration establishing clear organizational commitment to toxicological risk management within overarching corporate policies; responsibility definition clarifying specific roles at all organizational levels from executive leadership through frontline supervision; standardized processes embedding exposure considerations within routine operational decision-making; integrated metrics measuring both health protection and production performance within unified reporting systems; and coordinated improvement processes addressing toxicological risk reduction alongside productivity, quality, and efficiency enhancement rather than competing prioritization. Critical success factors include leadership commitment demonstrating consistent priority for health protection through resource allocation, personal involvement, and consequence management; middle management engagement translating high-level commitment into daily operational reality; effective communication ensuring understanding throughout organizational hierarchy; appropriate balancing between standardization ensuring consistent protection and flexibility accommodating operational diversity; and performance measurement providing objective evidence regarding management system effectiveness beyond policy declaration or program existence. Advanced approaches increasingly incorporate sophisticated methodologies including leading indicator development measuring activities predictive of future exposure control success rather than focusing exclusively on lagging outcome metrics; integrated risk assessment addressing toxicological hazards alongside other operational risks within unified decision frameworks; and sometimes external certification or verification providing independent assessment regarding management system effectiveness. These integrated management approaches transform toxicological risk management from specialized technical function operating parallel to core business activities toward embedded organizational process where exposure prevention becomes standard operating procedure rather than competing priority, creating sustainable protection through systematic organizational alignment rather than relying exclusively on individual expertise, initiative, or advocacy potentially vulnerable to personnel changes, budget fluctuations, or shifting organizational priorities.

EDUCATION PROGRAMS

Educational initiatives develop knowledge, skills, and motivation supporting toxicological risk reduction across diverse populations.

Professional Training

Healthcare provider education develops specialized toxicological knowledge among medical professionals, enhancing both diagnostic capability and treatment effectiveness across diverse practice settings. Comprehensive programs address multiple knowledge domains including exposure recognition supporting accurate identification of toxicological etiologies among presenting symptoms; diagnostic approach optimization including appropriate history elements, physical examination focus, and laboratory evaluation selection; management principles covering both supportive care and specific antidotal therapies; exposure-disease relationship understanding across acute, subacute, and chronic timeframes; and prevention guidance development helping patients reduce harmful exposures beyond immediate treatment. Implementation approaches vary across career stages, with medical school curricula typically providing foundational toxicology understanding through both dedicated coursework and integration within broader subjects like pharmacology, emergency medicine, and occupational health; residency training developing practical management skills through supervised clinical experience with toxicological cases; and continuing medical education maintaining and expanding knowledge throughout practice careers through various formats including conferences, online modules, journal articles, and case-based learning activities.

> **Remember**
>
> **Educational programs must be developmentally appropriate, culturally relevant, and delivered through multiple channels including schools, healthcare settings, community organizations, and media platforms to effectively reach target populations**

Content typically addresses both general principles and specific toxicant categories, with particular emphasis on substances commonly encountered in the provider's specific practice setting – emergency physicians focusing on acute poisonings and overdoses, primary care providers addressing environmental and occupational exposures, pediatricians covering common childhood exposures, and occupational medicine specialists developing detailed understanding of workplace toxicants. Specialized topics increasingly include emerging concerns like electronic cigarette associated lung injury, novel psychoactive substances, pharmaceutical adulterants, environmental justice dimensions affecting exposure distribution, and appropriate risk communication strategies helping patients understand exposure implications without creating unwarranted anxiety. Effectiveness evaluation examines both knowledge acquisition through testing and actual practice change through case management review, prescription pattern analysis, or referral appropriateness assessment. Implementation challenges include competition for curriculum time within already crowded medical education programs; limited toxicology expertise availability in many teaching institutions; rapidly evolving substance exposure patterns requiring continuous content updating; and sometimes limited perceived relevance among providers who may underestimate toxicological etiology prevalence within their patient populations. Despite these challenges, comprehensive healthcare provider education represents essential investment transforming medical practice from potential missed diagnosis or suboptimal management toward appropriate recognition and effective intervention addressing toxicological contributions to patient presentations across diverse clinical settings.

Industrial hygiene and safety professional development creates specialized technical expertise supporting workplace toxicant recognition, evaluation, and control. Comprehensive programs address multiple competency domains including hazard recognition developing capability identifying potential toxic exposures within complex industrial processes; sampling strategy development creating appropriate exposure assessment plans balancing comprehensiveness against practical resource limitations; control technology selection matching intervention approaches to specific hazard characteristics and operational constraints; regulatory compliance ensuring programs meet legal requirements across various jurisdictions; and management system implementation developing programs translating technical knowledge into organizational practice beyond individual assessments or interventions. Educational pathways typically include undergraduate or graduate degree programs providing foundational science including chemistry, biology, physics, and mathematics alongside specialized industrial hygiene and toxicology coursework; professional certification through organizations like the American Board of Industrial Hygiene (ABIH) or the Board of Certified Safety Professionals (BCSP) validating knowledge through standardized examination and experience requirements; and continuing education maintaining current knowledge through conferences, workshops, online learning, professional society participation, and technical publication review. Advanced specialization often develops through both formal education and professional experience in areas like analytical chemistry supporting complex exposure assessment; ventilation engineering designing effective control systems; exposure modeling predicting potential exposures when measurement proves impractical; epidemiological methods analyzing workplace health outcome patterns; and toxicological risk assessment integrating exposure and health effect information into comprehensive evaluation. Emerging competency areas increasingly include sensor technology application leveraging real-time monitoring developments; big data analytics examining large exposure datasets identifying patterns traditional analysis might miss; exposure visualization creating compelling communication tools beyond traditional numerical data presentation; and risk communication developing effective information transfer across diverse stakeholder groups from workers to management to surrounding communities. Implementation challenges include keeping pace with rapidly evolving scientific understanding requiring continuous knowledge updating; developing practical implementation skills beyond theoretical principles typically emphasized in academic programs; integrating technical expertise with business acumen supporting effective organizational implementation; and demonstrating value within organizations potentially viewing industrial hygiene as cost center rather than value-creating function. Despite these challenges, comprehensive professional development creates essential technical capability translating toxicological knowledge into practical workplace protection through specialized expertise development beyond general safety knowledge, enabling sophisticated exposure assessment, control technology implementation, and program management addressing complex toxicological hazards across diverse industrial environments.

Hazardous materials response training develops specialized capabilities for emergency personnel addressing chemical releases, spills, transportation incidents, and other scenarios creating potential toxic exposures beyond routine workplace operations. Comprehensive programs address multiple competency levels following established frameworks like OSHA's HAZWOPER (Hazardous Waste Operations and Emergency Response) standard or NFPA's Professional Competence of Responders to Hazardous Materials Incidents standards, with progressive development from awareness level understanding hazard recognition and notification procedures without direct intervention responsibility; operations level capability taking defensive actions containing releases without direct contact; technician level skills including risk assessment, material identification, and offensive control measures; specialist level expertise addressing specific chemical categories requiring unique approaches; and incident command competencies managing complex responses involving multiple agencies, disciplines, and hazard types. Content typically covers multiple knowledge domains including hazard recognition through shipping documentation, container identification, monitoring equipment, and physical property observation; personal protective equipment selection, use, and limitations across different ensembles from basic structural firefighting gear through fully encapsulating chemical suits; decontamination principles and techniques for both victims and responders; medical monitoring addressing both exposure victims and response personnel; hazard and risk assessment methodology supporting appropriate control strategy selection; and incident management systems establishing command structure, communication protocols, and coordination mechanisms during complex responses. Implementation methodology emphasizes practical skill development through hands-on training with actual equipment, realistic scenario exercises, and sometimes live agent training with controlled hazardous materials under carefully managed conditions. Refresher training maintains both knowledge and skills addressing natural decay over time, equipment or procedure changes, and emerging hazard awareness. Specialized modules increasingly address contemporary challenges including weapons of mass destruction response covering chemical warfare agents, biological threats, and radiological materials; drug laboratory hazards from both traditional methamphetamine production and emerging synthetic opioid manufacturing; alternative fuel vehicle incidents involving hydrogen, compressed natural gas, or high-voltage battery systems; and environmental crime investigation addressing illegal disposal or deliberate contamination scenarios. These comprehensive training programs transform general emergency response capability toward specialized hazardous materials competency, enabling appropriate risk assessment, protective measure implementation, exposure control, and scene management during incidents involving toxic materials where improper response could create substantial responder exposure, ineffective public protection, or environmental damage beyond the initial release through systematic development of both knowledge and practical skills necessary for effective hazardous materials incident management.

Environmental health specialist education develops professional capability addressing toxicant exposures across community settings beyond occupational environments. Comprehensive programs develop multidisciplinary expertise combining elements from public health, environmental science, toxicology, epidemiology, and risk assessment within specialized roles including public health department environmental health divisions, environmental protection agencies, academic research institutions, non-governmental organizations, and environmental consulting firms. Core competencies typically include exposure assessment measuring or modeling community exposures through various environmental media including air, water, soil, and food; environmental monitoring developing and implementing systematic sampling strategies addressing both routine surveillance and incident response; risk assessment integrating exposure data with toxicological information determining potential health implications; intervention development creating exposure reduction strategies through various approaches from regulatory enforcement to community education; and risk communication translating technical findings into understandable information supporting informed decision-making among affected populations. Educational pathways include undergraduate environmental health or environmental science degrees providing foundational understanding; graduate programs offering specialized focus in areas like environmental toxicology, exposure science, or environmental epidemiology; professional certification through organizations like the National Environmental Health Association validating knowledge through standardized examination; and continuing education maintaining current understanding through conferences, workshops, webinars, and professional literature review. Specialized knowledge areas increasingly include environmental justice addressing disproportionate exposure patterns across different demographic groups; climate change health implications as shifting patterns affect toxicant distribution, persistence, and human contact; cumulative risk assessment examining multiple exposure interactions rather than single-chemical evaluations; community-based participatory research engaging affected populations throughout assessment and intervention processes; and health impact assessment evaluating potential exposure implications from proposed projects or policies before implementation. Implementation challenges include addressing politically contentious issues where scientific findings may face resistance based on economic or ideological factors; developing effective interdisciplinary collaboration across diverse fields necessary for comprehensive environmental health protection; obtaining sufficient resources for appropriate monitoring and assessment within constrained public budgets; and sometimes navigating complex jurisdictional boundaries where exposure sources and affected populations cross administrative divides. Despite these challenges, comprehensive environmental health specialist development creates essential professional capability translating environmental toxicology knowledge into practical public protection through systematic professional development combining scientific expertise with implementation skills addressing community toxic exposures through evidence-based assessment, management, and communication approaches.

Professional ethics training addresses the complex value considerations arising when technical toxicological knowledge intersects with competing interests, confidentiality requirements, and public health responsibilities. Comprehensive programs develop ethical reasoning capability beyond simple rule compliance, addressing multiple dimensions including professional responsibility balancing obligations to employers against broader public health protection duties; appropriate risk communication avoiding both unwarranted reassurance and unnecessary alarm based on incomplete information; data integrity ensuring research and assessment findings remain unbiased despite potential pressure from stakeholders with predetermined conclusions; confidentiality management balancing legitimate proprietary information protection against appropriate hazard disclosure affecting public health; and conflict of interest recognition and management when professional judgment might be influenced by financial, organizational, or personal factors beyond technical assessment. Implementation approaches include case study examination analyzing complex scenarios without clear right/wrong answers developing nuanced reasoning capability; ethical framework introduction providing structured decision models integrating principles like beneficence, non-maleficence, justice, and autonomy within toxicological contexts; professional code of ethics review examining specific guidance from organizations like the American Industrial Hygiene Association, Society of Toxicology, or American College of Occupational and Environmental Medicine; and sometimes role-play exercises developing communication skills addressing ethical challenges through simulated stakeholder interactions. Content typically addresses both universal principles and situation-specific applications with examples including appropriate hazard communication when scientific uncertainty exists regarding exposure implications; whistleblower considerations when organizational practices potentially create unaddressed public health risks; research integrity when study findings may affect regulatory decisions with substantial economic impact; social justice dimensions when exposure distribution disproportionately affects vulnerable populations; and professional independence maintenance when employment or consulting relationships create pressure toward particular conclusions regardless of objective evidence. These ethical training programs transform technical professionals from narrowly focused specialists toward responsible practitioners balancing scientific expertise with appropriate ethical consideration, particularly important within toxicological fields where decisions often affect health protection for workers, communities, and consumers potentially unaware of their exposure circumstances and unable to independently evaluate complex technical information without professional interpretation and appropriate disclosure balancing multiple legitimate but sometimes competing values beyond purely technical assessment.

Public Education

School-based toxicology education integrates age-appropriate content within educational curricula, developing knowledge supporting both immediate safety behavior and foundational understanding for future decision-making. Comprehensive approaches address progressive development across educational levels: early elementary programs focusing on simple safety rules like "always ask first" before touching unknown substances, poison symbol recognition, and basic hygiene practices preventing incidental ingestion; later elementary content developing more sophisticated understanding including chemical safety reading labels, appropriate storage principles, and when to seek adult assistance; middle school curricula introducing basic toxicological concepts like dose-response relationships, exposure routes, and risk reduction strategies within science education; and high school content integrating more advanced topics including environmental health, occupational safety considerations for early employment experiences, and critical evaluation of health claims regarding chemical exposures. Implementation approaches include dedicated safety units within health education; integration within science curricula connecting toxicological principles with chemistry, biology, and environmental science content; service learning projects addressing community chemical safety concerns; and sometimes specialized programs addressing specific regional concerns like pesticide safety in agricultural communities, lead exposure in areas with older housing stock, or water quality issues in regions with specific contamination history. Pedagogical strategies emphasize active learning through hands-on activities, scenario-based problem solving, role play developing communication skills, and project-based approaches creating deeper engagement beyond passive information receipt. Resource development includes age-appropriate materials with visual design, reading level, and content complexity matched to developmental capabilities; teacher support materials providing background information addressing potential knowledge limitations among educators without specialized toxicology training; and sometimes community connection components linking classroom learning with home implementation through parent-child activities reinforcing educational content. Evaluation increasingly measures both knowledge acquisition through testing and actual behavior change through observation or parent reporting, with longitudinal assessment examining retention and application beyond immediate post-instruction periods. Successful programs recognize both the immediate safety value of appropriate toxicological knowledge and the long-term foundation these educational experiences create for future decision-making regarding chemical exposures across occupational, consumer, and environmental contexts as students mature into adults making independent choices affecting their exposure circumstances throughout life domains.

Community outreach initiatives extend toxicological education beyond formal educational settings, reaching diverse populations through various engagement approaches. Comprehensive programs employ multiple methodologies including public workshops providing interactive learning opportunities addressing specific toxicological concerns; informational materials distributed through community locations including healthcare facilities, libraries, community centers, and religious institutions; digital content delivery through websites, social media platforms, and mobile applications; media engagement through newspapers, local television, radio programming, and emerging digital channels; community health fairs offering direct engagement opportunities with educational activities, demonstrations, and personalized risk discussion; and train-the-trainer approaches developing local capacity through educating community members who subsequently share information throughout their social networks. Content typically addresses both general principles and community-specific concerns, with common topics including household chemical safety covering appropriate storage, usage, and disposal; environmental health literacy developing capability to understand exposure information from various sources; consumer product safety addressing potential toxic exposures through everyday products; emergency preparedness for chemical incidents including appropriate sheltering or evacuation responses; and sometimes specialized topics responding to community-specific concerns like particular industrial facilities, contaminated sites, or local environmental issues generating public interest or concern. Implementation effectiveness depends on several critical factors including cultural appropriateness addressing language preferences, communication norms, and relevant contextual examples; literacy level adjustment ensuring accessibility across diverse educational backgrounds; trust relationship development particularly important when historical experiences may have created skepticism regarding official information sources; practical applicability providing actionable guidance within realistic resource constraints rather than unrealistic recommendations; and meaningful community involvement throughout program development ensuring relevance to actual concerns rather than externally presumed educational needs. Evaluation increasingly employs outcome measures beyond simple participation counts, examining actual knowledge acquisition, reported behavior change, and sometimes environmental measurements assessing potential exposure reduction resulting from educational interventions. These comprehensive community outreach approaches transform toxicological knowledge from specialized technical information toward practical public understanding supporting informed decision-making across diverse populations who may never participate in formal educational programs but nevertheless make daily decisions affecting their potential toxic exposures through consumer choices, household practices, and environmental interactions.

Consumer education addresses toxicological considerations in purchasing decisions, product usage, and disposal practices through various information channels and engagement strategies. Comprehensive approaches provide both general principles and product-specific guidance across multiple dimensions including label interpretation developing capability to understand hazard communication, ingredient listings, and usage instructions on consumer products; appropriate usage practices minimizing exposure during normal product application; storage recommendations preventing accidental access, contamination, or degradation potentially increasing hazards; proper disposal guidance preventing environmental contamination or unintended exposure through inappropriate waste management; and sometimes alternative product information identifying potentially less toxic options for common household functions. Implementation utilizes diverse channels including point-of-sale materials providing information during purchase decision-making; product packaging communicating essential information through labels, package inserts, and sometimes QR codes linking to detailed digital content; media campaigns addressing broader awareness through advertising, public service announcements, and editorial content; retailer education initiatives developing knowledge among sales personnel providing customer guidance; digital resources including websites, mobile applications, and social media content providing accessible information ranging from general principles to specific product guidance; and sometimes direct education through workshops, demonstrations, or community presentations. Content increasingly addresses emerging consumer concerns including "green" product evaluation developing critical assessment beyond marketing claims; endocrine disruptor awareness regarding substances potentially affecting hormonal systems; nanomaterial presence in various consumer goods; fragrance component disclosure beyond generic "fragrance" listings; and appropriate interpretation of various certification programs making environmental or health claims about products. Implementation challenges include information complexity when complete toxicological details would overwhelm typical consumer decision processes; manufacturer resistance toward expanded disclosure potentially revealing proprietary formulations; varying literacy, language, and educational levels across consumer populations; competing priorities during purchase decisions where price, effectiveness, and convenience may outweigh potential toxicological considerations; and sometimes conflicting information from various sources creating consumer confusion rather than informed choice. Despite these challenges, effective consumer education initiatives transform purchasing and usage behavior through developing practical knowledge supporting informed decision-making within realistic constraints, enhancing consumer capability to make appropriate risk-benefit assessments regarding products containing potentially toxic components based on both hazard information and personal values rather than either uninformed selection or anxiety-driven avoidance resulting from incomplete or misunderstood information regarding chemical constituents and their potential health implications.

Specialized population education addresses groups with unique toxicological vulnerabilities, exposure circumstances, or communication needs through tailored approaches beyond general public education. Comprehensive programs develop targeted initiatives for various populations including pregnant women and new parents with specific content addressing developmental vulnerabilities during prenatal and early childhood periods; elderly individuals whose physiological changes may affect toxicant susceptibility alongside potential cognitive or sensory limitations affecting standard educational approaches; occupationally exposed workers receiving education beyond formal workplace training through unions, community organizations, or public health initiatives; limited English proficiency communities requiring culturally and linguistically appropriate materials beyond simple translation; low literacy populations needing specially designed communication employing visual elements, simplified language, and sometimes verbal delivery rather than text-dependent approaches; and specific cultural or ethnic groups whose exposure patterns, risk perception frameworks, or trusted information sources may differ significantly from majority populations. Implementation methodologies employ tailored approaches including appropriate communication channel selection matched to specific population media consumption patterns and trusted information sources; message development addressing group-specific concerns, values, and practical constraints; messenger selection identifying credible voices within particular communities; and sometimes participatory design engaging community members throughout program development ensuring relevance, appropriateness, and effectiveness. Content typically combines general toxicological principles with population-specific applications such as prenatal environmental exposure guidance for expectant mothers; medication management safety for elderly populations often managing multiple prescription regimens; take-home exposure prevention for workers who might inadvertently transport workplace toxicants to family members; culturally specific information addressing unique exposure scenarios like traditional medicines, cultural practices involving potential toxicants, or occupation-specific risks concentrated within particular communities. Evaluation employs culturally appropriate assessment methods measuring both program acceptance and effectiveness within the specific population context, sometimes utilizing community-based participatory research approaches involving community members throughout evaluation design, implementation, and interpretation. These specialized educational initiatives transform general toxicological information into contextually relevant guidance addressing the unique combinations of vulnerability, exposure circumstance, and communication needs characterizing diverse populations who might receive limited benefit from general educational approaches not specifically designed for their particular situation, creating more effective risk reduction through appropriate tailoring rather than one-size-fits-all approaches potentially missing critical population-specific considerations affecting both exposure patterns and effective communication strategies.

Media literacy development enhances critical evaluation capability regarding toxicological information encountered through news, social media, advertising, and entertainment sources. Comprehensive approaches address multiple skills including source evaluation assessing credibility, potential bias, and appropriate expertise behind toxicological claims; evidence assessment examining study design, sample size, and appropriate controls supporting specific conclusions; uncertainty recognition identifying appropriate distinction between established knowledge, emerging evidence, and speculation; risk contextualization understanding relative magnitude compared to other hazards rather than isolated focus on single risks; and recognition of common misrepresentation patterns including cherry-picked data, correlation-causation confusion, and dramatic individual anecdotes potentially mischaracterizing overall evidence. Implementation methodologies include formal educational modules within science or health curricula developing systematic evaluation skills; public workshops providing adults with practical frameworks for information assessment; digital resources offering guidance for evaluating online toxicological claims particularly important given social media's increasing role in information dissemination; and sometimes media partnership initiatives working with journalists to improve toxicological reporting accuracy and appropriate context inclusion. Content typically combines general scientific literacy principles with toxicology-specific applications addressing common challenges including sensationalistic reporting of preliminary animal studies as definitive human health evidence; misrepresentation of detection capability as proof of harm regardless of dose consideration; oversimplified "toxic"/"non-toxic" dichotomies ignoring fundamental dose-response relationships; and failure distinguishing between hazard (inherent toxicity potential) and risk (likelihood of actual harm under realistic exposure scenarios). Special attention increasingly addresses emerging information challenges including algorithmic content curation potentially creating information bubbles reinforcing existing beliefs regardless of evidence quality; visual information rapidly conveying emotional impact without nuanced context; influencer content potentially prioritizing engagement over accuracy; and sometimes deliberate misinformation regarding chemical exposures created for ideological, commercial, or engagement-driving purposes. These media literacy initiatives transform information consumption from passive acceptance toward active critical evaluation, developing public capability to distinguish between credible toxicological information and misleading, incomplete, or sensationalized content, particularly valuable within contemporary information environments where traditional gatekeeping functions have diminished while information volume has exponentially increased creating significant challenges for individuals attempting to make informed decisions regarding potential chemical exposures without specialized scientific training to independently evaluate complex toxicological evidence.

Risk Communication Training

Message development training builds capability to create effective toxicological risk communications balancing technical accuracy with recipient comprehension and appropriate action motivation. Comprehensive programs develop multiple skill dimensions including audience analysis identifying key characteristics affecting message reception including knowledge levels, concern patterns, information preferences, and practical constraints; content selection determining essential information supporting informed decision-making without overwhelming detail potentially reducing comprehension; appropriate framing establishing context helping recipients properly interpret technical information within their existing mental models; uncertainty communication honestly addressing knowledge limitations without undermining message credibility; action guidance connecting hazard information to specific protective measures within recipient capability; and evaluation techniques assessing message effectiveness before widespread dissemination. Implementation methodologies emphasize practical skill development through approaches including message development workshops with guided practice creating actual communications followed by expert and peer feedback; case study examination analyzing both successful and problematic real-world examples identifying specific elements contributing to effectiveness or failure; simulation exercises developing messaging under realistic time constraints and information limitations; and sometimes field testing opportunities where participants develop messages then evaluate actual recipient comprehension and reaction. Content typically addresses both general principles and specific applications across various scenarios including emergency communications during acute chemical releases requiring immediate protective action; ongoing exposure situations where behavior change might reduce chronic low-level contact; uncertain risk contexts where incomplete evidence creates communication challenges; and complex risk-benefit situations where simple "safe/unsafe" dichotomies prove inappropriate given legitimate trade-offs between various considerations. Specialized techniques include message mapping developing pre-structured content for anticipated scenarios enabling rapid yet comprehensive communication during time-sensitive situations; mental model elicitation identifying audience preconceptions requiring specific addressing within communication strategies; appropriate numeric risk presentation supporting comprehension through absolute risk, relative risk, or visual representations depending on specific communication goals; and message testing methodology incorporating both qualitative feedback addressing subjective comprehension and quantitative assessment measuring specific knowledge acquisition or intended behavior adoption. These communication development capabilities transform technical toxicological information into effective public guidance through systematic message creation processes addressing both scientific accuracy and human communication factors, particularly valuable for technical experts whose specialized training typically emphasizes content accuracy without equal attention to recipient-centered communication design necessary for effective information transfer beyond specialist audiences.

Spokesperson preparation develops individuals' capability to effectively deliver toxicological risk information through media interviews, public meetings, community presentations, and other direct communication channels. Comprehensive training addresses multiple skill dimensions including message organization creating clear, concise explanation of complex toxicological concepts; non-technical language usage finding appropriate alternatives for specialized terminology without oversimplification compromising accuracy; anticipated question management preparing for predictable inquiries with clear, consistent responses; confidence projection through verbal and non-verbal communication creating appropriate credibility without appearing defensive; emotional intelligence recognizing and appropriately addressing audience concerns, fears, or anger potentially affecting message reception; and specific technique application addressing different communication contexts from broadcast media interviews to community meetings to one-on-one conversations with concerned individuals. Implementation methodologies emphasize experiential learning through approaches including videotaped practice interviews with professional feedback identifying specific improvement opportunities; realistic scenario simulations recreating challenging communication situations like hostile questioning, emotional audience members, or complex technical explanation requirements; observation and analysis of effective and ineffective spokesperson examples identifying specific behaviors contributing to communication success or failure; and graduated exposure beginning with simple controlled practice progressing toward more challenging realistic scenarios building capability and confidence simultaneously. Content typically includes both general communication principles and toxicology-specific applications addressing common challenges including explaining dose-response relationships to audiences thinking in binary "safe/dangerous" categories; appropriately contextualizing detection limits and their significance without dismissing legitimate concerns; addressing scientific uncertainty without undermining overall message credibility; and effectively responding to emotionally charged questions about potential health effects, particularly those involving children, cancer risks, or reproductive concerns creating heightened emotional response.

Special attention increasingly addresses emerging communication challenges including social media environments where brief statements may be separated from crucial context; recorded interactions potentially reaching much broader audiences than originally anticipated; coordinated messaging importance across multiple communicators during complex incidents; and appropriate use of visual aids enhancing understanding of complex toxicological concepts through graphical representation rather than exclusively verbal explanation. These spokesperson preparation programs transform knowledgeable individuals into effective communicators capable of serving as credible information sources during situations involving toxicological concerns, particularly important given research consistently demonstrating that communication delivery characteristics significantly affect message reception, credibility perception, and ultimately protective action implementation regardless of technical content accuracy alone.

Community engagement facilitation develops capability to design and implement interactive risk communication processes beyond one-directional information provision. Comprehensive training addresses multiple skill dimensions including participatory process design creating structured engagement opportunities balancing open dialogue with productive focus; active listening demonstrating genuine interest in community perspectives beyond token consultation; conflict management addressing disagreements constructively without escalation or dismissal; power imbalance navigation creating meaningful participation despite disparities in technical knowledge, resources, or authority; collaborative problem-solving facilitating joint solution development rather than predetermined outcome presentation; and cross-cultural communication effectively engaging diverse community members despite varying communication styles, trust levels, or cultural frameworks. Implementation methodologies emphasize both conceptual understanding and practical skill development through approaches including facilitation practice with realistic scenarios followed by structured feedback; observation and analysis of experienced facilitators identifying specific techniques contributing to successful engagement; stakeholder role-play exercises developing perspective-taking beyond personal viewpoint; conflict simulation providing experience with productive management of disagreement; and sometimes actual community engagement experiences under mentorship providing supervised real-world application. Content typically addresses both general facilitation principles and specific applications to toxicological contexts including appropriate technical information provision supporting informed discussion without overwhelming participants or creating expert-dominated conversation; visualization techniques making complex exposure concepts accessible through graphical representation; structured approaches for eliciting community knowledge regarding local exposure patterns complementing technical assessment; and documentation methods capturing participation outcomes beyond meeting minutes alone. Special attention increasingly addresses challenging engagement scenarios including communities with historical distrust based on previous negative experiences; situations involving environmental justice concerns where socioeconomic, racial, or ethnic factors affect exposure distribution; contexts with significant technical uncertainty creating multiple legitimate interpretations; and highly polarized situations where underlying value differences rather than technical disagreements drive conflict. These facilitation capabilities transform toxicological risk communication from expert monologue toward collaborative dialogue, recognizing that effective risk management often requires integrating technical expertise with community knowledge, values, and perspectives through structured engagement processes rather than simply delivering predetermined technical information regardless of community concerns, questions, or contextual understanding.

Table 14.3: Evidence-Based Prevention Programs

Program Type	Target Population	Components
Poison Prevention Education	Parents/caregivers of children under 6	Safe storage, proper use, emergency response
Medication Safety	Older adults, medication users	Medication review, safe storage, disposal education
School-Based Programs	K-12 students	Age-appropriate curricula, take-home materials, teacher training
Healthcare Provider Training	Prescribers, pharmacists, nurses	Prescribing practices, patient education, risk recognition
Community-Based Initiatives	General population, high-risk communities	Multiple intervention levels, policy+education approach

Risk perception principles education develops understanding regarding psychological, social, and cultural factors influencing how individuals interpret and respond to toxicological information. Comprehensive programs address multiple knowledge domains including outrage factor recognition understanding characteristics beyond statistical probability significantly affecting risk perception including voluntariness, control, familiarity, equity, dread, and uncertainty; mental model awareness examining how pre-existing cognitive frameworks shape new information interpretation regardless of provided content; cultural cognition understanding how worldviews and group identity influence risk information reception beyond individual factors; social amplification recognition regarding how information flows through social systems potentially magnifying or minimizing risk perception independent of technical characteristics; trust determination factors including perceived competence, honesty, empathy, and commitment affecting information source credibility; and effective addressing strategies developing capability to acknowledge these factors rather than simply providing additional technical data unlikely to address underlying perception drivers. Implementation methodologies include case study examination analyzing perception patterns in historical toxicological incidents; structured exercises comparing expert versus public risk rankings with analysis of factors creating divergence; self-reflection activities examining personal risk perception patterns and potential professional biases; scenario analysis developing appropriate response strategies for various perception challenges; and sometimes field observation experiences examining actual public responses to toxicological information in community settings. Content typically combines theoretical frameworks with practical application across various contexts including emergency communication during acute chemical releases; ongoing environmental exposure situations requiring long-term community engagement; workplace risk communication addressing employee concerns about occupational exposures; and consumer product scenarios involving public risk-benefit decision-making. Special attention increasingly addresses emerging challenges including social media influence on risk perception through rapid information sharing, emotional content amplification, and algorithm-driven exposure potentially creating information bubbles; growing political polarization affecting risk perception through identity-protective cognition where factual interpretation aligns with group affiliation rather than objective evidence alone; and varying risk tolerance across different cultural contexts potentially creating miscommunication when technical experts assume universal perception patterns. These risk perception education programs transform communication approach from frustrated attempts aligning public perception with technical assessment through additional data provision toward more effective strategies acknowledging and appropriately addressing the legitimate psychological, social, and cultural factors fundamentally shaping risk perception regardless of technical information quality, creating more effective risk communication through human factor understanding rather than exclusively technical content focus.

POLICY DEVELOPMENT

Policy initiatives establish systematic approaches addressing toxicological risks through regulatory frameworks, organizational standards, and governance mechanisms.

Regulatory Guidelines

Chemical registration and evaluation systems establish pre-market assessment processes ensuring basic safety information availability before substances enter commerce. Comprehensive frameworks typically include new chemical notification requiring manufacturers to submit information regarding physical-chemical properties, toxicological testing results, and projected production volumes before marketing; tiered data requirements establishing proportional information needs based on exposure potential from production volume, application characteristics, and population vulnerability; evaluation processes where regulatory authorities assess submitted data determining whether additional information needs exist or risk management measures should apply; and continuous requirement adjustment as scientific understanding evolves regarding appropriate testing methods, endpoints of concern, or exposure assessment approaches. Implementation varies significantly across jurisdictions, with examples including the European Union's Registration, Evaluation, Authorization and Restriction of Chemicals (REACH) regulation establishing comprehensive requirements for both new and existing substances based on production volume thresholds; the United States Toxic Substances Control Act (TSCA) as amended by the Frank R. Lautenberg Chemical Safety for the 21st Century Act requiring EPA evaluation of new chemicals with enhanced authority addressing existing substances; and similar systems in Canada, Japan, South Korea, China, and other nations creating global patchwork of sometimes complementary, sometimes conflicting requirements. Modern systems increasingly incorporate alternative assessment principles supporting substitution with safer alternatives when feasible rather than simple risk management of inherently hazardous substances; enhanced vulnerability consideration for sensitive populations including children, pregnant women, and elderly individuals; transparent information sharing through public databases while protecting legitimate confidential business information; and international harmonization efforts reducing duplicative testing requirements across different national systems. Implementation challenges include administrative capacity limitations handling thousands of substances requiring evaluation with finite agency resources; determining appropriate balance between data requirements and innovation impacts; addressing substances already in commerce predating system implementation; and sometimes unexamined presumptions favoring international competitiveness over precautionary health protection. Despite these limitations, comprehensive chemical registration systems transform uncontrolled market introduction toward systematic evaluation ensuring basic hazard and exposure information availability before widespread use, creating foundation for appropriate risk management decisions based on evidence rather than reaction after problems manifest through detected health impacts following unexamined market introduction.

Workplace exposure standards establish maximum permissible airborne contaminant concentrations protecting worker health during occupational activities. Comprehensive frameworks define various limit types including time-weighted averages addressing typical full-shift exposures; short-term limits preventing adverse effects from brief high-concentration exposures; ceiling values never to be exceeded regardless of duration; and sometimes notation systems identifying special concerns like skin absorption potential, sensitization risk, or carcinogenic classification. Standard-setting methodologies vary across jurisdictions and substances, including health-based approaches establishing limits solely on toxicological evidence without feasibility consideration; feasibility-adjusted values modifying health-based determinations based on technical achievability and economic impact; technology-based standards requiring best available control technology regardless of specific concentration targets; and sometimes direct adoption of values from professional organizations like the American Conference of Governmental Industrial Hygienists (ACGIH) or research entities like the National Institute for Occupational Safety and Health (NIOSH). Implementation systems typically include monitoring requirements establishing when and how employers must assess workplace concentrations; control obligations when monitoring reveals standard exceedance; record-keeping provisions documenting both exposure measurements and control efforts; and sometimes medical surveillance requirements tracking potential health effects among exposed workers. Regulatory approaches vary significantly across global jurisdictions regarding both specific substance limits and overall framework characteristics, creating challenges for multinational operations navigating different requirements across various countries where facilities operate. Contemporary developments include expanding consideration beyond traditional occupational disease endpoints to address reproductive effects, developmental impacts, and endocrine disruption; greater attention to individual susceptibility variation rather than protection assumptions based solely on healthy worker populations; implementation of the globally harmonized system (GHS) standardizing hazard communication though not exposure limits themselves; and sometimes novel approaches like control banding providing structured risk management guidance when specific exposure limits remain unavailable for thousands of workplace chemicals beyond the several hundred with established regulatory values. While recognized limitations include inadequate coverage across the vast chemical landscape, limited update frequency creating significantly outdated values for many substances, and sometimes insufficient health protection when feasibility considerations substantially modify toxicologically-indicated limits, these standards nevertheless provide essential benchmarks establishing minimum acceptable workplace conditions and driving control technology implementation preventing occupational disease through systematic exposure limitation rather than uncontrolled workplace conditions potentially maximizing productivity at worker health expense.

Consumer product safety regulations establish frameworks addressing potential toxicological risks from items sold directly to the public through various approaches including banned ingredients prohibiting specific substances within particular product categories based on hazard characteristics and exposure patterns; concentration limits restricting potentially toxic components to levels deemed acceptable through risk assessment; performance standards establishing safety requirements without specifying particular formulations; labeling requirements ensuring appropriate hazard communication enabling informed consumer choice; and sometimes pre-market approval processes requiring demonstration of safety before commercial availability. Implementation varies substantially across product categories and jurisdictions, with examples including the European Union's Registration, Evaluation, Authorisation and Restriction of Chemicals (REACH) regulation and Cosmetic Products Regulation establishing comprehensive chemical management across consumer goods; the United States Consumer Product Safety Commission and Food and Drug Administration authorities addressing various product categories with significantly different requirements; and specialized frameworks for particular concerns like California's Proposition 65 requiring warning labels for products containing substances known to cause cancer or reproductive harm. Recent developments include increasing attention to vulnerable populations particularly children through specialized requirements for toys, childcare articles, and other child-specific products; enhanced disclosure requirements providing consumers more comprehensive ingredient information beyond minimum regulatory mandates; restricted substance lists developed by retailers exceeding regulatory requirements based on consumer preferences or corporate risk management decisions; and growing international harmonization efforts addressing global supply chain complexity. Emerging challenges include nanomaterial regulation when traditional toxicological approaches may inadequately address novel properties; endocrine disruptor identification and management when effects may occur at extremely low concentrations; cumulative exposure consideration when individual products meet standards while combined exposure across multiple sources may create concern; and appropriate balancing between legitimate confidential business information protection and consumer right-to-know principles. These comprehensive regulatory frameworks transform consumer protection from caveat emptor ("let the buyer beware") approaches toward systematic safety assurance, though with recognized limitations including resource constraints affecting enforcement coverage, global marketplace challenges creating uneven standards across different jurisdictions, and inevitably reactive components addressing newly recognized hazards only after market introduction due to practical limitations in anticipating all potential concerns before widespread use experience.

Environmental standards establish maximum allowable concentrations for toxic substances in air, water, soil, and other environmental media protecting both ecosystem integrity and human health through exposure pathway management. Comprehensive frameworks typically include ambient air quality standards establishing concentration limits for criteria pollutants and hazardous air pollutants protecting general population health; water quality criteria defining acceptable levels for drinking water, surface water supporting aquatic life, and groundwater protection; soil cleanup standards guiding remediation requirements for contaminated properties; and sometimes integrated multi-media approaches addressing total exposure across different environmental pathways. Standard-setting methodologies employ various approaches including health-based values derived from toxicological and epidemiological evidence using exposure assessment and risk characterization; technology-based standards requiring best available control technology regardless of specific concentration targets; cost-benefit analysis balancing protection benefits against economic implementation impact; and occasionally negotiated standards developed through stakeholder processes when scientific uncertainty creates multiple legitimate perspectives regarding appropriate levels. Implementation mechanisms include permitting systems establishing specific emission or discharge limits for industrial facilities; monitoring requirements tracking environmental concentrations across different media; enforcement provisions ensuring compliance with established limits; and remediation frameworks addressing situations where historical contamination exceeds current standards. Specific considerations within modern systems include cumulative impact assessment addressing combined effects from multiple sources particularly affecting environmental justice communities with concentrated industrial activity; background concentration accounting when natural levels or widespread anthropogenic contamination affects standard feasibility; developing contaminant inclusion addressing emerging substances like PFAS (per- and polyfluoroalkyl substances) lacking established standards despite widespread detection; and climate change interaction considering how shifting environmental conditions may affect contaminant transport, transformation, and exposure patterns. While implementation challenges include jurisdictional complexity when pollution crosses administrative boundaries; resource limitations affecting monitoring coverage and enforcement capacity; lag time between scientific recognition of hazards and regulatory standard development; and sometimes political influence potentially compromising health-protective standard establishment, these environmental frameworks nevertheless provide essential protection mechanisms establishing boundaries for acceptable environmental alteration through human activity, preventing uncontrolled release potentially creating significant public health impacts through systematic limitation rather than unrestricted discharge based solely on economic considerations without health protection constraints.

International agreements address cross-boundary toxicological concerns through multinational frameworks establishing coordinated approaches transcending individual national jurisdiction. Comprehensive examples include the Stockholm Convention on Persistent Organic Pollutants restricting production and use of substances demonstrating persistence, bioaccumulation, long-range transport, and toxicity; the Rotterdam Convention establishing prior informed consent procedures for hazardous chemical and pesticide international trade; the Basel Convention controlling transboundary movement and disposal of hazardous wastes; the Minamata Convention addressing mercury pollution throughout its lifecycle; the Montreal Protocol protecting stratospheric ozone through phasing out depleting substances; and various regional agreements addressing specific shared environmental resources like international water bodies or transboundary air pollution. Implementation mechanisms typically include national action plans translating international obligations into domestic regulations; reporting requirements documenting progress toward agreed objectives; technical and financial assistance supporting capacity development in nations with limited resources; and sometimes compliance mechanisms addressing situations where parties fail meeting obligations. Contemporary developments include increasing attention to vulnerable populations with specialized provisions addressing indigenous peoples, developing nations, and future generations potentially affected by persistent contamination; recognition of precautionary principles allowing protective action despite scientific uncertainty when potential harm appears significant; enhanced transparency provisions ensuring public access to information regarding chemical hazards and management activities; and growing integration between chemical management and sustainable development frameworks addressing interconnected environmental, social, and economic dimensions. Implementation challenges include sovereignty concerns occasionally limiting agreement scope or enforcement mechanisms; economic development tension when restrictions affect industrial activities or resource utilization; technical capacity limitations particularly in developing nations with restricted regulatory infrastructure; and sometimes excessive compromise during negotiation potentially undermining protective value through excessive exemptions, extended implementation timeframes, or inadequate compliance mechanisms. Despite these limitations, international agreements provide essential frameworks addressing inherently cross-boundary concerns where unilateral national action proves fundamentally inadequate regardless of individual country commitment, creating coordinated global approaches toward toxicological challenges transcending jurisdictional boundaries through shared responsibility recognition rather than fragmented responses potentially creating regulatory havens where hazardous activities migrate toward least-regulated environments without addressing fundamental risk reduction needs.

Program Evaluation

Compliance monitoring systems systematically assess adherence to regulatory requirements, providing essential feedback regarding implementation effectiveness beyond simple standard establishment. Comprehensive approaches employ multiple complementary techniques including self-reporting requiring regulated entities to regularly document compliance status through submissions like discharge monitoring reports, emissions inventories, or compliance certifications; agency inspections directly observing facilities, records, and operations through announced or unannounced visits; remote sensing utilizing aerial surveillance, satellite imagery, or continuous monitoring technologies providing data without physical presence; third-party verification engaging accredited independent evaluators assessing compliance through standardized protocols; and community monitoring involving local residents, advocacy organizations, or other stakeholders identifying potential violations through systematic observation. Implementation considerations include appropriate frequency balancing resource limitations against compliance verification needs; monitoring scope addressing all significant requirements rather than easily measured parameters alone; quality assurance ensuring data reliability through appropriate instrumentation calibration, methodology standardization, and occasional audit or split sampling; appropriate transparency balancing public right-to-know against confidentiality concerns including legitimate security considerations and proprietary information protection; and effective information management converting voluminous data into actionable intelligence identifying compliance patterns requiring attention. Analytical approaches extend beyond simple compliant/non-compliant determination to include trend analysis identifying improving or deteriorating performance over time; pattern recognition revealing potential systemic issues across multiple facilities or requirements; root cause examination determining underlying factors creating repeated non-compliance; performance benchmarking comparing different facilities, companies, or sectors identifying both concerning laggards and potential best practices; and sometimes predictive modeling estimating likely compliance status for facilities without recent direct assessment based on various risk factors. These comprehensive monitoring systems transform regulatory requirements from paper standards toward practical implementation drivers through systematic oversight creating actual compliance pressure rather than theoretical obligations without verification, while simultaneously generating valuable information supporting both individual facility intervention when problems appear and broader program evaluation identifying potential regulatory approach modifications when patterns suggest systemic rather than isolated implementation challenges.

Health outcome tracking evaluates whether regulatory and voluntary toxicant reduction efforts actually produce intended human health improvements beyond simple exposure reduction. Comprehensive approaches establish systematic connection between environmental interventions and health outcomes through various methodologies including disease surveillance monitoring condition prevalence associated with particular exposures like asthma, birth defects, or cancer; biomonitoring measuring toxicant levels in human specimens including blood, urine, or breast milk documenting actual body burden changes over time; health registries tracking condition development among exposed populations with particular attention to latency considerations for chronic effects; epidemiological studies examining associations between exposure changes and health outcomes accounting for potential confounding factors; environmental public health tracking systems integrating environmental monitoring, exposure assessment, and health outcome data identifying potential relationships; and occasionally health impact assessment prospectively evaluating intervention health implications before implementation. Implementation considerations include appropriate timeframe selection recognizing that health changes may manifest after considerable lag following exposure reduction, particularly for chronic conditions with extended latency periods; exposure reconstruction addressing historical conditions affecting current health outcomes when exposures occurred years or decades before health manifestation; appropriate comparison population identification creating valid reference groups for outcome evaluation; sufficient statistical power through adequate sample size detecting meaningful changes against background variation; and appropriate confounding control addressing non-exposure factors potentially affecting studied outcomes. Analytical approaches include time-series analysis examining outcome trends before and after specific interventions; geographical comparison evaluating outcome differences across areas with varying exposure profiles; dose-response assessment examining whether greater exposure reduction corresponds with larger health improvements; and benefit valuation quantifying intervention value through estimating prevented morbidity, mortality, and associated costs. These health outcome tracking approaches transform program evaluation beyond proximate indicators like emission reduction toward ultimate health improvement verification, providing crucial feedback regarding whether regulatory and voluntary efforts actually achieve their fundamental purpose protecting human health rather than assuming protection based on intermediate metrics potentially disconnected from eventual health outcomes due to complex exposure pathways, individual susceptibility variations, or multiple contributing factors beyond targeted interventions alone.

Economic impact analysis evaluates both costs and benefits of toxicological risk management programs, supporting evidence-based decision-making through systematic assessment rather than anecdotal claims or theoretical projection alone. Comprehensive approaches address multiple dimensions including compliance costs borne by regulated entities through equipment installation, operational changes, administrative requirements, and sometimes production constraints or reformulation needs; governmental implementation expenses covering regulatory development, compliance assistance, monitoring, and enforcement activities; broader economic effects including potential employment changes, competitiveness impacts, innovation consequences, and sometimes regional economic distribution considerations; monetized benefits quantifying avoided healthcare costs, productivity maintenance, property value protection, ecosystem service preservation, and other positive outcomes resulting from reduced toxic exposure; and occasionally distributional analysis examining how both costs and benefits distribute across different population segments, geographical regions, or economic sectors. Methodological approaches include retrospective studies examining actual measured impacts after implementation providing empirical validation of preliminary projections; prospective analysis estimating potential future effects before requirement implementation supporting informed regulatory decision-making; ex-post validation comparing actual outcomes with pre-implementation projections identifying systematic biases potentially affecting future assessments; and sometimes facility-level case studies examining specific implementation experiences providing detailed understanding beyond aggregate statistics alone. Technical considerations include appropriate scope encompassing all significant costs and benefits without artificial boundary constraints; reasonable timeframe capturing both short-term transition impacts and long-term steady-state effects; appropriate discount rate selection for future costs and benefits reflecting both investment opportunity costs and intergenerational equity considerations; uncertainty analysis explicitly addressing limitations in both cost and benefit quantification; and proper counterfactual development comparing intervention outcomes against realistic alternative scenarios rather than static baselines ignoring other potential changes. These comprehensive economic evaluations transform program assessment from ideological debate toward evidence-based analysis, supporting more informed decision-making by explicitly recognizing both protection benefits and implementation costs within systematic framework quantifying impacts across multiple dimensions. While acknowledging inherent limitations including monetization challenges for certain health and environmental benefits, methodological uncertainties in some assessments, and occasional data limitations restricting analytical comprehensiveness, these analyses nevertheless provide valuable structured evaluation supporting more transparent, rational decision-making regarding appropriate toxicological risk management compared to approaches lacking systematic economic dimension consideration.

Regulatory review processes systematically evaluate existing requirements identifying potential modifications enhancing effectiveness, efficiency, or scientific alignment. Comprehensive approaches include retrospective analysis examining whether established regulations achieve intended outcomes through monitoring compliance rates, exposure reduction, health improvement, or other success metrics; burden evaluation assessing administrative requirements, paperwork obligations, and implementation costs identifying potential streamlining opportunities; scientific review determining whether regulatory provisions remain aligned with current knowledge or require updating based on research developments; consistency assessment identifying potential conflicts or redundancies across different regulatory programs creating unnecessary compliance complexity; and sometimes sunset provisions requiring systematic reevaluation at predetermined intervals rather than indefinite continuation without review. Implementation typically follows structured methodology including clear review criteria establishing objective evaluation standards; stakeholder engagement collecting diverse perspectives regarding implementation experience; evidence gathering compiling relevant data regarding outcomes, costs, scientific developments, and implementation challenges; transparent documentation explaining analysis, findings, and recommended modifications; and appropriate decision-making balancing various considerations including health protection efficacy, implementation feasibility, economic efficiency, and distributional impacts. Specific review focuses include regulatory design examining whether chosen instruments optimally address identified hazards; administrative requirements assessing whether information collection, recordkeeping, or reporting obligations provide value justifying their burden; numerical standards evaluating whether established limits remain appropriate given current scientific understanding; and implementation approaches determining whether compliance promotion, monitoring, and enforcement strategies effectively translate requirements into actual practice. These regulatory review processes transform requirements from static, permanent impositions toward dynamic systems evolving based on implementation experience, scientific advancement, and changing societal conditions, creating ongoing improvement opportunity beyond initial development limitations through systematic assessment rather than maintaining original approaches regardless of identified shortcomings, changed circumstances, or emerging enhancement opportunities. While recognizing potential misuse when ideologically-driven reviews prioritize burden reduction above protection effectiveness, properly balanced processes provide valuable mechanisms ensuring regulations maintain both scientific relevance and implementation efficiency through appropriate modification based on structured evaluation rather than remaining unchanged despite identified improvement opportunities or demonstrated inadequacies in certain provisions.

Summary

Preventing toxic exposures requires integrated approaches spanning communication, engineering, education, and policy domains to address diverse hazards across populations and settings. Risk communication strategies employ principles of clarity, transparency, and cultural sensitivity to effectively convey toxicological information while addressing audience-specific needs, perceptions, and literacy levels. Effective communication balances technical accuracy with understandability, acknowledges uncertainty appropriately, provides concrete action recommendations, and maintains consistency across sources. Multiple channels including traditional media, social platforms, healthcare providers, and community organizations must deliver harmonized messaging tailored to diverse audiences. Safety measures follow a hierarchical framework prioritizing inherently safer chemical formulations and product designs, followed by engineering controls like child-resistant packaging, flow restrictors on liquid medications, automatic shut-off mechanisms, and physical barriers to hazardous materials. These technical interventions complement warning systems including standardized labeling, universal hazard symbols, and monitoring devices, alongside administrative measures such as storage regulations and handling protocols. Educational programs target developmentally appropriate content from simple poison recognition for young children to comprehensive hazard training for workers and specialized toxicology education for healthcare providers. School-based curricula, community workshops, healthcare encounters, and mass media campaigns deliver key prevention messages using evidence-based behavioral change techniques. Policy development completes the preventive framework through regulatory approaches including chemical testing requirements, exposure limits, reporting mandates, product restrictions or bans, and infrastructure supporting poison prevention. Implementation science principles guide adaptation of evidence-based interventions to specific communities and settings, with evaluation mechanisms measuring process indicators, knowledge and behavior changes, and ultimate outcomes in reduced poisoning incidence and severity. This comprehensive approach recognizes that effective prevention requires coordinated efforts across multiple sectors, addressing both individual behaviors and systemic factors contributing to toxic exposures.

Self-Assessment Questions

1. Analyze the key principles of effective risk communication about toxic hazards, explaining how message framing and delivery should differ when communicating with the general public versus healthcare professionals.
2. Describe the factors that influence risk perception regarding toxic exposures and explain how understanding these factors can improve the effectiveness of poison prevention messaging.
3. Evaluate the evidence regarding the effectiveness of child-resistant packaging in preventing pediatric poisonings, including its limitations and potential improvements to current designs.
4. Explain the concept of inherently safer design as applied to consumer products, pharmaceuticals, and industrial chemicals, providing specific examples of successful implementation.
5. Analyze how the Globally Harmonized System for Classification and Labeling of Chemicals addresses hazard communication needs, including its strengths and limitations for different audiences.
6. Design a comprehensive poison prevention education program for parents of young children, including key messages, delivery methods, behavioral change techniques, and evaluation strategies.
7. Discuss the role of healthcare providers in poison prevention across different clinical settings, identifying opportunities for intervention and education at various patient touchpoints.
8. Compare and contrast regulatory approaches to preventing toxic exposures in consumer products, workplace settings, and environmental contexts, discussing the strengths and limitations of each.
9. Describe how surveillance systems including poison center data, hospital records, and mortality statistics contribute to identifying emerging toxicological hazards and evaluating prevention measures.
10. Analyze the interrelationships between individual behaviors, product design, and policy approaches in comprehensive poison prevention, explaining how these elements must work together to effectively reduce poisoning incidence and severity.

Bibliography

1. Lovegrove MC, Weidle NJ, Budnitz DS. Trends in emergency department visits for unsupervised pediatric medication exposures, 2004-2013. Pediatrics. 2015;136(4):e821-e829.
2. Budnitz DS, Lovegrove MC. The last mile: taking the final steps in preventing pediatric pharmaceutical poisonings. J Pediatr. 2012;160(2):190-192.
3. Spiller HA, Beuhler MC, Ryan ML, Borys DJ, Aleguas A, Bosse GM. Evaluation of changes in packaging, labeling, and dosing of ipecac syrup in response to decreased use: understanding the effect of changes in ipecac use. Clin Toxicol (Phila). 2013;51(10):979-985.
4. Rodgers GB. The safety effects of child-resistant packaging for oral prescription drugs. Two decades of experience. JAMA. 1996;275(21):1661-1665.
5. Mrvos R, Dean BS, Krenzelok EP. Illiteracy: a contributing factor to poisoning. Vet Hum Toxicol. 1993;35(5):466-468.
6. Bronstein AC, Spyker DA, Cantilena LR Jr, Rumack BH, Dart RC. 2011 Annual report of the American Association of Poison Control Centers' National Poison Data System (NPDS): 29th Annual Report. Clin Toxicol (Phila). 2012;50(10):911-1164.
7. Kivistö JE, Arvola T, Parkkari J, Mattila VM. Paediatric poisonings treated in one Finnish main university hospital between 2002 and 2006. Acta Paediatr. 2008;97(6):790-794.
8. Morgan O, Griffiths C, Majeed A. Interrupted time-series analysis of regulations to reduce paracetamol (acetaminophen) poisoning. PLoS Med. 2007;4(4):e105.
9. Schmertmann M, Williamson A, Black D, Wilson L. Risk factors for unintentional poisoning in children aged 1-3 years in NSW Australia: a case-control study. BMC Pediatr. 2013;13:88.
10. Lee LK, Walia T, Forbes PW, Osganian SK, Samuels R, Cox JE, et al. Home safety practices in an urban low-income population: level of agreement between parental self-report and observed behaviors. Clin Pediatr (Phila). 2012;51(12):1119-1124.

ABOUT THE EDITORS

Dr. AMIT KUMAR

Dr. Amit Kumar is an Associate Professor at the Amity Institute of Pharmacy, Amity University, Lucknow. He received his Ph.D. in Pharmacy Practice from BPUT, Odisha, M.Pharm from Royal College of Pharmacy and Health Sciences, Berhampur, and B.Pharm from CNK Reddy College of Pharmacy, Bengaluru. He has over 40 research publications in prestigious journals, he has mentored 76 PharmD, 26 B.Pharm, and 10 M.Pharm scholars. He is a life member of the Association of Pharmaceutical Teachers of India (APTI) and the Indian Pharmaceutical Association (IPA).

Mrs. SHAIK ALEESHA

Mrs. Shaik Aleesha is currently working as Assistant Professor in the Department of Pharmacology and Clinical Toxicology at Dattakala College of Pharmacy, Pune. Currently pursuing her Ph.D. from Anurag School of Pharmacy, Hyderabad, she holds an M.Pharm in Pharmacology and B.Pharm from Rao's College of Pharmacy, JNTUA. During her six years of teaching and research experience, she has published over 15 papers in indexed journals, secured two patents, and actively participated in various national and international conferences.

Dr. NARASIMHA NAIK R

Dr. Narasimha Naik R is an Associate Professor at the Institute of Pharmaceutical Sciences and Research, Dattakala Sikshan Sanstha, Maharashtra. He holds a Ph.D. and M.Pharm from Andhra University, and a B.Pharm from Shri Vishnu College of Pharmacy. With 14 years of teaching experience, he has published 15 research papers in peer-reviewed journals and secured three patents.

Dr. RAMESH KUMAR GUPTA

Dr. Ramesh Kumar Gupta is an Associate Professor at the Amity Institute of Pharmacy, Amity University, Lucknow. He earned his Ph.D. in Pharmacology from Dr. A.P.J. Abdul Kalam Technical University, M.Pharm from Royal College of Pharmacy and Health Sciences, and B.Pharm from KIET School of Pharmacy. A prolific researcher with over 48 publications and 20 conference presentations, he has authored three books and guided 18 postgraduate students. He is a life member of the Association of Pharmaceutical Teachers in India.

Mr. SUMIT KUMAR GUPTA

Mr. Sumit Kumar Gupta is a Pharmacy graduate from RIMT University, Punjab. His research interests focus on contemporary medical developments, and he has published 10 papers in various national and international journals.

INDEX